MW00606789

J.V. Melo · J.M. Goldman

Hematologic Malignancies: Myeloproliferative Disorders

J.V. Melo · J.M. Goldman

Hematologic Malignancies: Myeloproliferative Disorders

With 69 Figures and 52 Tables

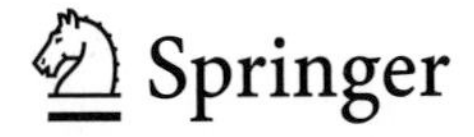

Junia V. Melo
Department of Haematology
Faculty of Medicine
Imperial College London
Hammersmith Hospital
Du Cane Road
London W12 0NN
UK

John M. Goldman
Hematology Branch
National Heart, Lung and Blood Institute
National Institutes of Health
Bethesda, MD 20892
USA

ISBN-10 3-540-34505-1 Springer Berlin Heidelberg New York
ISBN-13 978-3-540-34505-3 Springer Berlin Heidelberg New York

Library of Congress Control Number: 2006926428

A catalog record for this book is available from Library of Congress.

Bibliographic information published by Die Deutsche Bibliothek.
Die Deutsche Bibliothek lists this publication in the Deutsche Nationalbibliografie;
detailed bibliographic data is available in the Internet at http://dnb.ddb.de

Springer is a part of Springer Science+Business Media

springer.com

Editor: Dr. Ute Heilmann, Heidelberg, Germany
Desk editor: Meike Stoeck, Heidelberg, Germany
Production: LE-TEX Jelonek, Schmidt & Vöckler GbR, Leipzig, Germany
Typesetting: K+V Fotosatz GmbH, Beerfelden, Germany
Cover design: Erich Kirchner, Heidelberg, Germany

21/3100/YL – 5 4 3 2 1 0 – Printed on acid-free paper

Preface

"... To put together such apparently dissimilar diseases as chronic granulocytic leukemia, polycythemia, myeloid metaplasia and diGuglielmos's syndrome may conceivably be without foundation, but for the moment at least, this may prove useful and even productive. What more can one ask of a theory?"

So ended the editorial entitled "Some Speculations on the Myeloproliferative Syndomes" published in Blood in 1951 by the journal editor, William Dameshek. He speculated that these various conditions, which he had termed "myeloproliferative," were all somewhat variable manifestations of proliferative activity of the bone marrow cells, perhaps due to "a hitherto undiscovered stimulus." More than half a century later, Dameshek would probably have been pleased to learn that much has been learned about the cellular defects that cause these various disorders and that the term he coined has survived more or less intact. True, research focuses today as much on genetic abnormalities intrinsic in the clonal populations as on the dysregulation of cytokines or other stimulatory factors that contribute to features of these different diseases. However, in general his grouping of seemingly disparate diseases has stood the test of time. Chronic granulocytic leukemia has been renamed chronic myeloid leukemia or chronic myelogenous leukemia, and myeloid metaplasia is now idiopathic myelofibrosis – semantics only. On the other hand, erythroleukemia (diGuglielmos's syndrome) is now more usually classified as a form of acute leukemia, and the remaining myeloproliferative disorders are often referred to as the *chronic* myeloproliferative disorders, perhaps to distinguish them from the acute myeloid leukemias. One problem remains: Is chronic myeloid leukemia correctly included in this category of disease? For the purposes of this book we have elected to say that it is, though others might disagree.

We believe that recent advances in understanding the molecular and cellular biology of these disorders, taken in conjunction with the remarkable progress in treatment makes, this book especially timely. It would not be appropriate to attempt to summarize here all these advances, but clearly the gradual unraveling of the molecular basis of CML which led to the development and eventual clinical use of imatinib, all documented by various authors in this book, will come to be recognized as one of the great landmarks in the history of malignant disease. Many hope, not without good reason, that it may prove to be the model on which progress in understanding and treating other malignant hematological disorders and indeed solid tumors can be based. The major redirection of research efforts, both academic and pharmaceutical, bears eloquent testimony to this not unreasonable belief.

We do not regard this book as targeted to any particular audience. We believe it should be of interest to medical students who find the specialty of hematology truly fascinating, as we ourselves did some years ago and still do. We hope it will also attract the interest of established basic researchers and accredited hematologists, because we have stressed to our authors the need to up-date their stories to 2006, and this they have done. To many people who are no longer students but not yet established clinicians or scientists, this book should also appeal and, hopefully, be an inspiration for joining the teams of doctors and scientists who strive to understand the origins of the myeloproliferative disorders and to exploit the opportunities for improving therapy still further.

Finally, we are especially grateful to our authors who contributed excellent chapters – mostly on time – and who serenely accepted our detailed requests in some cases for further expansion or clarification of their manuscripts. We thank also our publishers for what in the end turned out to be an amazingly painless transition from manuscript to book.

London, July 2006

Junia V. Melo
John M. Goldman

Table of Contents

Contributors

Sonny O. Ang
St Jude Children's Research Hospital
332 N. Lauderdale St.
Memphis, TN 38103, USA

Jane Apperley
Department of Haematology
Faculty of Medicine
Imperial College London
Hammersmith Hospital
Du Cane Road
London W12 0NN, UK

David J. Barnes
Department of Haematology
Faculty of Medicine
Imperial College London
Hammersmith Hospital
Du Cane Road
London W12 0NN, UK

Susan Branford
Institute of Medical and Veterinary Science
University of Adelaide, North Terrace
Frome Road
Adelaide, 5000 SA, Australia

Daniela Cilloni
Department of Clinical and Biological Sciences
of the University of Turin
San Luigi Hospital, Gonzole 10
10043 Orbassano-Torino, Italy

Jan Cools
Department of Human Genetics
University of Leuven
Leuven, Belgium

Jorge Cortes
Department of Leukemia
The University of Texas
M.D. Anderson Cancer Center
1515 Holcombe Boulevard, Unit 428
Houston, TX 77030, USA

Charles Crawley
Department of Haematology
Addenbrooke's Hospital
Hills Road
Cambridge CB2 2QQ, UK

Nicholas C.P. Cross
Wessex Regional Genetics Laboratory
Salisbury District Hospital
Salisbury SP2 8BJ, UK

George Q. Daley
Division of Hematology/Oncology
Children's Hospital
300 Longwood Ave.
Boston, MA 02115, USA

Michael W.N. Deininger
Oregon Health & Science University
Center for Hematologic Malignancies
3181 SW Sam Jackson Park Road
Portland, OR 97239, USA

MIRA FARQUHARSON
Specialist Registrar in Haematology
Western General Hospital
Edinburgh EH4 2XU, Scotland

ROBERT P. GALE
Ziopharm, Inc.
11693 San Vicente Boulevard, Suite 335
Los Angeles, CA 90049-5105, USA

D. GARY GILLILAND
Howard Hughes Medical Institute
Harvard Medical School
Karp Family Research Laboratories
1 Blackfan Circle, Room 5210
Boston, MA 02115, USA

JOHN M. GOLDMAN
Hematology Branch
National Heart, Lung and Blood Institute
National Institutes of Health
Bethesda, MD 20892, USA

JASON GOTLIB
Stanford University School of Medicine
Stanford, CA, 94305, USA

ANDREAS HOCHHAUS
III. Medizinische Klinik
Fakultät für Klinische Medizin Mannheim
der Universität Heidelberg
Theodor-Kutzer-Ufer 1-3
68167 Mannheim, Germany

AXEL HOOS
Bristol-Myers Squibb
5 Research Parkway
Wallingford, CT 06492, USA

TIMOTHY HUGHES
Institute of Medical and Veterinary Science
University of Adelaide, North Terrace
Frome Road
Adelaide, 5000 SA, Australia

HAGOP KANTARJIAN
Department of Leukemia
The University of Texas
M.D. Anderson Cancer Center
1515 Holcombe Boulevard, Unit 428
Houston, TX 77030, USA

JUNIA V. MELO
Department of Haematology
Faculty of Medicine
Imperial College London
Hammersmith Hospital
Du Cane Road
London W12 0NN, UK

ALISON R. MOLITERNO
Johns Hopkins University School of Medicine
Ross Research 1025
720 Rutland Ave
Baltimore, MD 21205, USA

TARIQ I. MUGHAL
Division of Hematology
and Stem Cell Transplantation
University of Texas
Southwestern School of Medicine
Dallas, TX 75390, USA

EDUARDO OLAVARRIA
Consultant Haematologist
Catherine Lewis Centre
Haematology Department
Hammersmith Hospital
Du Cane Road
London W12 0NN, UK

JOSEF T. PRCHAL
University of Utah
Hematology Division
30 N. 1900 East, 4C416 SOM
Salt Lake City, UT 84132-2408, USA

ALFONSO QUINTÁS-CARDAMA
Department of Leukemia
The University of Texas
M. D. Anderson Cancer Center
1515 Holcombe Boulevard, Unit 428
Houston, TX 77030, USA

Jerald Radich
Clinical Research Division
Fred Hutchinson Cancer Research Center
1100 Fairview Ave. N.
Seattle, WA 98109, USA

John T. Reilly
Consultant Haematologist
Royal Hallamshire Hospital
Glossop Road
Sheffield S10 2JF, UK

Andreas Reiter
Medizinische Universitätsklinik
Fakultät für Klinische Medizin Mannheim
der Universität Heidelberg
68167 Mannheim, Germany

Giuseppe Saglio
Department of Clinical and Biological Sciences
of the University of Turin
San Luigi Hospital, Gonzole 10
10043 Orbassano-Torino, Italy

Patricia C. Shepherd
Consultant Haematologist
Western General Hospital
Edinburgh EH4 2XU, Scotland

Jerry L. Spivak
Johns Hopkins University School of Medicine
Traylor 924
720 Rutland Ave
Baltimore, MD 21205, USA

Elizabeth H. Stover
Division of Hematology
Department of Medicine
Brigham and Women's Hospital
Harvard Medical School
and the Howard Hughes Medical Institute
Boston, MA 02115, USA

Ayalew Tefferi
Division of Hematology
Mayo Clinic
200 First St. SW
Rochester, MN 55905, USA

Chronic Myeloid Leukemia – A Brief History

John M. Goldman and George Q. Daley

Contents

Abstract. Leukemia was first recognized as a distinct nosological entity in the early part of the 19th century and some of the early descriptions are highly suggestive of chronic myeloid leukemia (CML). The first important contribution to understanding the biological basis of CML was the discovery of the Philadelphia (Ph) chromosome in 1960. Almost equally important was the demonstration in 1973 that it resulted from a reciprocal translocation involving chromosomes 9 and 22. In the 1980s a "breakpoint cluster region" of the Ph chromosome was defined and this led fairly rapidly to the recognition that patients with CML had in their leukemia cells an acquired *BCR-ABL* fusion gene that was expressed as a protein with greatly enhanced tyrosine kinase activity. In 1990 *BCR-ABL* was shown to induce CML in murine models, thereby proving its central role in disease causation. Treatment for CML in the 19th century was rudimentary. The only agent known to be effective was arsenic. Radiotherapy and subsequently alkylating agents and hydroxyurea became the mainstay of therapy from the beginning of the 20th century until the advent of interferon-alfa in the early 1980s. During the 1980s it also became clear that allogeneic stem cell transplantation, though not without risk of mortality, could result in long-term disease-free survival and probably cure for selected patients. The introduction to the clinic of the original tyrosine kinase inhibitor (STI571, now imatinib) in 1998 has revolutionized approaches to the management of the newly diagnosed patient with CML in chronic phase.

1.1 Introduction

The history of leukemia and specifically of CML in the 19th century exemplifies beautifully the observational and deductive powers of some of the brilliant clinicians of the day, based as they were on technology that was developing only relatively slowly by today's standards. The major advances of the century were the increasingly widespread use of microscopy in medical research and the development of aniline dyes for staining biological tissues. The progress in the first half of the 20th century related mainly to evolving methods of treatment, and they in turn depended first on the discovery of ionizing radiation and the introduction of radiotherapy and later on the synthesis and clinical use of alkylating agents and antimetabolites. Progress in the second half of the 20th century depended critically on the application to leukemia of cytogenetics and molecular biology. Advances in chromosome analysis led in 1960 to the discovery of the cytogenetic abnormality that came to be known as the Philadelphia (Ph[1] or Ph) chromosome. Advances in molecular biology set the scene for the characterization in the early 1980s of the breakpoint cluster region of what was subsequently named the *BCR* gene, and led rapidly to the identification of the *BCR-ABL* fusion gene. Researchers in the 1990s provided convincing evidence that this fusion gene really was the "initiating event" in the chronic phase of CML and this molecular unravelling laid the foundations for work that led to the introduction of the first effective tyrosine kinase inhibitor, imatinib mesylate. Some of the highlights of this fascinating biomedical saga up to end of the last century are summarized in this chapter (for a chronology of events, see Tables 1.1 and 1.2).

Table 1.1. Milestones in unravelling the biology of CML

1845	Recognition of leukemia (probably CML) as a disease entity
1846	First diagnosis of leukemia in a live patient
1880s	Development of methods for staining blood cells
1951	Dameshek introduces the concept of myeloproliferative disorders
1960	Identification of the Philadelphia chromosome (22q-)
1973	Recognition of the reciprocal nature of the (9;22) translocation
1984	Description of the breakpoint cluster region (bcr) on chromosome 22
1985	Identification of the *BCR-ABL* fusion gene and p210-Bcr-Abl
1990	Demonstration that the *BCR-ABL* gene can induce a CML-like disease in mice
1996	Demonstration of selective blocking of Bcr-Abl kinase activity
1998	Blocking Bcr-Abl kinase activity reverses features of CML
2001	Recognition of nonrandom mutations in the Abl kinase domain

Table 1.2 Milestones in the treatment of CML

1865	First documented use of arsenic to treat CML (Fowler's solution)
1895	Discovery of x-irradiation and subsequent use in CML
1946	First effective chemotherapy for leukemia – nitrogen mustard
1956	Busulfan
1975	Hydroxyurea
1979	Identical twin transplants
1981	Allografting with sibling donors
1982	Clinical use of interferon-alfa
1984	Sokal's prognostic scoring system
1985	Allografting with unrelated donors
1990	Use of donor lymphocyte infusions and proof of a graft-versus-leukemia effect after allogeneic stem cell transplantation
1998	First clinical use of a Bcr-Abl tyrosine kinase (TK) inhibitor
2000	Launch of a prospective study comparing imatinib with IFN/Ara-C
2004	First clinical use of second-generation TK inhibitors

1.2 The 19th Century

1.2.1 Clinical Aspects and Biology

The first reasonably convincing description of leukemia was reported by Velpeau in France in 1827 (Velpeau 1827), although it is likely that forms of leukemia had been recognized as early as 1811 (Piller 1993, 2001). This was followed by the observations of Barth and Donne (Donne 1842) and of Craigie (Craigie 1845). Nevertheless, the definition of leukemia as a distinct entity is attributed to the virtually simultaneous autopsy reports in 1845 by John Hughes Bennett of a 28-year-old slater from Edinburgh and by Rudolph Virchow in Berlin of a 50-year-old cook (Bennett 1845; Virchow 1846, 1853) (Fig. 1.1). Both patients had been unwell for 1.5 to 2 years and their condition had progressively worsened with increasing weakness, bleeding, and other problems. In both cases the remarkable features at autopsy were the large size of the spleen and the consistency of the blood,

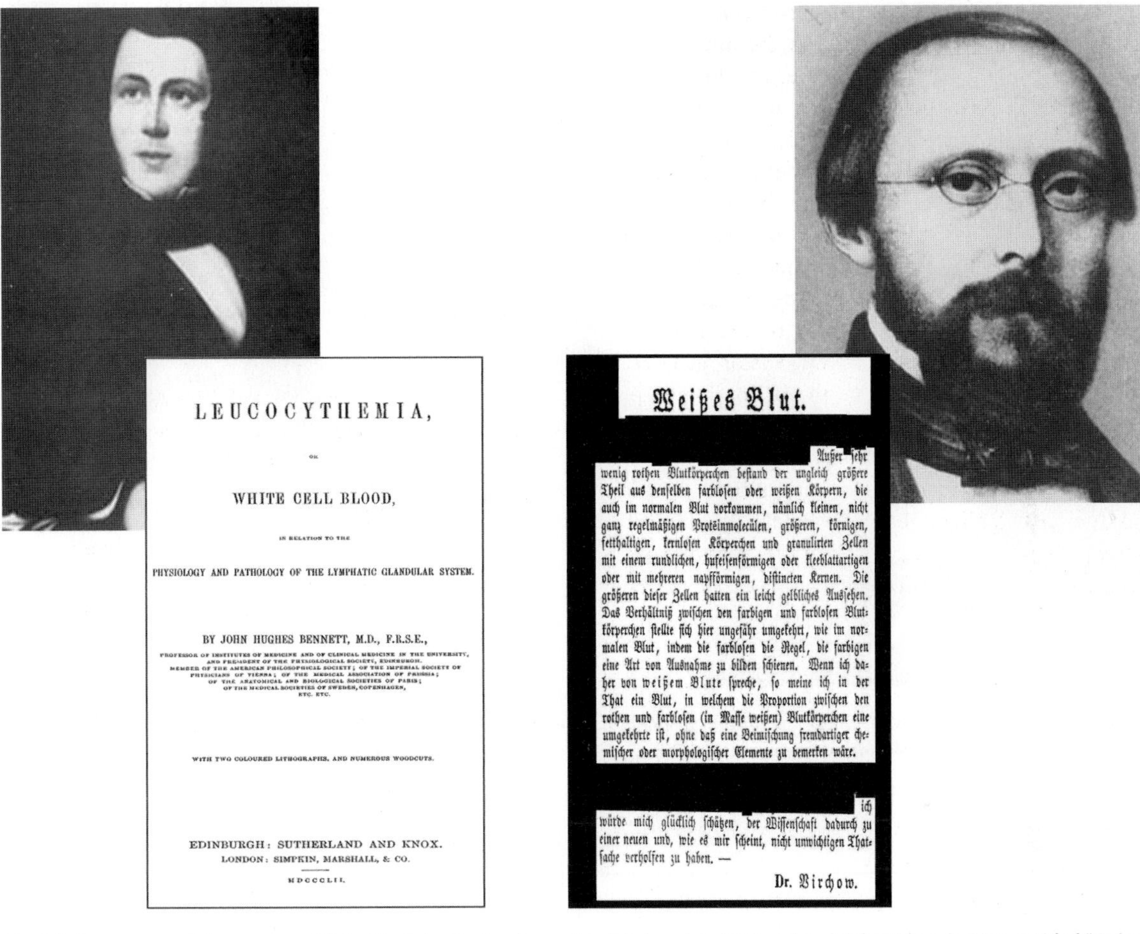

LEUCOCYTHEMIA,

OR

WHITE CELL BLOOD,

IN RELATION TO THE

PHYSIOLOGY AND PATHOLOGY OF THE LYMPHATIC GLANDULAR SYSTEM.

BY JOHN HUGHES BENNETT, M.D., F.R.S.E.,

PROFESSOR OF INSTITUTES OF MEDICINE AND OF CLINICAL MEDICINE IN THE UNIVERSITY, AND PRESIDENT OF THE PHYSIOLOGICAL SOCIETY, EDINBURGH. MEMBER OF THE AMERICAN PHILOSOPHICAL SOCIETY; OF THE IMPERIAL SOCIETY OF PHYSICIANS OF VIENNA; OF THE MEDICAL ASSOCIATION OF PRUSSIA; OF THE ANATOMICAL AND BIOLOGICAL SOCIETIES OF PARIS; OF THE MEDICAL SOCIETIES OF SWEDEN, COPENHAGEN, ETC. ETC.

WITH TWO COLOURED LITHOGRAPHS, AND NUMEROUS WOODCUTS.

EDINBURGH: SUTHERLAND AND KNOX.
LONDON: SIMPKIN, MARSHALL, & CO.

MDCCCLII.

Weißes Blut.

Außer sehr wenig rothen Blutkörperchen bestand der ungleich größere Theil aus denselben farblosen oder weißen Körpern, die auch im normalen Blut vorkommen, nämlich kleinen, nicht ganz regelmäßigen Proteïnmolecülen, größeren, körnigen, fetthaltigen, kernlosen Körperchen und granulirten Zellen mit einem rundlichen, hufeisenförmigen oder kleeblattartigen oder mit mehreren napfförmigen, distincten Kernen. Die größeren dieser Zellen hatten ein leicht gelbliches Aussehen. Das Verhältniß zwischen den farbigen und farblosen Blutkörperchen stellte sich hier ungefähr umgekehrt, wie im normalen Blut, indem die farblosen die Regel, die farbigen eine Art von Ausnahme zu bilden schienen. Wenn ich daher von weißem Blute spreche, so meine ich in der That ein Blut, in welchem die Proportion zwischen den rothen und farblosen (in Masse weißen) Blutkörperchen eine umgekehrte ist, ohne daß eine Beimischung fremdartiger chemischer oder morphologischer Elemente zu bemerken wäre.

ich würde mich glücklich schätzen, der Wissenschaft dadurch zu einer neuen und, wie es mir scheint, nicht unwichtigen Thatsache verholfen zu haben. —

Dr. Virchow.

Fig. 1.1. Front pages of the papers published by John Hughes Bennett in Edinburgh in 1852 and Rudolph Virchow in 1846, entitled "Weisses Blut," and pictures of the respective authors

in particular the white cell content. Bennett's case may have been CML and Virchow's chronic lymphocytic leukemia. Virchow used the term "Weisses Blut" to describe the predominance of white cells in the blood and later, in 1847, proposed the term "leukaemie." Bennett suggested "leucocythaemia." The first diagnosis of leukemia in a living patient was made by Fuller in 1846 (Fuller 1846), by which time Virchow had documented a further 9 cases. The first reported case of leukemia in America was of a 17-year-old seaman in Philadelphia in 1852 (Wood 1850); this was followed by several case reports, mainly from the Boston area. This sequence of events leading to the recognition of leukemia as a distinct entity, and in particular the competing claims of priority and the uncertain relationship that existed for many years between Virchow and Bennett, are well recounted in recent reviews of the topic (Geary 2000; Piller 2001).

The introduction of panoptic staining methods by Paul Ehrlich (Fig. 1.2) in the 1880s was a crucial contribution to the classification of the various major types of leukemia (Ehrlich 1891). He was able to characterize the differences in morphology between granulocytes and lymphocytes, a distinction which had previously been based only on microscopic examination of unstained granular and agranular cells with different nuclear shapes. This led in due course to better characterization of chronic granulocytic leukemia as a distinct nosological entity.

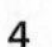

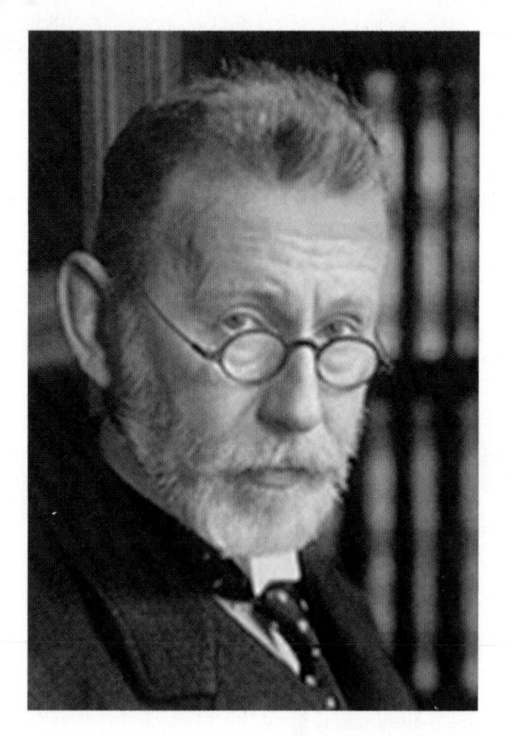

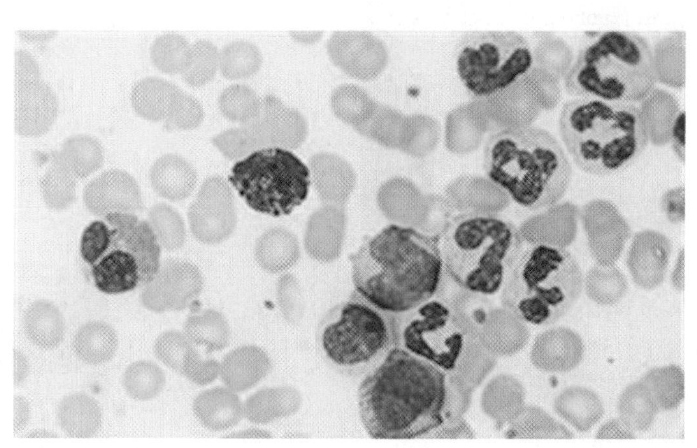

Fig. 1.2. Paul Ehrlich (1854–1915), whose application of panoptic staining methods to blood cells enabled clear visualization of the morphological features of the various types of leukocytes which are characteristically abnormal in the leukemias

1.2.2 Therapy

In the late 18th century Thomas Fowler was probably the first to use arsenic to treat patients with CML. A 1% solution of arsenic trioxide introduced as a general tonic for people and animals had been found to have a beneficial effect on the general health of horses, and was henceforth known as Fowler's solution (Forkner 1938). A German physician named Lissauer apparently treated a near-moribund patient with Fowler's solution and observed remarkable improvement in his well-being (Lissauer 1865). Arsenic was used intermittently throughout the second half of the 19th century in the treatment of CML and appropriate doses were found to control fever, reduce the white cell count, reduce the size of the spleen, relieve pruritus, and reduce the degree of anemia (Forkner 1938). It is interesting that a short letter appears in the Lancet in 1882 describing the use of arsenic to treat a patient with what was probably CML (Cowan Doyle 1882). The author is written as Arthur Cowan Doyle, but this is certainly a printer's error for Arthur Conan Doyle, rather more famous as author of the stories of Sherlock Holmes. He was known to have been working at the time as a general practitioner in the Birmingham (England) area.

1.3 First Half of the 20th Century

1.3.1 Clinical Aspects and Biology

The clinical features and natural history of CML were increasingly well characterized in the early part of the last century. Minot and colleagues reported the influence of specific clinical features on survival in 166 patients collected over a 10-year period and concluded that age was an important prognostic factor (Minot et al. 1926), a factor now incorporated into the Sokal prognostic scoring system. Patients treated with radiotherapy seemed to fare better than those treated by other means. Subsequently Hoffman and Craver confirmed the general benefit of radiotherapy to the spleen (Hoffman and Craver 1931). Dameshek made an important contribution in 1951 when he grouped chronic granulocytic leukemia (=CML) together with polycythemia vera, idiopathic myeloid metaplasia, and thrombocythemia under the general heading "myeloproliferative syndromes" (Dameshek 1951). He stressed the degree to which all myeloid lineages were to a greater or lesser degree involved in each of these conditions and foresaw the probability that they were disparate manifestations of a myeloid stem cell disorder, a thesis that has gained considerable support from the recent discovery of V617F JAK2 mutation in three of these disorders.

1.3.2 Therapy

Roentgen's discovery of x-rays in 1895 led to their enthusiastic use in the treatment of leukemias and lymphomas. Though initial attempts were unimpressive, it became gradually clear that irradiation directed to the spleen in patients with CML reduced the degree of splenomegaly with associated improvement in the blood picture and the patient's general state of health (Pusey 1902; Senn 1903). It was recommended at this stage that arsenic should not be given concurrently with x-irradiation but could be used as intermittent therapy. Remissions induced by x-ray therapy were often "complete" and while relapse was inexorable and life was not prolonged, the patient's quality of life was improved (Hoffman and Craver 1931; Minot et al. 1924). Internal irradiation with radioactive phosphorus also brought about satisfactory clinical and hematological remissions (Lawrence et al. 1939) but was not as effective as external x-rays in reducing organomegaly (Reinhard et al. 1946).

1.4 Latter Half of the 20th Century

1.4.1 Biology

Though Boveri had predicted as early as 1914 that human malignancies would prove to have a genetic basis (Boveri 1914), it was not until technology for examining human chromosomes developed sufficiently in the 1950s that cytogeneticists were able to confirm that normal human cells had 46 chromosomes and then to examine the chromosomal make-up of cells from cancers and leukemias. In 1960 Nowell and Hungerford were able to report the presence of a small abnormal acrocentric chromosome (from the G group) in the leukemia cells of 7 patients with chronic granulocytic leukemia (Nowell and Hungerford 1960 a, b); it resembled a Y chromosome but two of the patients were female (Fig. 1.3). Normal karyotypes were observed in nonleukemia cells. This observation was rapidly confirmed by others (Baikie et al. 1960). This was the first consistent cytogenetic abnormality in any form of human malignancy. It was termed the Philadelphia chromosome (initially abbreviated to Ph^1 because the early discovery of other consistent cytogenetic abnormalities was anticipated, but later modified to Ph). In practice it was some years before other cytogenetic changes were identified in human leukemia and there was in the interim spirited dispute as to whether the Ph chromosome was anything other than an interesting epiphenomenon. Nonetheless it provided a tool which Fialkow and colleagues were able to exploit to demonstrate that CML was probably a clonal disorder originating from a single hematopoietic stem cell (Fialkow et al. 1967); later they and others showed that this stem cell gave rise to cells of the granulocytic, erythroid, monocyte/macrophage, and megakaryocytic lineages (Fialkow et al. 1977)

In 1973 further advances in the technology of cytogenetics, notably the introduction of quinacrine fluorescence and Giemsa banding, enabled Janet Rowley (Fig. 1.4) in Chicago to observe that though the long arm of chromosome 22 was shortened (22q−), there was also consistent evidence of additional material on the long arm of chromosome 9 (9q+), from which she deduced that the Ph chromosome was the result of a reciprocal and balanced translocation involving chromosomes 9 and 22, [now designated t(9;22)(q23;q11)] (Rowley 1973). Thereafter nonrandom cytogenetic abnormalities were discovered in acute myeloid leukemia and the notion that chromosomal abnormalities must play a pivotal role in the pathogenesis of at least some leukemias gained much ground. Indeed, cytogenetic studies provided key evidence in support of the theory that malignancies were caused by genetic derangements in cells.

1.4.2 Therapy

Modern chemotherapy had its origins in secret research on agents for use in chemical warfare carried out during WWII. Thus, the fact that mustard gas or nitrogen mustard (HN2) was known to cause myelosuppression provided the rationale for its use in the treatment of leukemia (Goodman et al. 1946; Jacobson et al. 1946). Importantly, it was found that patients who were or who became resistant to x-ray therapy could still respond to ni-

Nowell & Hungerford, *Science*, 132: 1497, 1960

A Minute Chromosome in Human Chronic Granulocytic Leukemia

In seven cases thus far investigated (five males, two females), a minute chromosome has been observed replacing one of the four smallest autosomes in the chromosome complement of cells of chronic granulocytic leukemia cultured from peripheral blood. No abnormality was observed in the cells of four cases of *acute* granulocytic leukemia in adults or of six cases of acute leukemia in children. There have been several recent reports of chromosome abnormalities in a number of cases of human leukemia [including two of the seven cases reported here: Nowell and Hungerford, *J. Natl. Cancer Inst.* **25**, 85 (1960)], but no series has appeared in which there was a consistent change typical of a particular type of leukemia.

Cells of the five new cases were obtained from peripheral blood (and bone marrow in one instance), grown in culture for 24–72 hours, and processed for cytological examination by a recently developed air-drying technique (Moorhead, *et al.*, *Exptl. Cell Research*, in press). The patients varied from asymptomatic untreated cases to extensively treated cases of several years duration in terminal myeloblastic crisis. All seven individuals showed a similar minute chromosome, and none showed any other frequent or regular chromosome change. In most of the cases, cells with normal chromosomes were also observed. Thus, the minute is not a part of the normal chromosome constitution of such individuals.

The findings suggest a causal relationship between the chromosome abnormality observed and chronic granulocytic leukemia.

Peter C. Nowell
School of Medicine, University of Pennsylvania
David A. Hungerford
Institute for Cancer Research

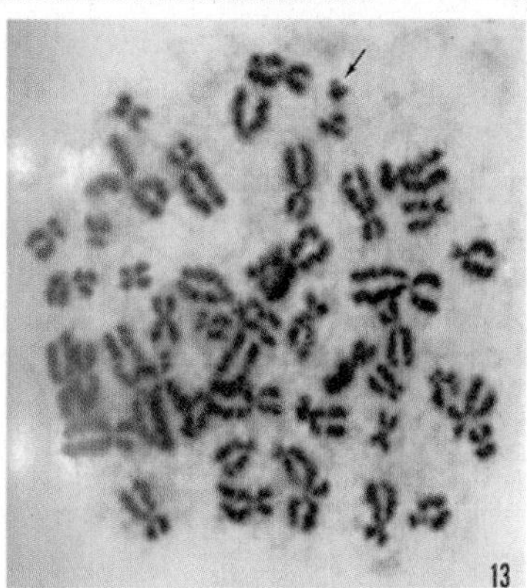

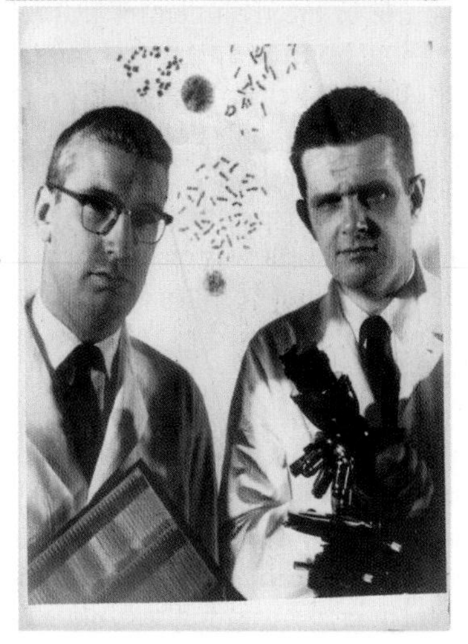

Fig. 1.3. The short paper published by Nowell and Hungerford in 1960 (reproduced with permission of the Science publishers) and a photograph of the authors, Peter Nowell (*left*) and David Hungerford (*right*), taken soon after their discovery of the Ph chromosome. The *top-right inset* shows a karyotype from a patient with CML showing a small acrocentric chromosome (*arrowed*) which was thought originally to be a Y chromosome (Nowell and Hungerford 1960a); however, a few months later, the authors had identified it as a unique abnormal chromosome "replacing one of the four smallest autosomes in the chromosome complement of cells of chronic granulocytic leukemia" (Nowell and Hungerford 1960 b)

trogen mustard (HN2). One related drug, urethane, was used in the treatment of CML and in the maintenance of x-ray-induced remission in the 1940s. In the 1950s Alexander Haddow in London spearheaded a program to produce a variety of alkylating agents based on HN2 which might prove more specific and less toxic than HN2 itself. A modified alkylating agent, busulfan, was introduced in 1953 and proved highly effective in controlling clinical features of CML for long periods of time, although it could induce irreversible marrow aplasia if given in excessive dosage (Galton 1953, 1959; Haddow and Timmis 1953). Later, a prospective comparison of busulfan and radiotherapy showed significant prolongation of life for the patients who received busulfan (Medical Research Council 1968) and it then rapidly became the treatment of choice for CML. Dibromomannitol, first investigated in 1961 (Eckhardt et al. 1963) became an alternative for patients in chronic phase who ceased to respond to busulfan. Hydroxyurea was first used in the 1960s and very gradually replaced busulfan as the first-line cytotoxic drug for newly diagnosed patients (Kennedy 1969).

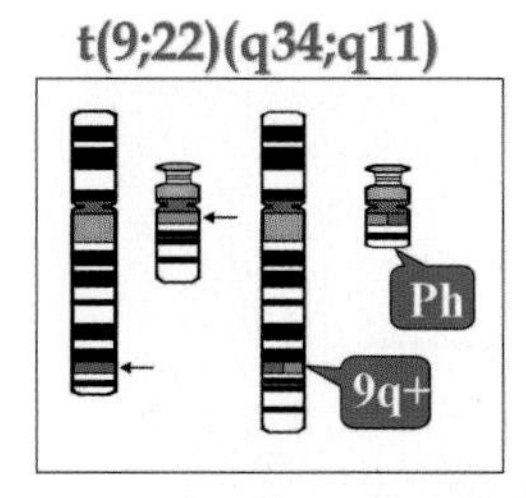

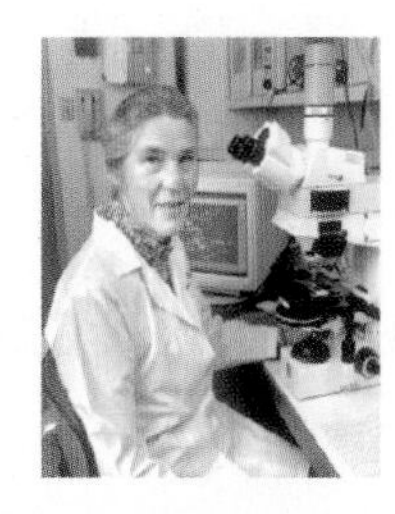

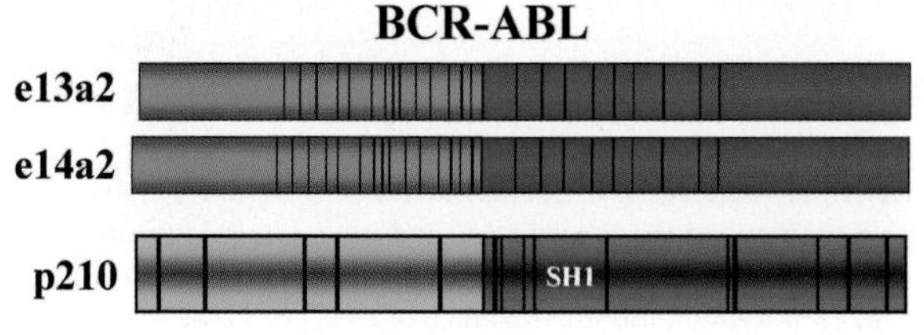

Fig. 1.4. The t(9;22)(q34;q11) translocation, first described by Janet Rowley (*photo*) in 1973, which generates the *BCR-ABL* fusion gene in the Ph chromosome, as well as a reciprocal *ABL-BCR* gene in the derivative 9q+ (Melo et al., 1993). In the last two decades of the 20th century, various groups were involved in demonstrating that *BCR-ABL* is transcribed into mRNA molecules with e13a2 and/or e14a2 junctions, and translated into a 210 KDa protein (p210) with enhanced tyrosine kinase due to constitutively activation of the SH1 region of its Abl portion

1.5 Last Quarter of the 20th Century

1.5.1 Biology

The starting point for the identification of the *BCR-ABL* fusion gene was the isolation by Abelson of a murine virus capable of inducing lymphosarcoma in mice (Abelson and Rabstein 1970), and the subsequent description of the Abl oncogene or v-*abl* (Goff et al. 1980; Reddy et al. 1983; Shields et al. 1979), a story recently very comprehensively reviewed by Wong and Witte (Wong and Witte 2004). The next important development was the report from the group in Rotterdam that the Ph translocation involved the translocation of the normal human counterpart of the murine v-*abl* proto-oncogene from chromosome 9 to chromosome 22 (de Klein et al. 1982). This seminal study suggested the hypothesis that the human *ABL* gene might be activated by the translocation in a manner that would cause it to malfunction like its oncogenic viral counterpart (Fig. 1.5). Exhaustive studies of the genomic structure of the Ph translocation established that the breakpoints occurred upstream of the *ABL* gene without disrupting the DNA that was homologous to v-*abl* (Heisterkamp et al. 1983). This apparent conundrum was later explained when the complete locus of the murine c-*abl* gene was characterized, and indeed showed that breakpoints typically disrupted a large first intron of the c-*abl* gene (Bernards et al. 1987). The major breakthrough leading to the identification of the *BCR-ABL* gene was the observation in 1984 that the chromosome 22 breakpoints that "produced" the Ph chromosome were clustered within a 5.8-kb region of DNA that was not unreasonably named the *bcr*, or breakpoint cluster region (Groffen et al. 1984). This proved later to be a centrally located sequence of the full gene which, despite attempts to find a more informative epithet, retained the name *BCR* (Goldman et al. 1990). At the same time Witte and colleagues showed that the Abl protein in the K562 cell line had abnormal size and greatly enhanced tyrosine kinase activity, from which they deduced that a structural abnormality resulting in enhanced enzymatic activity might play a central role in the pathogenesis of CML (Ben-Neriah et al. 1986; Konopka et al. 1984). Thereafter two groups showed independently that *BCR* and *ABL* sequences were linked to form a fusion transcript which characterizes the cells of all patients with Ph-positive CML (Canaani et al. 1984; Grosveld et al. 1986; Shtivelman et al. 1985). Thus the (9;22) translocation resulted in the formation of a fusion gene, *BCR-ABL*, on chromosome 22 (Fig. 1.4). In practice the breakpoint in the *BCR* gene occurs nearly always in the intron between exons e13 and e14 (previously b2 and b3) or in the intron between e14 and e15 (previously b3 and b4) while the *ABL* breakpoints occur upstream of *ABL* exon a2. Thus most patients have leukemia-specific transcripts with either e13a2 or e14a2 junctions; occasional patients have both transcripts. The consistency of these junctions at the RNA level means that it is now relatively easy to design disease-specific primers which can be used in the reverse transcriptase and polymerase chain reaction (RT-PCR) to amplify small quantities of residual disease-specific transcripts after effective treatment. This technique forms the basis for molecular monitoring of individual patients after stem cell transplant and in the present imatinib era (see Chap. 9 entitled Monitoring Disease Response).

The notion that more than one molecular event might be required to initiate chronic phase CML and that consequently the acquisition of a Ph chromosome might not be the primary event has been raised repeatedly over the years. In 1981 Fialkow and colleagues published results of cytogenetic studies of a series of EBV-induced B-cell lines established from a female CML pa-

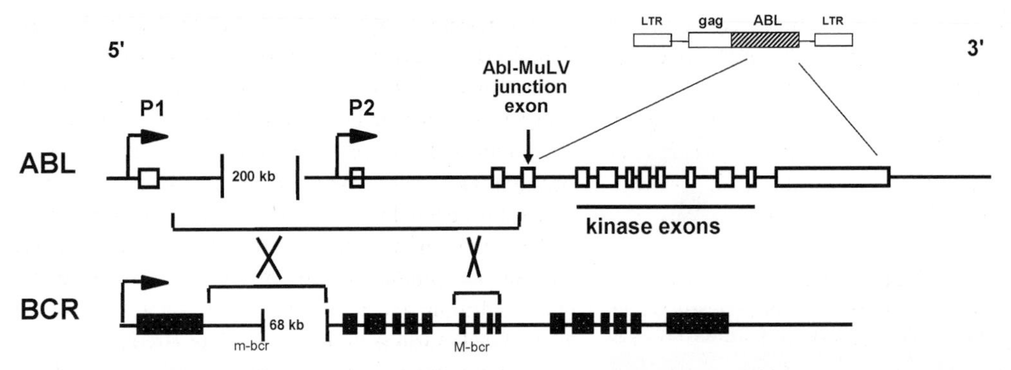

Fig. 1.5. Relationship of the murine v-*abl* oncogene to the human *ABL* proto-oncogene. The *top* diagram shows the Abelson variant of the Moloney murine leukemia virus with the LTR and *gag* sequences in relation to *Abl*. The two diagrams *below* represent the human *ABL* and *BCR* genes showing the relationship of *v-abl* to its humanhomologue. The *horizontal brackets* show the highly variable positions of the break in *ABL* and more localized positions of the break in *BCR*, which lead respectively to transcripts with the e1a2 (acute lymphoblastic leukemia) or e13a2 or e14a2 (CML) junctions

tient who was heterozygous for the A and B isozymes of G6PD (Fialkow et al. 1981). They concluded that the relatively high frequency of cytogenetic abnormalities in Ph-negative B-cell lines characterized by the same isozyme as the Ph-positive leukemia was evidence in favor of the concept that a clonal event leading to a proliferative advantage had preceded the origin of the Ph-positive clonal proliferation. For these and other reasons it was important to ascertain whether the *BCR-ABL* gene alone could induce the phenotype of CML. In 1990 Daley and colleagues reported that use of retroviral-mediated gene transfer to introduce a *BCR-ABL* gene into murine hematopoietic stem cells caused in a majority of the recipient animals a disease closely resembling CML in man (Daley et al. 1990). Analogous results were obtained by several groups using both retroviral and transgenic approaches to express *BCR-ABL* (Elephanty et al. 1990; Heisterkamp et al. 1990; Kelliher et al. 1990). As a consequence it seemed reasonably certain that the acquisition of a *BCR-ABL* fusion gene was indeed a sufficient initiating event for CML in man, although it remains entirely possible that in some cases the Ph translocation might be more likely to occur or be observed in the setting of a pre-existing clonal hematopoietic abnormality.

1.5.2 Therapy

Though busulfan and subsequently hydroxyurea were relatively effective at controlling the features of CML in chronic phase, neither drug reduced the proportion of Ph-positive cells in the bone marrow except on very rare occasions, and there remained the suspicion that their use did not prolong life significantly, if at all. Indeed it was possible that busulfan was mutagenic and even expedited the onset of blastic transformation. It was encouraging therefore when early studies with interferon-α demonstrated that a proportion of patients could achieve some degree of Ph-negative hematopoiesis and a smaller proportion became entirely Ph-negative (Talpaz et al. 1983). It also appeared that the frequency of Ph-negativity was increased at higher doses of the drug (Talpaz et al. 1986). Subsequent large scale prospective studies showed that interferon did indeed prolong life by 1–2 years compared with busulfan or hydroxyurea and the benefit seemed to be greatest in patients who achieved Ph-negativity (Allan et al. 1995; Italian Cooperative Study Group on CML 1994). Of great interest was the observation that small numbers of patients remained Ph-negative even after the drug was discontinued (Bonifazi et al. 2001). Thus for 20 years the drug was regarded as the treatment of choice for newly diagnosed patients with CML in chronic phase. A report from France suggested that the incidence of Ph-negativity was higher and survival was improved if interferon was used in conjunction with cytarabine compared with interferon alone (Guilhot et al. 1997), but superior survival for patients treated with the two-drug combination could not be confirmed in an Italian study (Baccarani et al. 2002).

Sporadic attempts were made throughout the 1970s to treat patients with CML in advanced phases by allogeneic stem cell transplantation (see Chap. 7, entitled Allogeneic Transplantation for CML); these were almost universally unsuccessful because patients died either of transplant complications or persistence of their leukemia. In 1979 the Seattle group reported the results of treating 4 patients with CML with high-dose chemoradiotherapy followed by transfusion of bone marrow cells from their genetically identical, normal twins (Fefer et al. 1979). At a median follow-up of 24 months these four patients were well without evidence of Ph-positive cells in their bone marrow. This very remarkable achievement considered in association with recent progress in defining the role of HLA in donor selection led a number of researchers on both sides of the Atlantic to initiate programs for treating CML patients by allogeneic stem cell transplantation using bone marrow from HLA-identical sibling donors (Champlin et al. 1982; Clift et al. 1982; Goldman et al. 1982; McGlave et al. 1982;).

By the mid-1980s a series of reports described the favorable results of allogeneic transplants performed for CML patients in chronic phase where the stem cell donor was a genetically HLA-identical sibling (Goldman et al. 1986; Speck et al. 1984; Thomas et al. 1986). The risk of morbidity and indeed mortality, attributable especially to graft-versus-host disease and to infection, were still appreciable but the majority of patients survived the procedure and relapses later than 3 years post-transplant were relatively infrequent. These results gave rise to the notion that allogeneic stem cell transplant could "cure" chronic myeloid leukemia, an extremely important prediction for a disease that for the preceding 140 years had been regarded as inexorably fatal. The mechanism underlying this cure was still enigmatic. Though it was easy to assume that the combination of cytotoxic drugs and radiotherapy that preceded the transplant eradicated all leukemia stem cells, the demonstration first that T cell depletion intended to reduce the risk of GvHD greatly increased the risk of leukemia relapse (Apperley et al. 1996; Horowitz et al. 1990) and second that patients in relapse could be restored to remission by transfusion of lymphocytes collected from the original transplant donor (Kolb et al. 1990) together implicated a graft-versus-leukemia effect as making an important contribution to the cure. This has renewed enthusiasm for the immunotherapy of CML which is manifest in the routine use of donor lymphocyte infusions (Mackinnon et al. 1995) and more recently in efforts to raise cytotoxic T cell clones restricted to killing cells expressing particular leukemia-associated antigens (Barrett 2003) (see Chap. 11, Immune Therapy of Chronic Myelogenous Leukemia)

The feasibility of leukapheresis as a method of tumor debulking in CML was established in the 1960s and depended on the development of continuous flow blood cell separators (Buckner et al. 1969; Morse et al. 1966). Indeed, repeated leukapheresis alone will induce complete hematological remission (Lowenthal et al. 1975). Today, there is probably little benefit in the long-term repeated leukapheresis of patients with CML but the procedure is valuable for producing a rapid initial reduction in the white cell count and as a means for collecting large numbers of cells for use in autografting (see below).

The concept that autografting might be valuable in the management of CML was developed in the 1970s (see Chap. 8, entitled Autografting in Chronic Myeloid Leukemia). Investigators in Seattle were the first to harvest bone marrow cells from patients in chronic phase. These cells were cryopreserved and stored in liquid nitrogen and then used as an autograft in conjunction with high dose chemotherapy when the patient began to show signs of transformation (Buckner et al. 1978). This was based on the hope that infusion of cells harvested at diagnosis would reinstate chronic phase hematopoiesis for a period equivalent to the length of the first chronic phase. Subsequently the Hammersmith Hospital (London) group was able to show that peripheral blood as well as bone marrow contained progenitor cells capable of re-establishing bone marrow function after "supralethal" irradiation (Goldman et al. 1979) and this observation provided support for the notion that stem cells might be present in the circulation of normal persons. The use of high dose cytoreduction followed by autografting did not however prove clinically valuable for patients in blastic transformation and attention switched to the possibility that the technique might prolong life for patients in chronic phase. At the Hammersmith Hospital in London results of using unmanipulated peripheral blood cells suggested the possibility that life might be prolonged (Hoyle et al. 1994); the use of this approach to autograft patients in chronic phase at 8 centers were summarized in the same year with similar conclusions (McGlave et al. 1994). Subsequently it was thought possible that results of autografting with peripheral blood stem cells might be improved using the strategy first reported by the group in Genoa (Carella et al. 1993, 1999) who demonstrated that recovery from chemotherapy was associated with the preferential release of Ph-negative, presumably normal, cells into the bloodstream and that these stem cells could be collected in sufficient numbers for reinfusion into the patient at a later date. In the light of the knowledge that normal stem cells co-exist with leukemic stem cells in the marrow of CML patients, and that CML stem cells survive poorly in culture, investigators in Vancouver cultured patient's marrow in vitro prior to autografting in the hope that the normal cells would become relatively enriched (Barnett et al. 1994). Other potential approaches to purging marrow for autografting included the use of antisense reagents designed to suppress the expression of p210$^{BCR\text{-}ABL}$ (Luger et al. 2002). Autografting has however fallen from favor since the advent of imatinib, but could again become important in the management of patients resistant to second-generation tyrosine kinase inhibitors.

1.5.3 Development of Imatinib Mesylate

The development of imatinib as a highly effective agent in the management of the chronic phase of CML illustrates very beautifully some of the basic principles and problems of medically orientated research (see Chap. 5, entitled Signal Transduction Inhibitors in Chronic Myeloid Leukemia). One of the biggest potential barriers to the eventual success of imatinib was the skepticism with which the notion of developing a potentially effective tyrosine kinase was viewed in the late 1980s and early 1990s (Druker and Lydon 2000; Lydon and Druker 2004). For example, there was grave doubt as to whether it would in fact be possible to develop compounds with action against specific protein kinases. Any such compound that was produced might also inhibit other kinases with unacceptable clinical toxicity. Some considered it unlikely that inhibiting a single kinase could be clinically useful if molecular lesions in individual tumors were multiple, and varied from patient to patient.

In the early 1990's Levitzki and colleagues studied a series of molecules, designated tyrphostins, that inhibited the tyrosine kinase activity of the Bcr-Abl oncoprotein and the proliferation of the CML cell line K562 at micromolar concentrations and also inhibited the tyrosine kinase activity of the BCR-ABL oncoprotein (Anafi et al. 1992; Kaur et al. 1994). These compounds were promising but only one tyrphostin, adaphostin, has recently proceeded to clinical trial. Another agent, herbimycin, was also studied at the time. Originally thought to inhibit the kinase activity of the Bcr-Abl, it was later shown to promote degradation of the Bcr-Abl oncoprotein (Okabe et al. 1992). Against this somewhat uncertain background, scientists working for Ciba-Geigy (now Novartis) in Basel showed that 2-phenylaminopyrimidine molecules could selectively inhibit the enzymatic activity of protein kinase C, Abl, and platelet-derived growth factor receptor (PDGFR) proteins and decided to modify their lead molecule to target more specifically PDGFR and Abl. The steps in medicinal chemistry that followed, the sequential introduction of a 3′ pyridyl group, the addition of a benzamide group to the phenyl ring, the attachment of a "flag-methyl" group ortho to the diaminophenyl ring, and the addition of an N-methylpiperazine, together improved the selectivity of the lead molecule and increased its water solubility and oral bioavailability (Deininger et al. 2005; Zimmermann et al. 1996). The resulting compound, designated CGP-57148B, was active against all forms of Abl, PDGFR A and B, and c-KIT. It was far less active against a wide variety of other kinases including EGF, Src family kinases, VEGF, JAK2, and RAF1.

The next stage was to test the new compound against a range of cell lines. It inhibited proliferation in a range of established Ph-positive cell lines but left Ph-negative lines unaffected (Beran et al. 1998; Deininger et al. 1997; Druker et al. 1996). The mechanism of action appeared to be induction of apoptosis (Deininger et al. 1997; Gambacorti-Passerini et al. 1997). Of very great importance was the observation that it selectively inhibited in vitro the proliferation of myeloid progenitor cells taken from the blood of patents with Ph-positive CML while leaving relatively unaffected residual Ph-negative progenitors (Deininger et al. 1997; Druker et al. 1996).

More or less simultaneously the compound was tested for its effects in animal model systems. Syngeneic control mice injected with BCR-ABL-transformed 32D cells developed tumors but intraperitoneal injection of the CGP 57148B caused dose-dependent inhibition of tumor growth (Druker et al. 1996). Similar results were obtained later with the BCR-ABL-positive KU812 cell line (Le Coutre et al. 1999). In another model system, lethally irradiated syngeneic mice received with bone marrow cells transfected with a BCR-ABL-containing retrovirus; treatment with the new compound prolonged survival in some but not all animals (Wolff and Ilaria 2001). In parallel with these experiments Ciba-Geigy/Novartis undertook extensive pharmacokinetic and toxicological studies in different species. Eventually the scene was set for initial clinical phase I studies, which began in Oregon in June 1998. The impressive clinical benefits associated with use of this agent are summarized in Chap. 6, entitled Treatment with Tyrosine Kinase Inhibitors. The remarkable activity of imatinib in inducing complete remissions in CML represents strong confirmation of the central role of the BCR-ABL oncoprotein in CML, and the culmination of almost 50 years of basic research, dating from the original description of the Philadelphia chromosome.

References

Abelson HT, Rabstein LS (1970) Lymphosarcoma: virus induced thymic-independent disease in mice. Cancer Res 30:2213–2222

Allan NC, Richards SM, Shepherd PCA et al (1995) Medical Research Council randomised multicentre trial of interferon-α1 for chronic myeloid leukaemia: Improved survival irrespective of cytogenetic response. Lancet 345:1392–1397

Anafi M, Gazit A, Gilon C, Ben Neriah Y, Levitzki A (1992) Selective interactions of transforming and normal Abl proteins with ATP, tyrosine copolymer substrates, and tyrphostins. J Biol Chem 267:4518–4523

Apperley JF, Jones L, Hale G, Waldmann H, Hows JM, Rombos Y, Tsatalas C, Goolden AWG, Gordon Smith EC, Catovsky D, Galton DAG, Goldman JM (1986) Bone marrow transplantation for patients with chronic myeloid leukaemia: T-cell depletion reduces the incidence of graft-versus-host disease but increases the risk of leukaemic relapse. Bone Marrow Transplant 1:53–66

Baccarani M, Rosti G, de Vivo A et al (2002) A randomized study of interferon-α versus interferon-α plus low dose arabinosyl cytosine in chronic myeloid leukemia. Blood 94:1527–1535

Baikie AG, Court-Brown WM, Buckton KE et al (1960) A possible specific chromosome abnormality in human chronic myeloid leukaemia. Nature 188:1165–1166

Barnett MJ, Eaves CJ, Phillips GL, Gascoigne RD, Hogge DE, Horseman DE, Humphries RK, Klingeman HG, Lansdorp PM, Nantel SH, Reece DE, Shepherd JD, Spinelli JJ, Sutherland HJ, Eaves AC (1994) Autografting with cultured marrow in chronic myeloid leukemia: Results of a pilot study. Blood 84:724–732

Barrett AJ (2003) Allogeneic stem cell transplantation for chronic myeloid leukemia. Semin Hematol 40:59–71

Bennett JH (1845) Case of hypertrophy of the spleen and liver in which death took place from suppuration of the blood. Edinb Med Surg J 64:413–423

Ben-Neriah Y, Daley GQ, Mes-Masson A-M, Witte ON, Baltimore D (1986) The chronic myelogenous leukemia specific p210 protein is the product of the bcr/abl hybrid gene. Science 223:212–214

Beran M, Cao X, Estrov Z et al (1998) Selective inhibition of cell proliferation and BCR-ABL phosphorylation in acute lymphoblastic leukemia cells expressing Mr 190 000 BCR-ABL protein by a tyrosine kinase inhibitor (CGP-57148). Clin Cancer Res 4:1661–1672

Bernards A, Rubin CM, Westbrook CA, Paskind M, Baltimore D (1987) The first intron in the human c-abl gene is at least 200 kilobases long and is a target for translocations in chronic myelogenous leukemia. Mol Cell Biol 7:3231–3236

Bonifazi F, de Vivo A, Rosti G et al (2001) Chronic myeloid leukemia and interferon-α: A study of complete cytogenetic responders. Blood 98:3074–3081

Boveri T (1914) Zur Frage der Entstehung maligner Tumoren. Verlag von Gustav Fischer, Jena, Germany

Buckner CD, Graw RG, Eisel RJ, Henderson ES, Perry S (1969) Leukapheresis by continuous flow centrifugation (CFC) in patients with chronic myelocytic leukemia (CML) Blood 33:353–369

Buckner CD, Stewart P, Clift RA, Fefer A, Neiman PE, Singer J, Storb R, Thomas ED (1978) Treatment of blastic transformation of chronic granulocytic leukemia by chemotherapy, total body irradiation and infusion of cryopreserved autologous marrow. Exp Hematol 6:96–109

Canaani E, Steiner-Saltz D, Aghai E, Gale RP, Berrebi A, Januszewicz E (1984) Altered transcription of an oncogene in chronic myeloid leukemia. Lancet 1:593–595

Carella AM, Pollicardo N, Pungolino E, Raffo MR Podesta M, Ferrero R, Pierluigi D, Nati S. Congui A (1993) Mobilization of cytogenetically normal blood progenitors by intensive chemotherapy for chronic myeloid and acute lymphoblastic leukemia. Leuk Lymphoma 9:477–483

Carella AM, Lerma E, Corsetti MT et al (1999) Autografting with Philadelphia chromosome negative mobilized hematopoietic progenitor cells in chronic myelogenous leukemia. Blood; 83:1534–1539

Champlin RE, Ho W, Arenson E, Gale RP (1982) Allogeneic bone marrow transplantation for chronic myelogenous leukemia in chronic or accelerated phase. Blood 60:1038–1041

Clift RA, Buckner CD, Thomas ED et al (1982) Treatment of chronic granulocytic leukemia in chronic phase by allogeneic marrow transplantation. Lancet 2:621–623

Cowan Doyle A (1882) Notes on a case of leucocythaemia. Lancet 25 March, 490

Craigie D (1845) Case of disease of the spleen in which death took place consequent on the presence of purulent matter in the blood. Edinb Med Surg J 64:400–413

Daley GQ, van Etten RA, Baltimore D (1990) Induction of chronic myelogenous leukemia in mice by the P210 BCR/ABL gene of the Philadelphia chromosome. Science 247:824–830

Dameshek W (1951) Some speculations on the myeloproliferative syndromes. [Editorial] Blood 6:372–375

Deininger M, Buchdunger E, Druker BJ (2005) The development of imatinib as a therapeutic agent for chronic myeloid leukemia. Blood 105:2640–2653

Deininger M, Goldman JM, Lydon NB, Melo JV (1997) The tyrosine kinase inhibitor CGP57148B selectively inhibits the growth of BCR-ABL positive cells. Blood 90:3691–3698

de Klein A, van Kessel A, Grosveld G, Bartram CR, Hagemeijer A, Bootsma D, Spurr NK, Heisterkamp N, Groffen J, Stephenson JR (1982) A cellular oncogene is translocated to the Philadelphia chromosome in chronic myelocytic leukaemia. Nature 300:765–767

Donne A (1842) De l'origine des globules du sang, de leur mode de formation, de leur fin. CR Acad Sci 4:366

Druker BJ, Lydon NB (2000) Lessons learned from the development of an Abl tyrosine kinase inhibitor for chronic myelogenous leukemia. J Clin Invest 105:3–7

Druker BJ, Tamura S, Buchdunger E et al (1996) Effects of a selective inhibitor of the Abl tyrosine kinase on the growth of Bcr-Abl positive cells. Nat Med 2:561–566

Eckhardt S, Sellei C, Horvath IP, Institorisz L (1963) Effect of 1,6-dibromo-1,6-dideoxy-D-mannitol on chronic granulocytic leukemia. Cancer Chemother Rep 33:57–71

Ehrlich P (1891) Farbenanalytische Untersuchungen zur Histologie und Klinik des Blutes. Hirschwald, Berlin

Elefanty AG, Hariharan IK, Cory S (1990) Bcr-abl, the hallmark of chronic myeloid leukemia in man, induces multiple haemopoietic neoplasms in mice. EMBO J 9:1069–1078

Fefer A, Cheever MA, Thomas ED et al (1979) Disappearance of Ph[1] positive cells in four patients with chronic granulocytic leukemia after chemotherapy, irradiation and marrow transplantation from an identical twin. New Engl J Med 300:333–337

Fialkow PJ, Gartler SM, Yoshida A (1967) Clonal origin of chronic myelocytic leukemia in man. Proc Natl Acad Sci USA 58:1468–1471

Fialkow PJ, Jacobson RJ, Papayannopoulou T et al (1977) Chronic myelocytic leukemia: clonal origin in a stem cell common to the granulocyte, erythrocyte, and platelet, and monocyte/macrophage. Am J Med 63:125–130

Fialkow PJ, Martin PJ, Najfeld V et al (1981) Evidence for a multistep pathogenesis of chronic myelogenous leukemia. Blood 58:158–163

Forkner CE (1938) Leukemia and allied disorders, 1st edn. Macmillan, New York

Fuller HW (1846) Particulars of a case in which enormous enlargement of the spleen and liver, together with dilatation of all vessels in the body were found coincident with a peculiarly altered condition of the blood. Lancet 2:43–44

Galton DAG (1953) Myleran in chronic myeloid leukaemia. Lancet i:208–213

Galton DAG (1959) Treatment of the chronic leukaemias. Brit Med Bull 15:79–86

Gambacorti-Passerini C, le Coutre P, Mologni L et al (1997) Inhibition of the ABL kinase activity blocks the proliferation of BCR/ABL+ cells and induces apoptosis. Blood Cells Mol Dis 23:380–384

Geary CG (2000) The story of chronic myeloid leukaemia. Br J Haematol 110:2–11

Goff SP, Gilboa E, Witte ON, Baltimore D (1980) Structure of the Abelson murine leukemia virus genome and the homologous cellular gene: studies with cloned viral DNA. Cell 22:777–785

Goldman JM, Catovsky D, Hows J, Spiers ASD, Galton DAG (1979) Cryopreserved peripheral blood cells functioning as autografts in patients with chronic granulocytic leukaemia. Brit Med J 1:1310–1313

Goldman JM, Baughan ASJ, McCarthy DM et al (1983) Marrow transplantation for patients in the chronic phase of chronic granulocytic leukaemia. Lancet 2:623–625

Goldman JM, Apperley JF, Jones L, et al (1986) Bone marrow transplantation for patients with chronic myeloid leukemia. N Engl J Med 314:202–207

Goldman JM, Grosveld G, Baltimore D, Gale RP (1990) Chronic myelogenous leukemia – the unfolding saga. Leukemia 4:163–167

Goodman LS, Wintrobe MM, Dameshek W, Goodman MJ, Gilman A, McLennan MT (1946) Nitrogen mustard therapy. JAMA 132:126–132

Groffen J, Stephenson JR, Heisterkamp N et al (1984) Philadelphia chromosome breakpoints are clustered within a limited region, bcr, on chromosome 22. Cell 36:93–99

Grosveld G, Verwoerd T, van Agthoven T et al (1986) The chronic myelocytic cell line K562 contains a breakpoint in *bcr* and produces a chimeric *bcr/abl* transcript. Mol Cell Biol 6:607–616

Guilhot F, Chastang C, Michallet M et al (1997) Interferon alfa-2b combined with cytarabine versus interferon alone in chronic myelogenous leukemia. New Engl J Med 337:223–229

Haddow A, Timmis GM (1953) Myleran in chronic myeloid leukaemia: chemical constitution and biological function. Lancet 1:207–208

Heisterkamp N, Stephenson JR, Groffen J, Hansen PF, de Klein A et al (1983) Localization of the c-abl oncogene adjacent to a translocation break point in chronic myelocytic leukaemia. Nature 306:239–242

Heisterkamp N, Jenster G, ten Hoeve J, Zovich D, Pattengale P, Groffen J (1990) Acute leukemia in BCR/ABL transgenic mice. Nature 344:251–253

Hoffman WJ, Craver LF (1931) Chronic myelogenous leukaemia: value of irradiation and its effect on duration of life. J Amer Med Ass 97:836–840

Horowitz MM, Gale RP, Sondel PM et al (1990) Graft-versus-leukemia reactions after bone marrow transplantation. Blood 75:555–562

Hoyle C, Gray R, Goldman JM (1994) Autografting for patients with CML in chronic phase: an update. Br J Haematol 86:76–81

Italian Cooperative Study Group on Chronic Myeloid Leukemia (1994) Interferon alfa-2a as compared with conventional chemotherapy for treatment of chronic myeloid leukemia. New Engl J Med 330:820–825

Jacobson LO, Spurr CL, Barron ESG, Smith T, Lushbaugh C, Dick GF (1946) Nitrogen mustard therapy. JAMA 132:263–271

Kaur G, Gazit A, Levitzki A et al (1994) Tyrphostin induced growth inhibition: correlation with effect on p210bcr-abl autokinase activitiy in K562 chronic myelogenous leukemia. Anticancer Drugs 5:213–222

Kelliher MA, McLaughlin J, Witte ON, Rosenberg N (1990) Induction of a chronic myelogenmous leukemia-like syndrome with v-abl and BCR/ABL. Proc Natl Acad Sci USA 87:6649–6653

Kennedy BJ (1969) Hydroxyurea in chronic myelogenous leukemia. Ann Intern Med 70:1084–1085

Kolb HJ, Mittermuller J, Clemm C et al (1990) Donor leukocyte transfusions for treatment of recurrent chronic myelogenous leukemia in marrow transplant patients. Blood 76:2462–2465

Konopka JB, Watanabe SM, Witte ON (1984) An alteration of the human c-abl protein in K562 leukemia cells unmasks associated tyrosine kinase activity. Cell 37:1035–1042

Lawrence JH, Scott KG, Tuttle LW (1939) Studies on leukaemia with the aid of radioactive phosphorus. Int Clin 3:33–58

le Coutre P, Mologni L, Cleris L et al (1999) In vivo eradication of human BCR/ABL positive leukemia with an Abl kinase inhibitor. J Natl Cancer Inst 91:163–168

Lissauer (initials unknown) (1865) Zwei Fälle von Leukämie. Berliner Klinische Wochenshrift 2:403–404

Lowenthal RM, Buskard NA, Goldman JM, Spiers ASD, Bergier N, Graubner M, Galton DAG (1975) Intensive leucapheresis as initial therapy of chronic granulocytic leukemia. Blood 46:835–840

Luger SM, O'Brien SG, Ratajczak J et al (2002) Oligodeoxynucleotide-mediated inhibition of c-myb gene expression in autografted bone marrow: a pilot study. Blood 99:1150–1158

Lydon NB, Druker BJ (2004) Lessons learned from the development of imatinib. Leuk Res 28S1:S29–S38

Mackinnon S, Papadopoulos E, Carabasi M et al (1995) Adoptive immunotherapy evaluating escalating doses of donor leukocytes for relapse of chronic myeloid leukemia after bone marrow transplantation: separation of graft-versus-leukemia from graft-versus-host disease. Blood 86:1261–1268

McGlave PB, Arthur DC, Kim TH et al (1982) Successful allogeneic bone-marrow transplantation for patients in the accelerated phase of chronic granulocytic leukaemia. Lancet 2 (8299):625–627

McGlave PB, de Fabritiis P, Deisseroth J et al (1994) Autologous transplants for chronic myelogenous leukaemia: results from eight transplant groups. Lancet 343:1486–1488

Medical Research Council's Working Party for Therapeutic Trials in Leukaemia (1968) Chronic granulocytic leukaemia: comparison of radiotherapy and busulphan therapy. Br Med J 1:201–208

Melo JV, Gordon DE, Cross NCP, Goldman JM (1993) The *ABL-BCR* fusion gene is expressed in chronic myeloid leukemia. Blood 81:158–165

Minot GR, Buckman TE, Isaacs R (1924) Chronic myelogenous leukaemia: age incidence, duration and benefit derived from irradiation. JAMA 82:1489–1494

Morse EE, Carbone PP, Freireich EJ, Bronson W, Kliman A (1966) Repeated leukapheresis of patients with chronic myelocytic leukemia. Transfusion 6:175–182

Nowell PC, Hungerford DA (1960 a) Chromosome studies on normal and leukemic leukocytes. J Natl Cancer Inst 25:85–109

Nowell PC, Hungerford DA (1960 b) A minute chromosome in human granulocytic leukemia. Science 132:1497

Okabe M, Uehara Y, Miyagishima T et al (1992) Effect of herbimycin A, an antagonist of tyrosine kinase, on *bcr/abl* oncoprotein-associated cell proliferations: abrogative effect on the transformation of murine hematopoietic cells by transfection of a retroviral vector expressing oncoprotein $P210^{bcr/abl}$ and preferential inhibition of Ph^1-positive leukemia cell growth. Blood 80:1330–1338

Piller G (1993) The history of leukemia: a personal perspective. Blood Cells 19:521–529

Piller GJ (2001) Leukaemia – a brief historical review from ancient times to 1950. Br J Haematol 112:282–292

Pusey WA (1902) Report of cases treated with Roentgen rays. JAMA 38:911–919

Reddy EP, Smith MJ, Srinivasan A (1983) Nucleotide sequence of the Abelson murine leukemia virus genome: structural similarity of its transforming gene product to other onc gene products with tyrosine kinase activity. Proc Natl Acad Sci USA 80:3623–3627

Reinhard EH, Moore CV, Bierbaum OS, Moore S (1946) Radioactive phosphorus as a therapeutic agent. A review of the literature and analysis of the results of treatment of 155 patients with various blood dyscrasias, lymphomas and other malignant neoplastic diseases. J Lab Clin Med 31:107–216

Rowley JD (1973) A new consistent chromosome abnormality in chronic myelogenous leukaemia identified by quinacrine fluorescence and Giemsa banding. Nature 243:290–293

Senn N (1903) Therapeutical value of Roentgen ray in treatment of pseudoleukemia. NY Med J 77:665

Shields A, Goff S, Paskind M, Otto G, Baltimore D (1979) Structure of the Abelson murine leukemia virus genome. Cell 18:955–962

Shtivelman E, Lifshitz B, Gale RP, Roe BA, Canaani E (1985) Fused transcript of bcr and abl genes in chronic myelogenous leukaemia. Nature 315:550–554

Speck B, Bortin M, Champlin RE et al (1984) Allogeneic bone marrow transplantation for chronic myelogenous leukaemia. Lancet 1 (8378):665–668

Talpaz M, McCredie KB, Malvigit GM, Gutterman JU (1983) Leukocyte interferon-induced myeloid cytoreduction in chronic myelogenous leukaemia. Ann Intern Med 62:689–692

Talpaz M, Kantarjian HM, McCredie K et al (1986) Hematologic remission and cytogenetic improvement induced by recombinant human interferon alpha-A in chronic myelogenous leukemia. New Engl J Med 314:1065–1069

Thomas ED, Clift RA, Fefer A et al (1986) Marrow transplantation for the treatment of chronic myelogenous leukemia. Ann Intern Med 104:155–163

Velpeau A (1827) Sur la resorption du pus et sur l'alteration du sang dans les maladies cliniques de persection nenemant. Premier observation. Rev Med 2:216–218

Virchow R (1846) Weisses Blut und Milztumoren. Med Z 15:157

Virchow R (1853) Zur pathologischen Physiologic des Bluts: Die Bedeutung der milz- und lymph-drusen-Krankheiten fur die Blutmischung (Leukaemia). Virchows Arch 5:43

Wolff NC, Ilaria RL (2001) Establishment of a murine model for therapy treated chronic myelogenous leukemia using the tyrosine kinase inhibitor STI571. Blood 98:2808–2816

Wong S, Witte ON (2004) The BCR-ABL story: Bench to bedside and back. Ann Rev Immunol 22:247–306

Wood GB (1850) Trans Coll Phys, Philadelphia, p 265

Zimmermann J, Buchdunger E, Mett H et al (1996) Phenylaminopyrimidine (PAP)-derivatives: A new class of potent and highly selective PDGF receptor autophosphorylation inhibitors. Bioorg Chem Med Lett 6:1221–1226

Bcr-Abl and Signal Transduction

Daniela Cilloni and Giuseppe Saglio

Contents

Abstract. The *BCR-ABL* oncogene is generated by the Philadelphia (Ph) chromosome translocation, fusing the *BCR* to the *ABL* gene. The Bcr-Abl fusion protein has constitutive and deregulated tyrosine kinase activity that is critical for transformation of hematopoietic cells. Different leukemia phenotypes are preferentially associated with the three fusion Bcr-Abl proteins (p190, p210, and p230) that may be expressed from the hybrid gene. Cells transformed by Bcr-Abl show activation of mitogenic signaling pathways, inhibition of apoptosis and altered cellular adhesion. CML is characterized by an inevitable progression from a chronic phase to an acute phase called blast crisis. Progression of the disease is related to the acquisition of additional genetic alterations probably associated with genomic instability. This can be a consequence of Bcr-Abl activation or may even represent an ancestral stem cell defect preceding the acquisition of the Ph-chromosome translocation, as recent observations seem to suggest. However, the mechanisms responsible for Bcr-Abl rearrangement remain elusive, although the chromosomal translocation seems to occur relatively frequently in the general population, as evidenced by the detection of rare *BCR-ABL* fusion transcripts in the leukocytes of healthy individuals.

2.1 Introduction

The discovery of the hybrid *BCR-ABL* genes was the final result of studies aimed at the identification of the molecular consequences of the translocation giving origin to the Philadelphia (Ph) chromosome. This chromosome was, for many years, the only cytogenetic abnormality known to be associated with a specific malignant disease in humans, namely chronic myeloid leukemia (CML) (Nowell and Hungerford 1960). Later it was recognized that the Ph-chromosome is the result of a reciprocal translocation, t(9;22)(q34;q11), between the long arms of chromosomes 9 and 22 (Rowley 1973), and that this translocation can be present also in other types of human leukemias (Catovsky 1979); namely in approximately 30% of adult acute lymphoblastic leukemias (ALL), in a small percentage of "de novo" acute myeloblastic leukemias (AML), in sporadic cases of other hematological malignancies, but not in other tumor types. Finally, in the 1980s, the molecular defect associated with this cytogenetic abnormality was identified and it was established that the Ph-chromosome results in the juxtaposition of parts of the *BCR* and *ABL* genes, which are normally located on chromosomes 22 and 9, respectively, to form a new hybrid gene, *BCR-ABL*, usually located on the derivative chromosome 22q- (the Ph-chromosome) (Groffen et al. 1984; Heisterkamp et al. 1985). A more detailed molecular dissection of the *BCR-ABL* genes present in CML and in other Ph-positive leukemias showed that hybrid genes with different types of junctions between *BCR* and *ABL* may be present and preferentially associated to specific leukemia phenotypes (Feinstein et al. 1987; Melo 1996), but that all the derived translated proteins share a common functional aspect: a constitutive tyrosine kinase (TK) activity (Konopka et al. 1984; Lugo et al. 1990).

Finally, through experiments with transfection of hematopoietic cells with retroviral vectors carrying *BCR-ABL* constructs in a mouse model, it was demonstrated that the expression of a functional Bcr-Abl protein was the primary and necessary factor for leukemic transformation (Daley et al. 1990).

The study of the *BCR-ABL* fusion gene has certainly played a pivotal role concerning the understanding of the role of TK activation in the development of neoplastic diseases. However, in spite of the fact that the structural organization and the molecular biology of *BCR-ABL* as well as of the normal *ABL* and *BCR* genes have been the subjects of intensive investigation in the last 20 years (Deininger et al. 2000; Melo and Deininger 2004), many questions concerning the normal functions of the two translocation partner genes, as well as the mechanisms by which the hybrid gene is formed and transforms hemopoietic cells still remains unanswered.

The unravelling of the molecular pathways activated in the Ph-positive leukemias has become of paramount importance also from the clinical point of view (Goldman and Melo 2004). Since the late 1990s, the data accumulated on the role of *BCR-ABL* in the onset and progression of CML indicated this oncoprotein as the most attractive target for molecular therapy. This finally led to the discovery of imatinib mesylate (Glivec, Novartis) (Buchdunger et al. 1996; Druker et al. 1996), whose importance goes well beyond its exceptional therapeutic value in CML and other Ph-positive leukemias, as it represents the real starting point of the so called molecularly targeted therapy.

This small chemical compound which, at micromolar concentrations, inhibits the kinase activity of Bcr-Abl by competing with ATP for its binding site, was shown to be able to inhibit cellular growth and to induce apoptosis of the leukemic cells both in vitro and in vivo (Deininger et al. 1997; Druker et al. 1996), producing a final proof of concept that Bcr-Abl TK activity is central to the pathogenesis of the leukemic process.

This chapter summarizes the most recent advances and also the outstanding questions regarding the *BCR-ABL* gene, and the functional consequences of its TK activation.

2.2 Structure and Function of the Normal *ABL* and *BCR* Genes

2.2.1 *ABL*

The *Abl* proto-oncogene belongs to the family of the nonreceptor tyrosine-kinases (Gu and Gu 2003; Robinson et al. 2000), which was originally identified for its homology with v-*abl*, a viral oncogene able to induce lymphoid tumors in the mouse (Abelson and Rabstein 1970). There are approximately 100 TK genes in the human genome which code for enzymes that transfer phosphate from ATP to tyrosine residues on specific cellular proteins, and which are deeply involved in controlling important cellular functions, including proliferation and differentiation (Robinson et al. 2000). Due to their key role in these vital processes, TKs are usually tightly controlled by various physiological mechanisms. However, alterations of the function of TKs are among the most frequent findings in human cancer and, in particular, seem to represent the common primary defect in most chronic myeloproliferative disorders (CMPDs), as extensively described on Chaps. 13–18 of this book.

TKs may become constitutively activated through at least two other mechanisms in addition to chromosomal translocations, which are overexpression and activating mutations (Blume-Jensen and Hunter 2001).

The *Abl* gene is ubiquitously expressed in cells of various tissues, and is transcribed into two types of transcripts that differ in the first alternative exons, named 1a and 1b, respectively (Chissoe et al. 1995). The main difference in the proteins encoded by these transcripts resides in the fact that only the Abl protein derived from the Abl 1b transcript contains a myristoylation site and can be anchored to the plasma membrane. Other relevant domains of Abl are those corresponding to the respective domains in Src (Courtneidge 2003; Harrison 2003): (1) the Src homologous (SH) 1 domain, which carries the tyrosine kinase function; (2) the SH2 domain which binds phosphotyrosine-containing sequences; (3) the SH3 domain which binds proline-rich consensus sequences. However, unlike Src, Abl has a long C-terminal portion that contains other important domains: an actin (McWhirter and Wang 1993) and DNA-binding sites (Kipreos and Wang 1992), three nuclear localization signals (NLS) (Wen et al. 1996), and one nuclear export signal (NES) (Taagepera et al. 1998). Due to the latter elements, the Abl protein may be found both in the cytoplasm and the nucleus, and it is able to shuttle continuously between these two compartments, where it may exert multiple and different functions, only in part elucidated so far (Zhu et al. 2004).

Unfortunately, the data derived from mouse knockout models in which the *abl* gene was inactivated have only in part contributed to understanding the physiological role of Abl. Mice with a homozygous disruption of the *abl* gene show an increased incidence of perinatal mortality, and surviving animals present phenotypes that include lymphopenia, osteoporosis, and abnormal head and eye development (Schwartzberg et al. 1991; Tybulewicz et al. 1991). The lack of more pronounced specific defects may also be due to the fact many of the Abl functions can be supplied by its homologue Arg. Indeed, mice deficient for both *abl* and *arg* suffer from defects in neurulation and die before embryonic day 11 (Koleske et al. 1998).

Nevertheless, the currently available data suggest that the normal Abl kinase can be implicated in essential cellular functions which involve control of cellular proliferation, signal transduction, apoptosis, and cell adhesion (Pendergast 2002).

Abl regulates these functions in response to extracellular signals like membrane receptor stimulation (Plattner et al. 1999, 2004) and cell adhesion (Woodring et al. 2003), as well as to internal signals like DNA damage and oxidative stress (Wang 2005; Welch et al. 1993). As Abl deregulation may have detrimental effects for cell survival, its TK activity is kept under strict control by several internal mechanisms. These rely on a complex set of intramolecular interactions involving the SH3 and SH2 domains, and other segments in the N-terminal portion of the protein (Hantschel and Superti-Furga 2004; Nagar et al. 2003; Pluk et al. 2002). In addition, external regulators such as Pag/ Msp23/ PrxI (Wen and Van Etten 1997), Abi1 (Ikeguchi et al. 2001; Shi et al. 1995), Abi2 (Dai and Pendergast 1995), Rb (Welch and Wang 1993), and F-actin (Woodring et al. 2001) have also been shown to bind to different domains of the Abl protein, directly downregulating its TK activity or maintaining the protein in an inactive conformation (Wang 2004).

Abl can act as both a positive and a negative regulator of cell growth, depending on its subcellular localisation (cytoplasmic or nuclear) (Zhu and Wang 2004), on its phosphorylation state (Pendergast 2002) and, maybe, also on its level of expression (Pendergast et al. 1991).

Several studies suggest a positive role of Abl in cell cycle regulation. In quiescent cells, nuclear Abl is kept in an inactive state by binding to the retinoblastoma (RB) protein (Welch and Wang 1993). Phosphorylation of pRB by cyclin D disrupts this complex and results in the activation of the Abl tyrosine kinase in S-phase (Welch and Wang 1995), during which Abl activates transcriptional factors such as CREB and E2F-1 as well as RNA polymerase II (Baskaran et al. 1993, 1996). Therefore, it appears that the Abl protein is part of the general mechanism of regulation of gene transcription during the cell cycle. This is consistent with the observation that fibroblasts derived from Abl knockout mice exhibit a consistent delay in S-phase entry in response to a PDGF stimulus (Plattner et al. 1999).

Cytoplasmic Abl also plays a key function in pathways regulating growth factor-induced proliferation. The existence of a signaling cascade involving receptor (PDGFR) and nonreceptor TKs (c-Src/Abl) important for mitogenesis and growth factor-induced Myc expression has been recently described (Plattner et al. 1999, 2004). Along this pathway, Abl is situated downstream of Src and contributes to transmitting the mitogenic signal activating Myc directly or through the Ras/Erk pathway (see below).

Within the context of cell proliferation and signal transduction, two other important aspects of Abl function have been recently discovered. The first is a complex functional interdependence between Abl and lipid signaling pathways involving phospholipase C-γ1 (PLC-γ1) (Plattner et al. 2003). This lipase is important in cell migration, membrane ruffling, and also mitogenesis (Rebecchi and Pentyala 2000). PLC-γ1 is also critically involved in cytoskeletal reorganization and cell adhesion and, similarly to Abl, localizes to membrane ruffles and translocates to the plasma membrane after growth factor stimulation (Rebecchi and Pentyala 2000). The recently uncovered bidirectional link between PLC-γ1 and Abl shows that PLC-γ1 is required for Abl activation by PDGFR and Src, and that Abl functions downstream of PLC-γ1, as Abl inactivation blocks PLC-γ1 function. PLC-γ1 and Abl form a complex that is enhanced by PDGF stimulation but, after activation, Abl phosphorylates PLC-γ1 and, in turn, negatively modulates its function (Plattner et al. 2003, 2004). The second recently described role for Abl in signaling is that involved in T-cell receptor (TCR) activation (Zipfel et al. 2004), where Abl seems to act downstream of Lck and upstream of ZAP-70, and to directly promote LAT phosphorylation (Wange 2004; Zipfel et al. 2004).

In contrast to the previously described positive role in stimulating proliferation, overexpression of wild-type Abl in fibroblasts can induce arrest in the G1 phase of the cell cycle (Sawyers et al. 1994). The growth inhibitory effect of Abl requires its TK activity and its nuclear localization, and is likely to relate to the ability of Abl to induce apoptosis in response to genotoxic stress such as that due to ionizing radiation, which is known to activate Abl (Wang 2000). Activation of the Abl kinase by DNA damage has been shown to require the function of ATM, which regulates cell cycle checkpoint, DNA repair, and apoptosis in response to DNA damage (Wang 2000). Cells lacking Abl can activate cell cycle checkpoints and DNA repair, but show defects in apoptosis. This Abl function is dependent on the presence of wild-type Rb and p73 (a functional homologue of the p53 tumor suppressor) proteins, although a proapoptotic activity of Abl independent from the presence of these factors has also been reported (Barila et al. 2000). Therefore, multiple and different signaling pathways may contribute to the induction of apoptosis through activation of Abl under cellular stress-conditions, but the complete scenario still lacks definition.

Another classical approach aimed at understanding the possible functions of Abl at both cytoplasmic and nuclear levels has been to consider the proteins able to bind and to interact with its structural domains. As in other nonreceptor TKs, the Abl protein possesses at its N-terminus SH3 and SH2 domains, which are docking sites for proteins that contain, respectively, proline-rich sequences interacting with the SH3 region and phosphotyrosine residues interacting with the SH2 region (Scheijen and Griffin 2002). Molecules like SOS which are capable of converting G-proteins (like Ras, Rho, Rac) from the inactive form, linked to GDP, to the active form linked to GTP, may bind to SH3. Molecules like Shc, Crkl, Nck, Bp-1, and Grb2, which lack enzyme activity but possess both phosphotyrosine and SH3 and SH2 sequences, may bind to SH2. These proteins may show complex interactions (Li et al. 2001) and may play a role of "adaptors," allowing the formation of complexes capable of putting enzymes and specific substrates in contact with each other. On the basis of these domains, it is deducible that Abl, like its oncogenic counterpart Bcr-Abl, is capable of activating a mitogenic signal through a pathway that sequentially involves Ras, Raf, Mek1 and Mek2, and Erk (Puil et al. 1994). This last kinase is capable of phosphorylating transcription factors such as Jun, triggering cellular proliferation (Raitano et al. 1995).

The C-terminal portion of the Abl protein contains a domain that interacts with F-actin (McWhirter and Wang 1993), as a consequence of which Abl plays a key role in the physiology of the cytoskeleton. Homozygous deletion of this region in transgenic mice is incompatible with life, resulting in a phenotype overlapping that induced by the deletion of the entire *ABL* gene (Schwartzberg et al. 1991). The exact function of this interaction is unknown; several data, however, suggest an important role for Abl in the mechanisms which regulate variations in cellular morphology and intercellular adhesion (Woodring et al. 2003). In addition, Abl has also been shown to inhibit migration of fibroblasts by phosphorylating Crk, which results in disruption of Crk-CAS complexes (Kain and Klemke 2001).

The Abl protein is the only nonreceptor tyrosine kinase to possess a DNA-binding domain in the C-terminal region of the molecule (Kipreos and Wang 1992). It also contains specific sequences which allow its nuclear localization (NLS) and nuclear export (NE) (Taagepera et al. 1998; Wen et al. 1996). These structural data are in agreement with the fact that Abl continuously shuttles between the nucleus and the cytoplasm. The mechanisms responsible for nuclear targeting of Abl have only recently been elucidated (Yoshida et al.

2005). Abl is sequestered in the cytoplasm by binding to 14-3-3 proteins and this binding requires phosphorylation of Abl on Thr 735. In response to DNA damage, activation of the Jun N-terminal kinase (Jnk) induces phosphorylation of 14-3-3 proteins and their release from Abl which, as a consequence, is able to translocate to the nucleus (Pendergast 2005; Yoshida and Miki 2005; Yoshida et al. 2005).

2.2.2 *BCR*

Unlike its partner, the *BCR* gene was first identified because of its rearrangement with *ABL* as a consequence of the t(9;22) translocation (Groffen et al. 1984). Named after its breakpoint cluster region, *BCR* contains 23 exons and maps to a region of about 135 kb on chromosome 22 (Chissoe et al. 1995). It is expressed as two 4.5 and 6.7 kb transcripts, which code for the same ubiquitously expressed cytoplasmic 160 kd protein (Chissoe et al. 1995). The Bcr protein contains several structural domains that underlie possible functions. The first large *BCR* exon encodes: (1) a serine–threonine kinase, whose substrates include Bap-1, a member of the 14-3-3 proteins (Reuther et al. 1994); (2) a coiled-coil domain which allows formation of dimers (McWhirter and Wang 1993); (3) a tyrosine residue at position 177 which, when phosphorylated in the Bcr-Abl hybrid protein, can bind Grb-2 (Pendergast et al. 1993), an adaptor molecule involved in the activation of the Ras pathway (Ma et al. 1997).

In the central part of Bcr there is a DBL-like pleckstrin-homology (PH) domain, able to stimulate Rho, and a GDP-GTP (guanidine diphosphate-triphosphate) exchange factor (Denhardt et al. 1996), which activates NF-kB and other transcription factors (Montaner et al. 1998). The C-terminal part of the molecule contains a GTPase activity domain for Rac (Diekmann et al. 1991), a small GTPase of the Ras family of proteins, which regulates also the activity of an NADPH oxidase in phagocytic cells (Diekmann et al. 1995). The latter finding may explain the increased oxidative burst observed in the neutrophils of *bcr*-knockout mice (Voncken et al. 1995). This is indeed the only relevant defect presented by these mice. Therefore, the significant cellular functions of the Bcr protein remain so far mostly elusive.

2.3 Molecular Anatomy of the *Bcr-Abl* Rearrangements and Their Preferential Association with Different Leukemia Phenotypes

Although generally regarded as the cytogenetic hallmark of CML, the Ph-chromosome may be associated with different leukemia phenotypes, ranging from very indolent chronic myeloproliferative disorders to acute leukemias of either lymphoid or myeloid lineage (Melo 1996).

CML is a myeloproliferative disease, initially characterized by an abnormal expansion of a clonal hematopoiesis still capable of achieving terminal differentiation (Goldman and Melo 2003). CML exhibits a characteristic biphasic clinical course: the initial chronic phase (CP), which can last for several years, originates as an indolent disease, but is invariably followed by an acute leukemia, termed blast crisis (BC). This is marked by the emergence within the clonal hematopoiesis of fully transformed subclones arrested at an early stage of differentiation, of either myeloid or lymphoid origin (Kantarjian et al. 1987). The latter finding provides evidence that the chromosome translocation occurs in a multipotent stem cell, able to give origin to cells of different hematopoietic lineages. Indeed, in CP CML patients, the erythroid, monocytic, and at least part of the B- and T-lymphoid lineages have been found to harbor the t(9;22) translocation (Fialkow et al. 1977; Haferlach et al. 1997; Tefferi et al. 1995). However, there is no evidence that these cells are functionally abnormal in CML and, during the CP, the disease phenotype is predominantly characterized by high WBC and platelet counts, with a variable increase in the percentage of the eosinophils and basophils (see Chap. 4, entitled Clinical Features of CML).

However, the Ph-chromosome, harboring the *BCR-ABL* gene, is not exclusive to CML because it is found in approximately 30% of adults (Saglio et al. 1991) and 5% of children (Priest et al. 1980) with ALL, as well as in 1–1.5% of cases of AML (Saglio et al. 2005) and in sporadic cases of lymphoma and myeloma. Furthermore, a hybrid *BCR-ABL* gene can also be found in patients who apparently lack a classical Ph-chromosome, which account for approximately 5% of all CML cases (Hagemejier 1987). In some of these Ph-negative cases, the absence of the hallmark chromosome is due to variant translocations involving other chromosomes in addition to 9 and 22 (Huret 1990; Vermaet al. 1989). In

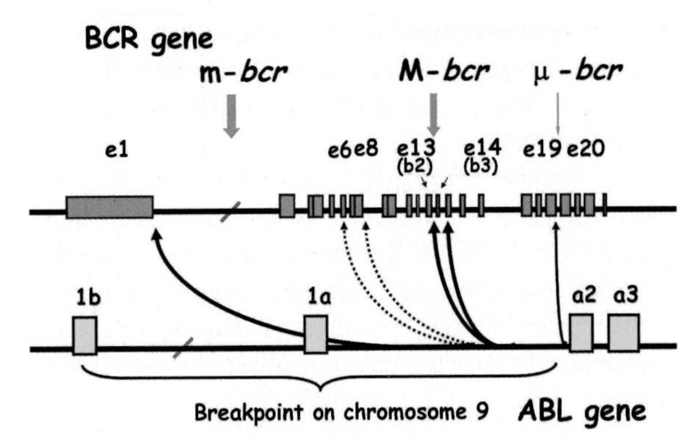

Fig. 2.1. Molecular anatomy of the BCR-ABL rearrangement. All *BCR-ABL* fusion genes contain a 5′ portion derived from *BCR* sequences and a 3′ portion which includes the bulk of the *ABL* gene. With the exception of sporadic cases, the breakpoint within the *ABL* gene falls always upstream of exon 2. In CML, the breakpoints within the *BCR* gene on chromosome 22 are predominantly restricted to a central region of the gene called major breakpoint cluster region (M-bcr). Two different types of *BCR-ABL* transcript may be expressed, joining respectively *BCR* exon 13 to *ABL* exon 2 (e13a2) or *BCR* exon 14 to *ABL* exon 2 (e14a2). In most Ph-positive acute lymphoid leukemias (ALL) the breakpoint on chromosome 22 is located in the first large intron of the *BCR* gene (minor breakpoint cluster region, or m-bcr), and, as a consequence, *BCR* exon 1 is joined to *ABL* exon 2 (e1a2 junction). In few cases, the breakpoint may take place at the very 3′ end of the *BCR* gene (micro breakpoint cluster region, or -bcr), producing a junction between *BCR* exon 19 and *ABL* exon 2 (e19a2). Rare types of *BCR-ABL* transcripts with junction between *BCR* exon 6 or exon 8 to *ABL* exon 2 have been occasionally identified in CML

others, however, the *BCR-ABL* fusion can be found by FISH (fluorescent in situ hybridization) in cells showing an apparently normal karyotype, and derives from a subcytogenetic translocation moving only a small portion of chromosome 9 containing the *ABL* gene to chromosome 22 or vice versa (Morel et al. 2003).

The rearrangement between *BCR* and *ABL* shows a certain degree of variability at the molecular level (Fig. 2.1), and the different types of *BCR-ABL* hybrid genes generate different types of fusion transcripts and proteins, which show a preferential but not exclusive association with different leukemia phenotypes (Melo 1996; Saglio et al. 1997).

All *BCR-ABL* fusion genes contain a 5′ portion derived from *BCR* sequences and a 3′ portion which includes the bulk of the *ABL* gene, most often devoid of the 1b alternative first exon and less frequently of exon 1a as well (Chissoe et al. 1995). In very rare cases, the breakpoint within the *ABL* gene falls downstream of exon 2, and in these cases the fusion transcripts encode a protein-lacking part of the SH3 domain. Although this domain in normal Abl is considered to exert the role of an internal negative regulator of the TK activity, its truncation in the Bcr-Abl fusion protein does not imply a different leukemia phenotype in the cases showing this peculiarity (Tiribelli et al. 2000).

In CML, the breakpoints on chromosome 22 are predominantly restricted to a central region of the *BCR* gene called "M-bcr" (major breakpoint cluster region), which contains 5 exons originally named b1 to b5, corresponding to *BCR* exons e10 to e14. Two different types of *BCR-ABL* transcript junction may be present (Groffen et al. 1984; Heisterkamp et al. 1985). In the first, *BCR* exon 13 is joined to *ABL* exon 2 (e13a2 junction, previously b2a2), whereas in the second, *BCR* exon 14 is spliced to *ABL* exon 2 (e14a2 junction, previously b3a2) (Shtivelman et al. 1985). The two chimeric mRNAs differ by 75 bp corresponding to the length of exon 14 sequences, and the corresponding P210 proteins differ by 25 amino acids.

Whereas approximately 30% of the Ph-positive ALL cases show the same types of Bcr-Abl rearrangements and express the same types of hybrid proteins found in CML; in the remaining 70%, a shorter Bcr-Abl hybrid protein (P190) is detected (Chan et al. 1987). In these cases the breakpoint is located in the first large intron of the *BCR* gene (the minor breakpoint cluster region, or m-bcr), and in this rearrangement the sequences of the first *BCR* exon are joined to *ABL* exon 2 (e1a2 junction) (Fainstein et al. 1987). Both in vitro (Lugo et al. 1990) and animal studies (Li et al. 1999; Quackenbush et al. 2000) suggest that P190 is characterized by a higher transforming activity than P210, and this could explain why P190 is preferentially associated with an acute leukemia phenotype.

However, the relationship between the type of Bcr-Abl fusion protein and the leukemia phenotype is an intriguing question which, at present, remains largely unsolved. Thus, whereas the P190 fusion protein is almost exclusively associated with acute leukemias, mainly lymphoid (Ph-positive ALL), there are also rare CML cases which, instead of P210, express exclusively P190 (Selleri et al. 1990). These P190 CMLs frequently appear to have a disease similar in many aspects to chronic myelomonocytic leukemia (Melo et al. 1994; Ravandi et al. 1999). The discovery that at diagnosis all CML patients also express a variable amount of transcripts with an e1a2 junction (encoding the P190 protein) as a consequence of an alternative splicing between *BCR* exon 1 and *ABL* exon 2 within the original e13a2 or e14a2 transcripts leading to P210, makes the question even more complex (Saglio et al. 1996; van Rhee et al. 1996).

Finally, a longer type of *BCR-ABL* transcript in which the breakpoint takes place at the very 3′ end of the *BCR* gene (at the micro breakpoint cluster region, or μ-bcr) and joins *BCR* exon 19 to *ABL* exon 2 (e19a2) is found in a small proportion of CML patients (Saglio et al. 1990). This transcript contains the same portion of *ABL* mRNA as the other more common types of *BCR-ABL* transcripts, but includes almost all the *BCR* coding sequence, and results in a fusion protein of 230 kd molecular weight (P230) (Verstovsek et al. 2002). Interestingly, this type of *BCR-ABL* rearrangement has been often associated with a very mild form of CML, denominated Ph-positive neutrophilic CML (Ph+ N-CML), showing clinical and hematological features overlapping those of classical CML and chronic neutrophilic leukemia (CNL) (Pane et al. 1996). However, p230 Bcr-Abl cases associated with a classical CML phenotype or even to acute leukemia have been also described (Pane et al. 2002)

Additional rare types of *BCR-ABL* transcripts have been occasionally identified in CML and Ph-positive leukemia patients. Among the other potential junctions with *ABL* exon 2 or exon 3 that can maintain the fusion sequences in frame, those involving *BCR* exon 6 (Hochhaus et al. 1996) or exon 8 (How et al. 1999) have been described but are rare, and the former are generally associated with a rather aggressive CML phenotype (Schultheis et al. 2003). In other cases, the correct reading frame between *BCR* exons and *ABL* exon2 is maintained through the presence of abnormal breakpoints within the *BCR* exons, or through the interposition of extraneous sequences derived from introns or even from other (and sometimes rather distant) genes (Melo 1997; Roman et al. 2000; Saglio et al. 2002). Although the number of these cases is small, it appears that many of these patients had a somewhat unusual and frequently aggressive clinical course (Melo 1997).

The latter findings and other observations, in particular those showing frequent deletions on the derivative chromosome 9q+ (see below) or unexpected duplications of *BCR* sequences present in both the *BCR-ABL* and the reciprocal *ABL-BCR* transcripts (Melo 1997; Melo et al. 1993; Litz et al. 1993; Zhang et al. 1995), suggest that the genesis of the Ph-chromosome and that of the consequent *BCR-ABL* rearrangement can be the result of rather complex events and the reason why certain types of rearrangement are more frequent than others is presently unknown.

In conclusion, whereas there is a clear preferential association between certain types of *BCR-ABL* transcripts and specific leukemia phenotypes, such association is not absolute. In cases in which the same fusion occurs in different types of leukemia (i.e., p210 in CML and in ALL, p190 in ALL and in CML) other still unknown factors, like different levels of expression, may play a significant role (Verstovsek et al. 2002).

2.4 Mechanisms Leading to Constitutive Activation of the Bcr-Abl Tk Activity

The Bcr-Abl fusion protein certainly plays a key role in the neoplastic transformation of the Ph-chromosome positive clone. Definitive evidence of this emerged from experiments with transfection of normal hemopoietic bone marrow progenitors of mice with retroviral vectors carrying the P210-type *BCR-ABL* gene (Daley et al. 1990; Pear et al. 1998; Zhang and Ren 1998). In this manner, it was possible to reproduce a CML-like disease, which frequently and rapidly switched into an acute lymphoid leukemia, thus mimicking at least in part the characteristic biphasic course of the human disease.

A substantial increase of the TK activity, compared to that of normal Abl, is the leading feature of all known forms of rearranged Abl proteins endowed with transforming properties, in all viruses, mice, and humans (Pendergast 2002). Moreover, there is a direct relationship between the level of TK activity and its transforming potential, suggesting that the Abl enzymatic activity is the key factor in inducing and maintaining the neoplastic phenotype (Wang 2004). However, more efficient and sophisticated mouse models of CML created more recently have been crucial for establishing a correct structure–function analysis of Bcr-Abl (Van Etten 2002). These models have clearly indicated that the activation of the tyrosine-kinase activity of Abl is necessary, but not sufficient per se to induce a CML-like disease. Domains/motifs of Bcr-Abl outside the Abl kinase catalytic site could be crucial determinants of both the severity and lineage specificity of Bcr-Abl-induced leukemogenesis (Ren 2005).

In the past years, considerable efforts have been devoted to understanding the critical sequences of the *BCR-ABL* gene whose mutations, deletions, or rearrangements might influence the enzymatic activity and trigger its oncogenic potential. As discussed, the central feature is certainly the fact that the normally regulated TK of the Abl protein is constitutively activated by the junction with the N-terminal portion of the *BCR* gene product. The presence of these sequences allows constitutive dimerization of the Bcr-Abl protein, thus promoting a transphosphorylation process (McWhirter and Wang 1993). The uncontrolled TK activity of Bcr-Abl somehow mimics the functions of the normal Abl by interacting with its effector proteins, and ultimately determines an uncontrolled cellular proliferation, a decreased adherence of the leukemia cells to the bone marrow stroma, and a reduced sensitivity to apoptotic stimuli.

However, to consider Bcr-Abl only a constitutively activated form of normal Abl is too simplistic: Bcr-Abl may have different binding properties with respect to its normal counterpart. For instance, Bcr-Abl binds directly to Grb2, and since this association involves the Bcr portion of the protein, which is absent in Abl, signaling through this pathway is unique to the human oncogene (Pendergast et al. 1993).

The kinase domain of Bcr-Abl is also regulated differently from that of Abl. The latter is tightly regulated (Hantschel and Superti-Furga 2004), as shown by the lack of oncogenic activity even following Abl overexpression (Pendergast 2002). Both intra- and intermolecular interactions are implicated in the tight control of Abl TK activity (Wang 2004). The crystal models of inactive Abl have shown that, as for Src, its autoinhibition relies on a complex set of intramolecular interactions that involve, besides the catalytic TK domain, the SH3 and SH2 domains (Barila and Superti-Furga 1998; Brasher and Van Etten 2000; Smith et al. 2003) and other segments in the N-terminal portion of the protein, such as the myristoyl group (Hantschel et al. 2003), the SH3–SH2 connector (Nagar et al. 2003), the SH2–kinase-domain linker, and the so-called Cap region, a domain of approximately 80 residues located immediately upstream of the SH3 domain (Hantschel and Superti-Furga 2004; Pluk et al. 2002). In the inactive conformation Abl resembles Src, in that the SH2 and SH3 domains bind to the kinase domain and this conformation is kept stable by the contact of the myristoyl group with a hydrophobic region on the C-terminal portion of the protein (Nagar et al. 2002). As a consequence, mutations or deletions able to disrupt the coordinated interaction of these domains may lead to activation of the Abl TK (Azam et al. 2003). In addition, several proteins that bind to the Abl SH3 domain and inhibit the kinase activity in vivo have been identified, such as Pag/Msp23/PrxI (Wen and Van Etten 1997), Abi1 (Ikeguchi et al. 2001; Shi et al. 1995), Abi2 (Dai and Pendergast 1995), and F-actin (Woodring et al. 2001). In the nucleus, the Rb protein binds to the ATP-binding portion of the Abl kinase domain during the G1 phase of the cell cycle and this interaction inhibits the Abl kinase activity (Welch and Wang 1993). At the moment, however, the physiologic relevance of the Abl binding proteins is not completely clear. Recently, an interesting hypothesis reconciling the self-imposed ability of Abl to maintain a latent conformation with the presence of Abl inhibitors has been proposed. According to this hypothesis the cellular inhibitors of Abl control and stabilize the autoinhibited conformation (Wang 2004).

In the Bcr-Abl fusion protein, the first few Abl residues are replaced by the N-terminal segment of Bcr. Since the major part of the SH3 region is intact, the mechanism of increased tyrosine-kinase activity is mainly due to the dimerization induced by the coiled-coil (CC) motif on the Bcr portion (Pendergast et al. 1993). Mutations or deletions in this CC motif abolishing the capacity of Bcr to dimerize abrogate the leukemogenic potential of Bcr-Abl in mice, at least on the myeloid lineage (He et al. 2002; Zhang et al. 2001). Therefore, dimerization through the CC-motif is essential for Bcr-Abl TK activation, allowing an initial transphosphorylation of a regulatory Tyr residue at position 1294 in the kinase domain, followed by phosphorylation of another Tyr residue at position 177 of the Bcr portion, that becomes a Grb2-binding site (Fig. 2.2). Grb2 in turn binds SOS and GAB2, and the formation of this complex, strictly dependent on phosphorylation at Tyr 177, leads to activation of RAS and recruitment of SHP2 and PI3K (Pendergast et al. 1993; Puil et al. 1994). The role of other sites of phosphorylation, such as a Tyr residue at position 245 of Abl in the linker between the SH2 and the kinase domain, is still matter of debate (Brasher and Van Etten 2000; Tanis et al. 2003). This sequence of phosphorylation events, in part similar to that occurring in the full activation of normal Abl, is important to understand the mechanism of action of imatinib, and may explain why certain mutations outside the ATP binding pocket may cause resistance to the drug (Azam et al. 2003). Since imatinib binds to the Bcr-Abl TK in its inactive conformation, mutations that favor the maintenance of an active state can cause resistance to the drug.

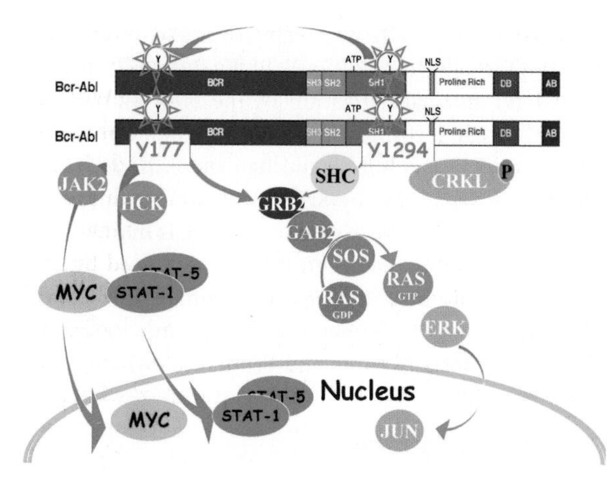

Fig. 2.2. Pathways activated by Bcr-Abl. The Bcr-Abl proteins can form dimers or tetramers and transautophosphorylate at Tyr residue 1294. Subsequent phosphorylation at the Tyr 177 residue in the Bcr portion generates a high-affinity binding site for growth factor receptor-bound protein 2 (Grb2). Grb2 binds to Bcr-Abl through its SH2 domain and to Sos and Grb2-associated binding protein 2 (Gab2) through its SH3 domains. Sos in turn activates Ras and its downstream effectors. The SH2 domain of Abl can bind SHC, which, following phosphorylation, can also recruit Grb2. Bcr-Abl proteins may also activate STATs either by direct association of Stat SH2 domains with phosphorylated tyrosines on Bcr-Abl or via the Src family kinase Hck. Finally, Myc is activated by Bcr-Abl activation through the SH2 and the C-terminus regions of the Abl portion and via Jak2

In addition to dimerization, the inability of cellular inhibitors of Abl to bind to the SH3 region of the Bcr-Abl protein may contribute to the mechanisms leading to the constitutive TK activity (Brasher et al. 2001). This could occur through the formation of oligomers which, in turn, might interfere with the SH3 binding of inhibitory proteins (Golub et al. 1996), and is thus in keeping with the observation that rare CML cases carrying *BCR-ABL* transcripts in which the SH3 domain is absent because of an unusual breakpoint position within the *ABL* gene, do not differ significantly in leukemia phenotype from those carrying the classical types of transcripts (Tiribelli et al. 2000). It has been shown that Bcr-Abl TK activity may induce the proteasome degradation of Abl cellular inhibitor proteins, such as Abi-2 (Dai et al. 1998).

Finally, the failure of normal mechanisms of inactivation may also play a role in maintaining Bcr-Abl activation. Whereas activated Abl is rapidly downregulated by ubiquitin-dependent proteasome machinery, and this prevents the unwarranted persistence of high levels of activated Abl kinase activity in the cells, this mechanism may fail to inactivate Bcr-Abl (An et al. 2000). It is also known that tyrosine phosphatases may counterbalance the effect of the TK proteins in the cells (Neel et al. 2003). Transcriptional or posttranscriptional deregulation of the tyrosine-phosphatases has been described to occur in Bcr-Abl transformed cells (Chien et al. 2003) and, although we still lack a comprehensive vision of all these aspects, an important possible role of these proteins to the leukemogenic process induced by Bcr-Abl can be envisaged.

2.5 Pathways Activated by Bcr-Abl

The molecular pathways by which the Bcr-Abl proteins induce transformation still remain rather elusive, in spite of the large body of data accumulated in recent years. This is in part a consequence of our incomplete knowledge of the physiological function of the *ABL* proto-oncogene product. Nevertheless, it is becoming progressively evident that a multiplicity of molecular interactions is implicated in the transforming activity of the Bcr-Abl hybrid proteins, inducing perturbations of various molecular pathways at different levels, from membrane to nucleus, and affecting three main functions: proliferation, adhesion, and apoptosis. In this context, however, two general aspects must be considered: (1) each activated pathway may be implicated in more than one function, as e.g., the PI3K/AKT pathway, which is relevant for both proliferation and apoptosis (Vivanco and Sawyers 2002); (2) the functional relevance of each activated pathway may vary in the context of lineage of the *BCR-ABL* positive cells (Hu et al. 2004).

2.5.1 Effects of Bcr-Abl on Signal Transduction

2.5.1.1 RAS Pathway

One of the critical signaling pathways constitutively activated in CML hematopoiesis is that controlled by Ras proteins and their relatives (Cortez et al. 1997) (Fig. 2.2). The TK activity of P210 maintains p21 Ras in an active state, bound to GTP. Ras activation results from interaction of P210 with other cytoplasmic proteins, which function as adaptor molecules, to create multiprotein signaling complexes. The amino-terminal *BCR*-encoded sequences of Bcr-Abl contains a tyrosine phosphorylated site at position 177 that binds the SH2 domain of the adaptor proteins Grb2 (Pendergast et al. 1997). The essential role of phosphorylation of this Tyr residue in the Bcr portion is underlined by the finding that mutation of tyrosine 177 to Phe abrogates the ability of Bcr-Abl to induce myeloid leukemia in a murine model of CML (He et al. 2002). The P210-Grb2 ligand recruits Sos, a Ras-guanine nucleotide-releasing-protein (GNRP), which is constitutively associated to the Grb2 SH3 domain (Cortez et al. 1997) (Fig. 2.2). In turn, Bcr-Abl-Grb2-Sos complex stimulates conversion of the inactive GDP-bound form of Ras to its active GTP-bound state (Cortez et al. 1997). In addition, the RAS-controlled pathway is enhanced by the phosphorylation of the Shc gene products p46 and p52 by the Bcr-Abl phospho-Tyr residue located at position 1294 of the TK domain, which, after the formation of a Shc-Grb2 complex, has the potential to further activate the RAS-mediated signaling (Pelicci et al. 1995). The critical role of intermediate adaptor proteins, consisting of SH2/SH3 domains, but lacking a catalytic domain, as potential substrates for P210 Bcr-Abl TK activity is substantiated by heavy phosphorylation of Crkl. This is the most prominent tyrosine phosphorylated protein in Ph-positive cells (Oda et al. 1994), where it binds Bcr-Abl and through p120CBL may link P210 to the PI-3 kinase pathway (Sattler et al. 1996), which is not only relevant for proliferation but also for the regulation of apoptosis. Finally, Bcr-Abl activates Raf1, Mek1, Mek2, and Erk kinases through p21 Ras, which elicits early nuclear events, such as transactivation of *JUN* (Raitano et al. 1995).

Another way to activate both the RAS and the PI3K/AKT pathways is represented by the activation of the scaffold protein Gab2 which is recruited and phosphorylated by Bcr-Abl through the formation of a complex with the adaptor protein Grb-2, that binds the phosphorylated Tyr residue at position 177 of the Bcr portion of Bcr-Abl (Sattler et al. 2002). The fundamental role of Gab2 activation in this pathway is underlined by the fact that Bcr-Abl was unable to confer cytokine-independent growth, a characteristic of *BCR-ABL*-positive leukemia cells, in primary myeloid cells isolated from Gab2^{-}/$^{-}$ mice (Sattler et al. 2002). Gab2 is also implicated in the activation of SHP2, a phosphatase also known as PTPN11, which is frequently found inactivated in many types of human cancer and in an autosomal-dominant genetic disorder, the Noonan syndrome. The subjects affected by this syndrome, besides other congenital defects, show a predisposition to develop leukemia (Tartaglia et al. 2004). PI3K and SHP2 are required for normal activation of the RAS pathway by most receptor tyrosine kinases and cytokine receptors (Sattler et al. 2002), but the mechanism of the activation of RAS–ERK pathway by SHP2 is at present unknown. The importance of Ras signaling in CML is mainly associated with the increased proliferation induced by Bcr-Abl activation but, through the stimulation of the PI3K/AKT pathway, it may also be relevant for inhibition of apoptosis (Kharas and Fruman 2005).

2.5.1.2 MYC Pathway

Another postulated nuclear "target" of the transforming activity of the P210 protein is the proto-oncogene *MYC*, which is expressed at high levels in CML cells. *MYC* activation, however, seems to be independent from the activation of the Ras pathway and, in fact, in vitro complementation studies reveal that the SH2 and the C-terminus regions of Abl are directly involved in the mechanism of *MYC* upregulation (Zou et al. 1997).

It has been recently demonstrated that Jak2 is implicated in Myc induction by Bcr-Abl (Xie et al. 2001, 2002). This is particularly relevant in light of the recent reports that Jak2 activation through a specific point mutation is responsible for a very high percentage of classic myeloproliferative disorders such as polycytemia vera (PV), essential thrombocythemia (ET) and idiopathic myelofibrosis (IM) (Baxter et al. 2005; James et al. 2005; Jones et al. 2005; Kralovics et al. 2005; Levine et al. 2005). This finding seems to establish a connection between the molecular pathogenesis of different myeloproliferative disorders. Myc seems also essential for Bcr-Abl-mediated transformation of both fibroblasts and hematopoietic cells, as dominant negative mutants of Myc were shown to be able to block this process (Sawyers et al. 1992). Although most of the Myc functions still lack a precise definition, it is known that this transcription factor induces the transcription of specific genes connected with cell cycle and apoptosis in response to mitogenic signals (Menssen and Hermeking 2002).

2.5.1.3 STAT Pathway

STAT1 and *STAT5* are constitutively activated in *BCR-ABL*-positive cell lines and in primary cells from CML patients (Carlesso et al. 1996; Ilaria and Van Etten

1996). P190 Bcr-Abl is also able to activate STAT6 (Ilaria and Van Etten 1996), and this may be relevant for the preferential association with the lymphoid phenotype shown by this type of Bcr-Abl protein.

Demonstration of STAT activation by Bcr-Abl led to the attractive model that this could explain the cytokine independence characteristic of the *BCR-ABL* positive cells. In normal cells, nuclear translocation of STATs occurs only after cytokine binding to receptor and is mediated by the activation of the receptor-associated Jak kinases (Sillaber et al. 2000). However, Bcr-Abl proteins activate STATs not by a Jak-dependent pathway, by but either direct association of Stat SH2 domains with phosphorylated tyrosines on Bcr-Abl or via the Src family kinase Hck (Schreiner et al. 2002). Furthermore, factor-independent growth may also derive from an autocrine loop (Sirard et al. 1994). The suggestion that Bcr-Abl induces secretion of growth factors such as IL-3 and G-CSF has been supported in some experimental systems (Humphries et al. 1988).

2.5.1.4 Other Signaling Pathways

Activation of the transcription factor NF-kB/Rel by Bcr-Abl has been demonstrated, but the mechanisms remain obscure. Bcr-Abl induces NFkB/Rel nuclear translocation, which is at least partially due to increased IkBa degradation (Kirchnera et al.2003). The p38 MAPK pathway has also been recently reported to show alterations in CML (Mayer et al. 2001). A hypothetic scenario is that this pathway, normally inhibited by Bcr-Abl, could be restored by interferon-alpha, explaining the antiproliferative effect of this drug on CML cells

Several other pathways activated by Bcr-Abl still lack a precise definition. For example, associations with the subunit of the IL-3 receptor (Wilson Rawls et al. 1996) and with the Kit receptor (Hallek et al. 1996) have been reported. More recently, however, the role of the Dok-1 and Dok-2 proteins, also known to be heavily phosphorylated by Bcr-Abl (Kashige et al. 2000), has been in part elucidated. Indeed, Dok-1 and Dok-2 negatively regulate Ras and MAP kinase activation and, therefore, seem to oppose the transformation induced by p210 Bcr-Abl (Di Cristofano et al. 2001). As a consequence, Dok-1 and Dok-2 functional loss could potentially contribute to disease progression (Niki et al. 2004; Yasuda et al.2004), but whether this really occurs in the natural history of the human disease still needs to be established.

2.5.2 Impaired Adhesion to Bone Marrow Stroma

An increasing set of data suggests that stromal proteins are also implicated in the well-known defective adhesion capacity of CML cells. This may derive from the fact that the Bcr-Abl protein forms multimeric complexes with adhesion proteins like Paxillin, and is able to bind to F-actin or focal adhesion kinase (FAK), thus suggesting a direct action on the cytoskeleton function (Salgia et al. 1995). Crkl, the most abundant phosphorylated protein in CML neutrophils, has roles in the regulation of cellular motility (Uemura et al. 2000) and may mediate these interactions by way of its association with focal adhesion proteins such as Fak and p130Cas (Salgia et al. 1996).

Since adhesive interactions are tools for extensive "cross talk" between cells, they ensure the regulated state of a large number of cell functions such as growth and differentiation. Part of the adhesion defect of Ph-positive hematopoiesis is mediated through abnormalities of the phosphatidyl-inositol (PI)-linked surface receptors, which are involved in the reduced adhesion capacity of CML progenitors to the bone marrow stromal compartment (Bathia et al. 1995). In particular, the deficient expression of one PI-linked cell surface cytoadhesion molecule, the lymphocyte-associated-antigen three (LFA 3), has been associated with the abrogation of the immuno-mediated control on the size of the Ph-positive clone (Upadhyaya et al. 1991). LFA 3 (identified by the monoclonal antibody CD58) is a widely expressed cell surface protein, whose only known function is to act as the binding ligand for the T cell surface protein CD2. CD2/LFA 3 adhesive interaction between a subset of human T cells and early (CD34+) hematopoietic progenitors plays a role in controlling the size of the actively cycling stem cell pool. Through LFA3-deficient expression, the Ph-positive stem cell compartment may escape this immune-mediated growth regulation.

However, the most relevant consequences of changes in the adhesion properties of CML cells arise from abnormal interactions of Ph-positive progenitors with the hematopoietic microenvironment. This was first described by Gordon et al., who observed the failure of the Ph-positive hematopoietic progenitors to adhere to preformed stromal layers (Gordon et al. 1987). Normally, adhesion of the hematopoietic stem cell to special "niches" within the bone marrow microenvironment is crucial for maintenance of its quiescent state. This phenomenon results from adhesive interactions between the $\beta 1$ integrins

VLA-4 and VLA-5, the homing lymphocyte receptor (CD44) and the cell surface proteoglycan receptor located on the cell surface, with distinct functional domains of fibronectin, a component of the hematopoietic microenvironment extracellular matrix (Verfaille et al. 1992, 1994, 1997). Hematopoietic inhibitory factors MIP1α and TGF-β have also been proposed as soluble messengers responsible for contact-mediated inhibitory effects on cell proliferation (Verfaille et al. 1994). As a consequence, impaired adhesion to the stromal microenvironment allows CML progenitors to cycle continuously, independently of physiological stimuli that induce cell cycle arrest on their normal counterparts (Eaves et al. 1986).

In conclusion, the complete biochemical pathway underlying the adhesion defect of Ph-positive progenitors has not yet been identified, and there are contrasting observations regarding the integrin function in cell lines as compared to primary cells. It seems to involve both direct interactions of Bcr-Abl with molecules playing a key role in cytoskeleton organization and indirect interactions mediated by other proteins. In relation to this, it is not presently known if the previously described interaction between PLC-γ1 and normal Abl (Plattner et al. 2003, 2004), is also deregulated in Bcr-Abl transformed cells thus underlying the adhesion defect observed in CML.

2.5.3 Inhibition of Apoptosis

Whereas the normal Abl protein plays a key role in the cellular response to genotoxic stress and has a proapoptotic function, the oncogenic Bcr-Abl tyrosine kinase is a potent inhibitor of apoptosis (Skorski 2002; Wang 2000). This may be in part explained by the fact that one of the most striking differences between the normal Abl and Bcr-Abl lies in their different subcellular localization. The Abl protein is found in both the nucleus and the cytoplasm and can shuttle between these two compartments because of the presence of nuclear localization and nuclear export domains. The mechanisms responsible for nuclear targeting of Abl have been recently elucidated (Pendergast 2005; Yoshida and Miki 2005; Yoshida et al. 2005). Abl is sequestered in the cytoplasm by binding to 14-3-3 proteins, and this binding requires phosphorylation of Abl on Thr 735. In response to DNA damage, activation of the c-Jun N-terminal kinase (Jnk) induces phosphorylation of 14-3-3 proteins and their release from Abl, which as a consequence is able to translocate to the nucleus, where it functions as it has been previously discussed. By contrast, Bcr-Abl is exclusively cytoplasmic and seems to be unable to enter the nucleus, where normal Abl exerts its pro-apoptotic activity (Wang 2000). Interestingly, Bcr-Abl is retained in the cytoplasm mainly because of its constitutively activated tyrosine kinase, but if the kinase is inhibited in vitro with imatinib and its nuclear export simultaneously blocked with leptomycin B, the oncoprotein may enter the nucleus. If imatinib is subsequently removed and the tyrosine kinase activity of the trapped nuclear Bcr-Abl is reactivated, apoptosis is induced (Vigneri and Wang 2001).

Furthermore, Bcr-Abl can inhibit apoptosis at the cytoplasmic level mainly by activating the PI3K/AKT pathway. Indeed, Bcr-Abl, but not Abl, associates with and activates PI3K (Varticovski et al. 1991). This is effected via more than one pathway, such as via Crk and Crkl (Sattler et al. 1996) or via p21Ras, as shown in other systems (Kauffmann-Zeh et al. 1997). Similarly, recent work suggests that the scaffolding adaptor protein Gab2, recruited to Tyr177 of Bcr-Abl via a Grb2/Gab2 complex, represents a fundamental factor in linking Bcr-Abl to PI3K activation (Sattler et al. 2002). Akt kinase is certainly an important effector of Bcr-Abl-activated PI3K (Skorski 1997), and its activation is dependent on the PI3K products, phosphatidylinositol 3,4 bisphosphate (PIP_2), and phosphatidylinositol 3,4,5 trisphosphate (PIP_3) (Jain et al. 1996). Once active, Akt exerts many cellular functions through the phosphorylation of downstream substrates such as mTOR, Bad, caspase 9, Ask1, Mdm2, and the forkhead transcription factor, FKHRL1 (Komatsu et al. 2003). The net result of Bcr-Abl activation of this pathway is the deregulation of the apoptotic machinery (Franke et al. 1997), ultimately leading to a prolonged survival and expansion of the abnormal clone.

Finally, downregulation of ICSBP (interferon consensus sequence binding protein) may also represent a way by which Bcr-Abl could inhibit apoptosis (Hao and Ren 2000). This is supported by the finding that ICSBP knockout mice show the development of a chronic myeloproliferative disease resembling CML (Holtschke et al. 1996).

In conclusion, multiple signals initiated by Bcr-Abl (in particular those transduced through the Ras and the PI3K/AKT pathways) have simultaneous proliferative and antiapoptotic consequences, and both these aspects may contribute to the expansion of a clone in which a proliferative stimulus is not counterbalanced (as it generally happens in normal clones) by increased apoptosis. Bcr-Abl acts on both fronts at the same time, promoting the expansion of the transformed clone.

2.6 Bcr-Abl and Genetic Instability

The same mechanisms responsible for inhibition of apoptosis could also be responsible for the rapid accumulation of those additional genetic mutations that may lead to disease progression, ending, in the great majority of cases, with an acute leukemia phase which is usually fatal in a few months (Skorski 2002b). Understanding the mechanisms which trigger the transition from chronic to acute phase is of utmost importance because the timing of this event is the major determinant of patient survival in CML. This is more extensively described and discussed in Chap. 3, entitled Chronic Myeloid Leukemia: Biology of Advanced Phase.

2.7 Mechanisms Leading to the t(9;22) Translocation and to *BCR-ABL* Rearrangement

Although we know that leukemogenesis in humans results from a number of recurrent chromosomal translocations, we still lack any substantial information on the mechanisms of many of these translocations, including the t(9;22) which gives origin to the Ph-chromosome. We know that ionizing radiation may have a role, since accidental exposure to radiation has been demonstrated to be significantly associated to an increased risk to develop CML (Preston et al. 1994), and high-dose irradiation of myeloid cell lines in vitro is able to induce the formation of transcriptionally active *BCR-ABL* fusion genes similar to those present in CML patients (Deininger et al. 1998). In addition, the t(9;22) translocation and the *BCR-ABL* fusion is probably a relatively frequent event that only very sporadically leads to the development of a leukemia, as suggested by the finding of small amounts of *BCR-ABL* transcripts in leucocytes from a high percentage of adult normal subjects (Biernaux et al. 1995; Bose et al. 1998). However, at present, no clear molecular basis favoring the rearrangement between the *BCR* and *ABL* genes has been identified, and only hypothetical mechanisms have been proposed. The close proximity of the *BCR* and *ABL* genes in hematopoietic cells in interphase has been suggested to be a potential mechanism that may favor translocations between the two genes (Neves et al. 1999). In addition, a 76-kd duplicon on chromosome 9 near to the *ABL* gene and on chromosome 22 near to *BCR* has been recently identified (Saglio et al. 2002). Duplicons are chromosome-specific duplications, ranging from few to 200 kb in length, which have been implicated in the formation of new genes over evolutionary time and that, due to misalignment during meiosis, can be responsible for genetic diseases known as "genomic disorders"(Ji et al. 2000). At present, the possible role of duplicons in triggering mitotic changes in somatic cells, finally leading to the genesis of recurrent chromosomal translocations like those present in human leukemias, is purely speculative. The duplicon identified on chromosomes 9 and 22 could have a role in the initial step of the t(9;22) translocation process, simply by drawing together the specific chromosomal regions containing the *BCR* and the *ABL* genes and favoring exchanges between them. Very sporadically, this exchange could result directly in the formation of a functional *BCR-ABL* rearrangement, encoding an oncogenic Bcr-Abl protein able to confer a growth advantage to the Ph-positive clone, and ultimately leading to its expansion (Saglio et al. 2002).

However, several findings suggest that the genesis of the Ph chromosome and the *BCR-ABL* rearrangement can be the final result of a complex and, in some instances, multistep event. These findings include: (1) the presence of variant translocations involving also other chromosomes in addition to chromosome 9 and 22 (Huret 1990; Verma et al. 1989); (2) the presence of sporadic cases with aberrant *BCR-ABL* transcripts showing the presence of sequences of different origin interposed between the *BCR* and *ABL* exons (Melo 1997); (3) the presence of large deletions on the derivative chromosome 9q+ surrounding the breakpoint position and involving in most cases both the Abl and the Bcr genes and their nearby regions (Sinclair et al. 2000). The origin of these deletions, which have been associated with a worse prognosis in interferon (IFN)-treated patients (Sinclair et al. 2000), and whose prognostic significance for imatinib-treated patients is still controversial (Huntly et al. 2004; Quintas-Cardama et al. 2005), is unknown.

Furthermore, another important observation made on the high percentage of CML patients able to reach partial or complete cytogenetic responses (CCR) to imatinib treatment was that karyotypic abnormalities were detectable in the Ph-chromosome negative cells of some (5–10%) of these patients, and that this phenomenon, in a minority of cases, was also associated with myelodysplastic features (Alimena et al. 2004; Bumm et al. 2003; Deininger 2003; Goldberg et al. 2003; Loriaux and Deininger 2004; Medina et al. 2003; O'Dwyer et al. 2003; Terre et al. 2004). Interestingly, these cytogenetic abnormalities are not random and are similar to those, such as trisomy 8, monosomy 7, and del(20q), found associated with CML progression in the Ph-positive clone (Andersen et al. 2002; Loriaux and Deininger 2004). The mechanism behind the formation of cytogenetic abnormalities in Ph-negative cells is unclear. Although we cannot formally exclude that imatinib may be directly or indirectly responsible for these abnormalities, it must be underlined that the same findings have been also reported in patients treated with interferon-alpha (Casali et al. 1992; Fayad et al. 1997; Izumi et al. 1996). The lower incidence of the phenomenon observed in the latter cases could be simply due to the fact that the interferon-alpha antiproliferative effect, being much less Bcr-Abl-specific than that of imatinib, could have also suppressed most of the Ph-negative clones, in addition to the Ph-positive cells.

Therefore, the possible scenario is that imatinib simply unmasks the presence of clones with Ph-negative cytogenetic abnormalities and that these may represent the consequence of a diffuse damage to the hematopoietic compartment or the collateral progeny of an abnormal stem cell with a predisposition to acquire additional mutations, including the formation of a Ph chromosome (Loriaux and Deininger 2004). According to this hypothesis, the t(9;22) translocation is not the primary, but a subsequent event in the pathogenesis of CML. This model for CML development had been proposed several years ago by Fialkow and his coworkers, based on the observation that Ph-negative EBV-transformed lymphoblastoid cell lines established from female CML patients heterozygous for G6PD isoenzymes, exhibited a pattern of G6PD expression skewed towards the pattern of the CML clone (Fialkow et al. 1981; Raskind et al. 1993). In addition, evidence in favor of a multistep pathogenesis of CML comes from epidemiological studies that observed that the frequency of CML in England and Wales was more compatible with 2 or 3 than with a single event (Vickers 1996).

Based on the reported observations, a model for the pathogenesis of CML can be envisaged, in which the formation of the Ph-chromosome represents a secondary event taking place in a genetically unstable stem cell and favored by genetic elements (like the described duplicon for example), able to boost frequent exchanges between chromosomes 9 and 22 (Spencer and Granter 1999). These exchanges may also occur less frequently in normal hematopoietic cells, as suggested by the finding of low levels of BCR-ABL fusion transcripts in the normal population. Fortunately enough, they are probably not able to trigger the expansion of a leukemic clone without the coexistence of other defects such as those that can be present in ancestral leukemic or preleukemic stem cells. For unknown reasons, these can predispose to the accumulation of specific genetic lesions, like the t(9;22) translocation and the other common cytogenetic abnormalities found associated with CML progression. In this case, the genetic instability characterizing the Ph-positive clone and determining blastic transformation of the leukemia could precede, rather than follow the acquisition of the Bcr-Abl rearrangement, although an "expediting" role for the latter defect cannot be excluded.

Acknowledgements. This work was supported by AIRC (Associazione Italiana per la Ricerca sul Cancro), by Regione Piemonte and by AIL (Associazione Italiana contro le Leucemie).

References

Abelson HT, Rabstein LS (1970) Lymphosarcoma: virus-induced thymic-independent disease in mice. Cancer Res 30:2213–2222

Alimena G, Breccia M, Mancini M, Ferranti G, De Felice L, Gallucci C, Mandelli F (2004) Clonal evolution in Philadelphia chromosome negative cells following successful treatment with Imatinib of a CML patient: clinical and biological features of a myelodysplastic syndrome. Leukemia 18:361–362

An WG, Schulte TW, Neckers LM (2000) The heat shock protein 90 antagonist geldanamycin alters chaperone association with p210bcr-abl and v-src proteins before their degradation by the proteasome. Cell Growth Differ 11:355–360

Andersen MK, Pedersen-Bjergaard J, Kjeldsen L, Dufva IH, Brondum-Nielsen K (2002) Clonal Ph-negative hematopoiesis in CML after therapy with imatinib mesylate is frequently characterized by trisomy 8. Leukemia 16:1390–1393

Azam M, Latek RR and Daley GQ (2003) Mechanisms of autoinhibition and STI-571/imatinib resistance revealed by mutagenesis of BCR-Abl. Cell 112:831–843

Barila D, Superti-Furga G (1998) An intramolecular SH3-domain interaction regulates c-Abl activity. Nat Genet 18:280–282

Barila D, Mangano R, Gonfloni S, Kretzschmar J, Moro M, Bohmann D, Superti-Furga G (2000) A nuclear tyrosine phosphorylation circuit:

c-Jun as an activator and substrate of c-Abl and JNK. EMBO J 19:273–281

Baskaran R, Chiang GG, Wang JY (1996) Identification of a binding site in c-Ab1 tyrosine kinase for the C-terminal repeated domain of RNA polymerase II. Mol Cell Biol 16:3361–3369

Baskaran R, Dahmus ME, Wang JY (1993) Tyrosine phosphorylation of mammalian RNA polymerase II carboxyl-terminal domain. Proc Natl Acad Sci 90:1167–1171

Baskaran R, Wood LD, Whitaker LL, Canman CE, Morgan SE, Xu Y et al (1997) Ataxia telangiectasia mutant protein activates c-Abl tyrosine kinase in response to ionizing radiation. Nature 387:516–519

Baxter EJ, Scott LM, Campbell PJ, East C, Fourouclas N, Swanton S, Vassiliou GS, Bench AJ, Boyd EM, Curtin N, Scott MA, Erber WN, Green AR (2005) Acquired mutation of the tyrosine kinase JAK2 in human myeloproliferative disorders. Lancet 365:1054–1061

Bhatia R, McGlave PB, Dewald GW, Blazar BR, Verfaillie CM (1995) Abnormal function of the bone marrow microenvironment in chronic myelogenous leukemia: role of malignant stromal macrophages. Blood 85:3636–645

Biernaux C, Loos M, Sels A, Huez G, Stryckmans P (1995) Detection of major bcr-abl gene expression at a very low level in blood cells of some healthy individuals. Blood 86:3118–3122

Blume-Jensen P, Hunter T (2001) Oncogenic kinase signalling. Nature 411:355–365

Bose S, Deininger M, Gora-Tybor J, Goldman JM, Melo JV (1998) The presence of typical and atypical BCR-ABL fusion genes in leukocytes of normal individuals: biologic significance and implications for the assessment of minimal residual disease. Blood 92:3362–3367

Brasher BB, Van Etten RA (2000) c-Abl has high intrinsic tyrosine kinase activity that is stimulated by mutation of the Src homology 3 domain and by autophosphorylation at two distinct regulatory tyrosines. J Biol Chem 275:35631–35637

Brasher BB, Roumiantsev S, Van Etten RA (2001) Mutational analysis of the regulatory function of the c-Abl Src homology 3 domain. Oncogene 20:7744–7752

Buchdunger E, Zimmermann J, Mett H, Meyer T, Muller M, Druker BJ, Lydon NB (1996) Inhibition of the Abl protein-tyrosine kinase in vitro and in vivo by a 2-phenylaminopyrimidine derivative. Cancer Res 56:100–104

Bumm T, Muller C, Al-Ali HK, Krohn K, Shepherd P, Schmidt E, Leiblein S, Franke C, Hennig E, Friedrich T, Krahl R, Niederwieser D, Deininger MW (2003) Emergence of clonal cytogenetic abnormalities in Ph-cells in some CML patients in cytogenetic remission to imatinib but restoration of polyclonal hematopoiesis in the majority. Blood 101:1941–1949

Carlesso N, Frank DA, Griffin JD (1996) Tyrosyl phosphorylation and DNA binding activity of signal transducers and activators of transcription (STAT) proteins in hematopoietic cell lines transformed by Bcr/Abl. J Exper Med 183:811–820

Casali M, Truglio F, Milone G, Di Raimondo F, Parrinello G, Maserati E, Pasquali F (1992) Trisomy 8 in Philadelphia chromosome (Ph1)-negative cells in the course of Ph1-positive chronic myelocytic leukemia. Genes Chromosomes Cancer 4:269–270

Catovsky D (1979) Ph-positive acute leukaemia and chronic granulocytic leukaemia. Br J Haematol 60:493–498

Chan LC, Karhi KK, Rayter SI, Heisterkamp N, Eridani S, Powles R (1987) A novel abl protein expressed in Philadelphia chromosome positive acute lymphoblastic leukaemia. Nature 325:635–637

Chien W, Tidow N, Williamson EA, Shih LY, Krug U, Kettenbach A, Fermin AC, Roifman CM, Koeffler HP (2003) Characterization of a myeloid tyrosine phosphatase, Lyp, and its role in the Bcr-Abl signal transduction pathway. J Biol Chem 278:27413–27420

Chissoe SL, Bodenteich A, Wang YF, Wang YP, Burian D, Clifton SW, Crabtree J, Freeman A, Iyer K, Jian L, Ma Y, McLaurie HJ, Pan HQ, Sahran OH, Toth S, Wang Z, Zhang G, Heisterkamp N, Groffen J, Roe BA (1995) Sequence and analysis of the human ABL gene, the BCR gene, and regions involved in the Philadelphia chromosomal translocation. Genomics 27:67–82

Cortez D, Reuther GW, Pendergast AM (1997) The BCR-ABL tyrosine kinase activates mitotic signaling pathways and stimulates G1-to-S phase transition in hematopoietic cells. Oncogene 15:2333–2342

Courtneidge SA (2003) Cancer: escape from inhibition. Nature 422:827–828

Cross NC, Reiter A (2002) Tyrosine kinase fusion genes in chronic myeloproliferative diseases. Leukemia 16:1207–1212

Dai Z, Pendergast AM (1995) Abi-2, a novel SH3-containing protein interacts with the c-Abl tyrosine kinase and modulates c-Abl transforming activity. Genes Dev 9:2569–2582

Dai Z, Quackenbush RC, Courtney KD, Grove M, Cortez D, Reuther GW, Pendergast AM (1998) Oncogenic Abl and Src tyrosine kinases elicit the ubiquitin-dependent degradation of target proteins through a Ras-independent pathway. Genes Dev 12:1415–1424

Daley GQ, Van Etten RA, Baltimore D (1990) Induction of chronic myelogenous leukemia in mice by the P210bcr/abl gene of the Philadelphia chromosome. Science 247:824–830

Deininger MW (2003) Cytogenetic studies in patients on imatinib. Semin Hematol 40:50–55

Deininger MW, Bose S, Gora-Tybor J, Yan XH, Goldman JM, Melo JV (1998) Selective induction of leukemia-associated fusion genes by high-dose ionizing radiation. Cancer Res 58:421–425

Deininger MW, Goldman JM, Melo JV (2000) The molecular biology of chronic myeloid leukemia. Blood 96:3343–3356

Denhardt DT (1996) Signal-transducing protein phosphorylation cascades mediated by Ras/Rho proteins in the mammalian cell: the potential for multiplex signalling. Biochem J 318:729–747

Di Cristofano A, Niki M, Zhao M, Karnell FG, Clarkson B, Pear WS, Van Aelst L, Pandolfi PP (2001) p62(dok), a negative regulator of Ras and mitogen-activated protein kinase (MAPK) activity, opposes leukemogenesis by p210(bcr-abl). J Exp Med 194:275–284

Diekmann D, Brill S, Garrett MD (1991) Bcr encodes a GTPase-activating protein for p21rac. Nature 351:400–402

Diekmann D, Nobes CD, Burbelo PD, Abo A, Hall A (1995) Rac GTPase interacts with GAPs and target proteins through multiple effector sites. EMBO J 14:5297–5305

Druker BJ, Tamura S, Buchdunger E, Ohno S, Segal GM, Fanning S, Zimmermann J, Lydon NB (1996) Effects of a selective inhibitor of the Abl tyrosine kinase on the growth of Bcr-Abl positive cells. Nat Med 2:561–566

Eaves AC, Cashman JD, Gaboury LA, Kalousek DK, Eaves CJ (1986) Unregulated proliferation of primitive chronic myeloid leukemia progenitors in the presence of normal marrow adherent cells. Proc Natl Acad Sci USA 83:5306–5310

Fainstein E, Marcelle C, Rosner A, Canaani E, Gale RP, Dreazen O, Smith SD, Croce CM (1987) A new fused transcript in Philadelphia chromosome positive acute lymphocytic leukaemia. Nature 330:386–388

Fayad L, Kantarjian H, O'Brien S, Seong D, Albitar M, Keating M, Talpaz M (1997) Emergence of new clonal abnormalities following interferon-alpha induced complete cytogenetic response in patients with chronic myeloid leukemia: report of three cases. Leukemia 11:761

Fialkow PJ, Jacobson RJ, Papayannopoulou T (1977) Chronic myelocytic leukemia: clonal origin in a stem cell common to the granulocyte, erythrocyte, platelet and monocyte/macrophage. Am J Med 63:125–130

Fialkow PJ, Martin PJ, Najfeld V, Penfold GK, Jacobson RJ, Hansen JA (1981) Evidence for a multistep pathogenesis of chronic myelogenous leukemia. Blood 58:158–163

Franke TF, Kaplan DR, Cantley LC (1997) PI3K: downstream AKTion blocks apoptosis. Cell 88:435–437

Goldberg SL, Madan RA, Rowley SD, Pecora AL, Hsu JW, Tantravahi R (2003) Myelodysplastic subclones in chronic myeloid leukemia: implications for imatinib mesylate therapy. Blood 101:781

Goldman JM, Melo JV (2003) Chronic myeloid leukemia-advances in biology and new approaches to treatment. N Engl J Med 349:1451–1464

Golub TR, Goga A, Barker GF, Afar DE, McLaughlin J, Bohlander SK, Rowley JD, Witte ON, Gilliland DG (1996) Oligomerization of the ABL tyrosine kinase by the Ets protein TEL in human leukemia. Mol Cell Biol 16:4107–4116

Gordon MY, Dowding CR, Riley GP, Goldman JM, Greaves MF (1987) Altered adhesive interactions with marrow stroma of haemopoietic progenitor cells in chronic myeloid leukemia. Nature 328:342–344

Greenberger JS (1989) Ras mutations in human leukemia and related disorders. Int J Cell Cloning 7:343–359

Groffen J, Stephenson JR, Heisterkamp N, de Klein A, Bartram CR, Grosveld G (1984) Philadelphia chromosome breakpoint are clustered within a limited region, bcr, on chromosome 22. Cell 33:93–99

Gu J, Gu X (2003) Natural history and functional divergence of protein tyrosine kinases. Gene 317:49–57

Haferlach T, Winkemann M, Nickenig C, Meeder M, Ramm-Petersen L, Schoch R (1997) Which compartments are involved in Philadelphia-chromosome positive chronic myeloid leukaemia? An answer at the single cell level by combining May-Grunwald-Giemsa staining and fluorescence in situ hybridization techniques. Br J Haematol 97:99–106

Hallek M, Danhauser-Riedl S, Herbst R, Warmuth M, Winkler A, Kolb HJ, Druker B, Griffin JD, Emmerich B, Ullrich A (1996) Interaction of the receptor tyrosine kinase p145c-kit with the p210bcr/abl kinase in myeloid cells. Br J Haematol 94:5–16

Hantschel O, Nagar B, Guettler S, Kretzschmar J, Dorey K, Kuriyan J, Superti-Furga G (2003) A myristoyl/phosphotyrosine switch regulates c-Abl. Cell 112:845–857

Hantschel O, Superti-Furga G (2004) Regulation of the c-Abl and Bcr-Abl tyrosine kinases. Nat Rev Mol Cell Biol 5:33–44

Hao SX, Ren R (2000) Expression of interferon consensus sequence binding protein (ICSBP) is downregulated in Bcr-Abl-induced murine chronic myelogenous leukemia-like disease, and forced coexpression of ICSBP inhibits Bcr-Abl-induced myeloproliferative disorder. Mol Cell Biol 20:1149–1161

Harrison SC (2003) Variation on an Src-like theme. Cell 112:737–740

Haskovec C, Ponzetto C, Polak J, Maritano D, Zemanova Z, Serra A, Michalova K, Klamova H, Cermak J, Saglio G (1998) P230 BCR/ABL protein may be associated with an acute leukaemia phenotype. Br J Haematol 103:1104–1108

He Y, Wertheim JA, Xu L, Miller JP, Karnell FG, Choi JK, Ren R, Pear WS (2002) The coiled-coil domain and Tyr177 of bcr are required to induce a murinE chronic myelogenous leukemia-like disease by bcr/abl. Blood 99:2957–2968

Heisterkamp N, Stam K, Groffen J, de Klein A, Grosveld G (1985) Structural organization of the BCR gene and its role in the Ph translocation. Nature 315:758–761

Holtschke T, Lohler J, Kanno Y, Fehr T, Giese N, Rosenbauer F, Lou J, Knobeloch KP, Gabriele L, Waring JF, Bachmann MF, Zinkernagel RM, Morse HC 3rd, Ozato K, Horak I (1996) Immunodeficiency and chronic myelogenous leukemia-like syndrome in mice with a targeted mutation of the ICSBP gene. Cell 87:307–317

How GF, Lim LC, Kulkarni S, Tan LT, Tan P, Cross NC (1999) Two patients with novel BCR/ABL fusion transcripts (e8/a2 and e13/a2) resulting from translocation breakpoints within BCR exons. Br J Haematol 105:434–436

Hu Y, Liu Y, Pelletier S, Buchdunger E, Warmuth M, Fabbro D, Hallek M, Van Etten RA, Li S (2004) Requirement of Src kinases Lyn, Hck and Fgr for BCR-ABL1-induced B-lymphoblastic leukemia but not chronic myeloid leukemia. Nat Genet 36:453–461

Humphries RK, Abraham S, Krystal G, Lansdorp P, Lemoine F, Eaves CJ (1988) Activation of multiple hemopoietic growth factor genes in Abelson virus-transformed myeloid cells. Exp Hematol 16:774–781

Huntly BJ, Guilhot F, Reid AG, Vassiliou G, Hennig E, Franke C, Byrne J, Brizard A, Niederwieser D, Freeman-Edward J, Cuthbert G, Bown N, Clark RE, Nacheva EP, Green AR, Deininger MW (2003) Imatinib improves but may not fully reverse the poor prognosis of patients with CML with derivative chromosome 9 deletions. Blood 102: 2205–2212

Huret JL (1990) Complex translocations, simple variant translocations and Ph-negative cases in chronic myelogenous leukaemia. Hum Genet 85:565–568

Ikeguchi A, Yang HY, Gao G, Goff SP (2001) Inhibition of v-Abl transformation in 3T3 cells overexpressing different forms of the Abelson interactor protein Abi-1. Oncogene 20:4926–4934

Ilaria RL, Van Etten RA (1996) P210 and P190(BCR/ ABL) induce the tyrosine phosphorylation and DNA binding activity of multiple specific STAT family members. J Biol Chem 271:31704–31710

Izumi T, Imagawa S, Hatake K, Miura Y, Ariyama T, Inazawa J, Abe T (1996) Philadelphia chromosome-negative cells with trisomy 8 after busulfan and interferon treatment of Ph1-positive chronic myelogenous leukemia. Int J Hematol 64:73–77

Jain SK, Susa M, Keeler ML, Carlesso N, Druker B, Varticovski L (1996) PI3-kinase activation in BCR/ABL-transformed hematopoietic cells does not require interaction of p85 SH2 domains with p210 BCR/ABL. Blood 88:1542–1550

James C, Ugo V, Le Couedic JP, Staerk J, Delhommeau F, Lacout C, Garcon L, Raslova H, Berger R, Bennaceur-Griscelli A, Villeval JL, Constantinescu SN, Casadevall N, Vainchenker W (2005) A unique clonal JAK2 mutation leading to constitutive signalling causes polycythaemia vera. Nature 434:1144–1148

Ji Y, Eichler EE, Schwartz S, Nicholls RD (2000) Structure of chromosomal duplicons and their role in mediating human genomic disorders. Genome Res 10:597–610

Jones AV, Kreil S, Zoi K, Waghorn K, Curtis C, Zhang L, Score J, Seear R, Chase AJ, Grand FH, White H, Zoi C, Loukopoulos D, Terpos E, Vervessou EC, Schultheis B, Emig M, Ernst T, Lengfelder E, Hehlmann R, Hochhaus A, Oscier D, Silver RT, Reiter A, Cross NC (2005) Widespread occurrence of the JAK2 V617F mutation in chronic myeloproliferative disorders. Blood 106:2162–2168

Kain K, Klemke R (2001) Inhibition of cell migration by Abl family tyrosine kinases through uncoupling of Crk-CAS complexes. J Biol Chem 276:16185–16192

Kantarjian HM, Keating MJ, Talpaz M, Walters RS, Smith TL, Cork A, McCredie KB, Freireich EJ (1987) Chronic myelogenous leukemia in blast crisis. Analysis of 242 patients. Am J Med 83:445–454

Kantarjian HM, O'Brien S, Cortes J, Giles F, Shan J, Rios MB, Faderl S, Verstovsek S, Garcia-Manero G, Wierda W, Kornblau S, Ferrajoli A, Keating M, Talpaz M (2004) Survival advantage with imatinib mesylate therapy in chronic-phase chronic myelogenous leukemia (CML-CP) after IFN-alpha failure and in late CML-CP, comparison with historical controls. Clin Cancer Res 10:68–75

Kashige N, Carpino N, Kobayashi R (2000) Tyrosine phosphorylation of p62dok by p210 bcr-abl inhibits RasGAP activity. Proc Natl Acad Sci USA 97:2093–2098

Kauffmann-Zeh A, Rodriguez-Viciana P, Ulrich E, Gilbert C, Coffer P, Downward J, Evan G (1997) Suppression of c-Myc-induced apoptosis by Ras signalling through PI 3-kinase and PKB. Nature 385:544–548

Kharas MG and Fruman DA (2005) ABL oncogenes and phosphoinositide 3-kinase: mechanism of activation and downstream effectors. Cancer Res 65:2047–2053

Kipreos ET, Wang JY (1992) Cell cycle-regulated binding of c-Abl tyrosine kinase to DNA. Science 256:382–5

Kirchner D, Duysterc J, Ottmannd O, Roland M, Schmid T, Bergmanna LD, Munzerta G (2003) Mechanisms of Bcr-Abl-mediated NF-kB/Rel activation. Exp Hematol 31:504–511

Koleske AJ, Gifford AM, Scott ML, Nee M, Bronson RT, Miczek KA, Baltimore D (1998) Essential roles for the Abl and Arg tyrosine kinases in neurulation. Neuron 21:1259–1272

Komatsu N, Watanabe T, Uchida M, Mori M, Kirito K, Kikuchi S, Liu Q, Tauchi T, Miyazawa K, Endo H, Nagai T, Ozawa K (2003) A member of Forkhead transcription factor FKHRL1 is a downstream effector of STI571-induced cell cycle arrest in BCR-ABL-expressing cells. J Biol Chem 278:6411–6419

Konopka JB, Watanabe SM, Witte ON (1984) An alteration of the human c-abl protein in K562 leukemia cells unmasks associated tyrosine kinase activity. Cell 37:1035–1042

Kralovics R, Passamonti F, Buser AS, Teo SS, Tiedt R, Passweg JR, Tichelli A, Cazzola M, Skoda RC (2005) A gain-of-function mutation of JAK2 in myeloproliferative disorders. N Engl J Med 352:1779–1790

Levine RL, Wadleigh M, Cools J, Ebert BL, Wernig G, Huntly BJ, Boggon TJ, Wlodarska I, Clark JJ, Moore S, Adelsperger J, Koo S, Lee JC, Gabriel S, Mercher T, D'Andrea A, Frohling S, Dohner K, Marynen P, Vandenberghe P, Mesa RA, Tefferi A, Griffin JD, Eck MJ, Sellers WR, Meyerson M, Golub TR, Lee SJ, Gilliland DG (2005) Activating mutation in the tyrosine kinase JAK2 in polycythemia vera, essential thrombocythemia, and myeloid metaplasia with myelofibrosis. Cancer Cell 7:387–397

Li S, Ilaria RL Jr, Million RP, Daley GQ, Van Etten RA (1999) The P190, P210, and P230forms of the BCR/ABL oncogene induce a similar chronic myeloid leukemia-like syndrome in mice but have different lymphoid leukemogenic activity. J Exp Med 189:1399–1412

Li S, Couvillon AD, Brasher BB, Van Etten RA (2001) Tyrosine phosphorylation of Grb2 by Bcr/Abl and epidermal growth factor receptor: a novel regulatory mechanism for tyrosine kinase signaling. EMBO J 20:6793–6804

Litz CE, McClure JS, Copenhaver CM, Brunning RD (1993) Duplication of small segments within the major breakpoint cluster region in chronic myelogenous leukemia. Blood 81:1567–1572

Loriaux M, Deininger M (2004) Clonal cytogenetic abnormalities in Philadelphia chromosome negative cells in chronic myeloid leukemia patients treated with imatinib. Leuk Lymphoma 45:2197–2203

Lugo TG, Pendergast AM, Muller AJ, Witte ON (1990) Tyrosine kinase activity and transformation potency of bcr-abl oncogene products. Science 247:1079–1082

Ma G, Lu D, Wu Y, Liu J, Arlinghaus RB (1997) Bcr phosphorylated on tyrosine 177 binds Grb2. Oncogene 14:2367–2372

Mauro MJ, Maziarz RT, Braziel RM (2003) Demonstration of Philadelphia chromosome negative abnormal clones in patients with chronic myelogenous leukemia during major cytogenetic responses induced by imatinib mesylate. Leukemia 17:481–487

Mayer IA, Verma A, Grumbach IM, Uddin S, Lekmine F, Ravandi F, Majchrzak B, Fujita S, Fish EN, Platanias LC (2001) The p38 MAPK pathway mediates the growth inhibitory effects of interferon-alpha in BCR-ABL-expressing cells. J Biol Chem 276:28570–28577

McWhirter JR, Wang JY (1993) An actin-binding function contributes to transformation by the Bcr-Abl oncoprotein of Philadelphia chromosome-positive human leukemias. EMBO J 12:1533–1546

McWhirter JR, Galasso DL, Wang JY (1993) A coiled-coil oligomerization domain of Bcr is essential for the transforming function of Bcr-Abl oncoproteins. Mol Cell Biol 13:7587–7595

Medina J, Kantarjian H, Talpaz M, O'Brien S, Garcia-Manero G, Giles F, Rios MB, Hayes K, Cortes J (2003) Chromosomal abnormalities in Philadelphia chromosome-negative metaphases appearing during imatinib mesylate therapy in patients with Philadelphia chromosome-positive chronic myelogenous leukemia in chronic phase. Cancer 98:1905–1911

Melo JV (1996) The diversity of Bcr-Abl fusion proteins and their relationship to leukemia phenotype. Blood 88:2375–2384

Melo JV (1997) BCR-ABL gene variants. Baillieres Clin Haematol 10:203–222

Melo JV, Deininger MW (2004) Biology of chronic myelogenous leukemia-signaling pathways of initiation and transformation. Hematol Oncol Clin North Am 18:545–568

Melo JV, Gordon DE, Cross NC, Goldman JM (1993) The ABL-BCR fusion gene is expressed in chronic myeloid leukemia. Blood 81:158–165

Melo JV, Myint H, Galton DA, Goldman JM (1994) p190 BCR-ABL chronic myeloid leukemia: the missing link with chronic myelomonocytic leukemia? Leukemia 8:208–211

Menssen A, Hermeking H (2002) Characterization of the c-MYC-regulated transcriptome by SAGE: identification and analysis of c-MYC target genes. Proc Natl Acad Sci USA 99:6274–6279

Montaner S, Perona R, Saniger L, Lacal JC (1998) Multiple signaling pathways lead to the activation of the nuclear factor kB by the Rho family of GTPases. J Biol Chem 273:12779–12785

Morel F, Herry A, Le Bris MJ, Morice P, Bouquard P, Abgrall JF, Berthou C, De Braekeleer M (2003) Contribution of fluorescence in situ hybridization analyses to the characterization of masked and complex Philadelphia chromosome translocations in chronic myelocytic leukemia. Cancer Genet Cytogenet 147:115–120

Nagar B, Bornmann WG, Pellicena P, Schindler T, Veach DR, Miller WT, Clarkson B, Kuriyan J (2002) Crystal structures of the kinase domain of c-Abl in complex with the small molecule inhibitors PD173955 and imatinib (STI-571). Cancer Res 62:4236–4243

Nagar B, Hantschel O, Young MA, Scheffzek K, Veach D, Bornmann W, Clarkson B, Superti-Furga G, Kuriyan J (2003) Structural basis for the autoinhibition of c-Abl tyrosine kinase. Cell 112:859–871

Neel BG, Gu H, Pao L (2003) The "Shp"ing news: SH2 domain-containing tyrosine phosphatases in cell signaling. Trends Biochem Sci 28:284–293

Neves H, Ramos C, da Silva MG, Parreira A, Parreira L (1999) The nuclear topography of ABL, BCR, PML, and RARalpha genes: evidence for gene proximity in specific phases of the cell cycle and stages of hematopoietic differentiation. Blood 93:1197–1207

Niki M, Di Cristofano A, Zhao M, Honda H, Hirai H, Van Aelst L, Cordon-Cardo C, Pandolfi PP (2004) Role of Dok-1 and Dok-2 in leukemia suppression. J Exp Med 200:1689–1695

Nowell PC, Hungerford DA (1960) A minute chromosome in human chronic granulocitic leukemia. Science 32:1497–1501

Oda T, Heaney C, Hagopian JR, Okuda K, Griffin JD, Druker BJ (1994) Crkl is the major tyrosine-phosphorylated protein in neutrophils from patients with chronic myelogenous leukemia. J Biol Chem 269:22925–22928

O'Dwyer ME, Gatter KM, Loriaux M, Druker BJ, Olson SB, Magenis RE, Lawce H, Mauro MJ, Maziarz RT, Braziel RM (2003) Demonstration of Philadelphia chromosome negative abnormal clones in patients with chronic myelogenous leukemia during major cytogenetic responses induced by imatinib mesylate. Leukemia 17:481–487

Pane F, Frigeri F, Sindona M, Luciano L, Ferrara F, Cimino R, Meloni G, Saglio G, Salvatore F, Rotoli B (1996) Neutrophilic-chronic myeloid leukemia: a distinct disease with a specific molecular marker (BCR/ABL with C3/A2 junction) Blood 88:2410–2414

Pane F, Intrieri M, Quintarelli C, Izzo B, Muccioli GC, Salvatore F (2002) BCR/ABL genes and leukemic phenotype: from molecular mechanisms to clinical correlations. Oncogene 21:8652–8667

Pear WS, Miller JP, Xu L, Pui JC, Soffer B, Quackenbush RC, Pendergast AM, Bronson R, Aster JC, Scott ML, Baltimore D (1998) Efficient and rapid induction of a chronic myelogenous leukemia-like myeloproliferative disease in mice receiving P210 bcr/abl-transduced bone marrow. Blood 92:3780–3792

Pelicci G, Lanfrancone L, Grignani F, McGlade J, Cavallo F, Forni G, Nicoletti I, Grignani F, Pawson T, Pelicci PG (1995) Constitutive phosphorylation of Shc proteins in human tumors. Oncogene 11:899–907

Pendergast AM (2002) The Abl family kinases: mechanisms of regulation and signalling. Adv Cancer Res 85:51–100

Pendergast AM (2005) Stress and death: breaking up the c-Abl/14–3–3 complex in apoptosis. Nat Cell Biol 7:213–214

Pendergast AM, Muller AJ, Havlik MH, Clark R, McCormick F, Witte ON (1991) Evidence for regulation of the human ABL tyrosine kinase by a cellular inhibitor. Proc Natl Acad Sci 88:5927–5931

Pendergast AM, Quilliam LA, Cripe LD, Bassing CH, Dai Z, Li N, Batzer A, Rabun KM, Der CJ, Schlessinger J, Witte ON (1993) BCR-ABL-induced oncogenesis is mediated by direct interaction with the SH2 domain of the GRB-2 adaptor protein. Cell. 75:175–185

Plattner R, Kadlec L, DeMali KA, Kazlauskas A, Pendergast AM (1999) c-Abl is activated by growth factors and Src family kinases and has a role in the cellular response to PDGF. Genes Dev 13:2400–2411

Plattner R, Irvin BJ, Guo S, Blackburn K, Kazlauskas A, Abraham RT, York JD, Pendergast AM (2003) A new link between the c-Abl tyrosine kinase and phosphoinositide signaling through PLC-gamma1. Nat Cell Biol 5:309–319

Plattner R, Koleske AJ, Kazlauskas A, Pendergast AM (2004) Bidirectional signaling links the Abelson kinases to the platelet-derived growth factor receptor. Mol Cell Biol 24:2573–2583

Pluk H, Dorey K, Superti-Furga G (2002) Autoinhibition of c-Abl. Cell 108:247–254

Preston DL, Kusumi S, Tomonaga M, Izumi S, Ron E, Kuramoto A (1994) Cancer incidence in atomic bomb survivors. III. Leukemia, lymphoma and multiple myeloma, 1950–1987. Radiat Res 137(Suppl): S68–S97

Priest JR, Robinson LL, McKenna RW, Lindquist LL, Warkentin PI, LeBien TW, Woods WG, Kersey JH, Coccia PF, Nesbit ME (1980) Philadelphia chromosome positive childhood acute lymphoblastic leukemia. Blood 56:15–22

Puil L, Liu J, Gish G, Mbamalu G, Bowtell D, Pelicci PG, Arlinghaus R, Pawson T (1994) BCR-ABL oncoproteins bind directly to activators of Ras signalling pathway. EMBO J 13:764–773

Quackenbush RC, Reuther GW, Miller JP, Courtney KD, Pear WS, Pendergast AM (2000) Analysis of the biologic properties of p230 Bcr-Abl reveals unique and overlapping properties with the oncogenic p185 and p210 Bcr-Abl tyrosine kinases. Blood 95:2913–2921

Quintas-Cardama A, Kantarjian H, Talpaz M, O'brien S, Garcia-Manero G, Verstovsek S, Rios MB, Hayes K, Glassman A, Bekele BN, Zhou X, Cortes J (2005) Imatinib mesylate therapy may overcome the poor prognostic significance of deletions of derivative chromosome 9 in patients with chronic myelogenous leukemia. Blood 105:2281–2286

Raitano AB, Halpern JR, Hambuch TM, Sawyers CL (1995) The Bcr-Abl leukemia oncogene activates Jun kinase and requires Jun for transformation. Proc Natl Acad Sci USA 92:11746–11750

Raskind WH, Ferraris AM, Najfeld V, Jacobson RJ, Moohr JW, Fialkow PJ (1993) Further evidence for the existence of a clonal Ph-negative stage in some cases of Ph-positive chronic myelocytic leukaemia. Leukemia 7:1163–1167

Ravandi F, Cortes J, Albitar M, Arlinghaus R, Qiang Guo J, Talpaz M, Kantarjian HM (1999) Chronic myelogenous leukaemia with p185(BCR/ABL) expression: characteristics and clinical significance. Br J Haematol 107:581–586

Rebecchi MJ, Pentyala SN (2000) Structure, function and control of phosphoinositide-specific phospholipase C. Physiol Rev 80: 1291–1335

Ren R (2005) Mechanisms of BCR-ABL in the pathogenesis of chronic myelogenous leukaemia. Nat Rev Cancer 5:172–183

Reuther GW, Fu H, Cripe LD, Collier RJ, Pendergast AM (1994) Association of the protein kinases c-Bcr and Bcr-Abl with proteins of the 14–3–3 family. Science 266:129–133

Robinson DR, Wu YM, Lin SF (2000) The protein tyrosine kinase family of the human genome. Oncogene 19:5548–5557

Roman J, Parziale A, Gottardi E, De Micheli D, Cilloni D, Tiribelli M, Gonzalez MG, del Carmen Rodriguez M, Torres A, Saglio G (2000) Novel type of BCR-ABL transcript in a chronic myelogenous leukaemia patient relapsed after bone marrow transplantation. Br J Haematol 111:644–646

Rowley JD (1973) A novel consistent chromosome abnormality in chronic myelogenous leukemia detected by quinacrine fluorescence and Giemsa staining. Nature 243:290–293

Salgia R, Brunkhorst B, Pisick E, Li JL, Lo SH, Chen LB, Griffin JD (1995) Increased tyrosine phosphorylation of focal adhesion proteins in myeloid cell lines expressing p210BCR/ABL. Oncogene 11:1149–1155

Salgia R, Pisick E, Sattler M, Li JL, Uemura N, Wong WK, Burky SA, Hirai H, Chen LB, Griffin JD (1996) p130CAS forms a signaling complex with the adapter protein CRKL in hematopoietic cells transformed by the BCR/ABL oncogene. J Biol Chem 271:25198–25203

Saglio G, Guerrasio A, Rosso C, Lo Coco F, Frontani M, Annino L, Mandelli F (1991) Detection of Ph1-positive acute lymphoblastic leukaemia by PCR. GIMEMA Cooperative Study Group. Lancet 338:958

Saglio G, Pane F, Gottardi E, Frigeri F, Buonaiuto MR, Guerrasio A, de Micheli D, Parziale A, Fornaci MN, Martinelli G, Salvatore F (1996) Consistent amounts of acute leukemia-associated P190BCR/ABL transcripts are expressed by chronic myelogenous leukemia patients at diagnosis. Blood 87:1075–1080

Saglio G, Pane F, Martinelli G, Guerrasio A (1997) BCR/ABL transcripts and leukemia phenotype: an unsolved puzzle. Leuk Lymphoma 26:281–286

Saglio G, Storlazzi CT, Giugliano E, Surace C, Anelli L, Rege-Cambrin G, Zagaria A, Jimenez Velasco A, Heiniger A, Scaravaglio P, Torres Gomez A, Roman Gomez J, Archidiacono N, Banfi S, Rocchi M (2002) A 76-kb duplicon maps close to the BCR gene on chromosome 22 and the ABL gene on chromosome 9: possible involvement in the genesis of the Philadelphia chromosome translocation. Proc Natl Acad Sci USA 99:9882–9887

Saglio G, Lo Coco F, Cuneo A, Pane F, Rege Cambrin G, Diverio D, Mancini M, Testoni N, Vignetti M, Fazi P, Iacobelli P, Bardi P, Izzo B, Bolli N, La Starza R, Amadori S, Mandelli F, Pelicci PG, Mecucci C, Falini B (2005) Prognostic Impact of Genetic Characterization in the GIMEMA LAM99P Study for Newly Diagnosed Adult AML. Relevance of Combined Analysis of Conventional Karyotyping, FLT3 and NPM Mutational Status. Blood 106:69a, abstract no. 226

Sattler M, Salgia R, Okuda K, Uemura N, Durstin MA, Pisick E, Xu G, Li JL, Prasad KV, Griffin JD (1996) The proto-oncogene product p120CBL and the adaptor proteins CRKL and c-CRK link c-ABL, p190BCR/ABL and p210BCR/ABL to the phosphatidylinositol-3′ kinase pathway. Oncogene 12:839–846

Sattler M, Mohi MG, Pride YB, Quinnan LR, Malouf NA, Podar K, Gesbert F, Iwasaki H, Li S, Van Etten RA, Gu H, Griffin JD, Neel BG (2002) Critical role for Gab2 in transformation by BCR/ABL. Cancer Cell 1:479–492

Sawyers CL, Callahan W, Witte ON (1992) Dominant negative MYC blocks transformation by ABL oncogenes. Cell 70:901–910

Sawyers CL, McLaughlin J, Goga A, Havlik M, Witte O (1994) The nuclear tyrosine kinase c-Abl negatively regulates cell growth. Cell 77:121–131

Sawyers CL, McLaughlin J, Witte ON (1995) Genetic requirement for RAS in the trasformation of fibroblasts and hematopoietic cells by the BCR-ABL oncogene. J Exp Med 181:307–313

Scheijen B, Griffin JD (2002) Tyrosine kinase oncogenes in normal hematopoiesis and hematological disease. Oncogene 21:3314–3333

Schreiner SJ, Schiavone AP, Smithgall TE (2002) Activation of STAT3 by the Src family kinase Hck requires a functional SH3 domain. J Biol Chem 277:45680–45687

Schultheis B, Wang L, Clark RE, Melo JV (2003) BCR-ABL with an e6a2 fusion in a CML patient diagnosed in blast crisis. Leukemia17:2054–2055

Schwartzberg PL, Stall AM, Hardin JD, Bowdish KS, Humaran T, Boast S, Harbison ML, Robertson EJ, Goff SP (1991) Mice homozygous for the ablm1 mutation show poor viaility and depletion of selected B and T cell populations. Cell 65:1165–1175

Selleri L, von Lindern M, Hermans A, Meijer D, Torelli G, Grosveld G (1990) Chronic myeloid leukemia may be associated with several bcr-abl transcripts including the acute lymphoid leukemia-type 7 kb transcript. Blood 75:1146–1153

Shi Y, Alin K, Goff SP (1995) Abl-interactor-1, a novel SH3 protein binding to the carboxy-terminal portion of the Abl protein, suppresses v-abl transforming activity. Genes Dev 9:2583–2597

Shtivelman E, Lifshitz B, Gale RP, Roe BA, Canaani E (1985) Fused transcript of abl and bcr genes in chronic myeloid leukaemia. Nature 315:550–554

Sillaber C, Gesbert F, Frank DA, Sattler M, Griffin JD (2000) STAT5 activation contributes to growth and viability in Bcr/Abl- transformed cells. Blood 95:2118–2125

Sinclair PB, Nacheva EP, Leversha M, Telford N, Chang J, Reid A, Bench A, Champion K, Huntly B, Green AR (2000) Large deletions at the t(9;22) breakpoint are common and may identify a poor-prognosis subgroup of patients with chronic myeloid leukemia. Blood 95:738–743

Sirard C, Laneuville P, Dick JE (1994) Expression of bcr-abl abrogates factor-dependent growth of human hematopoietic M07E cells by an autocrine mechanism. Blood 83:1575–1585

Skorski T (2002a) Oncogenic tyrosine kinases and the DNA-damage response. Nat Rev Cancer 2:351–360

Skorski T (2002b) BCR/ABL regulates response to DNA damage: the role in resistance to genotoxic treatment and in genomic instability. Oncogene 21:8591–8604

Skorski T, Bellacosa A, Nieborowska-Skorska M, Majewski M, Martinez R, Choi JK, Trotta R, Wlodarski P, Perrotti D, Chan TO, Wasik MA, Tsichlis PN, Calabretta B (1997) Transformation of hematopoietic cells by BCR/ABL requires activation of a PI-3k/Akt-dependent pathway. EMBO J 16:6151–6161

Smith KM, Yacobi R, Van Etten, RA (2003) Autoinhibition of Bcr–Abl through its SH3 domain. Mol Cell 12:27–37

Spencer A, Granter N (1999) Leukemia patient-derived lymphoblastoid cell lines exhibit increased induction of leukaemia associated transcripts following high-dose irradiation. Exp Hematol 27:1397–1401

Taagepera S, McDonald D, Loeb JE, Whitaker LL, McElroy AK, Wang JY et al (1998) Nuclearcytoplasmic shuttling of C-ABL tyrosine kinase. Proc Natl Acad Sci USA 95:7457–7462

Tanis KQ, Veach D, Duewel HS, Bornmann WG, Koleske AJ (2003) Two distinct phosphorylation pathways have additive effects on abl family kinase activation. Mol Cell Biol 23:3884–3896

Tartaglia M, Niemeyer CM, Shannon KM, Loh ML (2004) SHP-2 and myeloid malignancies. Curr Opin Hematol 11:44–50

Tefferi A, Schad CR, Pruthi RK, Ahmann GJ, Spurbeck JL, Dewald GW (1995) Fluorescent in situ hybridization studies of lymphocytes and neutrophils in chronic granulocytic leukemia. Cancer Genet Cytogenet 83:61–64

Terre C, Eclache V, Rousselot P, Imbert M, Charrin C, Gervais C, Mozziconacci MJ, Maarek O, Mossafa H, Auger N, Dastugue N, Talmant P, Van den Akker J, Leonard C, Khac FN, Mugneret F, Viguie F, Lafage-Pochitaloff M, Bastie JN, Roux GL, Nicolini F, Maloisel F, Vey N, Laurent G, Recher C, Vigier M, Yacouben Y, Giraudier S, Vernant JP, Salles B, Roussi J, Castaigne S, Leymarie V, Flandrin G, Lessard M; France Intergroupe pour la Leucemie Myeloide Chronique (2004) Report of 34 patients with clonal chromosomal abnormalities in Philadelphia-negative cells during imatinib treatment of Philadelphia-positive chronic myeloid leukemia. Leukemia 18:1340–1346

Tiribelli M, Tonso A, Ferro D, Parziale A, Rege-Cambrin G, Scaravaglio P, Saglio G (2000) Lack of SH3 domain does not imply a more severe clinical course in Ph+ chronic myeloid leukemia patients. Blood 95:4019–4020

Tybulewicz VLJ, Crawford CE, Jackson PK, Bronson RT, Mulligan RC (1991) Neonatal lethality and lymphopenia in mice with a homozygous disruption of the c-abl proto-oncogene. Cell 65:1153–1163

Uemura N, Salgia R, Ewaniuk DS, Little MT, Griffin JD (1999) Involvement of the adapter protein CRKL in integrin-mediated adhesion. Oncogene 18:3343–3353

Upadhyaya G, Guba SC, Sih SA, Feinberg AP, Talpaz M, Kantarjian HM, Deisseroth AB, Emerson SG (1991) Interferon-alpha restores the deficient expression of the cytoadhesion molecule lymphocyte function antigen-3 by chronic myelogenous leukemia progenitor cells. J Clin Invest 88:2131–2136

Van Etten RA (2002) Studying the pathogenesis of BCR-ABL+ leukemia in mice. Oncogene 21:8643–8651

van Rhee F, Hochhaus A, Lin F, Melo JV, Goldman JM, Cross NC (1996) p190 BCR-ABL mRNA is expressed at low levels in p210-positive chronic myeloid and acute lymphoblastic leukemias. Blood 87:5213–5217

Varticovski L, Daley GQ, Jackson P, Baltimore D, Cantley LC (1991) Activation of phosphatidylinositol 3-kinase in cells expressing abl oncogene variants. Mol Cell Biol 11:1107–1113

Verfaillie CM (1997) Stem cells in chronic myelogenous leukemia. Hemat Oncol Clin North Am 11:1079–1114

Verfaillie CM, McCarthy JB, McGlave PB (1992) Mechanisms underlying abnormal trafficking of malignant progenitors in chronic myelogenous leukemia. Decreased adhesion to stroma and fibronectin but increased adhesion to the basement membrane components laminin and collagen type IV. J Clin Invest 90:1232–1241

Verfaillie CM, Benis A, Iida J, McGlave PB, McCarthy JB (1994) Adhesion of committed human hematopoietic progenitors to synthetic peptides from the C-terminal heparin-binding domain of fibronectin: cooperation between the integrin 41 and the CD44 adhesion receptors. Blood 84:1802–1811

Verma RS, Macera MJ, Benn P, Groffen J (1989) Molecular characterization of variant translocations in chronic myelogenous leukemia. Oncogene 4:1145–1148

Verstovsek S, Lin H, Kantarjian H, Saglio G, De Micheli D, Pane F, Garcia-Manero G, Intrieri M, Rotoli B, Salvatore F, Guo JQ, Talpaz M, Specchia G, Pizzolo G, Liberati AM, Cortes J, Quackenbush RC, Arlinghaus RB (2002) Neutrophilic-chronic myeloid leukemia: low levels of p230 BCR/ABL mRNA and undetectable BCR/ABL protein may predict an indolent course. Cancer 94:2416–2425

Vickers M (1996) Estimation of the number of mutations necessary to cause chronic myeloid leukaemia from epidemiological data. Br J Haematol 94:1–4

Vigneri P, Wang JY (2001) Induction of apoptosis in chronic myelogenous leukemia cells through nuclear entrapment of BCR-ABL tyrosine kinase. Nat Med 7:228–234

Vivanco I, Sawyers CL (2002) The phosphatidylinositol 3-Kinase AKT pathway in human cancer. Nat Rev Cancer 2:489–501

Voncken JW, van Schaick H, Kaartinen V, Deemer K, Coates T, Landing B, Pattengale P, Dorseuil O, Bokoch GM, Groffen J, Heisterkamp N (1995) Increased neutrophil respiratory burst in bcr-null mutants. Cell 80:719–728

Wang JY (2000) Regulation of cell death by the Abl tyrosine kinase. Oncogene 19:5643–5650

Wang JY (2004) Controlling Abl: auto-inhibition and co-inhibition? Nat Cell Biol 6:3–7

Wang JY (2005) Nucleo-cytoplasmic communication in apoptotic response to genotoxic and inflammatory stress. Cell Res 15:43–8

Wange RL (2004) TCR signaling: another Abl-bodied kinase joins the cascade. Curr Biol 14:562–564

Welch PJ, Wang JY (1993) A C-terminal protein-binding domain in the retinoblastoma protein regulates nuclear c-Abl tyrosine kinase in the cell cycle. Cell 75:779–790

Welch PJ, Wang JY (1995) Disruption of retinoblastoma protein function by coexpression of its C pocket fragment. Genes Dev 9:31–46

Wen ST, Van Etten RA (1997) The PAG gene product, a stress-induced protein with antioxidant properties, is an Abl SH3-binding protein and a physiological inhibitor of c-Abl tyrosine kinase activity. Genes Dev 11:2456–2467

Wen ST, Jackson PK, Van Etten RA (1996) The cytostatic function of c-Abl is controlled by multiple nuclear localization signals and requires the p53 and Rb tumor suppressor gene products. EMBO J 15:1583–1595

Wilson Rawls J, Xie S, Liu J, Laneuville P, Arlinghaus RB (1996) P210 Bcr-Abl interacts with the interleukin 3 receptor beta(c) subunit and constitutively induces its tyrosine phosphorylation. Cancer Res 56:3426–3430

Woodring PJ, Hunter T, Wang JY (2001) Inhibition of c-Abl tyrosine kinase activity by filamentous actin. J Biol Chem 276:27104–27110

Xie S, Wang Y, Liu J, Sun T, Wilson MB, Smithgall TE, Arlinghaus RB (2001) Involvement of Jak2 tyrosine phosphorylation in Bcr-Abl transformation. Oncogene 20:6188–6195

Xie S, Lin H, Sun T, Arlinghaus RB (2002) Jak2 is involved in c-Myc induction by Bcr-Abl. Oncogene 21:7137–7146

Yasuda T, Shirakata M, Iwama A, Ishii A, Ebihara Y, Osawa M, Honda K, Shinohara H, Sudo K, Tsuji K, Nakauchi H, Iwakura Y, Hirai H, Oda H, Yamamoto T, Yamanashi Y (2004) Role of Dok-1 and Dok-2 in myeloid homeostasis and suppression of leukemia. J Exp Med 200:1681–1687

Yoshida K, Miki Y (2005) Enabling death by the Abl tyrosine kinase: mechanisms for nuclear shuttling of c-Abl in response to DNA damage. Cell Cycle 4:777–779

Yoshida K, Yamaguchi T, Natsume T, Kufe D, Miki Y (2005) JNK phosphorylation of 14-3-3 proteins regulates nuclear targeting of c-Abl in the apoptotic response to DNA damage. Nat Cell Biol 7:278–785

Zhang JG, Goldman JM, Cross NC (1995) Characterization of genomic BCR-ABL breakpoints in chronic myeloid leukaemia by PCR. Br J Haematol 90:138–146

Zhang X, Ren R (1998) Bcr-Abl efficiently induces a myeloproliferative disease and production of excess interleukin-3 and granulocyte-macrophage colony-stimulating factor in mice: a novel model for chronic myelogenous leukemia. Blood 92:3829–3840

Zhang X, Subrahmanyam R, Wong R, Gross AW, Ren R (2001) The NH2-terminal coiled-coil domain and tyrosine 177 play important roles in induction of a myeloproliferative disease in mice by Bcr–Abl. Mol Cell Biol 21:840–853

Zhu J, Wang JY (2004) Death by Abl: a matter of location. Curr Top Dev Biol 59:165–192

Zipfel PA, Zhang W, Quiroz M, Pendergast AM (2004) Requirement for Abl kinases in T cell receptor signaling. Curr Biol 14:1222–1231

Zou X, Calame K (1999) Signaling pathways activated by oncogenic forms of Abl tyrosine kinase. J Biol Chem 274:18141–18144

Zou X, Rudchenko S, Wong K, Calame K (1997) Induction of c-myc transcription by the v-Abl tyrosine kinase requires Ras, Raf1, and cyclin-dependent kinases. Genes Dev 11:654–662

Chronic Myeloid Leukemia: Biology of Advanced Phase

Junia V. Melo and David J. Barnes

Contents

Abstract. Chronic myeloid leukemia (CML) usually starts with an indolent chronic phase characterized by the overproduction of mature granulocytes, but inevitably evolves to a terminal blastic phase in which excessive numbers of undifferentiated blasts are produced. The molecular mechanisms underlying disease progression are still very poorly understood. Whereas the *BCR-ABL* oncogene has a central role in disease etiology, it is not sufficient by itself to precipitate the transition to blast crisis. Other secondary genetic events are presumed to be essential for this process but the number required for blastic transformation is still unknown. Although various genetic abnormalities have been identified in blast crisis samples, the significance of these for disease progression is far from certain. Candidate genes, suggested by their induced cellular phenotype, have been investigated, usually in in vitro models of CML. Several of these genes have also proven to have abnormal expression or activity in small numbers of CML blast crisis samples. At the cytogenetic level, disease progression in CML is often accompanied by the appearance of nonrandom chromosomal abnormalities. These are the microscopically visible manifestations of an underlying genomic instability and increased tolerance of genetic aberrations. Here we summarize the current state of knowledge concerning the biology of advanced phase CML.

3.1 Introduction

Chronic myeloid leukemia (CML) is a clonal myeloproliferative disorder originating in a single hematopoietic stem cell. The course of the disease generally involves three phases: an initial chronic phase (CP), an intermediate accelerated phase (AP), and a terminal blast crisis (BC). Common symptoms of CP include fatigue, weight loss, excessive sweating, and splenic discomfort, although many patients are asymptomatic and it has been estimated that an incidental diagnosis is made in at least 20% of cases of CML (Savage et al. 1997). In almost all cases of CP CML, the neoplastic expansion involves a leukemic clone that retains a capacity for differentiation. Consequently, there is excessive production of mature granulocytes that function normally despite being derived from malignant progenitors. The "mild" or "indolent" phenotype of CP CML typically used to last for 3–7 years from diagnosis and rarely posed major problems for clinical management, though its duration may be considerably longer since the introduction of tyrosine kinase inhibitors. The evolution of CML, however, to a more aggressive disease used to be inexorable and may still be so. Disease progression is heralded by the appearance of numerous immature blasts, a sign that differentiation is being arrested in the leukemic clone, leading to the exuberant production of undifferentiated precursors rather than terminally differentiated cells. As CML progenitors lose their capacity for differentiation, the disease either enters the transitional AP or transformation to BC occurs. When present, the AP precedes BC by 2–15 months (Sawyers et al. 2002). Blastic transformation is characterized by the development of a marked refractoriness to treatment (Wadhwa et al. 2002) but the formal diagnosis of BC requires there to be 20%, or more, blasts in the peripheral blood (PB) or bone marrow (BM) (Sawyers et al. 2002). In 25% of cases, blasts are derived from the lymphoid lineage but the majority of patients have blasts which are either myeloid or undifferentiated (Kantarjian et al. 1987; Vardiman et al. 2001). Clinical indications of BC include: fever, sweating, pain, weight loss, cytopenia, hepatosplenomegaly, enlarged lymph nodes, and extramedullary disease (Sawyers et al. 2002). The clinical outcome of blastic transformation is dismal: median survival after onset of myeloid BC used to be no more than 3–6 months (Wadhwa et al. 2002) but may today be somewhat longer since the introduction of tyrosine kinase inhibitors. The unravelling of the biological causes and mechanisms of disease evolution is therefore of paramount importance for defining effective therapeutic approaches in advanced phase CML.

3.2 The BCR-ABL Oncogene and Its Role in Determining Disease Phenotype

A consistent chromosomal abnormality, the Philadelphia chromosome (Ph), is associated with over 90% of all cases of CML (Nowell and Hungerford 1960). The Ph is a partially deleted chromosome 22 that is produced as a result of a reciprocal translocation involving the long arms of chromosomes 9 and 22, the t(9;22q)(q34;q11) (Rowley 1973). As a result of this translocation, 3′ sequences from the *ABL1* (Abelson) proto-oncogene on chromosome 9 (Bartram et al. 1983) are juxtaposed with 5′ sequence from the *BCR* (breakpoint cluster region) gene on chromosome 22 (Groffen et al. 1984). The fusion gene, *BCR-ABL*, encodes a protein tyrosine kinase, Bcr-Abl, which is necessary and sufficient for the transformation of cells (Daley and Baltimore 1988; Lugo et al. 1990; McLaughlin et al. 1987). In fact, mice transplanted with BM cells retrovirally transduced with the *BCR-ABL* gene develop a myeloproliferative syndrome that recapitulates features of CML (Daley et al. 1990). Depending upon the break points within the *BCR* gene, three variants of the *BCR-ABL* oncogene may be generated which are transcribed and translated into 190, 210, and 230 kDa species (Melo 1996; Shtivelman et al. 1985). Of these, by far the most common is $p210^{Bcr\text{-}Abl}$ which is the form of the oncoprotein associated with "classical" CML (Ben Neriah et al. 1986).

CML progenitors are characterized by defective adhesive properties (Gordon et al. 1987), increased resistance to multiple anticancer agents (Bedi et al. 1995), and increased resistance to apoptosis (Bedi et al. 1994). This last property may be a feature predominantly of advanced phase CML since it has been reported that CP progenitors are no more resistant to apoptosis, upon growth factor withdrawal, than normal progenitors (Amos et al. 1995). Hence, complete growth factor-independence and resistance to apoptosis may require other mutations in addition to formation of the *BCR-ABL* oncogene. Other phenotypic characteristics associated with blastic transformation include the aforementioned increased rate of proliferation and the loss of differentiation in cells that comprise the leukemic clone. Recently, the role of self-renewal of CML-committed progenitors in disease progression has been highlighted; progression to blast crisis has been reported to originate in the granulocyte-macrophage "pool" rather than in the pool of hematopoietic stem cells (Jamieson et al. 2004). Elevated levels of *BCR-*

ABL mRNA transcripts were detected in this subpopulation which was also found to possess self-renewal capacity in vitro. In addition, these authors demonstrated that *β*-catenin may be important in disease evolution, since it was activated in granulocyte-macrophage progenitors from patients with CML in AP or BC. These findings are novel and somewhat controversial (Huntly and Gilliland 2004; Huntly et al. 2004); it remains for other investigators to confirm the importance of self-renewal of the granulocyte-macrophage pool in BC.

The molecular signaling in CML is highly complex, and the cytoplasmic location of the Bcr-Abl (Wetzler et al. 1993) oncoprotein affords it access to numerous cellular substrates that are unavailable to the predominantly nuclear proto-oncogene, Abl (Van Etten et al. 1989). The signal transduction pathways affected by Bcr-Abl have been extensively reviewed in Chap. 2, entitled Bcr-Abl and Signal Transduction, and elsewhere (Deininger et al. 2000). The relevance of Bcr-Abl itself in disease progression is uncertain (Calabretta and Perrotti 2004). Whereas it has been demonstrated in cell lines that secondary mutations causing activation of the STAT5 (signal transducer and activator of transcription 5) pathway can maintain the transformed phenotype in the absence of Bcr-Abl (Klucher et al. 1998), it is notable that in CML patients' *BCR-ABL* expression is retained by the leukemic clone throughout the course of the disease. This suggests that Bcr-Abl must be important for the continued maintenance of the neoplastic phenotype, even in advanced phase CML, and that a selection pressure favors the continued existence of the oncogene. Moreover, Bcr-Abl expression increases with disease progression (Elmaagacli et al. 2000; Gaiger et al. 1995; Guo et al. 1991; Lin et al. 1996), a phenomenon that has recently been shown to occur at the mRNA and protein levels in $CD34^+$ progenitors (Barnes et al. 2005a). Elevated expression of Bcr-Abl is likely to contribute to the phenotype of advanced phase disease since studies using cell line models of CP and BC CML suggest that this oncoprotein exerts dose-dependent effects upon growth factor dependence (Barnes et al. 2005b; Cambier et al. 1998; Issaad et al. 2000), clonogenicity (Barnes et al. 2005b; Cambier et al. 1998), migration (Barnes et al. 2005b), and the rate at which cells develop resistance to imatinib (Barnes et al. 2005a).

3.3 Cytogenetic Aspects of Blast Crisis

The t(9; 22) translocation is the sole chromosomal abnormality detected in most cases of CP CML. In BC, however, additional chromosomal anomalies are found in 60–80% of patients (Johansson et al. 2002). Many of these abnormalities are not random (Alimena et al. 1987; Mitelman et al. 1976) and a subset of them occur with high frequency in BC karyotypes. In a survey of the 1,674 cases of secondary chromosomal changes reported in the literature up to 2002, Johansson et al. (Johansson et al. 2002) list the most common (with their frequency of occurrence) as being: trisomy 8 (+8; 33%), an additional Ph chromosome (+Ph; 30%), isochromosome 17 (i(17q); 20%), trisomy 19 (+19; 12%), loss of the Y chromosome (−Y; 8% of males), trisomy 21 (+21; 7%), and monosomy 7 (−7; 5%). In addition, they propose that these represent the major evolutionary "routes" by which disease progression proceeds. Combinations of these abnormalities are often seen in BC patients and this has led to speculation concerning their order of appearance within the leukemic clone. A putative temporal sequence beginning with i(17q) followed by +8, +Ph, and +19 has been assigned to their occurrence (Johansson et al. 2002). Although the source of the nonrandom nature of the chromosomal abnormalities is unknown, a correlation between centrosome aberrations and disease stage in CML has recently been identified (Giehl et al. 2005). An examination of the distribution of breakpoints has revealed that certain chromosome regions must be particularly susceptible to breakage. These include: 1p36, 1q12–32, 3q21, 3q26, 7p15, 11q23, 12p13, 12q24, 13q14, 14q32, 17p11–13, 17q10–11, 21q22, and 22q10 (Johansson et al. 2002). A majority of the secondary chromosomal changes in CML are unbalanced since they consist of trisomies, monosomies, and deletions. Rare exceptions do exist, however, such as the presence of t(15; 17)(q22;q12–21) in addition to t(9; 22), which has been described in less than 10 cases of CML and which is associated with promyelocytic BC (Johansson et al. 2002). Other balanced rearrangements are characteristic of acute myeloid leukemia (AML) or myelodysplastic syndromes (MDS) but are infrequently found in CML BC. These include inv(3)(q21q26)/t(3; 3)(q21;q26), t(3; 21)(q26;q22), t(7; 11)(p15; p15), t(8; 21)(q22;q22), and inv(16)(p13q22) (Johansson et al. 2002).

With regard to the phenotype of BC, cytogenetic evolution patterns are not especially informative. In reviewing the available data, Johansson et al. (Johansson et al.

2002) concluded that the only significant differences in the patterns seen between myeloid and lymphoid BC are a slightly higher prevalence of +8 and i(17)q in myeloid BC and a higher frequency of –7 and hypodiploidy in lymphoid BC. Moreover, the type of treatment employed affects the frequency of occurrence of certain secondary abnormalities. Busulphan, for instance, appears to be associated with a particularly high incidence of +8 (44%) compared with the frequency observed after hydroxyurea therapy (12%) (Johansson et al. 2002). Conversely, the incidences of +8, +Ph, i(17q), +19, +21 and +17 are lower in patients treated with interferon α (IFN-α) than in those receiving busulphan or hydroxyurea (Johansson et al. 2002). At present, it is unknown whether imatinib mesylate is associated with particular secondary chromosomal abnormalities, although one study (Fabarius et al. 2005) has linked this drug to centrosome and chromosome aberrations in in vitro cultures of cell lines.

The prognostic impact of secondary abnormalities in CML is complex. Trisomy 8 and +Ph occurring in BC have been linked to a poor prognosis, and i(17)q or other changes causing the loss of 17p predict a poor outcome (Johansson et al. 2002). The presence of an additional secondary chromosomal abnormality is not always a sign of disease progression. Very rarely, patients present with an inherited chromosomal abnormality in addition to the t(9; 22), as was the case in a recent report of a woman with an inherited inv(16)(p13q22) (Silva et al. 2005). Finally, it should be remembered that a significant proportion of patients enter blast crisis without detectable secondary chromosomal abnormalities indicating that these gross changes, though common, are not by themselves necessary for blastic transformation.

3.4 Molecular Genetic Aspects of Blast Crisis

The search for genes whose loss or altered function contributes to disease evolution has been guided by knowledge of both the genotype and phenotype of blast crisis cells (Shet et al. 2002). Visible cytogenetic changes such as the chromosomal abnormalities discussed previously suggest the loci for genes that are lost, mutated, duplicated, or otherwise altered by the disease process (Fig. 3.1). Changes in cellular phenotype associated with blast crisis have implicated genes which are subject to cytogenetically cryptic abnormalities (Table 3.1). The correct functioning of these candidate genes is often essential for the regulation of cell signaling in the untransformed cell.

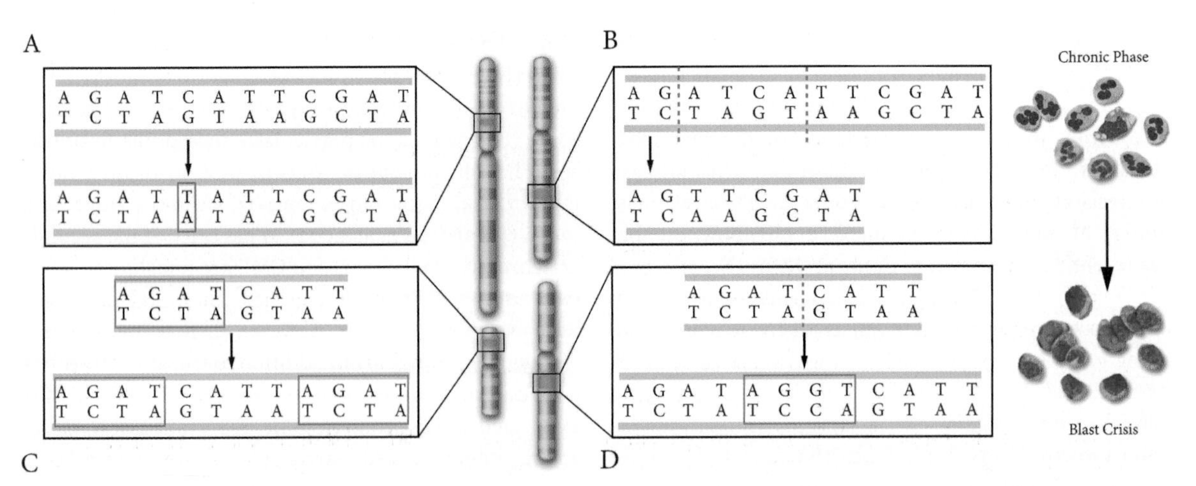

Fig. 3.1. Transformation of CML CP to CML BC is driven by the acquisition of secondary mutations. BC occurs when the leukemic clone has undergone multiple genetic changes (secondary to formation of the *BCR-ABL* oncogene) including loss, gain, and mutation of genes essential for normal cell physiology. These mutations may occur on different chromosomes and confer a selective advantage on the cells harboring them. Examples include: (**A**) point mutation of single base pairs, (**B**) deletion of DNA sequences, (**C**) amplification of DNA sequences, and, (**D**) interstitial insertion of "foreign" DNA from another chromosome (translocation) or another region of the same chromosome (isochromosome). The deleted, amplified and inserted sequences shown in (**B**), (**C**) and (**D**) are not to scale; the actual lesions may be much larger and, in the case of amplification, involve whole genes. The cumulative effect is transition from an indolent to an aggressive disease phenotype. CP progenitors continue to undergo differentiation to become mature granulocytes, whereas BC cells experience a differentiation arrest

Table 3.1. Mechanisms and gene abnormalities involved in blastic transformation

Mechanisms of disease progression	Genes implicated	References
Loss of leukemia tumor suppressor function	*TP53*	Ahuja et al. 1989; Feinstein et al. 1991; Bi et al. 1992, 1993, 1994a, b; Skorski et al. 1996; Honda et al. 2000; Fioretos et al. 1999
	INK4/ARF	Sill et al. 1995
	p16 *INK4A(CDKN2)*	Serra et al. 1995
	p14 *ARF*	Hernandez-Boluda et al. 2003; Nagy et al. 2003; Serrano et al. 1993; Sharpless and DePinho 1999; Pomerantz et al. 1998
	RB1	Towatari et al. 1991; Ahuja et al. 1991; Beck et al. 2000
	PP2A	Neviani et al. 2005
Overexpression of protooncogenes	*MYC*	McCarthy et al. 1984; Blick et al. 1987; Jennings and Mills 1998; Sawyers et al. 1992; Notari et al. 2005
Differentiation arrest	*C/EBP* α	Perrotti et al. 2002; Zhang et al. 1997
Mutator phenotype	*POLB* (DNA polymerase β)	Canitrot et al. 1999
	MLH1,PMS2,MSH2	Stoklosa et al. 2005
Deficiencies of DNA repair	*DNA-PKcs*	Deutsch et al. 2001; Gaymes et al. 2002; Brady et al. 2003
	RAD51	Slupianek et al. 2001; Nowicki et al. 2004
	FANCD2	Slupianek et al. 2005b; Koptyra et al. 2005
	WRN	Slupianek et al. 2005a
	NBS1	Rink et al. 2005
	XPB	Takeda et al. 1999; Canitrot et al. 2003
Failures of genome surveillance	*BRCA1*	Deutsch et al. 2003
	ATR	Dierov et al. 2004, 2005; Nieborowska et al. 2005
Loss of hematopoietic homeostasis	*DOK-1/DOK-2*	Niki et al. 2004
Unknown but present in 2% of cases of myeloid BC	*AML-1/EVI-1*	Mitani et al. 1994; Mitani 2004; Ogawa et al. 1996
Unknown – present infrequently in BC	*NUP98/HOXA9*	Yamamoto et al. 2000; Dash et al. 2002; Grand et al. 2005
Unknown – gene expression profiling candidates	*PIASy*	Ohmine et al. 2001
	RUNX1 AML-1, AF1Q, ETS2, LYL-1, PLU-1, GBDR1, NME1, GRO2, CA4, SNC73,	Nowicki et al. 2003
	MSF, CREBBP KNSL1EG5	Nowicki et al. 2003; Carter et al. 2005
	CD7, PR-3, ELA2	Yong et al. 2005

3.5 Gene Abnormalities Suggested by Chromosomal Abnormalities

3.5.1 Trisomy 8

Trisomy 8 is the most common (33%) (Johansson et al. 2002) secondary chromosomal abnormality observed in CML BC. Trisomies have pathological consequences for cellular physiology, but the mechanisms by which the occurrence of a third chromosome translates into pathophysiology are poorly understood. In the case of +8, whereas gene dosage effects are the probable underlying cause, enumerating and identifying the duplicated genes that are responsible have proven to be extremely difficult. It is unlikely that duplication of the entire complement of genes on chromosome 8 is necessary for the selective advantage of cells with this genotype since many genes will be "irrelevant", having no involvement with cell signaling in hematopoietic cells. Conversely, the hypothesis that the +8 clone persists and contributes to disease evolution because of duplication of a single essential gene has been criticized as simplistic (Johansson et al. 2002). Nevertheless, one candidate gene on chromosome 8, the proto-oncogene *MYC* located at 8q24, has been implicated in disease progression in CML.

Overexpression of *MYC* – in which state it functions as an oncogene – has been observed in CML patients due to an increase in its copy number (McCarthy et al. 1984) and in BC with +8 (Blick et al. 1987). In a survey of fourteen CML patients, Jennings et al. (Jennings and Mills 1998) found that only one of eleven patients demonstrating +8 had evidence of increased dosage of *MYC*. In a further two patients without +8, increased copy numbers for *MYC* were detected as a result of gene amplification. These findings led the authors to propose +8 and gene amplification as representing alternative mechanisms for increasing *MYC* gene dosage (Jennings and Mills 1998). However, evidence to contradict the link between increased expression of *MYC* and +8 has been provided by a microarray gene expression profiling study in which acute myeloid leukemia (AML) samples with +8 were compared with normal $CD34^+$ progenitors (Virtaneva et al. 2001). As is to be expected with microarray profiles, a complex pattern of up- and downregulated genes was revealed in the leukemic samples relative to the normal samples. Perhaps surprisingly, *MYC* was found to be downregulated in AML +8 samples relative to $CD34^+$ samples (Virtaneva et al. 2001). These findings, however, remain to be confirmed in CML samples with +8. Moreover, reduced expression of *MYC* in CML cells would be expected to attenuate the oncogenic "signal" that originates from Bcr-Abl. This was demonstrated by Sawyers et al. (Sawyers et al. 1992) who showed that transformation by v-Abl and Bcr-Abl of rat fibroblasts and primary mouse BM cells could be blocked by functionally inhibiting *MYC* expression with dominant negative mutants of *MYC*. Bcr-Abl has recently been shown to regulate *MYC* expression via a pathway involving $MAP^{ERK1/2}$ and the translational regulator, heterogeneous nuclear ribonucleoprotein K (hnRNP K) (Notari et al. 2005). Upon phosphorylation by Bcr-Abl, $MAP^{ERK1/2}$ stimulates transcription of hnRNP K which, in turn, promotes the translation, but not the transcription, of *MYC* mRNA.

If overexpression of *MYC* is not the primary reason for disease progression associated with +8, then it is possible that other genetic abnormalities involving the additional chromosome 8 could be responsible. Moreover, structural alteration of chromosome 8 genes can occur via subtle and microscopically cryptic chromosomal rearrangements. In addition to the common secondary chromosomal abnormalities described previously, "marker" chromosomes resulting from highly complex rearrangements are found in 20% of cases of CML BC (Gribble et al. 1999). Conventional Giemsa banding (G-banding) techniques lack sufficient resolution to discern the rearrangements involved in the formation of marker chromosomes, but newer cytogenetic methods such as comparative genomic hybridization (CGH) and multicolor fluorescence in situ hybridization (M-FISH) have proven effective in resolving some of these abnormalities (Gribble et al. 2003). In a cytogenetic study in which eleven BC samples were analyzed by G-banding and CGH (Gribble et al. 1999), overrepresentation of the long arm of chromosome 8 was found to be the commonest anomaly and was present in five patients. Furthermore, in a subsequent cytogenetic analysis of ten CML-derived cell lines (Gribble et al. 2003), overrepresentation of 8q23/q24 was the most frequent genomic imbalance. Overrepresentation was not associated with a unique chromosomal abnormality but was the result of numerous complex structural rearrangements. An especially highly rearranged chromosome 8 was detected in the cell line MEG-01 which contained no less than five different 8q amplicons. On the basis of the evidence from these cytogenetic studies, overrepresentation of 8q, and hence overrepresentation of the genes contained within this region, would seem to have a strong association with disease progression. It is expected that further fine mapping of the regions involved in amplifications of chromosome 8 will reveal the gene(s) which, in triple dose, underlie the association with disease transformation.

3.5.2 Loss of 17p

Loss of the short arm of chromosome 17 (17p) occurs frequently in CML BC, most often associated with isochromosome 17 (i(17q)) which is found in 20% of patients (Johansson et al. 2002). Since the *TP53* gene which encodes the vital tumor suppressor protein, p53, is located on 17p, it is not surprising that abnormalities of chromosome 17 have been linked to mutations or deletions of *TP53*. These are found in up to 30% of cases of BC, but not CP CML (Ahuja et al. 1989; Feinstein et al. 1991). In addition, inactivating mutations of *TP53* are common in CML cell lines (all of which have been isolated from BC patients) (Bi et al. 1992, 1993), and both alleles of this gene are absent in the myeloid BC cell line, K562 (Bi et al. 1992). Retroviral transduction of progenitors from CP patients with mutant *TP53* has been shown to promote their proliferation and to lead to the growth of factor-independent colonies (Bi et al. 1994b). Similarly, treatment of CP cells with *TP53* antisense oligonucleotides caused a significant increase in the number of granulocyte-macrophage colony-forming unit colonies (Bi et al. 1994a).

The effects of loss of p53 function on disease progression in CML have been studied in animal models (Honda et al. 2000; Skorski et al. 1996). In the first of these, mice injected with Bcr-Abl-expressing cells lacking p53 were found to develop a more aggressive disease than mice injected with cells expressing both Bcr-Abl and p53 (Skorski et al. 1996). In the second, more refined model, transgenic mice expressing $p210^{Bcr\text{-}Abl}$ under the control of the *Tec* promoter were bred with mice heterozygous for p53 ($p53^{+/-}$) (Honda et al. 2000). The $Bcr\text{-}Abl^{+/-}$ $p53^{+/-}$ mice resulting from this crossing developed a myeloproliferative disorder resembling CML and ultimately died after the disease underwent blastic transformation. An unexpected finding of this work was that the residual, normal *TP53* allele was frequently lost in Bcr-Abl-expressing blasts. This implies that a Bcr-Abl-dependent mechanism causes loss of the remaining allele. On balance, however, the cytogenetic evidence linking abnormalities of chromosome 17 with mutations of *TP53* is rather weak. Fioretos et al. (Fioretos et al. 1999) carried out a detailed FISH analysis of samples from 21 hematological malignancies and found that the majority of cases of i(17)q were dicentric, containing two centromeres, and had breakpoints clustering in 17p11. They proposed that these cases should be redesignated idic(17)(p11). Furthermore, these authors sequenced the *TP53* coding region in 16 cases of CML reported to have i(17q) and could find no mutations. Based on current knowledge, Johansson et al. (Johansson et al. 2002) suggest that whereas *TP53* mutations are undoubtedly involved in the progression of some CML cases, the mutation or loss of other, as yet unidentified, genes on 17p which result from idic(17)(p11) are likely to be of greater pathogenetic significance in cases of CML associated with this chromosomal abnormality.

3.5.3 Additional Chromosomal Translocations

Fusion genes generated by secondary chromosomal translocations in addition to the t(9; 22)(q34;q11) are known to contribute to disease progression in CML (Table 3.1). The most common of these, found in 2% of cases of myeloid BC, is *AML-1/EVI-1* generated by the t(3; 21)(q26;q22) (Mitani et al. 1994). The molecular mechanisms by which the product of the *AML-1/EVI-1* fusion accelerates disease evolution are complex (reviewed by Mitani 2004). Four processes have been suggested: a dominant-negative effect upon transcriptional activation of *AML-1(RUNX1)*, antagonism of the growth-inhibitory signals transduced by transforming growth factor α (TGF-α), blockade of signaling by Jun N-terminal kinase (JNK), and stimulation of AP-1 activity (Mitani 2004). In addition, it is of note that the *EVI-1* (ecotropic viral integration site) partner gene in this fusion is frequently overexpressed in CML BC cases lacking any cytogenetic evidence of 3q26 involvement (Ogawa et al. 1996). Another fusion gene, *NUP98/HOXA9*, is found infrequently in cases of CML BC and is generated by the t(7; 11)(p15; 15) (Yamamoto et al. 2000). In a mouse model, *NUP98/HOXA9* has been shown to co-operate with Bcr-Abl to induce "blast crisis" (Dash et al. 2002). A recent report (Grand et al. 2005) describes a case of CML with a *NUP98/LEDGF* (Lens epithelium derived growth factor) fusion generated by a t(9;11) (p21; p15). The condition of this patient deteriorated rapidly, consistent with the notion that the appearance of these rare fusion genes precipitates disease progression (Grand et al. 2005).

3.6 Gene Abnormalities Suggested by Disease Phenotype

3.6.1 Loss of Tumor Suppressor Function

Both the expression of oncogenes and the inactivation of tumor suppressor genes contribute to the process of transformation in human malignancies (Table 3.1). In CML, whereas a potent oncogene, *BCR-ABL*, has a central role in causing the malignant phenotype, the importance of inactivated tumor suppressor genes is less clear. The evidence regarding *TP53* has already been considered. Mutations of another locus for the tumor suppressor genes *INK4/ARF* have been implicated in disease progression in cases of lymphoid BC. This locus, located on 9p21, encodes two tumor suppressor proteins by means of two distinct promoters and alternative reading frames. Both proteins share a common second exon but are translated from alternative reading frames. One of these, $p16^{INK4A}$, also known as CDKN2, is a cyclin-dependent kinase inhibitor which has an RNA transcript comprising exons 1*α*, 2, and 3 (Serrano et al. 1993). The other product, $p14^{ARF}$ (*a*lternative *r*eading *f*rame), has a smaller transcript containing exons 1*β*, 2, and 3 (Stott et al. 1998). The expression of $p16^{INK4A}$ prevents the Ds-cdk4/6 complex from phosphorylating Rb, leading to an arrest of the cell cycle at late G1 (Sharpless and DePinho 1999). When overexpressed, $p14^{ARF}$ stabilizes p53 in the nucleus by preventing its MDM2-mediated cytoplasmic export and degradation (Pomerantz et al. 1998). Sill et al. (Sill et al. 1995) used a semiquantitative multiplex polymerase chain reaction (PCR) to look for deletions of p16 in 34 CML BC patients. Homozygous deletions of p16 exons were found in 5 of 10 (50%) of patients with lymphoid BC but no deletions could be detected in BC samples of nonlymphoid phenotype. Results from another mutational study using PCR corroborated the restriction of these mutations to the lymphoid lineage (Serra et al. 1995). Homozygous deletion of this locus was present in 3 of 8 (40%) cases of lymphoid BC but no losses were detected in 9 cases of myeloid BC or in 22 CML CP cases. Similarly, in a sequential study of 42 patients (Hernandez-Boluda et al. 2003), homozygous deletions of the *INK4/ARF* locus were found in 6 of 21 (29%) patients with lymphoid BC but none could be detected in 21 myeloid BC patients. None of the samples from these patients taken when they were still in CP had detectable deletions. Apart from the correlation with a lymphoid BC phenotype, these deletions were not associated with any clinico-hematological feature and had no bearing on the therapeutic response and survival of the lymphoid BC patients. Homozygous deletion of the *INK4/ARF* locus undoubtedly contributes to disease progression in some cases of BC with a lymphoid phenotype. However, the role of promoter methylation at the *INK4/ARF* locus in disease progression is somewhat controversial. Whereas Hernández-Boluda et al. found no hypermethylation of the *p16* gene in lymphoid BC samples, Nagy et al. (Nagy et al. 2003) detected aberrant methylation of the $p16^{INK4A}$ or $p14^{ARF}$ promoters in 14 of 30 accelerated phase samples. Further studies will be needed to resolve these discrepancies. Promoter methylation at this locus could have important clinical implications since this would be expected to lead to transcriptional silencing.

Normal cell physiology requires tight regulation of kinase and phosphatase activities. Where a kinase transduces an oncogenic signal, as is the case with Bcr-Abl, then phosphatases that share the same protein substrates as the kinase can function as tumor suppressors. A phosphatase which has recently been shown to act as a tumor suppressor by antagonizing Bcr-Abl is protein phosphatase 2A (PP2A) (Neviani et al. 2005). In $CD34^+$ cells from CML CP patients, the phosphatase activity of PP2A was found to be only moderately impaired but in those from BC patients, PP2A had negligible activity (Neviani et al. 2005). Inactivation of PP2A was mediated via SET, a phosphoprotein which functions as a physiological inhibitor of PP2A and which is frequently overexpressed in solid tumors and leukemias (Neviani et al. 2005). SET transcription was shown to be regulated by Bcr-Abl in a dose-dependent manner, and its increased expression in BC $CD34^+$ progenitors correlated with the increased expression of Bcr-Abl, which is a feature of advanced phase disease (Barnes et al. 2005a; Elmaagacli et al. 2000; Gaiger et al. 1995; Guo et al. 1991; Lin et al. 1996). In addition, Bcr-Abl may inhibit PP2A via a second mechanism involving the Jak2-dependent or Src-dependent phosphorylation of its catalytic subunit (PP2Ac) on tyrosine 307 (Neviani et al. 2005). Significantly, Bcr-Abl and PP2A were found to share protein substrates, including MAPK, STAT5, and Akt. In the recombinant murine cell line 32D/

BCR-ABL, phosphorylation of these proteins by Bcr-Abl was reduced by inhibiting SET expression or through the forced expression of PP2Ac (Neviani et al. 2005). It is probable that the expression of active PP2A is incompatible with disease progression in CML, since Bcr-Abl is itself a substrate for this phosphatase. Inhibition of SET expression by short hairpin RNA interference or overexpression of PP2A by retroviral transduction led to a reduction in Bcr-Abl expression in 32D/*BCR-ABL* cells. Furthermore, pharmacological stimulation of PP2A using forskolin resulted in reduced Bcr-Abl expression in CML BC $CD34^+$ cells, a CML cell line (K562) and in murine cell lines expressing imatinib-resistant mutants of Bcr-Abl. Downregulation of Bcr-Abl was shown to involve proteasomal degradation of the nonphosphorylated oncoprotein via a mechanism mediated by the tyrosine phosphatase, SHP-1 (Neviani et al. 2005). Reactivation of PP2A in imatinib-sensitive and resistant Bcr-Abl-expressing cells led to growth suppression, impaired clonogenicity, restored differentiation capacity, enhanced apoptosis and decreased their in vivo leukemogenic properties (Neviani et al. 2005). In view of the mutual antagonism of Bcr-Abl and PP2A, inhibition of the latter tumor suppressor protein may be a prerequisite for disease progression in CML.

Loss of function of another tumor suppressor gene, the retinoblastoma-susceptibility (*RB1*) gene, located on 13q14, may be involved in disease evolution in some cases of CML. Reports differ as to the frequency with which it is mutated or deleted in CML. In one study (Towatari et al. 1991) abnormalities of *RB1* were detected in five cases of megakaryoblastic CML but not in seventeen cases with either a lymphoid or myeloid phenotype. In other reports (Ahuja et al. 1991; Beck et al. 2000), abnormalities were not confined to megakaryoblastic BC but were also found in cases with myeloid and lymphoid lineages. Overall, *RB1* mutations and deletions are found in up to 20% of cases of CML BC, and most of these will be submicroscopic, as cytogenetically identifiable deletions of 13q are rare in CML (Johansson et al. 2002).

3.6.2 Differentiation Arrest

Advanced phase CML is characterized by the excessive production of immature, undifferentiated blasts. It follows, therefore, that blastic transformation must involve a failure of hemopoietic differentiation. The genes responsible for normal differentiation, together with their attendant transcription factors, represent candidate molecules for investigators studying this process in CML. An important candidate transcription factor which is essential for granulocytic differentiation is the CCAAT/enhancer binding protein α (C/EBP α) (Zhang et al. 1997). C/EBP α, a member of the basic region leucine zipper (bZIP) family of transcription factors, is actively expressed in myeloid cells where it activates transcription of granulocyte colony-stimulating factor receptor (G-CSF-R) from the *CSF3R* gene (Smith et al. 1996). Mice which are null for the *C/EBP α* gene have monocytes but lack neutrophils and eosinophils (Zhang et al. 1997). Perrotti et al. (Perrotti et al. 2002) have shown that whereas C/EBP α protein was expressed in normal BM and CML CP samples, it was undetectable in BC BM cells. In one case, this differential expression of C/EBP α could be demonstrated in paired CP/BC samples from the same patient. Interestingly, the levels of C/EBP α mRNA were similar in all samples suggesting that this transcription factor, similarly to *MYC* (Notari et al. 2005), is downregulated at the translational, rather than the transcriptional level in the CML BC cells. An upstream open reading frame (uORF) is present in mRNA transcripts of C/EBP α which is separated from the AUG initiation codon of the second open reading frame (ORF) by a spacer of seven nucleotides. Mutational analysis revealed that a CCC nucleotide triplet within this spacer was necessary for the repression of C/EBP α translation. A protein that bound to this motif was subsequently isolated and was identified as being the heterogeneous nuclear ribonucleoprotein E2 (hnRNP E2) (Perrotti et al. 2002). The expression of hnRNP E2 inversely correlated with that of C/EBP α in CML cells and was readily detected, by immunoblotting, in CML BC samples but was either low or undetectable in normal and CML CP BM cells. Induction of hnRNP E2 required the tyrosine kinase activity of Bcr-Abl and expression of this ribonucleoprotein could be inhibited by treating cells with imatinib mesylate. Abrogation of translation of C/EBP α resulting from the induction of hnRNP E2 by Bcr-Abl may be one of the key events responsible for the arrest of differentiation that characterizes CML BC. Significantly, *BCR-ABL* expression per se does not appear to be sufficient to completely inhibit C/EBP expression since it was readily detectable in CML CP cells. These authors demonstrate a dose-dependent effect of Bcr-Abl expression on depletion of C/EBP α and speculate that the elevated levels of Bcr-Abl seen in advanced phase disease (Barnes et al. 2005 a) may be required for the complete suppression of translation of this transcription factor (Perrotti et al. 2002). Mutation of the *CEBPA* gene, which is observed in 10–15% of AML patients preferentially of M1/M2 subtype, has recently been discounted as a factor in disease evolution in CML (Pabst et al. 2006). In this study, no mutations could be detected in the coding region of *CEBPA* in 64 CP samples, 95 myeloid BC samples, and 15 *BCR-ABL*-expressing cell lines.

3.6.3 Mutator Phenotype

Malignant cells commonly have mutations which are present at a frequency and number that cannot be accounted for by the spontaneous mutation rate of normal cells. This disparity led to the proposal of the "mutator phenotype" hypothesis (reviewed in Loeb 2001). The mutator phenotype arises due to mutation of genes that are critical for maintaining genomic stability. The increased rates of mutation and genetic evolution associated with tumor progression are cited as being manifestations of this phenotype (Loeb 2001). Evidence that Bcr-Abl can induce a mutator phenotype in hemopoietic cell lines is provided by a study in which Ba/F3 cells were transfected with $p190^{Bcr\text{-}Abl}$ and $p210^{Bcr\text{-}Abl}$ (Canitrot et al. 1999). Mutation rates for two loci, hypoxanthine guanine phosphoribosyl transferase (*HPRT*) and Na-K-ATPase, were determined for transfected and untransfected cells. Expression of either form of Bcr-Abl resulted in mutation rates that were three to fivefold higher than those observed for untransfected cells. Moreover, the presence of Bcr-Abl was associated with a twofold ($p210^{Bcr\text{-}Abl}$) or fourfold ($p190^{Bcr\text{-}Abl}$) increase in expression of DNA polymerase β (Canitrot et al. 1999), the most error-prone of the DNA polymerases responsible for base excision repair (BER) of damaged DNA (Hoeijmakers 2001) (Fig. 3.2 C). Although this finding has yet to be confirmed in primary cells, upregulation of this polymerase has been reported for other cancer cell lines (Scanlon et al. 1989), including ovarian and colon lines. Increased expression of the least accurate DNA polymerase, at the expense of others with greater fidelity, might be expected to create an imbalance that would contribute to genomic instability.

Failure of proof-reading by DNA polymerases leads to the incorporation of incorrect nucleotides into DNA sequences (misincorporation). This leads to mismatches between the misincorporated nucleotide and the correct nucleotide on the second DNA strand. A recent preliminary report (Stoklosa et al. 2005), suggests that the mismatch repair (MMR) mechanism responsible for the detection and removal of misincorporated nucleotides may be compromised in Bcr-Abl-expressing cells. Colocalization of the MMR proteins MLH1 and PMS2 could be detected in untransformed, but not in Bcr-Abl-expressing leukemic cells. MLH1 was also found to colocalize with MSH2 in normal but not Bcr-Abl-positive cells following treatment with *N*-methylyl-*N*′-nitro-*N*-nitrosoguanine. The apparent inability of these proteins to form the required heterodimers in the presence of Bcr-Abl implies that MMR may be deficient in CML cells. These findings, although yet to be confirmed in a greater number of patient samples, suggest another mechanism by which Bcr-Abl may induce a mutator phenotype.

3.6.4 Deficiencies of DNA Repair

Another DNA repair protein, the catalytic subunit of the DNA-dependent protein kinase (DNA-PKcs) has been shown to have abnormal expression in primary CML progenitors and in human and murine hemopoietic cell lines expressing different amounts of Bcr-Abl (Deutsch et al. 2001) (Fig. 3.2 A). DNA-PKcs was found to be downregulated in human (UT-7) and murine (Ba/F3) cell lines in inverse proportion to the amount of expressed Bcr-Abl protein. Such inverse correlation was confirmed in Ba/F3 cells containing the *BCR-ABL* transgene under the control of a tetracycline-inducible promoter. Levels of DNA-PKcs mRNA were found to be consistently high in all of the UT-7 clones despite the fact that DNA-PKcs was virtually undetectable by immunoblotting in cells with high Bcr-Abl expression. This finding prompted the authors to conclude that Bcr-Abl was exerting a negative effect on DNA-PKcs expression by a posttranscriptional mechanism. Treatment of Bcr-Abl-expressing UT-7 cells with a tyrosine kinase inhibitor or either of two proteasome inhibitors resulted in the restoration of expression of DNA-PKcs to levels comparable to those seen in clones which did not express Bcr-Abl. Significantly, DNA-PKcs protein was abundant in nonleukemic $CD34^{+}$ cells but was almost undetectable in $CD34^{+}$ cells obtained from two CML patients. In agreement with the findings in cell lines, upregulation of DNA-PKcs expression in CML

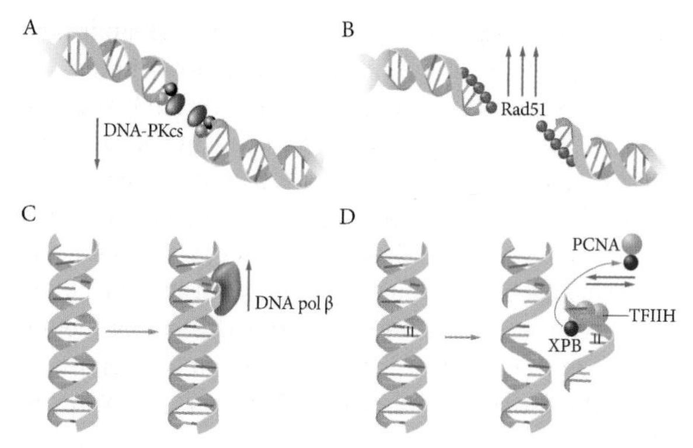

Fig. 3.2. Bcr-Abl-induced defects in DNA repair that may contribute to genomic instability in advanced-phase CML. The two main mechanisms for repair of DNA double-strand breaks (DSB) are (**A**) nonhomologous end-joining (NHEJ) and (**B**) homologous recombination (HR). (**A**) The expression of the catalytic subunit of DNA-dependent protein kinase (DNA-PKcs) is downregulated (*red arrow*) in inverse relation to the expression of Bcr-Abl in cells. DNA-PKcs binds to the free ends of DSBs where it forms a complex with the Ku70/Ku80 heterodimer. Ligation of the broken strands also requires DNA ligase IV, x-ray cross complementation group 4 protein (XRCC4) and the nuclease, Artemis (not shown). (**B**) The transcription, activation, and stability of the DNA repair protein Rad51 are all stimulated (*three red arrows*) by Bcr-Abl expression. Rad51 associates with exposed strands of DNA at a DSB to form a nucleoprotein filament. Repair by HR also requires numerous other proteins including Rad51-paralogs and the Rad50/Mre11/Nbs1 complex (not shown). The fidelity of Bcr-Abl-stimulated HR has been reported to be worse than that of untransformed cells leading to unfaithful repair and genomic instability. (**C**) Point mutations or "abasic" sites caused by depurination are repaired by base excision repair (BER). Bcr-Abl stimulates the expression (*red arrow*) of DNA polymerase β (DNA pol β), the most "error-prone" DNA polymerase involved in BER. The gap-filling reaction in BER also requires an XRCC1-/DNA ligase 3 complex (not shown). Insertion of incorrect nucleotides into DNA by DNA pol β may contribute to the mutator phenotype of CML cells. (**D**) Exposure to UV radiation causes "bulky" or helix-altering DNA lesions in which covalent bonds form between adjacent pyrimidines. These are resolved by nucleotide excision repair (NER) in which the lesion is excised within a section of DNA spanning 25–30 nucleotides. In myeloid cells, Bcr-Abl stimulates and, in lymphoid cells, inhibits (*red arrows*) the association of xeroderma pigmentosum group B (XPB) protein with proliferating cell nuclear antigen (PCNA). XPB functions as a helicase as part of the TFIIH complex which is essential for recognition of the DNA lesion and its excision. PCNA forms part of a second complex (not shown) which is responsible for DNA repair synthesis following excision of the lesion-containing segment. Defects in NER in CML cells may contribute to genomic instability and may account for why advanced phase cells are resistant to cytotoxic drugs that induce lesions similar to those caused by UV irradiation

$CD34^+$ cells was achieved by treatment with a proteasome inhibitor implying a major role for the proteasomal-ubiquitin pathway in the inhibition of DNA-PKcs by Bcr-Abl. It remains to be confirmed how prevalent downregulation of DNA-PKcs is in the CML patient population and this must await studies with larger cohorts of patients. Loss of this protein would be expected to have severe consequences for genomic stability since DNA-PKcs has an essential role in the nonhomologous end-joining (NHEJ) pathway by which mammalian cells repair DNA double-strand breaks (DSBs) (reviewed by Collis et al. 2005). In this capacity, DNA-PKcs forms a complex with a heterodimer of the Ku proteins (Ku70 and Ku80) (Gottlieb and Jackson 1993; Suwa et al. 1994), DNA ligase IV (Nick McElhinny et al. 2000), x-ray cross complementation group 4 protein (XRCC4) (Grawunder et al. 1997), and Artemis, a nuclease (Ma et al. 2002). DSBs are the most difficult form of DNA damage to repair and are also the most insidious since they pose a severe threat to the integrity of the genome if they are left unrepaired (Khanna and Jackson 2001). Furthermore, there is evidence that the NHEJ mechanisms in CML cells are "error-prone" and capable of "misrepair" when challenged with excessive DSBs (Brady et al. 2003; Gaymes et al. 2002). This situation is likely to exacerbate genomic instability contributing to disease progression.

An alternative mechanism for the repair of DSBs, homologous recombination (HR), has been shown to be enhanced in cell lines transfected with *BCR-ABL* (Slupianek et al. 2001) (Fig. 3.2 B). The process of HR requires Rad51, one of six human homologs of the RecA protein of *E.coli* (Rad51-paralogs). Unusually, Bcr-Abl was implicated in controlling the transcription, activation, and degradation of Rad51 (Slupianek et al. 2001). Transcriptional regulation of Rad51 was found to involve the *src* homology (SH) 2 and SH3 domains of Bcr-Abl and signaling via activation of STAT5. Elevated levels of Rad51 protein could be detected in BM cells from six CML patients (three in CP and three in BC) relative to the level found in normal BM cells. No correlation between disease phase and expression level of Rad51 was apparent. Activation of Rad51 by Bcr-Abl was shown to occur via phosphorylation of the HR repair protein on tyrosine residue 315. Degradation of Rad51 can be mediated via proteolysis catalyzed by caspase-3. In agreement with its known role in blocking the activation of caspase-3 (Amarante et al. 1998; Dubrez et al. 1998), Bcr-Abl was found to prevent the activation of this enzyme, which in turn led to abrogation of Rad51 proteolysis. The collective effects of Bcr-Abl on the transcription, activation, and stability of Rad51 are manifest as a drug-resistant phenotype whereby lesions caused by the cytotoxic agents, mitomycin C and cisplatin, are rapidly repaired by enhanced HR activity. It is unclear whether the fidelity of the Bcr-Abl-stimulated HR repair mechanism is the same or worse than that of untransformed cells. If the latter possibility were the case, then regulation of Rad51 by Bcr-Abl would be expected to contribute to the genomic instability of CML cells in addition to its effect upon repair of drug-induced DNA lesions.

Subsequent reports by the same group found that HR and NHEJ mechanisms activated in response to DSBs caused by reactive oxygen species (ROS) (Nowicki et al. 2004) or γ-irradiation (Slupianek et al. 2005b) were indeed less faithful in Bcr-Abl-expressing cells than in normal cells. In addition, these workers have recently identified two Rad51-interacting proteins, Fanconi D2 protein (FANCD2) (Koptyra et al. 2005) and the Werner syndrome protein (WRN) (Slupianek et al. 2005a) whose expression and activity are stimulated by Bcr-Abl kinase activity in CML cells. In the former case activation involves monoubiquitination, whereas tWRN is activated by tyrosine phosphorylation. Additional and more detailed studies will be required to determine the consequences of these altered molecular interactions for the repair of DSBs. It should be noted that other groups (Deutsch et al. 2003; Dierov et al. 2003) have failed to find elevated expression of Rad51 in other cell line models of CML. Furthermore, it remains to be seen whether regulation of Rad51-paralogs by Bcr-Abl is common in CML, and this will require a larger sample size.

Although DSBs are undoubtedly the most lethal form of DNA damage, other genetic lesions, such as the so-called bulky or helix-altering lesions, may contribute to the underlying genomic instability that characterizes the advanced phase of CML. There is growing evidence that the p210 form of Bcr-Abl may interfere with mechanisms responsible for the repair of such damage. An interaction between the CDC24 homology domain of Bcr-Abl and the xeroderma pigmentosum group B protein (XPB) was identified following a yeast two-hybrid screen (Takeda et al. 1999). The CDC24 homology domain is present within $p210^{Bcr\text{-}Abl}$ but not $p190^{Bcr\text{-}Abl}$, and the purpose of the screen was to functionally characterize this region by isolating proteins capable of interacting with it. In the event, XPB emerged as the only positive "hunter" protein to target the CDC24 "bait." XPB, a subunit of the basal transcription factor TFIIH, is mutated in the hereditary condition xeroderma pigmentosum group B, which predisposes sufferers to skin cancer upon exposure to ultraviolet (UV) light. When expressed in the 27-1 cell line (a UV-sensitive mutant of the Chinese hamster ovary-9 cell line), XPB corrected its DNA repair-deficient phenotype. Coexpression of $p210^{Bcr\text{-}Abl}$ (but not $p190^{Bcr\text{-}Abl}$) with XPB abrogated this effect (Takeda et al. 1999). Intriguing differences in the ability of $p210^{Bcr\text{-}Abl}$-expressing lymphoid and myeloid cell lines to repair short-wave UV (UVC)-damaged DNA were observed by Canitrot et al. (Canitrot et al. 2003). In an in vitro repair assay, extracts from lymphoid Ba/F3-p210 cells expressing $p210^{Bcr\text{-}Abl}$ were twofold less active in repairing UVC-damaged DNA than parental Ba/F3 cells. In contrast, the opposite was the case for myeloid cell lines where the DNA repair activity of extracts from 32D-p210 cells was more than twofold that of parental 32Dcl3 cells. Similarly, increased (twofold) activity for repair of UVC-damaged DNA was obtained from primary murine BM cells infected with a *BCR-ABL*-containing retrovirus compared with their untransduced counterparts. Sensitivity to UVC-induced cytotoxicity was increased by $p210^{Bcr\text{-}Abl}$ expression in Ba/F3 cells whereas $p210^{Bcr\text{-}Abl}$ rendered 32Dcl3 cells more resistant to UVC. Both effects could be reversed by treatment with imatinib indicating that the influence of Bcr-Abl on DNA repair was mediated via its tyrosine kinase activity. In addition, Bcr-Abl was found to regulate the colocalization of XPB with proliferating cell nuclear antigen (PCNA), stimulating this reaction in myeloid and inhibiting it in lymphoid cell lines (Canitrot et al. 2003) (Fig. 3.2 D). Lesions generated by UVC, including cyclobutane pyrimidine dimers and (6-4) photoproducts, are repaired by nucleotide excision repair (NER) (de Laat et al. 1999). This mechanism involves recognition of the lesion, excision of between 25 to 30 nucleotides spanning it, and DNA synthesis to repair the excised region using the opposite, undamaged strand as a template. Two multiprotein complexes are required for NER: one is involved in recognition and excision, and contains TFIIH, XPA, XPG proteins and replication protein A (RPA); the second, essential for DNA repair synthesis, contains PCNA, replication factor C (RFC), RPA, DNA polymerase δ/ε and DNA ligase I (Aboussekhra et al. 1995). The findings of Canitrot et al. not only suggest a means by which Bcr-Abl-expression may contribute to genomic instability by interfering with NER, but may explain, in part, why advanced phase CML cells are resistant to cytotoxic drugs that induce lesions in DNA similar to those caused by UV irradiation (Canitrot et al. 2003). The observation that p210$^{\text{Bcr-Abl}}$-expression has opposite effects upon NER in lymphoid and myeloid cell lines is novel, but remains to be confirmed in primary cells from CML patients in lymphoid and myeloid BC.

3.6.5 Failures of Genome Surveillance

A feature of advanced phase CML is the acquisition of additional genetic changes. The presence of such changes implies a failure of the mechanisms that have evolved to detect aberrations that threaten the integrity of the genome. These mechanisms constitute a system for "genome surveillance." A key component of this system is the nuclear protein kinase, ataxia telangiectasia mutated (ATM), which functions as a DNA damage "sensor," initiating a signaling cascade in response to the detection of DSBs (Hoeijmakers 2001). Inactivating mutations of the *ATM* gene cause ataxia telangiectasia, a recessive disorder characterized by x-ray hypersensitivity, genomic instability and a predisposition to both solid tumors and hematological malignancies. Since blastic transformation is associated with complex karyotypes, many of which involve DSBs, *ATM* would seem to be a logical candidate for a gene which is likely to be mutated or deleted in CML BC. However, a mutational analysis of *ATM* involving 59 CML BC patients and 14 CML cell lines failed to find any clearly deleterious mutations (Melo et al. 2001). Mutation of histidine to tyrosine at amino acid position 1380 was detected in the NALM1 cell line, and two patients were found to have a mutation of leucine to phenylalanine at position 1420. Both of these mutations corresponded to polymorphisms present at almost identical frequencies in normal individuals. This negative result strongly suggests that mutations of *ATM* are unlikely causes of disease progression in CML.

Downstream of ATM is *br*east *ca*ncer 1 (*BRCA1*), a gene first identified as being mutated in hereditary breast cancer (Miki et al. 1994), and which has been reported as being expressed at abnormally low levels in CML cells (Deutsch et al. 2003). In mononuclear cells obtained from one patient in CP, two in AP, and two in BC, BRCA1 was almost undetectable by immunoblotting (Deutsch et al. 2003). Disease phase had no bearing on BRCA1 expression since levels of protein were equally low in all five samples. In contrast, BRCA1 was highly expressed in three samples from mobilized PB. Immunoblotting revealed that BRCA1 expression was also severely reduced in Bcr-Abl-transfected human UT-7 and murine Ba/F3 cell lines, relative to their parental counterparts. A reciprocal relationship between expression of p210$^{\text{Bcr-Abl}}$ and BRCA1 was confirmed in Ba/F3 cells containing a tetracycline-inducible *BCR-ABL* transgene. Negative regulation of BRCA1 expression by Bcr-Abl was shown to involve a posttranscriptional mechanism, since mRNA levels were not significantly different in UT-7 cells which expressed different amounts of Bcr-Abl. The phenomenon depends upon the tyrosine kinase activity of Bcr-Abl and may involve the ubiquitin-proteasomal pathway. The latter point could not be demonstrated conclusively, since a prolonged exposure to proteasome inhibitors was required to reverse the downregulation of BRCA1 but this, in turn, caused a reduction in the levels of Bcr-Abl within cells (Deutsch et al. 2003). A precise role for BRCA1 has yet to be defined, but it is believed to act as part of a DNA damage sensor that moves to sites of repair within the nucleus (Wang et al. 2000). BRCA1 acts in conjunction with other proteins involved in genome surveillance and DNA repair including Rad51 (Scully et al. 1997), the Rad50/MRE11/NBS1 complex (Zhong et al. 1999), ATM (Cortez et al. 1999), and BLM (Wang et al. 2000). A recent report (Rink et al. 2005), describes enhanced expression of Mre11 and Nbs1, but not Rad50, as a consequence of Bcr-Abl kinase activity. In addition, Nbs1 exhibited increased phosphorylation on serine 343 in mitomycin-c-treated CML progenitors and cell lines relative to normal cells. The consequences of these findings for genome surveillance remain to be determined but these authors hypothesize that the enhanced phosphorylation of Nbs1 may contribute to the resistance of Bcr-Abl-positive cells to genotoxic agents (Rink et al. 2005). Consistent with the notion of Bcr-Abl acting to abrogate or compromise genome surveillance, is the finding that the frequency of ionizing radiation-induced sister chromatid exchange in a UT-7 cell line expressing Bcr-Abl was substantially higher than in the parental cells (Deutsch et al. 2003).

The process of genome surveillance activates discrete checkpoints within the cell cycle. The fate of cells with damaged DNA is determined at each cell cycle checkpoint. Activated checkpoints either delay the cell cycle to provide additional time for DNA repair, or initiate cell death by apoptosis, if the damage proves irreparable (reviewed in Bartek and Lukas 2003). Recent evidence suggests that a checkpoint within the synthesis phase (S-phase) of the cell cycle may be compromised in CML cells by the direct involvement of Bcr-Abl with nuclear proteins (Dierov et al. 2004). Although Bcr-Abl has a predominantly cytoplasmic localization (Wetzler et al. 1993) it can be induced to "shuttle" to the nucleus in response to treatment of cells with imatinib mesylate (Vigneri and Wang 2001). In a series of elegant experiments performed by Dierov et al. (Dierov et al. 2004), Bcr-Abl was shown to undergo a rapid (within 10 min) translocation to the nucleus in response to etoposide-induced genotoxic "insult." This effect, which was demonstrated in both NIH 3T3 fibroblasts with ectopic expression of $p210^{Bcr\text{-}Abl}$ and mononuclear cells from a CML patient in BC, was transient, and Bcr-Abl was found to return to the cytoplasm within 2 h of the etoposide having been washed away. Cell lines expressing Bcr-Abl, including 3T3 cells and Ba/F3 cells containing tetracycline-inducible $p210^{Bcr\text{-}Abl}$ (Ba/F3 pTet-on p210), exhibited enhanced DNA damage, as measured by the "comet" assay, in response to etoposide insult. These cell lines exhibited a radioresistant DNA synthesis (RDS) phenotype, since the DNA damage was rapidly repaired and the cells were found to have passed through S-phase more rapidly than etoposide-treated control cells. Immunoprecipitation studies revealed that Bcr-Abl associated with the two main DNA damage sensor proteins, ataxia-telangiectasia mutated (ATM), and rad 3-related protein (ATR). ATM function was unaltered by this interaction, as assessed by the phosphorylation of its substrate Chk2 (Matsuoka et al. 2000). In contrast, the kinase activity of ATR was inhibited by Bcr-Abl as evidenced by a significant reduction in the phosphorylation of its substrate, Chk1 (Liu et al. 2000; Sanchez et al. 1997). The failure to phosphorylate, and hence activate, Chk1 in turn leads to a protein complex, cdc7/Dbf4, remaining active and DNA replication proceeding inappropriately. Normally, activated Chk1 mediates the intra-S phase checkpoint by disrupting the cdc7/Dbf4 complex, which in turn causes decreased loading of cdc45 in the prereplication complex (Costanzo et al. 2003). The association of Bcr-Abl with ATR, in response to etoposide treatment, and the concomitant reduction in Chk1 phosphorylation were demonstrated in both Ba/F3 pTet-on p210 cell lines and in primary cells from two CML patients (Dierov et al. 2004). These findings led the authors to speculate that disruption of ATR-signaling by Bcr-Abl should predispose cells to increased translocations and deletions following DSBs, and that this is the increased DNA damage that they are detecting in their comet assays. The same group have recently confirmed that this is indeed the case, as these chromosomal abnormalities have been observed in etoposide-treated Bcr-Abl-expressing cell lines and Ph^+ cells from CML patients when spectral karyotyping (SKY) was used to visualize chromosomes (Dierov et al. 2004, 2005). A picture is emerging of DNA damage in Bcr-Abl-expressing cells, which may take the form of increased sister chromatid exchange as a result of downregulation of BRCA1 (Deutsch et al. 2003) or may involve large numbers of chromosomal translocations due to the abrogation of ATR-Chk1 signaling (Dierov et al. 2004, 2005). Neither mechanism is mutually exclusive, and it is of note that inactivation of Chk1 may be a common theme in the erosion of genome surveillance in Bcr-Abl-expressing cells, since this kinase has also been reported as being a substrate for BRCA1 (Yarden et al. 2002). Recently, however, Skorski's group have reported contrary findings in which ATR-signaling is enhanced in Bcr-Abl-positive CML cells and Chk1 is strongly activated by phosphorylation on serine 345 (Nieborowska et al. 2005). Further studies should resolve this controversy, but it is clear that Bcr-Abl alters normal cellular responses to DNA damage via an interaction with ATR.

3.6.6 Loss of Hemopoietic Homeostasis

Mechanisms responsible for maintaining homeostasis in the hemopoietic compartment, involving two Dok (downstream of tyrosine kinase) proteins, may be compromised in advanced phase CML (Niki et al. 2004). This finding was unexpected since neither of the Dok proteins, $p62^{dok}$ (Dok-1) (Carpino et al. 1997; Yamanashi and Baltimore 1997) and $p56^{dok\text{-}2}$ (Dok-2) (Di Cristofano et al. 1998) had been considered as essential tumor suppressor genes. Both Dok proteins, however, are known substrates of $p210^{Bcr\text{-}Abl}$ (Carpino et al. 1997; Di Cristofano et al. 1998; Yamanashi and Baltimore 1997). Upon phosphorylation by Bcr-Abl, Dok-1 and Dok-2 associate with the p120 rasGTPase-activating protein (rasGAP) (Cong et al. 1999; Lemay et al. 2000). In a recent report by Niki et al. (Niki et al. 2004), single and double knockout (KO) Dok-1 and Dok-2 mutant mice were generated. Whereas mice with a single KO had normal hemopoiesis, inactivation of both Dok-1 and Dok-2 caused a transplantable, CML-like myeloproliferative disorder with complete penetrance. Cells from these mice displayed increased proliferation and reduced apoptosis. Moreover, Ras-signaling was implicated in this phenotype since the double Dok-1 and Dok-2 KO cells were found to have elevated Ras activation. This finding is understandable in light of the known role of these proteins in the negative regulation of Ras. By crossing Dok-1$^{-/-}$ and Dok-2$^{-/-}$ mice with a transgenic mouse model of CML, *Tec-p210*$^{bcr/abl}$ (Honda et al. 2000), these authors additionally demonstrated that inactivation of these proteins reduced the latency of disease and accelerated the onset of blastic transformation of the myeloproliferative disorder. It remains to be seen how the animal data are related to the actual expression of Dok-1 and Dok-2 in human cells and how relevant these findings prove to be for CML.

3.7 Candidate Genes from Expression Profiling

Expression profiling studies have identified candidate genes that are differentially regulated in CML BC relative to CP samples (Table 3.1). Consistent with the idea that CML BC is a very heterogeneous disorder, few "universal" genes have been found that show consistent differences between CP and BC. Ohmine et al. (Ohmine et al. 2001) carried out a background-matched population screening in which cRNA from the AC133^{+} blasts of 7 CP, 2 AP, and 4 myeloid BC patients, together with a control mixture from healthy individuals, was hybridized to oligonucleotide microarrays representing 3,456 human genes. They found 17 genes which were upregulated and 9 which were downregulated in CML BC. Of the latter group, the protein inhibitor of activated STAT (*PIASy*) was considered the most worthy of further study. Nowicki et al. (Nowicki et al. 2003) performed expression profiling of mononuclear cells of 5 CP patients (BM), 5 myeloid BC patients (BM and PB) and 7 normal individuals (4 PB and 3 BM). After hybridization of this cRNA to an Affymetrix (Affymetrix, Santa Clara, CA, USA) human genome U95Av2 microarray, they found only 13 genes, amongst those considered as being potentially relevant for malignant transformation, that were consistently deregulated by fourfold or more in all of their CML samples. These were: transcription factors (*RUNX1(AML-1)*, *AF1Q*, *ETS2*, *LYL-1*), a chromatin binding protein (*PLU-1*), an enzyme (inosine-5-monophosphate dehydrogenase), genes associated with other malignancies (*GBDR1*, *NME1*, *GRO2*, *CA4*, *SNC73*, *MSF*), and a gene which causes Rubinstein-Taybi malformation syndrome upon inactivation (*CREBBP*). Another gene identified in this profiling study, although not one of the 13 consistently deregulated genes, was *EG5* (*KNSL1*). *EG5* encodes a microtubule-associated motor protein required for generation of the mitotic spindle (Blangy et al. 1995) and was found to be highly expressed in BC. Recently, the Eg5 protein has been shown to be expressed in CML cell lines and BC patient samples (Carter et al. 2005). Eg5 expression was downregulated by treatment of the BC cell line, KBM5, with imatinib but not of the imatinib-resistant KBM5 derivative or the Bcr-Abl-negative HL-60 cells. These findings implicate Eg5 as being a downstream effector of Bcr-Abl. Knock-down of Eg5 expression using antisense oligonucleotides induced a G2/M cell cycle block followed by cell death in both imatinib-sensitive and imatinib-resistant KBM5 cells. Moreover, the survival of *Scid* mice which had been injected with KBM5 cells was significantly improved by Eg5-antisense treatment (Carter et al. 2005). Excessive expression of Eg5 in BC may contribute to the disease process by facilitating mitosis, but additional studies, involving a greater number of patient samples, will be required to ascertain whether this is the case, and if this gene product is required for the proliferation and survival of BC CML cells.

Using cDNA subtractive hybridization, Janssen et al. (Janssen et al. 2005) identified 8 genes which may be relevant to disease progression in CML: genes related to apoptosis (*YWHAZ*, *GAS2*), cytokines (*IL8*, *IL6*, *PBEF1*, *CCL4*), a cell cycle-associated gene (SAT), and a specific factor V/Va-binding protein (*MMRN*). The relevance of each of these candidate genes to disease progression in CML will need to be further clarified in follow-up studies.

Gene expression profiling studies which compare CP and BC samples by microarray are open to criticism because this experimental design does not take account of the extreme heterogeneity of the disease. In particular, no distinction is made regarding the rate of disease progression between individuals. The duration of CP in different CML patients is highly variable. Considering patients in the extreme "tails" of the frequency distribution for the onset of BC raises important questions. Why do some patients enter BC within months of diagnosis while others take years to do so? What is the source of this heterogeneity? Two main explanations may be envisaged. The first is that all patients develop CML with an equal chance of their disease undergoing transformation to BC. In this scenario, the genetic makeup of the patient has no bearing upon their susceptibility to subsequent disease progression. Heterogeneity of CP duration may be explained as being due to the timing of the appearance of deleterious mutations in essential genes. Individuals whose disease progresses more rapidly than others have acquired early on sufficient mutations in the "constellations" of proto-oncogenes and tumor suppressor genes required to precipitate BC. According to this explanation, disease evolution should be entirely stochastic. The second explanation is that patients develop CML with an unequal chance of their disease undergoing blastic transformation. In this scenario, differences in gene expression at presentation of CP determine the susceptibility of individuals to disease progression. Heterogeneity of CP duration reflects the heterogeneity in the patterns of genes expressed by different patients. This heterogeneity will be present from the outset and should be detectable in samples taken at diagnosis.

To investigate this latter hypothesis, Yong et al. (Yong et al. 2005) carried out gene expression profiling using samples from CP patients that had been stored within 3 months of diagnosis and before the start of treatment. The CP samples were retrospectively stratified according to whether the patients had entered BC within 3 years of diagnosis, in which case they were defined as having had "aggressive disease," or whether the patients had survived for over 7 years prior to the onset of BC, with an "indolent disease." Unlike other studies (Nowicki et al. 2003) where RNA was extracted from the heterogeneous pool of mononuclear cells, Yong et al. used $CD34^+$ progenitors, which constitute the majority of immature cells in chronic phase. cRNA was synthesized from 19 (aggressive = 10, indolent = 9) patients and hybridized to Affymetrix HG-U133A GeneChip microarrays. This study identified 20 genes with a pattern of expression that was significantly different between patients with aggressive disease and patients with indolent disease. These findings were confirmed by quantitative real-time PCR (Q-RT/PCR) and gene expression was correlated with patient survival using a multivariate Cox regression model on 68 patients. The combination of a low expression of *CD7*, with high expression of proteinase 3 (*PR-3*) or elastase (*ELA2*) was found to be highly predictive of longer survival. Although these results have yet to be confirmed in a larger cohort of patients, this expression profile may represent an important prognostic marker for predicting the onset of blast crisis in different individuals.

3.8 Conclusion

Disease progression in CML is complex and multifactorial. No single cytogenetic or molecular genetic event can be responsible for the heterogeneous nature of BC. In reviewing the biology of advanced phase CML a few patterns may be discerned amongst the general chaos. Nonrandom chromosomal abnormalities are common in disease progression in CML. These are mainly gross markers of an underlying genomic instability and an increased tolerance of genetic aberrations due to compromised "genome surveillance" mechanisms. The nonrandom nature of these cytogenetic patterns is probably a consequence of certain chromosome regions being innately more "break-prone" than others. Gross chromosomal changes, such as trisomies, rarely yield useful clues concerning changes at the molecular level. However, in the case of *MYC*, its duplication, either by +8 or as a result of more complex rearrangements, may be important for disease progression.

It remains an open question as to how many secondary mutations need to be combined in order for blastic transformation to occur. It is unlikely that this number is the same for all patients and, conversely, it is likely that in some cases BC is precipitated by fewer mutations than in others because these mutations are in more critical genes. Data (some of them conflicting) are available concerning the frequency of loss of the tumor suppressor genes *TP53* and *INK4/ARF*. Due to the high frequency of inactivating mutations of *TP53* it seems likely that loss of p53 function has an important role in disease progression. However, it is also possible that there are other genes located on 17p whose loss is as significant, if not more so, for disease progression than p53. The correlation of loss of heterozygosity of *INK4/ARF* with lymphoid BC is well established and it seems certain that this mutation is important in driving the process of disease evolution in some cases of BC with a lymphoid phenotype. Deletion of this locus may be equivalent to two "hits" at other loci since it encodes two tumor suppressor proteins. In addition, transcriptional silencing via promoter methylation may be an alternative mechanism for functionally removing these tumor suppressors.

In the absence of a general "handle" on how to uncover the specific causative abnormality in each individual patient, much of the investigation to date has concentrated on analyzing candidate genes which, by nature of their function, are suspected as underlying the phenotype of CML blasts. In some cases, such as the mutational analyses of *ATM* (Melo et al. 2001), *ABL* (v-*abl* transforming mutations) (Melo and Goldman 1992), *ABL-BCR* (Melo et al. 1993), *JunB* (Yang et al. 2003), *N-ras* (Garicochea et al. 1998; Watzinger et al. 1994), neurofibromatosis gene (*NF1*) (Garicochea et al. 1998), *BCL10* (a proapoptotic gene) (Bose et al. 1999), Wilms tumor predisposing gene (*WT1*) (Carapeti et al. 1997), granulocyte colony-stimulating factor receptor (*G-CSF-R*) (Carapeti et al. 1997), *p57Kip2* (Guran et al. 1998), type II transforming growth factor-β receptor(*TGF-β* RII) (Rooke et al. 1999), *FHIT* (Carapeti et al. 1998), and Fms-like tyrosine kinase 3 (*FLT3*) (Wang et al. 2005) the results are negative, but in others this approach has proven fruitful (Table 3.1). An epigenetic mechanism for the differentiation arrest of CML progenitors has been proposed involving induction of *hnRNP E2* which, in turn, inhibits translation of the transcription factor C/EBP α. The impaired genome surveillance of CML cells may result from direct binding of Bcr-Abl to ATR in the nucleus or it may result from loss of *BRCA1*. Such mechanisms are not mutually exclusive and both may operate together. A recurring theme is that of deficient or error-prone repair of DNA damage. Several mechanisms have been implicated including: BER (overexpression of error-prone DNA polymerase β, NER (stimulation and inhibition of colocalization of XPB with PCNA), NHEJ (downregulation of DNA-PKcs), and HR (upregulation of Rad51). Finally, loss of homeostasis of the hemopoietic compartment may be important in disease progression following the unexpected discovery that Dok-1 and Dok-2 may function as essential tumor suppressor genes. The relevance of these mechanisms to disease progression in CML will need to be tested by sequential analyses, ideally with paired CP and BC material, on larger cohorts of patients. It seems likely that the approach of studying candidate genes will continue and that many of these will be suggested by microarray expression profiling.

References

Aboussekhra A, Biggerstaff M, Shivji MK, Vilpo JA, Moncollin V, Podust VN, Protic M, Hubscher U, Egly JM, Wood RD (1995) Mammalian DNA nucleotide excision repair reconstituted with purified protein components. Cell 80:859–868

Ahuja H, Bar-Eli M, Advani SH, Benchimol S, Cline MJ (1989) Alterations in the p53 gene and the clonal evolution of the blast crisis of chronic myelocytic leukemia. Proc Natl Acad Sci USA 86: 6783–6787

Ahuja HG, Jat PS, Foti A, Bar Eli M, Cline MJ (1991) Abnormalities of the retinoblastoma gene in the pathogenesis of acute leukemia. Blood 78:3259–3268

Alimena G, De Cuia MR, Diverio D, Gastaldi R, Nanni M (1987) The karyotype of blastic crisis. Cancer Genetics and Cytogenetics 26:39–50

Amarante MG, Naekyung KC, Liu L, Huang Y, Perkins CL, Green DR, Bhalla K (1998) Bcr-Abl exerts its antiapoptotic effect against diverse apoptotic stimuli through blockage of mitochondrial release of cytochrome C and activation of caspase-3. Blood 91:1700–1705

Amos TA, Lewis JL, Grand FH, Gooding RP, Goldman JM, Gordon MY (1995) Apoptosis in chronic myeloid leukaemia: normal responses by progenitor cells to growth factor deprivation, X-irradiation and glucocorticoids. Br J Haematol 91:387–393

Barnes DJ, Palaiologou D, Panousopoulou E, Schultheis B, Yong AS, Wong A, Pattacini L, Goldman JM, Melo JV (2005a) Bcr-Abl expression levels determine the rate of development of resistance to imatinib mesylate in chronic myeloid leukemia. Cancer Res 65:8912–8919

Barnes DJ, Schultheis B, Adedeji S, Melo JV (2005b) Dose-dependent effects of Bcr-Abl in cell line models of different stages of chronic myeloid leukemia. Oncogene 24:6432–6440

Bartek J, Lukas J (2003) Chk1 and Chk2 kinases in checkpoint control and cancer. Cancer Cell 3:421–429

Bartram CR, de Klein A, Hagemeijer A, van Agthoven T, Geurts vK, Bootsma D, Grosveld G, Ferguson-Smith MA, Davies T, Stone M et al (1983) Translocation of c-ab1 oncogene correlates with the presence of a Philadelphia chromosome in chronic myelocytic leukaemia. Nature 306:277–280

Beck Z, Kiss A, Toth FD, Szabo J, Bacsi A, Balogh E, Borbely A, Telek B, Kovacs E, Olah E, Rak K (2000) Alterations of P53 and RB genes and the evolution of the accelerated phase of chronic myeloid leukemia. Leuk Lymphoma 38:587–597

Bedi A, Barber JP, Bedi GC, el Deiry WS, Sidransky D, Vala MS, Akhtar AJ, Hilton J, Jones RJ (1995) BCR-ABL-mediated inhibition of apoptosis with delay of G2/M transition after DNA damage: a mechanism of resistance to multiple anticancer agents. Blood 86:1148–1158

Bedi A, Zehnbauer BA, Barber JP, Sharkis SJ, Jones RJ (1994) Inhibition of apoptosis by BCR-ABL in chronic myeloid leukemia. Blood 83:2038–2044

Ben Neriah Y, Bernards A, Paskind M, Daley GQ, Baltimore D (1986) Alternative 5′ exons in c-abl mRNA. Cell 44:577–586

Bi S, Lanza F, Goldman JM (1993) The abnormal p53 proteins expressed in CML cell lines are non-functional. Leukemia 7:1840–1845

Bi S, Lanza F, Goldman JM (1994a) The involvement of "tumor suppressor" p53 in normal and chronic myelogenous leukemia hemopoiesis. Cancer Res 54:582–586

Bi S, Hughes T, Bungey J, Chase A, De Fabritiis P, Goldman JM (1992) p53 in chronic myeloid leukemia cell lines. Leukemia 6:839–842

Bi S, Barton CM, Lemoine NR, Cross NC, Goldman JM (1994b) Retroviral transduction of Philadelphia-positive chronic myeloid leukemia cells with a human mutant p53 cDNA and its effect on in vitro proliferation [see comments]. Exp Hematol 22:95–99

Blangy A, Lane HA, d'Herin P, Harper M, Kress M, Nigg EA (1995) Phosphorylation by p34cdc2 regulates spindle association of human Eg5, a kinesin-related motor essential for bipolar spindle formation in vivo. Cell 83:1159–1169

Blick M, Romero P, Talpaz M, Kurzrock R, Shtalrid M, Andersson B, Trujillo J, Beran M, Gutterman J (1987) Molecular characteristics of chronic myelogenous leukemia in blast crisis. Cancer Genet Cytogenet 27:349–356

Bose S, Goldman JM, Melo JV (1999) Mutations of the BCL10 gene are not associated with the blast crisis of chronic myeloid leukaemia. Leukemia 13:1894–1896

Brady N, Gaymes TJ, Cheung M, Mufti GJ, Rassool FV (2003) Increased error-prone NHEJ activity in myeloid leukemias is associated with DNA damage at sites that recruit key nonhomologous end-joining proteins. Cancer Res 63:1798–1805

Calabretta B, Perrotti D (2004) The biology of CML blast crisis. Blood 103:4010–4022

Cambier N, Chopra R, Strasser A, Metcalf D, Elefanty AG (1998) BCR-ABL activates pathways mediating cytokine independence and protection against apoptosis in murine hematopoietic cells in a dose-dependent manner. Oncogene 16:335–348

Canitrot Y, Lautier D, Laurent G, Frechet M, Ahmed A, Turhan AG, Salles B, Cazaux C, Hoffmann JS (1999) Mutator phenotype of BCR-ABL transfected Ba/F3 cell lines and its association with enhanced expression of DNA polymerase beta. Oncogene 18:2676–2680

Canitrot Y, Falinski R, Louat T, Laurent G, Cazaux C, Hoffmann JS, Lautier D, Skorski T (2003) p210 BCR/ABL kinase regulates nucleotide excision repair (NER) and resistance to UV radiation. Blood 102: 2632–2637

Carapeti M, Goldman JM, Cross NC (1997a) Dominant-negative mutations of the Wilms' tumour predisposing gene (WT1) are infrequent in CML blast crisis and de novo acute leukaemia. Eur J Haematol 58:346–349

Carapeti M, Soede-Bobok A, Hochhaus A, Sill H, Touw IP, Goldman JM, Cross NC (1997b) Rarity of dominant-negative mutations of the G-CSF receptor in patients with blast crisis of chronic myeloid leukemia or de novo acute leukemia. Leukemia 11:1005–1008

Carapeti M, Aguiar RC, Sill H, Goldman JM, Cross NC (1998) Aberrant transcripts of the FHIT gene are expressed in normal and leukaemic haemopoietic cells. Br J Cancer 78:601–605

Carpino N, Wisniewski D, Strife A, Marshak D, Kobayashi R, Stillman B, Clarkson B (1997) p62(dok): a constitutively tyrosine-phosphorylated, GAP-associated protein in chronic myelogenous leukemia progenitor cells. Cell 88:197–204

Carter BZ, Mak D, Shi YX, Schober WD, Wang RY, McQueen T, Konopleva M, Koller E, Dean NM, Andreeff M (2005) Regulation and targeting of Eg5 in blast crisis CML: Overcoming imatinib resistance. Blood 106:806A

Collis SJ, DeWeese TL, Jeggo PA, Parker AR (2005) The life and death of DNA-PK. Oncogene 24:949–961

Cong F, Yuan B, Goff SP (1999) Characterization of a novel member of the DOK family that binds and modulates Abl signaling. Mol Cell Biol 19:8314–8325

Cortez D, Wang Y, Qin J, Elledge SJ (1999) Requirement of ATM-dependent phosphorylation of brca1 in the DNA damage response to double-strand breaks. Science 286:1162–1166

Costanzo V, Shechter D, Lupardus PJ, Cimprich KA, Gottesman M, Gautier J (2003) An ATR- and Cdc7-dependent DNA damage checkpoint that inhibits initiation of DNA replication. Mol Cell 11: 203–213

Daley GQ, Baltimore D (1988) Transformation of an interleukin 3-dependent hematopoietic cell line by the chronic myelogenous leukemia-specific P210bcr/abl protein. Proc Natl Acad Sci USA 85: 9312–9316

Daley GQ, Van Etten RA, Baltimore D (1990) Induction of chronic myelogenous leukemia in mice by the P210bcr/abl gene of the Philadelphia chromosome. Science 247:824–830

Dash AB, Williams IR, Kutok JL, Tomasson MH, Anastasiadou E, Lindahl K, Li S, Van Etten RA, Borrow J, Housman D, Druker B, Gilliland DG (2002) A murine model of CML blast crisis induced by cooperation between BCR/ABL and NUP98/HOXA9. Proc Natl Acad Sci USA 99:7622–7627

de Laat WL, Jaspers NG, Hoeijmakers JH (1999) Molecular mechanism of nucleotide excision repair. Genes Devel 13:768–785

Deininger MW, Goldman JM, Melo JV (2000) The molecular biology of chronic myeloid leukemia. Blood 96:3343–3356

Deutsch E, Dugray A, AbdulKarim B, Marangoni E, Maggiorella L, Vaganay S, M'Kacher R, Rasy SD, Eschwege F, Vainchenker W, Turhan AG, Bourhis J (2001) BCR-ABL down-regulates the DNA repair protein DNA-PKcs. Blood 97:2084–2090

Deutsch E, Jarrousse S, Buet D, Dugray A, Bonnet ML, Vozenin-Brotons MC, Guilhot F, Turhan AG, Feunteun J, Bourhis J (2003) Down-regulation of BRCA-1 in BCR-ABL-expressing hematopoietic cells. Blood 101:4583–4588

Di Cristofano A, Carpino N, Dunant N, Friedland G, Kobayashi R, Strife A, Wisniewski D, Clarkson B, Pandolfi PP, Resh MD (1998) Molecular cloning and characterization of p56dok-2 defines a new family of RasGAP-binding proteins. J Biol Chem 273:4827–4830

Dierov J, Dierova R, Carroll M (2004) BCR/ABL translocates to the nucleus and disrupts an ATR-dependent intra-S phase checkpoint. Cancer Cell 5:275–285

Dierov JK, Schoppy DW, Carroll M (2005) CML progenitor cells have chromsomal instability and display increased DNA damage at DNA fragile sites. Blood 106:563A

Dubrez L, Eymin B, Sordet O, Droin N, Turhan AG, Solary E (1998) BCR-ABL delays apoptosis upstream of procaspase-3 activation. Blood 91:2415–2422

Elmaagacli AH, Beelen DW, Opalka B, Seeber S, Schaefer UW (2000) The amount of BCR-ABL fusion transcripts detected by the real-time quantitative polymerase chain reaction method in patients with Philadelphia chromosome positive chronic myeloid leukemia correlates with the disease stage. Ann Hematol 79:424–431

Fabarius A, Giehl M, Frank O, Duesberg P, Hochhaus A, Hehlmann R, Seifarth W (2005) Induction of centrosome and chromosome aberrations by imatinib in vitro. Leukemia 19:1573–1578

Feinstein E, Cimino G, Gale RP, Alimena G, Berthier R, Kishi K, Goldman J, Zaccaria A, Berrebi A, Canaani E (1991) p53 in chronic myelogenous leukemia in acute phase. Proc Natl Acad Sci USA 88:6293–6297

Fioretos T, Strombeck B, Sandberg T, Johansson B, Billstrom R, Borg A, Nilsson PG, Van den BH, Hagemeijer A, Mitelman F, Hoglund M (1999) Isochromosome 17q in blast crisis of chronic myeloid leukemia and in other hematologic malignancies is the result of clustered breakpoints in 17p11 and is not associated with coding TP53 mutations. Blood 94:225–232

Gaiger A, Henn T, Horth E, Geissler K, Mitterbauer G, Maier-Dobersberger T, Greinix H, Mannhalter C, Haas OA, Lechner K (1995) Increase of bcr-abl chimeric mRNA expression in tumor cells of patients with chronic myeloid leukemia precedes disease progression. Blood 86:2371–2378

Garicochea B, Giorgi R, Odone VF, Dorlhiac-Llacer PE, Bendit I (1998) Mutational analysis of N-RAS and GAP-related domain of the neurofibromatosis type 1 gene in chronic myelogenous leukemia. Leuk Res 22:1003–1007

Gaymes TJ, Mufti GJ, Rassool FV (2002) Myeloid leukemias have increased activity of the nonhomologous end-joining pathway and concomitant DNA misrepair that is dependent on the Ku70/86 heterodimer. Cancer Res 62:2791–2797

Giehl M, Fabarius A, Frank O, Hochhaus A, Hafner M, Hehlmann R, Seifarth W (2005) Centrosome aberrations in chronic myeloid leukemia correlate with stage of disease and chromosomal instability. Leukemia 19:1192–1197

Gordon MY, Dowding CR, Riley GP, Goldman JM, Greaves MF (1987) Altered adhesive interactions with marrow stroma of haematopoietic progenitor cells in chronic myeloid leukaemia. Nature 328:342–344

Gottlieb TM, Jackson SP (1993) The DNA-dependent protein kinase: requirement for DNA ends and association with Ku antigen. Cell 72:131–142

Grand FH, Koduru P, Cross NC, Allen SL (2005) NUP98-LEDGF fusion and t(9;11) in transformed chronic myeloid leukemia. Leuk Res 29:1469–1472

Grawunder U, Wilm M, Wu X, Kulesza P, Wilson TE, Mann M, Lieber MR (1997) Activity of DNA ligase IV stimulated by complex formation with XRCC4 protein in mammalian cells. Nature 388:492–495

Gribble SM, Sinclair PB, Grace C, Green AR, Nacheva EP (1999) Comparative analysis of G-banding, chromosome painting, locus-specific fluorescence in situ hybridization, and comparative genomic hybridization in chronic myeloid leukemia blast crisis. Cancer Genet Cytogenet 111:7–17

Gribble SM, Reid AG, Roberts I, Grace C, Green AR, Nacheva EP (2003) Genomic imbalances in CML blast crisis: 8q24.12-q24.13 segment identified as a common region of over-representation. Genes Chromosomes Cancer 37:346–358

Groffen J, Stephenson JR, Heisterkamp N, de Klein A, Bartram CR, Grosveld G (1984) Philadelphia chromosomal breakpoints are clustered within a limited region, bcr, on chromosome 22. Cell 36:93–99

Guo JQ, Wang JY, Arlinghaus RB (1991) Detection of BCR-ABL proteins in blood cells of benign phase chronic myelogenous leukemia patients. Cancer Res 51:3048–3051

Guran S, Bahce M, Beyan C, Korkmaz K, Yalcin A (1998) P53, p15INK4B, p16INK4A and p57KIP2 mutations during the progression of chronic myeloid leukemia. Haematologia (Budap) 29:181–193

Hernandez-Boluda JC, Cervantes F, Colomer D, Vela MC, Costa D, Paz MF, Esteller M, Montserrat E (2003) Genomic p16 abnormalities in the progression of chronic myeloid leukemia into blast crisis: a sequential study in 42 patients. Exp Hematol 31:204–210

Hoeijmakers JH (2001) Genome maintenance mechanisms for preventing cancer. Nature 411:366–374

Honda H, Ushijima T, Wakazono K, Oda H, Tanaka Y, Aizawa S, Ishikawa T, Yazaki Y, Hirai H (2000) Acquired loss of p53 induces blastic transformation in p210(bcr/abl)- expressing hematopoietic cells: a transgenic study for blast crisis of human CML. Blood 95:1144–1150

Huntly BJ, Gilliland DG (2004) Blasts from the past: new lessons in stem cell biology from chronic myelogenous leukemia. Cancer Cell 6:199–201

Huntly BJP, Shigematzu H, Deguchi K, Lee B, Mizuno S, Duclos N, Rowan R, Amaral S, Curley D, Williams IR, Akashi K, Gilliland G (2004) MOZ-TIF2, but not BCR-ABL, confers properties of leukemic stem cells to committed murine hematopoietic progenitors. Blood 104:21a

Issaad C, Ahmed M, Novault S, Bonnet ML, Bennardo T, Varet B, Vainchenker W, Turhan AG (2000) Biological effects induced by variable levels of BCR-ABL protein in the pluripotent hematopoietic cell line UT-7. Leukemia 14:662–670

Jamieson CH, Ailles LE, Dylla SJ, Muijtjens M, Jones C, Zehnder JL, Gotlib J, Li K, Manz MG, Keating A, Sawyers CL, Weissman IL (2004) Granulocyte-macrophage progenitors as candidate leukemic stem cells in blast-crisis CML. New Engl J Med 351:657–667

Janssen JJ, Klaver SM, Waisfisz Q, Pasterkamp G, de Kleijn DP, Schuurhuis GJ, Ossenkoppele GJ (2005) Identification of genes potentially involved in disease transformation of CML. Leukemia 19:998–1004

Jennings BA, Mills KI (1998) c-myc locus amplification and the acquisition of trisomy 8 in the evolution of chronic myeloid leukaemia. Leuk Res 22:899–903

Johansson B, Fioretos T, Mitelman F (2002) Cytogenetic and molecular genetic evolution of chronic myeloid leukemia. Acta Haematol 107:76–94

Kantarjian HM, Keating MJ, Talpaz M, Walters RS, Smith TL, Cork A, McCredie KB, Freireich EJ (1987) Chronic myelogenous leukemia in blast crisis. Analysis of 242 patients. Am J Med 83:445–454

Khanna KK, Jackson SP (2001) DNA double-strand breaks: signaling, repair and the cancer connection. Nat Genet 27:247–254

Klucher KM, Lopez DV, Daley GQ (1998) Secondary mutation maintains the transformed state in BaF3 cells with inducible BCR/ABL expression. Blood 91:3927–3934

Koptyra M, Houghtaling S, Grompe M, Skorski T (2005) Fanconi anemia D2 protein contributes to BCR/ABL-mediated transformation of hematopoietic cells. Blood 106:806A–807A

Lemay S, Davidson D, Latour S, Veillette A (2000) Dok-3, a novel adapter molecule involved in the negative regulation of immunoreceptor signaling. Mol Cell Biol 20:2743–2754

Lin F, van Rhee F, Goldman JM, Cross NC (1996) Kinetics of increasing BCR-ABL transcript numbers in chronic myeloid leukemia patients who relapse after bone marrow transplantation. Blood 87:4473–4478

Liu Q, Guntuku S, Cui XS, Matsuoka S, Cortez D, Tamai K, Luo G, Carattini-Rivera S, DeMayo F, Bradley A, Donehower LA, Elledge SJ (2000) Chk1 is an essential kinase that is regulated by Atr and required for the G(2)/M DNA damage checkpoint. Genes Devel 14:1448–1459

Loeb LA (2001) A mutator phenotype in cancer. Cancer Res 61:3230–3239

Lugo TG, Pendergast AM, Muller AJ, Witte ON (1990) Tyrosine kinase activity and transformation potency of bcr-abl oncogene products. Science 247:1079–1082

Ma Y, Pannicke U, Schwarz K, Lieber MR (2002) Hairpin opening and overhang processing by an Artemis/DNA-dependent protein kinase complex in nonhomologous end joining and V(D)J recombination. Cell 108:781–794

Matsuoka S, Rotman G, Ogawa A, Shiloh Y, Tamai K, Elledge SJ (2000) Ataxia telangiectasia-mutated phosphorylates Chk2 in vivo and in vitro. Proc Natl Acad Sci USA 97:10389–10394

McCarthy DM, Rassool FV, Goldman JM, Graham SV, Birnie GD (1984) Genomic alterations involving the c-myc proto-oncogene locus during the evolution of a case of chronic granulocytic leukaemia. Lancet 2:1362–1365

McLaughlin J, Chianese E, Witte ON (1987) In vitro transformation of immature hematopoietic cells by the P210 BCR/ABL oncogene product of the Philadelphia chromosome. Proc Natl Acad Sci USA 84:6558–6562

Melo JV (1996) The diversity of BCR-ABL fusion proteins and their relationship to leukemia phenotype [editorial]. Blood 88:2375–2384

Melo JV, Goldman JM (1992) Specific point mutations that activate v-abl are not found in Philadelphia-negative chronic myeloid leukaemia, Philadelphia-negative acute lymphoblastic leukaemia or blast transformation of chronic myeloid leukaemia. Leukemia 6:786–790

Melo JV, Gordon DE, Cross NC, Goldman JM (1993) The ABL-BCR fusion gene is expressed in chronic myeloid leukemia. Blood 81:158–165

Melo JV, Kumberova A, van Dijk AG, Goldman JM, Yuille MR (2001) Investigation on the role of the ATM gene in chronic myeloid leukaemia. Leukemia 15:1448–1450

Miki Y, Swensen J, Shattuck-Eidens D, Futreal PA, Harshman K, Tavtigian S, Liu Q, Cochran C, Bennett LM, Ding W et al (1994) A strong candidate for the breast and ovarian cancer susceptibility gene BRCA1. Science 266:66–71

Mitani K (2004) Molecular mechanisms of leukemogenesis by AML1/EVI-1. Oncogene 23:4263–4269

Mitani K, Ogawa S, Tanaka T, Miyoshi H, Kurokawa M, Mano H, Yazaki Y, Ohki M, Hirai H (1994) Generation of the AML1-EVI-1 fusion gene in the t(3;21)(q26;q22) causes blastic crisis in chronic myelocytic leukemia. EMBO J 13:504–510

Mitelman F, Levan G, Nilsson PG, Brandt L (1976) Non-random karyotypic evolution in chronic myeloid leukemia. Int J Cancer 18:24–30

Nagy E, Beck Z, Kiss A, Csoma E, Telek B, Konya J, Olah E, Rak K, Toth FD (2003) Frequent methylation of p16INK4A and p14ARF genes implicated in the evolution of chronic myeloid leukaemia from its chronic to accelerated phase. Eur J Cancer 39:2298–2305

Neviani P, Santhanam R, Trotta R, Notari M, Blaser BW, Liu S, Mao H, Chang JS, Galietta A, Uttam A, Roy DC, Valtieri M, Bruner-Klisovic R, Caligiuri MA, Bloomfield CD, Marcucci G, Perrotti D (2005) The tumor suppressor PP2A is functionally inactivated in blast crisis CML through the inhibitory activity of the BCR/ABL-regulated SET protein. Cancer Cell 8:355–368

Nick McElhinny SA, Snowden CM, McCarville J, Ramsden DA (2000) Ku recruits the XRCC4-ligase IV complex to DNA ends. Mol Cell Biol 20:2996–3003

Nieborowska M, Stoklosa T, Datta M, Czechowska A, Rink L, Blasiak J, Skorski T (2005) ATR-Chk1 axis is activated, but the function of Chk1 is disrupted in BCR/ABL leukemia cells responding to DNA damage. Blood 106:808A

Niki M, Di Cristofano A, Zhao M, Honda H, Hirai H, Van Aelst L, Cordon-Cardo C, Pandolfi PP (2004) Role of Dok-1 and Dok-2 in leukemia suppression. J Exp Med 200:1689–1695

Notari M, Neviani P, Santhanam R, Bradley BW, Chang JS, Galietta A, Willis AE, Roy DC, Caligiuri MA, Marcucci G, Perrotti D (2005) A MAPK/HNRPK pathway controls BCR/ABL oncogenic potential by regulating MYC mRNA translation. Blood (in press)

Nowell PC, Hungerford DA (1960) A minute chromosome in human chronic granulocytic leukemia. Science 132:1497

Nowicki MO, Pawlowski P, Fischer T, Hess G, Pawlowski T, Skorski T (2003) Chronic myelogenous leukemia molecular signature. Oncogene 22:3952–3963

Nowicki MO, Falinski R, Koptyra M, Slupianek A, Stoklosa T, Gloc E, Nieborowska-Skorska M, Blasiak J, Skorski T (2004) BCR/ABL oncogenic kinase promotes unfaithful repair of the reactive oxygen species-dependent DNA double-strand breaks. Blood 104:3746–3753

Ogawa S, Mitani K, Kurokawa M, Matsuo Y, Minowada J, Inazawa J, Kamada N, Tsubota T, Yazaki Y, Hirai H (1996) Abnormal expression of Evi-1 gene in human leukemias. Hum Cell 9:323–332

Ohmine K, Ota J, Ueda M, Ueno S, Yoshida K, Yamashita Y, Kirito K, Imagawa S, Nakamura Y, Saito K, Akutsu M, Mitani K, Kano Y, Komatsu N, Ozawa K, Mano H (2001) Characterization of stage progression in chronic myeloid leukemia by DNA microarray with purified hematopoietic stem cells. Oncogene 20:8249–8257

Pabst T, Mueller BU, Stillner E, Nimer S, Gilliland G, Melo JV, Tenen DG (2006) Mutations of the myeloid transcription factor CEBPA are not associated with the blast crisis of chronic myeloid leukemia. Br J Haematol (in press)

Perrotti D, Cesi V, Trotta R, Guerzoni C, Santilli G, Campbell K, Iervolino A, Condorelli F, Gambacorti-Passerini C, Caligiuri MA, Calabretta B (2002) BCR-ABL suppresses C/EBPalpha expression through inhibitory action of hnRNP E2. Nat Genet 30:48–58

Pomerantz J, Schreiber-Agus N, Liegeois NJ, Silverman A, Alland L, Chin L, Potes J, Chen K, Orlow I, Lee HW, Cordon-Cardo C, DePinho RA (1998) The Ink4a tumor suppressor gene product, p19Arf, interacts with MDM2 and neutralizes MDM2's inhibition of p53. Cell 92:713–723

Rink L, Stoklosa T, Skorski T (2005) Enhanced phosphorylation of Nbs1, a member of the DNA repair/checkpoint activation complex Rad50/Mre11/Nbs1, prolongs cell cycle S phase and contributes to drug resistance in BCR/ABL-positive leukemias. Blood 106:804A

Rooke HM, Vitas MR, Crosier PS, Crosier KE (1999) The TGF-beta type II receptor in chronic myeloid leukemia: analysis of microsatellite regions and gene expression. Leukemia 13:535–541

Rowley JD (1973) Letter: A new consistent chromosomal abnormality in chronic myelogenous leukaemia identified by quinacrine fluorescence and Giemsa staining. Nature 243:290–293

Sanchez Y, Wong C, Thoma RS, Richman R, Wu Z, Piwnica-Worms H, Elledge SJ (1997) Conservation of the Chk1 checkpoint pathway in mammals: linkage of DNA damage to Cdk regulation through Cdc25. Science 277:1497–1501

Savage DG, Szydlo RM, Goldman JM (1997) Clinical features at diagnosis in 430 patients with chronic myeloid leukaemia seen at a referral centre over a 16-year period. Br J Haematol 96:111–116

Sawyers CL, Callahan W, Witte ON (1992) Dominant negative MYC blocks transformation by ABL oncogenes. Cell 70:901–910

Sawyers CL, Hochhaus A, Feldman E, Goldman JM, Miller CB, Ottmann OG, Schiffer CA, Talpaz M, Guilhot F, Deininger MW, Fischer T, O'Brien SG, Stone RM, Gambacorti-Passerini CB, Russell NH, Reiffers JJ, Shea TC, Chapuis B, Coutre S, Tura S, Morra E, Larson RA, Saven A, Peschel C, Gratwohl A, Mandelli F, Ben Am M, Gathmann I, Capdeville R, Paquette RL, Druker BJ (2002) Imatinib induces hematologic and cytogenetic responses in patients with chronic myelogenous leukemia in myeloid blast crisis: results of a phase II study. Blood 99:3530–3539

Scanlon KJ, Kashani-Sabet M, Miyachi H (1989) Differential gene expression in human cancer cells resistant to cisplatin. Cancer Invest 7:581–587

Scully R, Chen J, Plug A, Xiao Y, Weaver D, Feunteun J, Ashley T, Livingston DM (1997) Association of BRCA1 with Rad51 in mitotic and meiotic cells. Cell 88:265–275

Serra A, Gottardi E, Della RF, Saglio G, Iolascon A (1995) Involvement of the cyclin-dependent kinase-4 inhibitor (CDKN2) gene in the pathogenesis of lymphoid blast crisis of chronic myelogenous leukaemia. Br J Haematol 91:625–629

Serrano M, Hannon GJ, Beach D (1993) A new regulatory motif in cell-cycle control causing specific inhibition of cyclin D/CDK4. Nature 366:704–707

Sharpless NE, DePinho RA (1999) The INK4A/ARF locus and its two gene products. Curr Opin Genet Dev 9:22–30

Shet AS, Jahagirdar BN, Verfaillie CM (2002) Chronic myelogenous leukemia: mechanisms underlying disease progression. Leukemia 16:1402–1411

Shtivelman E, Lifshitz B, Gale RP, Canaani E (1985) Fused transcript of abl and bcr genes in chronic myelogenous leukaemia. Nature 315:550–554

Sill H, Goldman JM, Cross NC (1995) Homozygous deletions of the p16 tumor-suppressor gene are associated with lymphoid transformation of chronic myeloid leukemia. Blood 85:2013–2016

Silva PM, Lourenco GJ, Bognone RA, Delamain MT, Pinto-Junior W, Lima CS (2005) Inherited pericentric inversion of chromosome 16 in chronic phase of chronic myeloid leukaemia. Leuk Res (in press)

Skorski T, Nieborowska-Skorska M, Wlodarski P, Perrotti D, Martinez R, Wasik MA, Calabretta B (1996) Blastic transformation of p53-deficient bone marrow cells by p210bcr/abl tyrosine kinase. Proc Natl Acad Sci USA 93:13137–13142

Slupianek A, Schmutte C, Tombline G, Nieborowska-Skorska M, Hoser G, Nowicki MO, Pierce AJ, Fishel R, Skorski T (2001) BCR/ABL regulates mammalian RecA homologs, resulting in drug resistance. Mol Cell 8:795–806

Slupianek A, Jozwiakowski S, Gurdek E, Nowicki MO, Skorski T (2005a) BCR/ABL regulates the expression and interacts with Werner syndrome helicase/exonuclease to modulate its biochemical properties. Blood 106:805A

Slupianek A, Nowicki MO, Skorski T (2005b) BCR/ABL modifies the kinetics and fidelity of DNA double-strand breaks repair in leukemia cells. Blood 106:561A

Smith LT, Hohaus S, Gonzalez DA, Dziennis SE, Tenen DG (1996) PU.1 (Spi-1) and C/EBP alpha regulate the granulocyte colony-stimulating factor receptor promoter in myeloid cells. Blood 88:1234–1247

Stoklosa T, Slupianek A, Basak G, Skorski T (2005) BCR/ABL kinase disrupts formation of mismatch repair complex to induce genomic instability. Blood 106:803A

Stott FJ, Bates S, James MC, McConnell BB, Starborg M, Brookes S, Palmero I, Ryan K, Hara E, Vousden KH, Peters G (1998) The alternative product from the human CDKN2A locus, p14(ARF), participates in a regulatory feedback loop with p53 and MDM2. EMBO J 17:5001–5014

Suwa A, Hirakata M, Takeda Y, Jesch SA, Mimori T, Hardin JA (1994) DNA-dependent protein kinase (Ku protein-p350 complex) assembles on double-stranded DNA. Proc Natl Acad Sci USA 91:6904–6908

Takeda N, Shibuya M, Maru Y (1999) The BCR-ABL oncoprotein potentially interacts with the xeroderma pigmentosum group B protein. Proc Natl Acad Sci USA 96:203–207

Towatari M, Adachi K, Kato H, Saito H (1991) Absence of the human retinoblastoma gene product in the megakaryoblastic crisis of chronic myelogenous leukemia. Blood 78:2178–2181

Van Etten RA, Jackson P, Baltimore D (1989) The mouse type IV c-abl gene product is a nuclear protein, and activation of transforming ability is associated with cytoplasmic localization. Cell 58:669–678

Vardiman JW, Pierre R, Thiele J, Imbert J, Brunning RD, Flandrin G (2001) Chronic myelogenous leukaemia. In: Jaffe ES et al (eds) World Health Organization Classification of Tumours: Tumours of Haematopoietic and Lymphoid Tissues. IARC Press, Lyon pp 20–26

Vigneri P, Wang JY (2001) Induction of apoptosis in chronic myelogenous leukemia cells through nuclear entrapment of BCR-ABL tyrosine kinase. Nat Med 7:228–234

Virtaneva K, Wright FA, Tanner SM, Yuan B, Lemon WJ, Caligiuri MA, Bloomfield CD, de La CA, Krahe R (2001) Expression profiling reveals fundamental biological differences in acute myeloid leukemia with isolated trisomy 8 and normal cytogenetics. Proc Natl Acad Sci USA 98:1124–1129

Wadhwa J, Szydlo RM, Apperley JF, Chase A, Bua M, Marin D, Olavarria E, Kanfer E, Goldman JM (2002) Factors affecting duration of survival after onset of blastic transformation of chronic myeloid leukemia. Blood 99:2304–2309

Wang L, Lin D, Zhang X, Chen S, Wang M, Wang J (2005) Analysis of FLT3 internal tandem duplication and D835 mutations in Chinese acute leukemia patients. Leuk Res 29:1393–1398

Wang Y, Cortez D, Yazdi P, Neff N, Elledge SJ, Qin J (2000) BASC, a super complex of BRCA1-associated proteins involved in the recognition and repair of aberrant DNA structures. Genes Devel 14:927–939

Watzinger F, Gaiger A, Karlic H, Becher R, Pillwein K, Lion T (1994) Absence of N-ras mutations in myeloid and lymphoid blast crisis of chronic myeloid leukemia. Cancer Res 54:3934–3938

Wetzler M, Talpaz M, Estrov Z, Kurzrock R (1993) CML: mechanisms of disease initiation and progression. Leuk Lymphoma 11, Suppl 1: 47–50

Yamamoto K, Nakamura Y, Saito K, Furusawa S (2000) Expression of the NUP98/HOXA9 fusion transcript in the blast crisis of Philadelphia chromosome-positive chronic myelogenous leukaemia with t(7;11)(p15;p15). Br J Haematol 109:423–426

Yamanashi Y, Baltimore D (1997) Identification of the Abl- and rasGAP-associated 62 kDa protein as a docking protein, Dok. Cell 88:205–211

Yang MY, Liu TC, Chang JG, Lin PM, Lin SF (2003) JunB gene expression is inactivated by methylation in chronic myeloid leukemia. Blood 101:3205–3211

Yarden RI, Pardo-Reoyo S, Sgagias M, Cowan KH, Brody LC (2002) BRCA1 regulates the G2/M checkpoint by activating Chk1 kinase upon DNA damage. Nat Genet 30:285–289

Yong AS, Szydlo RM, Goldman JM, Apperley JF, Melo JV (2005) Molecular profiling of CD34+ cells identifies low expression of CD7 with high expression of proteinase 3 or elastase as predictors of longer survival in CML patients. Blood (in press)

Zhang DE, Zhang P, Wang ND, Hetherington CJ, Darlington GJ, Tenen DG (1997) Absence of granulocyte colony-stimulating factor signaling and neutrophil development in CCAAT enhancer binding protein alpha-deficient mice. Proc Natl Acad Sci USA 94:569–574

Zhong Q, Chen CF, Li S, Chen Y, Wang CC, Xiao J, Chen PL, Sharp ZD, Lee WH (1999) Association of BRCA1 with the hRad50-hMre11-p95 complex and the DNA damage response. Science 285:747–750

Clinical Features of CML

Mira Farquharson and Pat Shepherd

Contents

Abstract. This chapter describes the incidence and clinical features of CML at diagnosis and the required investigations to evaluate patients with *BCR-ABL*-positive chronic myeloid leukemia. Some rarer presentations or features at diagnosis are highlighted. It describes prognostic indicators for evaluating outcome both in the preimatinib and imatinib era. Response to therapy is now a more powerful predictor of outcome than the traditional risk groupings derived from diagnostic data. The IRIS Trial shows 93% of patients treated with imatinib free of progression to accelerated phase or blast crisis at 54-month follow-up. For patients in complete cytogenetic and major molecular responses at 12 months, the figures are even better. Criteria associated with disease progression are evaluated. There is a general consensus for definition of blast crisis but definitions for accelerated phase still vary. The outcome for patients who have progressed to these stages is poor, although the impact of newer kinase inhibitors is still to be evaluated. It is likely that definitions of progression will change to take into account failure to obtain an adequate response to kinase inhibitor therapy. Despite the efficacy demonstrated with imatinib so far, resistance does occur and, in addition, sudden transformation to blast phase, particularly of lymphoid lineage, may occur. The outlook for patients with transformed disease remains poor even with intensive therapy including allogeneic transplantation.

4.1 Clinical Features of CML

Chronic myeloid leukemia (CML) is a clonal disorder of a pluripotent stem cell (Fialkow et al. 1997). It is characterized by the presence of a reciprocal translocation between chromosomes 9 and 22, t(9;22)(q34;q11) known as the Philadelphia chromosome (Nowell and Hungerford 1960). The translocation breakpoints involve two genes, a shortened *BCR* gene on chromosome 22 and a translocated *ABL* gene from chromosome 9 to form a fusion *BCR-ABL* gene on chromosome 22.

The resultant aberrant protein has dysregulated tyrosine kinase activity and is thought to be the initiating event in the chronic phase of CML (Daley et al. 1990). There are no known factors predisposing to CML other than ionizing radiation (Bizzozero et al. 1966; Corso et al. 1995). Ph positive CML has a worldwide incidence of 1–1.5 cases per 100,000 population per year (Faderl et al. 1999). Data from the Scottish Cancer Registry 1997–2001 show an incidence of 0.9–1.2 per 100,000 person-years at risk (Scottish Cancer Registry, ISD). Early data may not take into account only those persons with a Ph chromosome or an aberrant *BCR-ABL* fusion gene necessary for a diagnosis of CML. Despite the consistent molecular events in CML, the disease is heterogeneous in both presentation and clinical course. The disease is bi- or triphasic with patients typically presenting in the chronic phase (CP). The disease usually transforms to one or both of the advanced phases–accelerated phase (AP) and blast transformation (BT). Around 20% of patients will die in chronic phase of unrelated conditions (Kluin-Nelemans, et al. 2004).

In this chapter we discuss clinical features at disease diagnosis as well as the natural history of each phase of disease, prognostic risk grouping, and some of the side effects encountered with treatment.

4.1.1 Diagnosis

Most patients are easily diagnosed from the typical findings on an examination of the blood count and film and the demonstration of the typical Ph chromosome. While some cases are diagnosed incidentally, the majority of patients are symptomatic at presentation. The disease usually presents in the CP, which generally has an insidious onset. Occasional patients may present in more advanced stages of the disease. There are a number of investigations which should be performed at diagnosis:

- Full blood count (FBC) with manual differential of at least 300 cells for percent of blasts, eosinophils, and basophils. This is necessary for the parameters required by the Sokal and Hasford Prognostic Risk scores. Automated counters do not give a sufficiently accurate differential count. It should be performed before any therapy has been given.
- Demonstration of a Ph chromosome and/or a *BCR-ABL* fusion gene. This can be done on peripheral blood or marrow. Standard cytogenetics should be done on a minimum of 20 metaphases. If cytogenetics fail fluorescence in situ hybridization (FISH) analysis using dual fusion probes spanning the breakpoints on both chromosome 9 and 22 is helpful. The FISH report should also include the deletion status of chromosome 9 as this may have prognostic significance (Huntly et al. 2001; Quintas-Cardama et al. 2005), as discussed later. The presence or absence of additional cytogenetic changes should be noted.
- Measurement of spleen size on quiet breathing in centimeters below the costal margin, again for prognostic indices.
- Quantitative RT-PCR analysis of blood or marrow for type and level of *BCR-ABL* transcript.

4.1.2 Laboratory Features

In CP CML, the peripheral blood typically shows significant leukocytosis. Typical levels from the multicenter randomized trials in CML show levels of around 100–150×10^9/l (Allan et al. 1995; Kluin-Nelmans et al. 2004; The Benelux CML Study Group 1998; The Italian Cooperative Study Group 1994). This leukocytosis is largely due to myeloid cells in varying stages of maturation, predominantly myelocytes and segmented neutrophils. Blasts usually account for <2% of the WBC. Basophilia is invariably present and there is often eosinophilia. The platelet count may be normal or increased with thrombocytopenia rarely occurring during CP. There is often a mild normocytic anemia (Spiers et al. 1977). Some cases may present with predominant thrombocytosis with little if any elevation of the white cell count (Morris et al. 1988). Thus all patients with high platelet counts consistent with a myeloproliferative disorder should have cytogenetic or molecular analysis to detect a *BCR-ABL* fusion gene.

The bone marrow aspirate and biopsy are typically markedly hypercellular with a high myeloid:erythroid ratio. Blasts are usually less than 10% but often these are fewer than 5% of cells. Megakaryocytes are small with hypolobulated nuclei. They may be increased, normal or slightly decreased in number, but increased numbers are the most common finding with up to 50% of patients having moderate to extensive proliferation of megakaryocytes (Thiele et al. 2000). An increased amount of reticulin fibers in the marrow correlates with increased numbers of megakaryocytes, extent of splenomegaly, and severity of anemia (Thiele et al. 2000). Pseudo-Gaucher cells and sea-blue histiocytes are seen in approximately one third of specimens. They reflect the increased bone marrow cell turnover and are derived from the malignant clone (Bhatia et al. 1991; Golde et al. 1977; Thiele et al. 1998).

4.1.3 Clinical Features at Diagnosis

The median age at diagnosis is 55–60 years, with fewer than 10% of cases occurring under age 20 years. The disease occurs in both sexes with a male:female ratio of 1.3:1 (Faderl et al. 1999). Data from the Scottish Can-

Table 4.1. Findings at diagnosis by allocated treatment in Ph-positive CML patients (n=513) (with permission from Hehlmann et al. 1994)

	IFN (n=133)	Bu (n=186)	HU (n=194)
Age years median(range)	47.4±14.9/47(18–85)	48.5±15.5/4.9(17–84)	46.9±15.3/47(15–84)
Sex (% male)	66.2	61.3	50.5
Fatigue, general ill-feeling (%)	61.8	68.8	57.9
Symptoms due to organomegaly (%)	28.8	36.0	34.9
Weight loss (%)	17.4	23.9	19.5
Fever (%)	3.8	9.7	3.7
Extramedullary manifestations (skin, lymph nodes (%))	9.2	8.2	3.7
Splenomegaly (%)	68.3	72.1	72.6
Hepatomegaly (%)	47.9	53.2	46.3
Spleen size (cm below costal margin)	6.2±6.4	6.4±6.7	6.5±6.5
Liver size (cm in mid clavicular line)	12.7±2.3	12.8±2.6	12.6±2.7

IFN=Interferon-α; Bu=Busulfan; HU=Hydroxyurea

cer Registry over 1997–2001 show a median age of 64 years and a rising incidence with age. Only 5% of cases were <25 years (Scottish Cancer Registry, ISD).

About 20–45% of patients are asymptomatic at diagnosis and are picked up incidentally from examination of the peripheral blood (Faderl et al. 1999; Savage et al. 1997). Clinical features include weight loss, sweats, symptoms of anemia, abdominal discomfort secondary to splenic enlargement, bruising, epistaxis, or other hemorrhagic sequelae. The only recent description of symptoms comes from the multicenter randomized trials of therapy from the German Study Group (Table 4.1). They found fatigue to be common in about 60% of cases, symptoms of organomegaly in around 30% of patients, and fever and weight loss in about 20% (Hehlmann et al. 1994). In the UK CML V trial comparing low and high dose interferon (247 patients), symptoms at diagnosis were present in 66% of patients. The major symptoms were malaise/fatigue 54%, weight loss 30%, organomegaly symptoms 37%, fever/sweats 25%, and hyperviscosity symptoms 8%. However, these symptoms were generally mild as the WHO performance status was >1 in only 4% (personal communication, P. Shepherd). The median age for the German Study Group was 47 years and 60 years for the UK CML V Trial. The incidence of symptoms is not dissimilar in these two trials.

Savage, Szydlo, and Goldman (Savage et al. 1997) have reported on the major presenting features of CML. They reviewed the records of 430 patients with CML referred to the Hammersmith Hospital in London for allogeneic bone marrow transplantation between 1981 and 1997. This was obviously a selected population of relatively young patients with a median age of 34 years (range 5 to 62 years). However, it is the most descriptive series to report on signs and symptoms at diagnosis of CML. Less than 10% were diagnosed in advanced phase. Male patients outnumbered female patients (58% vs. 42% respectively). The median duration of symptoms was 3 months (range 0 to 36 months). Table 4.2 summarizes the various clinical features and their relative frequencies.

Some similarities and differences are evident if we compare this series to the initial patient characteristics reported in the German CML-1 trial – see Table 4.1 (Hehlmann et al. 1994). Fatigue was the most common symptom in both groups although the incidence was lower in Savage's study, perhaps reflecting a younger cohort of patients. The incidence of weight loss was similar. However, hepatomegaly was more common in the German group. In the UK study, the frequency of weight loss, sweats, and bone pain did not differ between those diagnosed in CP and AP. The authors observed that symptoms improved or resolved following treatment in patients diagnosed in CP but often persisted in those treated for AP. Laboratory features for this study are given in Table 4.3. The WBC count was >100 in over

Table 4.2. Clinical features at diagnosis of CML (n = 430) (with permission from Savage, Szydlo and Goldman 1997)

Clinical feature	n	%
Symptoms		
Fatigue or lethargy	140	33.5
Bleeding	89	21.3
Weight loss	84	20.0
Splenic discomfort	76	18.6
Abdominal mass or fullness	62	14.8
Sweats	61	14.6
Bone pain	31	7.4
Infection	26	6.2
Headache	21	5.8
Dyspnea	19	4.5
Visual disturbances	18	4.4
Weakness	18	4.4
Arthralgia	17	4.0
Cough	13	3.1
Malaise	13	3.1
Dizziness	9	2.2
Nausea/vomiting	9	2.2
Ankle edema	9	2.2
Priapism	8	1.9
Mental changes	7	1.6
Signs		
Spleen palpable:	314	75.8
1–10 cm	153	36.9
>10 cm	161	38.9
Spleen not palpable	100	24.2
Purpura	66	15.8
Palpable liver	9	2.2
Incidental diagnosis	85	20

70% of patients and the platelet count >450 in 50% of cases. Low platelet counts <150 are uncommon at diagnosis, being present in around 10% only. Anemia, generally mild, was present in about 60% of patients.

Bleeding was reported in 21% of cases in the study by Savage, et al. 1997. Purpura was the most common hemorrhagic sign, occurring in 15.8% of patients. This is somewhat surprising given that <1% had platelets $<50\times10^9$/l. Seven women (3.7%) presented with menorrhagia. Retinal hemorrhages occurred in 11 patients, of whom six had WBC count $>250\times10^9$/l. Other patients presented with prolonged bleeding after dental extraction, epistaxis, bleeding duodenal ulcer, oozing gums, rectal bleeding, and one patient had a subdural hematoma. Splenic discomfort was reported in 19% of cases. This was usually felt in the left upper abdomen but could be referred to the left shoulder or left lower chest in a minority of patients. Splenic rupture was seen in one patient. Avascular necrosis of the femoral head has been reported rarely. Gout was also rarely seen. Other reported symptoms included skin rash in three patients, including one with leukocytoclastic vasculitis. One patient presented with acute dizziness and unilateral hearing loss suggestive of hemorrhage or ischemia in the inner ear. Laboratory findings at diagnosis from this series are shown in Table 4.3. Male patients were reported to have higher WBC counts, larger spleens, and lower platelet counts than females. These differences persisted after exclusion of patients diagnosed incidentally. Duration of symptoms did not differ between male and female patients. Patients <40 years of age had greater degrees of leukocytosis, anemia, and splenomegaly than older patients. One could speculate that this could be because they tolerate these symptoms better and took longer to seek medical attention. Male patients were slightly older than female patients (ages 33.7 years and 31.6 years respectively, $P=0.06$). The WBC count correlated with spleen size. Both WBC and spleen size correlated inversely with hemoglobin level, but neither correlated with platelet count. With respect to hemostasis, the median platelet count of bleeding patients was lower than that of nonbleeding patients (median values 319 and 485, respectively, $P=0.0002$). However, thrombocytopenia ($<150\times10^9$/l) was present in <10% of patients with hemorrhage. The median WBC was higher in patients with than in those without bleeding manifestations (217 and 170×10^9/l, $P=0.004$). These observations suggest that platelet dysfunction rather than thrombocytopenia is the major cause of the bleeding and that high numbers of circulating granulocytes contribute to impaired platelet function. Since hemorrhagic manifestations abate with treatment, platelet dysfunction is likely related to disease activity.

A large variety of platelet dysfunctions have been described in chronic myeloproliferative disorders. These abnormalities may be due to a decrease in the

Table 4.3. Hematological findings at diagnosis in CML (with permission from Savage, Szydlo and Goldman 1997)

Laboratory Measurement	Median	Range
WBC ($\times 10^9$/l) (n=400)	174	5.0–850.0
Hb (g/dl) (n=344)	10.3	4.9–16.6
Platelets ($\times 10^9$/l) (n=337)	430	17–3182
WBC ($\times 10^9$/l)	**n**	**%**
<20	18	4.5
20–99	92	23.0
100–249	145	36.2
250–350	69	17.2
>350	76	19.0
Hb (g/dl)	**n**	**%**
<7.5	38	11.0
7.6–9.4	81	23.5
9.5–11.4	95	27.6
≥11.5	130	37.8
Platelets ($\times 10^9$/l)	**n**	**%**
<50	3	6.9
50–149	12	3.6
150–449	155	46.0
450–599	55	16.3
600–999	73	21.7
>1000	39	11.6

platelet content of serotonin and adenine nucleotides, decreased platelet density, an abnormal ultrastructure with paucity of granules, platelet membrane glycoprotein abnormalities, defective arachidonic acid metabolism, and reduced aggregation response with epinephrine (Holme and Murphy 1990; Pareti et al. 1982; Wehmeier et al. 1989; Yamamoto et al. 1984).

Decreased intraplatelet levels of vWF:Ag and fibrinogen have also been reported in CML (Meschengieser et al. 1987). However, this was more frequently observed in essential thrombocythemia and polycythemia vera and was thought to be secondary to platelet activation and in vivo release of both antigens.

Despite the fact that some patients in the UK series had a marked thrombocytosis, none presented with classic ischemic events such as stroke or myocardial infarction. These complications have, however, been described in CML and were related to hyperleukocytosis (Hild and Myers 1980). The UK investigators suggested that the lack of ischemic symptoms may have been due to their relatively young study population. However, they also acknowledge that thrombosis has not been a clinical feature of previous large unselected series which included older patients (Mason et al. 1974; MRC Working Party 1968; Rowe 1983). In addition, it has not been noted as a presenting feature of the randomized trials of interferon therapy. This suggests that platelet-related ischemia is rare in CP CML compared with other myeloproliferative disorders.

Priapism was present in 3% of male patients. Ponniah and colleagues reported successful management of this urological emergency with prompt leukapheresis in a previously fit 19-year-old man with previously undiagnosed CML who presented with a WBC count of 513×10^9/l (Ponniah et al. 2004). Aseptic necrosis of the femoral head complicating severe leukostasis has also been reported (Kraemer et al. 2003).

The benefits of leukapheresis in the treatment of other symptoms of hyperviscosity and thrombocytosis in CML are well documented. These reports include rapid improvement in cases of impaired visual acuity secondary to a "hyperleukocytic retinopathy" (Mehta et al. 1984) and recovery from digital gangrene due to thrombocytosis (Win and Mitchell 2001).

4.1.4 Prognostic Risk Grouping

The clinical course of CML is variable and survival is related to the phase of the disease and the risk characteristics of the patient. Prognostic risk grouping based on the diagnostic blood film and clinical features can delineate subgroups with varying survival. The response to therapy, especially cytogenetic and molecular responses, either to interferon (Hasford et al. 2005) or to imatinib (Hughes et al. 2003; Kantarjian et al. 2004) is also of prognostic significance. The Sokal (Sokal et al. 1984) and Hasford scores (Hasford et al. 1998) are widely used "staging" systems which can predict, at diagnosis, statistically significant differences in median survival for busulfan/hydroxyurea or interferon-treated patients, respectively. Until the advent of imatinib, these scoring systems were helpful for informing patient choice on whether to proceed directly to allograft if a donor was available or to first consider a trial of drug therapy, reserving transplantation for those with an inadequate clinical response. Sokal, et al. evaluated the prognostic significance of disease features recorded at diagnosis among 813 patients with Ph-positive CP CML. They identified three different cohorts of patients within this population, most of which were treated with single-agent busulfan or hydroxyurea. The disease features found to have prognostic significance included spleen size, age, percent of circulating blasts, and platelet count. Only the platelet count did not have progressive influence on risk over its entire range of values; it did not influence survival significantly at values below $700 \times 10^9/l$. However, above this threshold it behaved as a continuous variable. The following hazard ratio function was derived:

$$\lambda_i(t)/\lambda_o(t) = \text{Exp } 0.0116 \text{ (Age} - 43.4) + 0.0345 \text{ (Spleen} - 7.51) + 0.188 \text{ [(platelets/700)}^2 - 0.563 + 0.0887 \text{ (Blasts} - 2.10)$$

The Sokal score divided patients into three approximately equal groups scoring as low <0.8, intermediate 0.8–1.2, and high-risk >1.2. Median survivals were roughly twice as high in the low-risk group compared to the high-risk group, 60 vs. 32 months (Sokal et al. 1984). In the 1980s interferon-alpha was shown to be effective therapy in CML and in particular was able to induce cytogenetic remissions when used as therapy for CML (Talpaz et al. 1986). Multicenter prospective randomized trials comparing interferon to hydroxyurea or busulfan showed improvement in survival with interferon regimens. A meta-analysis of these randomized trials showed an improvement in survival by 15% at 5 years for interferon-treated patients from 41.8 to 56.8% (Chronic Myeloid Leukemia Trialists' Collaborative Group 1997). Major cytogenetic responses were seen in the randomized trials of 11–21%, and from 11–43% in single center studies (reviewed by Shepherd 2001). Major cytogenetic response rates were predominantly seen in Sokal low-risk patients and to a lesser extent in intermediate-risk patients. Where they occurred in high-risk patients they were frequently not durable. Clinical features associated with improved cytogenetic response to interferon-alpha included asymptomatic disease at diagnosis, smaller spleen size, lower leukocyte and peripheral blast counts, normal platelet count, and hemoglobin level (Kantarjian et al. 1995; The Italian Cooperative Study Group 1994). These are the patients who fall into low and intermediate Sokal risk groups. A cooperative study of complete cytogenetic responders (CCyR) to interferon showed low-risk patients achieving CCyR to have a 10-year survival of >80% (Bonifazi et al. 2001). High-risk patients with CCyR did not obtain durable responses. However, while the Sokal score worked well for patients treated with busulfan or hydroxyurea, it was reported by some authors to be a poor prognostic discriminator for patients treated with interferon-alpha (Hasford et al. 1996; Ohnishi et al. 1995; Ozer et al. 1993). The Collaborative CML Prognostic Factors Study Group analyzed 1,303 newly diagnosed patients with CML and used statistical methods to identify independent prognostic factors for patients treated with interferon-alpha (Hasford et al. 1998). They described a new scoring system, which in addition to the Sokal variables included percent eosinophils and basophils:

$$\text{Prognostic score} = ([0.6666 \times \text{age}] + [0.042 \times \text{spleen size}] + [0.0584 \times \% \text{ blasts}] + [0.0413 \times \% \text{ eosinophils}] + [0.2039 \times \% \text{ basophils}] + [1.0956 \times \text{platelets}]) \times 1000$$

where age equals 0 when the patient is <50 years or equals 1 when patient ≥50 years old; spleen size is measured as centimeters below costal margin; basophils equals 0 when basophil count <3% or equals 1 when is ≥3%; and platelets equals 0 when platelet count is $<1500 \times 10^9/l$ or equals 1 when $\geq 1500 \times 10^9/l$. Three groups were identified by the score:

- Low-risk – 41% of all patients; score ≤780
- Intermediate-risk – 45% of all patients; score >780 and ≤1480
- High-risk – 15% of all patients; score >1480

They showed on this database that the Sokal score failed to discriminate between intermediate- and high-risk groups for survival. The new proposed staging system showed better discrimination between the risk groups with median survivals of 96 months vs. 65 months vs. 42 months for low-, intermediate-, and high-risk groups, respectively. Five-year survival probabilities were 75%, 56%, and 28%, respectively. In addition, this scoring system has been combined with an analysis of major cytogenetic response rates to assess survival for patients on interferon alpha (Hasford et al. 2005). Major cytogenetic response within the low- and intermediate-risk groups had a marked influence on survival within these groups; however, major cytogenetic response within the high-risk group, admittedly rare, did not confer any advantage.

With the advent of imatinib, a selective *BCR-ABL* kinase inhibitor, and other agents, the prognostic value of the Sokal or Hasford scores needs to be reassessed. However, the data on interferon-treated patients can serve as a benchmark for the assessment of the long-term effectiveness of imatinib. Imatinib is now first-line therapy for CML, except for those (few) who proceed directly to allograft. Around 60% of patients treated with imatinib 400 mg in CP after failing interferon-alpha therapy will achieve a major cytogenetic response. This is complete in 41% (Kantarjian et al. 2002a). CCyR is reached in 75% of those treated with imatinib as first-line therapy (O'Brien et al. 2003). This study, the IRIS study, is the only study that has at least some details of the Sokal risk score for the patients entered. The IRIS study did not initially show a significant difference in progression-free survival among the different Sokal risk-group categories (O'Brien et al. 2003). However, with further follow-up, the Sokal classification was shown to differentiate three groups with distinct progression-free survival probabilities (Cervantes et al. 2003). A further update of these results at 54 months of follow-up was presented at ASH 2005 (Simonsson et al. 2005). They confirm the prognostic significance of Sokal Risk Group (Fig. 4.1). However, in addition they show that if high-risk patients do achieve CCyR on imatinib, their survival to date seems as good as other patients achieving CCyR (Simonsson et al. 2005). Details of Hasford scores are not available for the IRIS study. Hence, these "traditional" prognostic models need to be re-examined and possibly revised in this new era of treatment for CML.

The major prognostic indicator now appears to be the depth and quality of cytogenetic and molecular responses to imatinib. There is good evidence from the IRIS Trial (O'Brien et al. 2003) and indeed from the earlier studies in interferon-resistant and interferon-intolerant patients (Kantarjian et al. 2002a,b; Marin et al. 2003) that the achievement of a major or complete cytogenetic response is associated with improved prognosis. If CCyR is achieved at 12 months, a >3 log reduction in BCR-ABL transcript levels is associated with improved progression-free survival (Hughes et al. 2003). A further update with 54 months of follow-up was presented at ASH 2005 (Simonsson et al. 2005). These confirm the prognostic importance of achieving a cytogenetic response and a >3 log reduction in transcript level for those in CCyR (Figs. 4.2, 4.3). There is also some evidence that higher doses of imatinib, i.e., 800 mg daily, are associated with improved rates of CCyR, major molecular response, and transcript undetectability com-

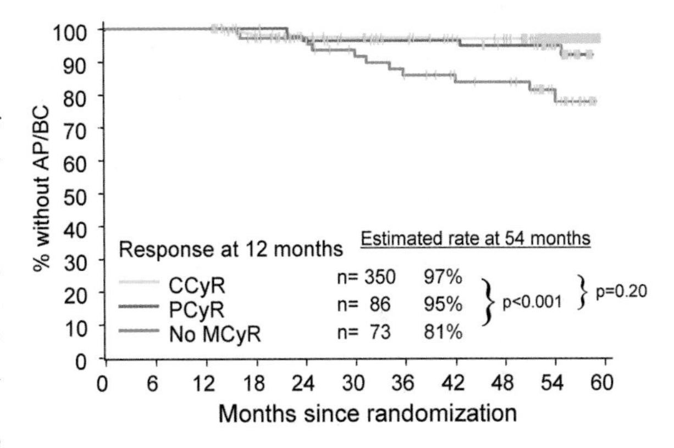

Fig. 4.2. Survival without accelerated phase or blast crisis by the level of cytogenetic response at 12 months in the imatinib arm of the IRIS trial: 54-month follow-up. CCyR – complete cytogenetic response; PCyR – partial cytogenetic response; MCyR – major cytogenetic response

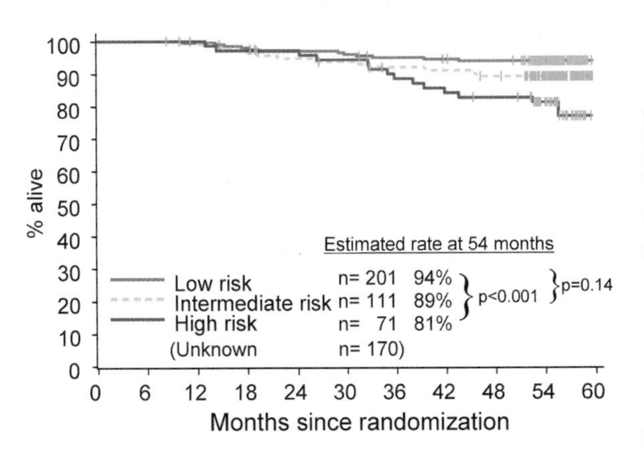

Fig. 4.1. Survival by Sokal Group in patients on the imatinib arm of the IRIS trial: 54-month follow-up

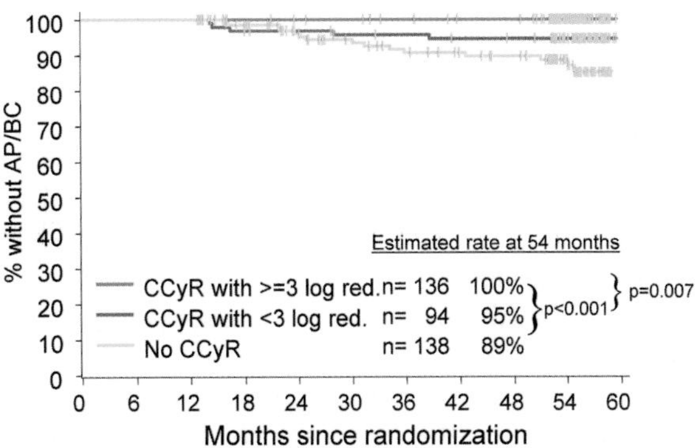

Fig. 4.3. Survival without accelerated phase or blast crisis by the level of molecular response at 12 months in the imatinib arm of the IRIS trial: 54-month follow-up

pared with standard dosage, i.e., 400 mg daily (Kantarjian et al. 2004).

Other traditional prognostic variables are now challenged by the advent of imatinib. Older age has been a consistent poor prognostic factor in patients with CML and as such is a feature of the Sokal and Hasford risk scores. However, with imatinib therapy older age appears to have lost much of its prognostic relevance (Cortes et al. 2003). Cortes, et al. reported that among 187 patients in early CML-CP, a complete cytogenetic response was achieved in 87% of patients aged 60 years as compared to a rate of 79% in younger patients (P = 0.28). This suggests that the previous poor prognosis amongst older patients was related to comorbidity or treatment-associated toxicity rather than to an intrinsically worse disease biology.

The development of FISH techniques led to the discovery of deletions of derivative chromosome 9 [der(9)] in 10–15% of patients with Ph-positive CML (Grand et al. 1999; Sinclair et al. 2000). These deletions are thought to occur at the same time as the Ph translocation, and are usually large and located in the regions flanking the translocation breakpoint of the der(9). They have been associated with a poor prognosis, with patients having earlier disease progression and reduced survival (Cohen et al. 2001; Huntly et al. 2001, 2003; Kolomietz et al. 2001; Sinclair et al. 2000). However, it has recently been reported that imatinib overcomes the adverse prognostic significance of der(9) deletions; the rates of major (82% vs. 79%, P = 0.82) and complete cytogenetic response (76% vs. 66%, P = 0.33) with imatinib therapy were similar in patients with and without der (9) deletions, respectively (Quintas-Cardama et al. 2005). Twenty-eight-month median follow-up revealed no difference in overall survival or response duration.

An additional clinical variable to be considered in imatinib-treated patients is the development of myelosuppression. Grade 3 or 4 neutropenia has been reported in 35–45% of patients treated with standard-dose imatinib (Kantarjian et al. 2002 a; Sneed et al. 2004). In a multivariate analysis of 143 patients with late CML-CP, Sneed, et al. reported that any myelosuppression ≥ grade 3 was associated with a lower rate of major (P = 0.04) or complete (P = 0.01) cytogenetic responses (Sneed et al. 2004). This was more pronounced with myelosuppression that lasted more than 2 weeks. A low neutrophil count and poor cytogenetic response at 3 months were found to have poor prognostic significance (Marin et al. 2003). However, a similar analysis failed to find these to have prognostic significance (Kantarjian and Cortes 2004). Myelosuppression is commoner when imatinib was used later in the course of the disease. It may reflect reduced numbers of surviving Ph-negative stem cells. It may also in part contribute to reduced dose intensity and this may impact unfavorably on prognosis.

The toxicity profile of imatinib is very much more favorable when compared with interferon. This was demonstrated in the International Randomized Study of Interferon and STI 571 (IRIS) trial (O'Brien et al. 2003) where intolerance to treatment in the combination-therapy group resulted in a high rate of crossover to imatinib. Quality of life was also significantly better with imatinib compared to interferon (Hahn et al. 2003). Imatinib-related nonhematological side effects occurred in less than 10% of patients and included nausea, vomiting, edema, weight gain, muscle cramps, diarrhea, and cutaneous reactions (Druker et al. 2001; O'Brien et al. 2003). These skin reactions represent 7–21% of all toxic events (Brouard and Saurat 2001), and are usually dose dependent. The spectrum of skin reactions includes pruritus, dermatitis, hypopigmentation, and an occasional severe form, including one report of Steven-Johnson syndrome (Hsiao et al. 2002), and in two cases, squamous cutaneous carcinoma (Baskaynak et al. 2003). Grade 3 and 4 adverse events usually require cessation of imatinib and possible reintroduction at lower doses once resolved. Many Grade 1 and 2 reactions can be treated symptomatically. The practical management of patients on imatinib therapy has been comprehensively reviewed (Deininger et al. 2003; Marin et al. 2002).

The outlook for CML patients has improved remarkably in recent years. When treated with conventional chemotherapy (busulfan or hydroxyurea), the median survival was 45 months and 58 months, respectively (Hehlmann et al. 1993). Median survival for interferon-treated patients was 59% at 5 years (Chronic Myeloid Leukemia Trialists' Collaborative Group 1997). However, patients who achieved a CCyR on interferon-alpha had an expected survival probability at 10 years of 78% (Bonifazi et al. 2001). Preliminary data suggest that the long-term survival of patients who receive imatinib as first line therapy may prove to be substantially longer.

4.1.5 Accelerated Phase (AP)

After a variable period of time, the majority of patients with CP CML treated in the preimatinib era progressed through an AP to BT. It is generally thought to be associated with further instability of the CML stem cell that confers resistance to therapy. To what extent the same sequence of events will apply to imatinib-treated patients is still uncertain. The earliest stage of this progression from CP is difficult to determine and may (with the aid of the retrospectoscope) be suspected by an increase in white cell count, the presence of >5% circulating immature cells, or by an increase in platelet count requiring a higher dose of drug, be it imatinib, interferon, or hydroxyurea, than was previously required to maintain good control of the disease. Anemia may develop or the spleen size may increase. The patient does not fulfil the required criteria for complete hematological response. There are no universally accepted definitions to accurately gauge the precise time when AP occurred but a number of different criteria for defining AP have been published. Kantarjian, et al. in 1988 performed multivariate analysis on features reported to be associated with AP in 357 patients. They identified 5 characteristics with independent prognostic importance, namely clonal (cytogenetic) evolution, peripheral blasts >15%, blood basophilia >20%, peripheral blasts + promyelocytes >30%, and thrombocytopenia $<100\times10^9$/l. Marked thrombocytosis ($>2000\times10^9$/l), eosinophilia, or nucleated red cells were not found to have adverse prognostic significance. Features such as increasing splenomegaly, resistance to therapy or systemic symptoms could not be evaluated due to the retrospective nature of the study. The criteria for advanced stage disease proposed by the International Bone Marrow Transplant Registry (IBMTR) have been used for defining outcomes after allogeneic transplantation (Speck et al. 1984; www.ibmtr.org). These include the degree of control of the white cell count, the doubling time of the WBC, and thrombocytosis $>1000\times10^9$/l, in addition to clonal evolution, and (different) % of basophils, blasts and promyelocytes as given above (see Table 4.4). In practice, the use of these differing criteria to define AP may well identify different patient groups with different outcomes. This was well exemplified in a study of CML patients undergoing transplant at the Hammersmith Hospital. The investigators compared survival according to their original criteria for CP and AP with survival after the patients were recategorized retrospectively according to the IBMTR criteria. This resulted in "stage migration" – some patients previously classified as CP were now allocated to the AP category. This led to an apparent improvement in survival for both CP patients and for AP patients as the worst of the CP group had been transferred to the AP group and they improved the survival of that group as they were then the best of the worst (the so-called Will Rogers phenomenon) (Savage et al. 1997). This serves to underline the necessity for well-defined objective criteria to specify disease phase so that appropriate comparisons can be made when looking at outcomes of therapeutic interventions. The World Health Organisation (WHO) classification of tumors (WHO Classification of Tumours 2001; and reviewed by Vardiman et al. 2002) introduced a new classification of AP disease. This is also the classification used by European Group for Blood and Marrow Transplantation (EBMT) for its Med-B forms, (www.ebmt.org). The various criteria with the various classifications are summarized in Table 4.4.

A recent analysis of the WHO classification (presented thus far only in abstract form) for patients treated with imatinib suggests that the criteria defined by the WHO are valid, although they noted that those patients with 20–29% blasts had cytogenetic response rates more similar to those in AP than to those in BT. They conclude that the threshold for defining BT should remain at ≥30% (Cortes et al. 2004). However, since the criteria for de novo acute leukemia is >20% blasts in the widely used WHO classification, it makes sense perhaps to use the same cut off to separate AP and BT CML.

4.1.6 Clonal Evolution

The development of additional chromosome abnormalities in addition to the Ph chromosome is seen in about 10% of cases at diagnosis (Kantarjian et al. 1990) and develops in 30–50% of cases before BT, often associated with other features of AP (Majlis et al. 1996; Sessarego et al. 1987; Swolin et al. 1985). In the series by Kantarjian et al. (1988) referred to above, the percent of patients with clonal evolution was lower at 24%. The usual abnormalities are trisomy 8, double Ph, and isochromosome 17 either alone or in combination. Other abnormalities involving other chromosomes are frequently seen (Majlis et al. 1996). These authors analyzed 264 patients who developed clonal evolution during the course of their disease. The majority of these patients were treated in the interferon era when cytogenetic analysis

Table 4.4. Criteria for accelerated and blast phase by various groups

	Multivariate analysis of prognostic factors (Kantarjian et al. 1987, 1988)	IBMTR criteria (www.ibmtr.org) Advanced stage disease (AP or BT not specified)	WHO classification of tumors (Vardiman et al. 2002) and EBMT criteria for Med-B (www.ebmt.org)
Accelerated phase (one or more present)			
PB/BM blasts	≥15%	≥10%	10–19%
PB blasts+promyelocytes	≥30%	≥20%	N/A
PB basophils	≥20%	≥20% plus eosinophils	≥20%
Platelets	$<100\times10^9$/l Unrelated to therapy	$<100\times10^9$/l Unrelated to therapy	$<100\times10^9$/l Unrelated to therapy
Platelets	N/A	$>1000\times10^9$/l Unresponsive to therapy	$>1000\times10^9$/l Unresponsive to therapy
Increasing spleen size and increasing WBC unresponsive to therapy	N/A	WBC $>100\times10^9$/l unresponsive to BU or HU Palpable splenomegaly	Yes
Cytogenetic clonal evolution	Yes	Yes	Yes
Anemia	N/A	<8 g/dl	N/A
Blast phase (one or more present)			
PB/BM blasts	≥30%		≥20%
Extramedullary blast proliferation	Yes		Yes
BM biopsy	N/A		Large foci or clusters of blasts

was performed on a regular basis. The median survival after development of clonal evolution was 19 months. However, this was not uniform and they could discriminate different groups with differing survival according to the type of chromosome involved, the percentage of abnormal metaphases, the time to clonal evolution, and whether other features of AP were present. They identified a good-risk group – no chromosome 17 abnormality, <16% abnormal metaphases, and time to clonal evolution <24 months – with a median survival of 54 months. In contrast, a poor-risk group – chromosome 17 abnormalities and >36% abnormal metaphases or the presence of other AP features, and >16% abnormal metaphases – had a median survival of 6 and 7 months, respectively. The remainder had an intermediate survival of 13–24 months.

4.1.7 Outcome for Patients in Accelerated Phase

In the interferon era, median survival after progression to AP was around 20 months (Kantarjian et al. 1988; Majlis et al. 1996). The majority of patients will transform to BT but about 25% of patients will die while in AP. With the introduction of imatinib into clinical use, Phase II trials were initiated in late CP patients resistant to or intolerant of interferon, in AP patients, or in BT patients. The Phase II study of imatinib in AP evaluated 181 patients in AP according to the Kantarjian criteria with the exception that clonal evolution without the presence of any of the other features of AP was not included (Talpaz et al. 2002). The initial 62 patients were treated at a dose of 400 mg daily. Subsequent patients were started at a dose of 600 mg daily after Phase I dose escalation studies. Those patients who were treated with imatinib at a dose of 600 mg did better than those treated with a dose of 400 mg, both in terms of cytogenetic response rate and survival. Estimated progression-free survival and overall survival were 78% and 67%, respectively, at 12 months. A recent update showed 3-year, progression-free survival and overall survival of 55% and 45%, respectively. Those achieving a major cytogenetic response by 3 months had significantly improved 3-year survival compared to those who did not achieve this – 85% vs. 52% (Silver et al. 2004). These would seem to be better outcomes than previous historical data for this phase of disease. A subsequent study from Oregon Health and Science University studied 71 patients with AP disease but included clonal evolution in addition to the criteria for AP of the Phase II study. They found that they could separate patients with different prognosis depending upon whether clonal evolution alone as a criterium for AP was present (AP-CE) or whether other signs of acceleration were present without (HEM-AP) or with clonal evolution (HEM-AP + CE). Those with AP-CE had major cytogenetic response rates of 73% vs. 31% vs. 12.5% and overall survival of 100%, 85%, and 67.5%, respectively at 12 months (O'Dwyer et al. 2002). This was confirmed by a further study which showed that patients with clonal evolution who were otherwise in CP performed worse than the remaining patients in CP but their survival was better than patients with AP without clonal evolution and significantly better than AP with clonal evolution (Cortes et al. 2003). A further study in patients in CP intolerant of or refractory to interferon confirmed clonal evolution and lack of cytogenetic response at 6 months to be adverse prognostic factors for hematologic relapse (O'Dwyer et al. 2004).

Clonal evolution should probably thus be considered as a marker for more aggressive disease, warranting earlier intervention either with higher doses of imatinib or alternative therapy. Detection of clonal evolution is dependent on regular BM examination. Many patients now are followed only by peripheral blood Q-RT-PCR for transcript levels once they achieve a complete cytogenetic response. However, increasing levels of BCR-ABL transcripts should prompt bone marrow examination for cytogenetic analysis to look for clonal evolution. In addition, cytogenetic abnormalities have been found in Ph-ve cells of patients who have achieved a cytogenetic remission (reviewed by Loriaux and Deininger 2004). The significance of these is not clear but many centers recommend yearly cytogenetic analyses for this reason.

The current definitions of progressive disease may now be becoming obsolete. Most patients are now treated with imatinib as first-line therapy and the majority will enter complete cytogenetic remission (O'Brien et al. 2003). For patients who fail to achieve an adequate response at the cytogenetic or molecular level or who lose their response, early intervention with higher doses of imatinib, combination therapy, or the newer kinase inhibitors could be planned, which would be for most patients while they remain in chronic phase. Branford, et al. (Branford et al. 2004) have shown that for patients treated from diagnosis with imatinib, increasing levels of BCR-ABL transcripts in the majority of patients who have achieved complete cytogenetic response are associated with an increased incidence of mutations of the tyrosine kinase domain of BCR-ABL. They suggest mutation screening where a twofold increase in transcript level is found (Branford et al. 2004). If mutations are detected, this is an indication for increasing the dose of imatinib or switching to alternative therapeutic strategies. One can then envisage a situation where definitions of progressive disease could include molecular markers and prompt a change in therapy at an earlier stage than before traditional markers of acceleration are present. If acceleration were to occur despite these interventions, then the outcome may be poorer given that resistance to currently employed therapeutic strategies is present. Hopefully, the second generation of kinase inhibitors with increased binding to their target or multiple targets could delay progress to AP and BT.

4.1.8 Blast Transformation (BT)

Characteristics of the terminal phase of CML were initially described in a seminal paper by Karanas and Silver in 1968. They identified the adverse prognostic impact of >30% blasts+promyelocytes in the peripheral blood on overall survival. Blast transformation from CML is now still defined by the presence of >30% blasts in the peripheral blood or bone marrow or the presence of extramedullary blastic disease (Enright and McGlave 2000; Kantarjian et al. 1987). One study suggests that >20% lymphoid blasts may be sufficient to diagnose lymphoid blast crisis (Arlin et al. 1990) and the WHO classification suggests >20% blasts for both myeloid and lymphoid transformations (Vardiman et al. 2002; WHO Classification of Tumours 2001). For the reasons given earlier, particularly for consistency with the nomenclature for acute leukemia and the prevalence of the use of the WHO Classification, this should probably be the regular cut off. It usually occurs after a period of AP but may occasionally, particularly in lymphoid BT, occur directly from CP without other features suggesting AP. The likelihood of this happening has been estimated at 0.4% in the first year, 1.8% in the second year, and 2.6% in the third year (Kantarjian et al. 2003). These data were based on predominantly interferon-treated patients. The risk for imatinib-treated patients is not yet known. Immunophenotyping shows myeloid BT in about 70–75% of patients and lymphoid BT in 25–30% of cases, but there is frequent cell lineage heterogeneity (Bettelheim et al. 1985; Khalidi et al. 1998; Saikia et al. 1988). Myeloid BT may involve cells of myelomonocytic, megakaryocytic, or erythroid lineage. Lymphoid BT is usually precursor B cell type, but may occasionally be of T cell lineage (Advani et al. 1991; Ye et al. 2002). A few are truly biphenotypic with coexpression of myeloperoxidase and one other myeloid marker (Cervantes et al. 1998). In addition, phenotypic changes may occur as the disease progresses. Immunoglobulin gene studies have shown that the majority of lymphoid BT show this rearrangement but it is also seen in about a third of cases with myeloid BT (Khalidi et al. 1998). Bone marrow trephine often shows increasing fibrosis. Clinical features associated with BT include anemia, bone pain, increasing splenomegaly, weight loss, and systemic symptoms. Extramedullary disease may involve the skin and subcutaneous tissues, lymph nodes bone, testis, CNS, ileum, and liver (Terjanian et al. 1987; Kumar et al. 1990; Suh and Shin 2000). Bone abnormalities on scanning or on plain radiographs are frequent (Valimaki et al. 1981). Bone necrosis has rarely been reported (Macheta et al. 1991).

The majority of patients will have evidence of cytogenetic evolution at BT (Johansson et al. 2002). The most frequent nonrandom cytogenetic features seen involve duplication of the Philadelphia chromosome (+Ph), trisomy 8, isochromosome 17, +19, and +21, but many other chromosomes may be involved either in combination with the above or separately. The presence of an isochromosome 17q is particularly associated with the myeloid phenotype.

The blast phase of CML differs from de novo acute leukemia in response to therapy and remission duration. Responses are less frequent, often of short duration, and median survival is usually less than 6 months (Kantarjian et al. 1987). Lymphoid transformation has a higher response rate to therapy and improved survival compared to myeloid transformation with standard chemotherapy regimes (Cervantes et al. 1998; Derderian et al. 1993). Imatinib has been investigated for use in this phase of the disease. In a recent phase II study in patients with myeloid BT, imatinib induced sustained (>4 weeks) hematologic response in 31% of patients. The median duration of this response was 10 months. However, median survival for all patients was only 6.9 months (Sawyers et al. 2002). The results in patients with lymphoid BT were worse. Although initial response in reducing the percentage of blood blasts was quite high, around 70%, this was usually not sustained – the median duration was around 2 months (Druker et al. 2001). A single center publication on CML patients in blast crisis showed a median survival of only 8 months despite intensive therapy including AML/ALL regimens, imatinib, and autografting or allografting (Wadhwa et al. 2002). Patients with lymphoid BT had a higher response to therapy (42% vs. 31%) and a longer median survival than those with myeloid BT (11 months vs. 7 months). Patients with cytogenetic evolution and those with >50% blood blasts did poorly. Achieving a response to therapy was associated with improved outcome (13 months vs. 6 months). The use of imatinib, although initially promising in providing a response rate of about 30%, did not translate into improved duration of survival. However, imatinib and other combination chemotherapy regimens may provide a window in which allogeneic transplant may be performed, although again, overall survival is only of the order of 15% at 2 years. The advent of second-generation tyrosine kinase inhibitors or combinations of these with other cytotoxic drugs may perhaps improve the current dismal prognosis of patients with BT, especially if they have not previously received treatment with imatinib.

References

Advani SH, Malhotra H, Kadam P, Iyer RS, Nanjangud G, Balsara B, Saikia T, Gopal R, Nair CN (1991) T-lymphoid blast crisis in chronic myeloid leukemia. Am J Hematol 36:86–92

Allan NC, Richards SM, Shepherd PCA (1995) UK Medical Research Council randomised, multicentre trial of interferon-αn1 for chronic myeloid leukemia: improved survival irrespective of cytogenetic response. Lancet 345:1392–1397

Arlin ZA, Silver RT, Bennett JM (1990) Blastic phase of chronic myeloid leukemia (blCML): a proposal for standardization of diagnostic and response criteria. Leukemia 4:755–757

Baskaynak G, Kreuzer KA, Schwarz M, Zuber J, Audring H, Riess H, Dorken B, le Coutre P (2003) Squamous cutaneous epithelial cell carcinoma in two CML patients with progressive disease under imatinib treatment. Eur J Haematol 70:231–234

Bettelheim P, Lutz D, Majdic O, Paietta E, Haas O, Linkesch W, Neumann E, Lechner K, Knapp W (1985) Cell lineage heterogeneity in blast crisis of chronic myeloid leukaemia. Br J Haematol 59:395–409

Bhatia R, McGlave PM, Dewald GW, Blaza BR, Verfaillie CM (1991) Abnormal function of the bone marrow microenvironment in chronic myelogenous leukemia: role of malignant stromal macrophages. Blood 85:3636–3645

Bizzozero OJ Jr, Johnson KG, Ciocco A (1966) Radiation-related leukemia in Hiroshima and Nagasaki, 1946–1964. Distribution incidence and appearance time. N Engl J Med 274:1095–1101

Bonifazi F, de Vivo A, Rosti G, Guilhot F, Guilhot J et al (2001) Chronic myeloid leukemia and interferon-α: a study of complete cytogenetic responders. Blood 98:3074–3081

Branford S, Rudzki Z, Parkinson I, Grigg A, Taylor K et al (2004) Real-time quantitative PCR analysis can be used as a primary screen to identify patients with CML treated with imatinib who have BCR-ABL kinase domain mutations. Blood 104:2926–2932

Brouard M, Saurat JH (2001) Cutaneous reactions to STI571. N Engl J Med 345:618–619

Cervantes F, Villamor N, Esteve J, Montoto S, Rives S, Rozman C, Montserrat E (1998) "Lymphoid" blast crisis of chronic myeloid leukaemia is associated with distinct clinicohaematological features. Br J Haematol 100:123–128

Cervantes F, on behalf of the IRIS Study Group (2003) Durability of responses to imatinib in newly diagnosed chronic-phase chronic myeloid leukemia (CML): 24-month update from the IRIS Study. Blood 102:181a

Chronic Myeloid Leukaemia Trialists' Collaborative Group (1997) Interferon alpha versus chemotherapy for chronic myeloid leukemia: a meta-analysis of seven randomized trials. J Natl Cancer Inst 89:1616–1620

Cohen N, Rozenfeld-Granot G, Hardan I et al (2001) Subgroup of patients with Philadelphia-positive chronic myelogenous leukemia characterised by a deletion of 9q proximal to ABL gene: expression profiling, resistance to interferon therapy and poor prognosis. Cancer Genet Cytogenet 128:114–119

Corso A, Lazzarino M, Morra E, Merante S, Astoni C, Bernasconi P, Boni M, Berusconi C (1995) Chronic myelogenous leukemia and exposure to ionizing radiation – a retrospective study of 443 patients. Ann Haematol 70:79–82

Cortes J, Talpaz, O'Brien S et al (2003) Effects of age on prognosis with imatinib mesylate therapy for patients with Philadelphia chromosome-positive chronic myelogenous leukemia. Cancer 98:1105–1113

Cortes J, Talpaz M, Giles F, O'Brien S, Rios MB et al (2003) Prognostic significance of cytogenetic clonal evolution in patients with chronic myelogenous leukemia on imatinib mesylate therapy. Blood 101:3794–3800

Cortes J, O'Brien S, Garcia-Manero G et al (2004) Is the proposed World Health Organisation (WHO) classification for chronic myeloid leukemia (CML) of clinical value in the imatinib era. Blood 104: abstract#1014

Daley GQ, Van Etten RA, Baltimore D (1990) Induction of chronic myelogenous leukemia in mice by the P210 bcr/abl gene of the Philadelphia chromosome. Science 24:824–830

Deininger M, O'Brien S, Ford J, Druker B (2003) Practical management of patients with chronic myeloid leukemia receiving imatinib. J Clin Oncol 21:1637–1647

Derderian PM, Kantarjian HM, Talpaz M, O'Brien S, Cork A, Estey E, Pierce S, Keating M (1993) Chronic myelogenous leukemia in the lymphoid blastic phase: characteristics, treatment response, and prognosis. Am J Med 94:69–74

Druker BJ, Talpaz M, Resta DJ et al (2001) Efficacy and safety of a specific inhibitor of the BCR-ABL tyrosine kinase in chronic myeloid leukemia. N Engl J Med 34:1031–1037

Druker BJ, Sawyers CL, Kantarjian H, Resta DJ, Reece SF, Ford JM, Capdeville R, Talpaz M (2001) Activity of a specific inhibitor of the bcr-abl tyrosine kinase in the blast crisis of chronic myeloid leukemia and acute lymphoblastic leukemia with the Philiadelphia chromosome. N Engl J Med 344:1038–1042

Enright H, McGlave P (2000) Chronic myelogenous leukemia. In: Hoffman R, Benz EJ, Shattil SJ (eds) Hematology: basic principles and practice. Churchill Livingstone, New York, pp 1155–1171

Faderl S, Talpaz M, Estrov Z et al (1999) Chronic myelogenous leukemia: biology and therapy. Ann Intern Med 131:207–219

Fialkow PJ, Jacobson RJ, Papayannopoulou T (1997) Chronic myelocytic leukemia: clonal origin in a stem cell common to the granulocyte, erythrocyte, platelet and monocytes/macrophage. Am J Med 63:125–130

Golde DW, Burgaleta C, Sparkes RS, Cline MJ (1977) The Philadelphia chromosome in human macrophages. Blood 49:367–370

Grand F, Kulkarni S, Chase A, Goldman JM, Gordon M, Cross NC (1999) Frequent deletion of hSNF5/INI1, a component of the SWI/SNF complex, in chronic leukemia. Cancer Res 59:3870–3874

Hahn E, Glendenning G, Sorensen M et al (2003) Quality of life in patients with newly diagnosed chronic phase chronic myeloid leukemia on imatinib versus interferon alfa plus low-dose cytarabine: results from the IRIS Study. J Clin Oncol 21:2138–2146

Hasford J, Ansari H, Pfirrman M et al (1996) Analysis and validation of prognostic factors for CML. German CML Study Group. Bone Marrow Transplant 17 (Suppl 3): 549–554

Hasford J, Pfirrmann M, Hehlmann R, Allan N, Baccarani M et al (1998) A new prognostic score for survival of patients with chronic myeloid leukemia treated with interferon-alpha. J Natl Cancer Inst 90:850–858

Hasford J, Pfirrmann M, Shepherd P, Guillot J, Hehlmann R, Mahon F, Kluin-Nelemans H, Ohnishi K, Steegmann J, Thaler J (2005) The impact of the combination of baseline risk group and cytogenetic response on the survival of patients with chronic myeloid leukemia treated with interferon-α. Haematologica 90:335–340

Hehlmann R, Heimpel H, Hasford J, Kolb H, Pralle H et al (1993) Randomised comparison of busulfan and hydroxyurea in chronic myelogenous leukemia: prolongation of survival by hydroxyurea. Blood 82:398–407

Hehlmann R, Heimpel H, Hasford J et al (1994) Randomised comparison of interferon-alpha with busulfan and hydroxyurea in chronic myelogenous leukemia. Blood 84:4064–4077

Hild DH, Myers TJ (1980) Hyperviscosity in chronic granulocytic leukemia. Cancer 46:1418–1421

Holme S, Murphy S (1990) Platelet abnormalities in myeloproliferative disorders. Clin Lab Med 10:873–888

Hsiao LT, Chung HM, Lin JJ, Chion TJ, Lin JH, Fan FS, Wang WS, Yen CC, Chen PM (2002) Stevens-Johnson syndrome after treatment with STI571: a case report. Br J Haematol 117:620–622

Hughes TP, Kaeda J, Branford S, Rudzki Z, Hochhaus A, Hensley M, Gathmann I, Bolton A, van Hoomissen I, Goldman J and Radich J for the International Randomised Study of Interferon versus STI571 (IRIS) Study Group (2003) Frequency of major molecular responses to imatinib or interferon alfa plus cytarabine in newly diagnosed chronic myeloid leukemia. N Engl J Med 349:1423–1432

Huntly BJP, Reid AG, Bench AJ, Campbell LJ, Telford N, Shepherd P, Szer J, Prince HM, Turner P, Grace C, Nocheva EP, Green AR (2001) Deletions of the derivative chromosome 9 occur at the time of the Philadelphia chromosome translocation and provide a powerful and independent prognostic indicator in chronic myeloid leukemia. Blood 98:1832–1738

Huntly BJP, Bench A, Green AR (2003) Double jeopardy from a single translocation: deletions of the derivative chromosome 9 in chronic myeloid leukemia. Blood 102:1160–1168

Jaffe ES, Harris NL, Stein H, Vardiman JW (eds) (2001) World Health Organisation classification of tumours: pathology and genetics of tumours and haematopoetic and lymphoid tissues. IARC Press, Lyon

Johansson B, Fioretas T, Mitelman F (2002) Cytogenetic and molecular genetic evolution of chronic myeloid leukemia. Acta Haematologica 107:76–94

Kantarjian H, Cortes J (2004) Testing the prognostic model of Marin et al in an independent chronic myelogenous leukemia study group. Leukemia 18:650

Kantarjian HM, Keating MJ, Talpaz M, Walters RS, Smith TL, Cork A, McCredie KB, Freireich EJ (1987) Chronic myelogenous leukemia in blast crisis. Am J Med 83:445–454

Kantarjian H, Dixon D, Keating M, Talpaz M, Walters R, McCredie K, Freireich E (1988) Characteristics of accelerated disease in chronic myelogenous leukemia. Cancer 61:1441–1446

Kantarjian HM, Keating MJ, Smith TL, Talpaz M, McCredie KB (1990) Proposal for a simple synthesis prognostic staging system in chronic myelogenous leukaemia. Am J Med 88:1–8

Kantarjian HM, Smith T, O'Brien S et al (1995) Prolonged survival in chronic myelogenous leukemia after cytogenetic response to interferon-alpha therapy. Ann Intern Med 122:254–261

Kantarjian H, Sawyers C, Hochhaus A et al (2002a) Hematological and cytogenetic responses to imatinib mesylate in chronic myelogenous leukemia. N Engl J Med 346:645–652

Kantarjian HM, Talpaz M, O'Brien S et al (2002b) Imatinib mesylate for Philadelphia chromosome – positive, chronic-phase myeloid leukemia after failure of interferon-alpha: follow up results. Clin Cancer Res 8:2177–2187

Kantarjian H, O'Brien S, Cortes J, Giles F, Thomas D, Kornblau S, Shan J, Rios MB, Keating M, Freireich E, Talpaz M (2003) Sudden onset of the blastic phase of chronic myelogenous leukemia. Patterns and implications. Cancer 98:81–85

Kantarjian H, Talpaz M, O'Brien S et al (2004) High dose imatinib mesylate therapy in newly diagnosed Philadelphia chromosome-positive chronic phase chronic myeloid leukemia. Blood 103:2873–2878

Karanas A, Silver R (1968) Characteristics of the terminal phase of chronic granulocytic leukemia. Blood 32:445–459

Khalidi HS, Brynes RK, Medeiros LJ, Chang KL, Slovak ML, Snyder DS, Arber DA (1998) The immunophenotype of blast transformation of chronic myelogenous leukemia: a high frequency of mixed lineage phenotype in "lymphoid" blasts and a comparison of morphologic, immunophenotypic, and molecular findings. Mod Pathol 11:1211–1221

Kluin-Nelemans HC, Buck G, le Cessie S, Richards S, Beverloo HB et al (2004) Randomized comparison of low-dose versus high-dose interferon-alpha in chronic myeloid leukemia: prospective collaboration of 3 joint trials by the MRC and HOVON groups. Blood 103:4408–4415

Kolomietz E, Al-Maghrabi J, Brannan S et al (2001) Primary chromosomal rearrangements of leukemia are frequently accompanied by extensive submicroscopic deletions and may lead to altered prognosis. Blood 97:3581–3588

Kraemer M, Weissinger F, Kraus R et al (2003) Aseptic necrosis of both femoral heads as first symptom of chronic myelogenous leukemia. Ann Hematol 82:44–46

Kumar L, Majhi U, Shanta V (1990) Destructive bone lesions in chronic granulocytic leukemia. Indian J Cancer 27:208–210

Loriaux M, Deininger M (2004) Clonal cytogenetic abnormalities in Philadelphia chromosome negative cells in chronic myeloid leukemia patients treated with imatinib. Leuk Lymphoma 45:2197–2203

Macheta A, Cinkotai K, Geary C, Liu Yin J (1996) Bone marrow necrosis complicating chronic myeloid leukaemia. Clin Lab Haematol 13:163–167

Majlis A, Smith TL, Talpaz M, O'Brien S, Rios MB, Kantarjian HM (1996) Significance of cytogenetic clonal evolution in chronic myelogenous leukemia. J Clin Oncol 14:196–203

Marin D, Marktel S, Bua M et al (2002) The use of imatinib (STI571) in chronic myeloid leukemia: some practical considerations. Haematologica 87:979–988

Marin D, Marktel S, Bua M et al (2003) Prognostic factors for patients with chronic myeloid leukemia in chronic phase treated with imatinib mesylate after failure of interferon-alpha. Leukemia 17:1448–1453

Mason JE Jr, DeVita VT, Canellos GP (1974) Thrombocytosis in chronic granulocytic leukemia: incidence and clinical significance. Blood 44:483–487

Medical Research Council's Working Party for Therapeutic Trials in Leukaemia (1968) Chronic granulocytic leukaemia: a comparison of radiotherapy and busulphan therapy. Br Med J i:201–208

Mehta AB, Goldman JM, Kohner E (1984) Hyperleukocytic retinopathy in chronic granulocytic leukaemia: the role of intensive leukapheresis. Br J Haematol 56:661–667

Meschengieser S, Blanco A, Woods A et al (1987) Intraplatelet levels of vWF:Ag and fibrinogen in myeloproliferative disorders. Throm Res 48:311–319

Morris C, Fitzgerald P, Hollings P et al (1988) Essential thrombocythaemia and the Philadelphia chromosome. Br J Haematol 70:13–19

Nowell PC, Hungerford DA (1960) A minute chromosome in human chronic granulocytic leukaemia. Science 132:1497–1501

O'Brien SG, Guilhot F, Larson R, Gathmann I, Baccarini M, Cervantes F, Cornelissen JJ, Fischer T, Hochhaus A, Hughes T, Lechner K, Nielson J, Rousselot P, Reiffers J, Saglio G, Shepherd J, Simonsson B, Gratwohl A, Goldman JM, Kantarjian H, Taylor K, Verhoef G, Bolton

AE, Capdeville R, Druker BJ for the IRIS investigators (2003) Imatinib compared with Interferon and low dose cytarabine for newly diagnosed chronic phase chronic myeloid leukemia. N Engl J Med 348:994–1004

O'Dwyer ME, Mauro MJ, Kurilik G, Mori M Balleison S et al (2002) The impact of clonal evolution on response to imatinib mesylate (STI571) in accelerated phase CML. Blood 100:1628–1633

O'Dwyer ME, Mauro MJ, Blasdel C, Famsworth M, Kurilik G et al (2004) Clonal evolution and lack of cytogenetic response are adverse prognostic factors for hematologic relapse of chronic phase CML patients treated with imatinib mesylate. Blood 103:451–455

Ohnishi K, Ohno R, Tomonaga M et al (1995) A randomised trial comparing interferon-alpha with busulfan for newly diagnosed chronic myelogenous leukemia in chronic phase. Blood 86:906–916

Ozer H, George SL, Schiffer CA et al (1993) Prolonged subcutaneous administration of recombinant alpha 2b interferon in patients with previously untreated Philadelphia chromosome-positive chronic-phase chronic myelogenous leukemia. Effect on remission duration and survival: Cancer and Leukemia Group B Study 8593. Blood 82:2975–2984

Pareti FI, Gugliotta L, Mannucci L, Guarini A, Mannucci PM (1982) Biochemical and metabolic aspects of platelet dysfunction in chronic myeloproliferative disorders. Throm Haemost 47:84–89

Ponniah A, Brown CT, Taylor P (2004) Priapism secondary to leukemia: Effective management with prompt leukapheresis. Int J Urol 11:809–810

Quintas-Cardama A, Kantarjian H, Talpaz M, O'Brien S, Garcia-Manero G, Verstovsek S, Rios MB, Hayes K, Glassman A, Betele BN, Zhon X, Cortes J (2005) Imatinib mesylate therapy may overcome the poor prognostic significance of deletions of derivative chromosome 9 in patients with chronic myelogenous leukemia. Blood 105:2281–2286

Rowe JM (1983) Clinical and laboratory features of the myeloid and lymphocytic leukemias. Am J Med Technol 49:103–109

Saikia T, Advani S, Dasgupta A, Ramakrishnan G, Nair C, Gladstone B, Kumar MS, Badrinath Y, Dhond S (1988) Characterization of blast cells during blastic phase of chronic myeloid leukaemia by immunophenotyping – experience in 60 patients. Leuk Res 12:499–506

Savage DG, Szydlo RM, Goldman JM (1997) Clinical features at diagnosis in 430 patients with chronic myeloid leukaemia seen at a referral centre over a 16-year period. Br J Haematol 96:111–116

Savage DG, Szydlo RM, Chase A, Apperley JA, Goldman JM (1997) Bone marrow transplantation for chronic myeloid leukaemia: the effects of differing criteria for defining chronic phase on probabilities of survival and relapse. Br J Haematol 99:30–35

Sawyers L, Hochhaus A, Feldman E, Goldman J, Miller C, Ottmann O, Schiffer C, Talpaz M, Guilhot F, Deininger M, Fischer T, O'Brien S, Stone R, Gambacorti-Passerini C, Russell N, Reiffers J, Shea T, Chapuis B, Coutre S, Tura S, Morra E, Larson R, Saven A, Peschel C, Gratwohl A, Mandell F, Ben-am M, Gathmann I, Capdeville R, Paquette R, Druker B (2002) Imatinib induces haematological and cytogenetic responses in patients with chronic myelogenous leukemia in myeloid blast crisis: results of a phase II study. Blood 99:3530–3539

Scottish Cancer Registry, ISD www.isdscotland.org/cancer_information

Sessarego M, Panarello C, Coviello DA et al (1987) Karyotype evolution in CML: high frequency of translocations other than the Ph. Cancer Genet Cytogenet 25:73–80

Shepherd P (2001) IFN dosage regimens in CML. In: Carella A, Daley G, Eaves C, Goldman J, Hehlmann R (eds) Chronic myeloid leukaemia: biology and treatment. Martin Dunitz Publishers, London

Silver R, Talpaz M, Sawyers C et al (2004) Four years follow-up of 1027 patients with late chronic phase (L-CP), accelerated phase (AP) or blast crisis (BC) chronic myeloid leukemia (CML) treated with imatinib in three large Phase II trials. Blood 104: abstract no. 23

Simonsson B on behalf of the IRIS Study Group (2005) Beneficial effects of cytogenetic and molecular response on long-term outcome in patients with newly diagnosed chronic myeloid leukaemia in chronic phase (CML-CP) treated with imatinib (IM): update from the IRIS Study. Blood 106:52a

Sinclair PB, Nacheva EP, Leversha M, Telford N, Chang J, Reid A et al (2000) Large deletions at the t(9;22) breakpoint are common and may identify a poor prognosis subgroup of patients with chronic myeloid leukemia. Blood 95:738–743

Sneed TB, Kantarjian HM, Talpaz M et al (2004) The significance of myelosuppression during therapy with Imatinib mesylate in patients with chronic myelogenous leukemia in chronic phase. Cancer 100:116–121

Sokal JE, Cox EB, Baccarani M, Tura S, Gomez S et al (1984) Prognostic discrimination in good-risk chronic granulocytic leukemia. Blood 63:789–799

Speck B, Bortin M, Champlin R, Goldman J, Herzig R, McGlave P, Messner H, Weiner R, Rimm A (1984) Allogeneic bone marrow transplant for chronic myelogenous leukaemia. Lancet 1:665–668

Spiers AS, Bain BJ, Turner JE (1977) The peripheral blood in chronic granulocytic leukaemia. Study of 50 untreated Philadelphia-positive cases. Scand J Haematol 18:25–38

Suh YK, Shin HJ (2000) Fine needle aspiration biopsy of granulocytic sarcoma: a clinicopathologic study of 27 cases. Cancer 90:364–372

Swolin B, Weinfeld A, Westin J et al (1985) Karyotypic evolution in Ph-positive chronic myeloid leukemia in relation to management and disease progression. Cancer Genet Cytogenet 18:65–79

Talpaz M, Kantarjian H, McCredie K et al (1986) Hematologic remission and cytogenetic improvement induced by recombinant human interferon-alpha A in chronic myelogenous leukemia. N Engl J Med 314:1065–1069

Talpaz M, Silver RT, Druker BJ, Goldman JM, Gambacorti-Passerini C et al (2002) Imatinib induces durable hematologic and cytogenetic responses in patients with accelerated phase chronic myeloid leukemia: results of a phase 2 study. Blood 99:1928–1937

Terjanian T, Kantarjian H, Keating M et al (1987) Clinical and prognostic features of patients with Philadelphia chromosome-positive chronic myelogenous leukemia and extramedullary disease. Cancer 59:297–300

The Benelux CML Study Group (1998) Randomized study on hydroxyurea alone versus hydroxyurea combined with low-dose interferon-α2b for chronic myeloid leukemia. Blood 91:2713–2721

The Italian Cooperative Study Group on Chronic Myeloid Leukemia (1994) Interferon-alpha 2a as compared with conventional chemotherapy for the treatment of chronic myeloid leukemia. The Italian Cooperative Study Group on Chronic Myeloid Leukemia. N Engl J Med 330:820–825

Thiele J, Schmitz B, Fuchs R et al (1998) Detection of the bcr/abl gene in bone marrow macrophages in CML and alterations during interferon therapy – a fluorescence in situ hybridization study on trephine biopsies. J Pathol 186:331–335

Thiele J, Kvasnicka HM, Schmitt-Graeff A, Zirbis TK, Birnbaum F, Kressman C, Melquizo-Graham M, Frackenpohl H, Springmann C, Leder LD, Diehl V, Zankovick R, Schaefer HE, Niederle N, Fischer R (2000) Bone marrow features and clinical findings in chronic myeloid leukemia – a comparative, multicenter, immunohistological and morphometric study on 614 patients. Leuk Lymphoma 36:295–308

Valimaki M, Vuopio P, Liewendahl K (1981) Bone lesions in chronic myelogenous leukaemia. Acta Med Scand 210:403–408

Vardiman JW, Harris NL, Brunning RD (2002) The World Health Organization (WHO) classification of the myeloid neoplasms. Blood 100:2292–2302

Wadhwa J, Szydlo R, Apperley J, Chase A, Bua M et al (2002) Factors affecting duration of survival after onset of blastic transformation of chronic myeloid leukemia. Blood 99:2304–2309

Wehmeier A, Scharf RE, Fricke S, Schneider W (1989) Bleeding and thrombosis in chronic myeloproliferative disorders: relation of platelet disorders to clinical aspects of the disease. Haemostasis 19:251–259

Win N, Mitchell DC (2001) Platelet apheresis for digital gangrene due to thrombocytosis in chronic myeloid leukaemia. Clin Lab Haematol 23:65–66

Yamamoto K, Sekiguchi E, Takatani O (1984) Abnormalities of epinephrine-induced platelet aggregation and adenine nucleotides in myeloproliferative disorders. Throm Haemost 52:292–296

Ye CC, Echeverri C, Anderson JE, Smith JL, Glassman A, Gulley ML, Claxton D, Craig FE (2002) T-cell blast crisis of chronic myelogenous leukemia manifesting as a large mediastinal tumor. Hum Pathol 33:770–773

Signal Transduction Inhibitors in Chronic Myeloid Leukemia

Michael W. N. Deininger

Contents

Abstract. Chronic myeloid leukemia (CML) is caused by Bcr-Abl, a constitutively active tyrosine kinase that activates multiple signaling pathways and is central to disease pathogenesis. Efforts to develop small molecule Bcr-Abl inhibitors led to the discovery of imatinib, a 2-phenylaminopyrimidine that inhibits Bcr-Abl with high selectivity and has rapidly become standard therapy for CML. Responses in newly diagnosed chronic phase patients tend to be durable, but there is a high relapse rate in advanced disease, which is mostly due to point mutations in critical residues that interfere with drug binding, thereby reactivating Bcr-Abl. The fact that Bcr-Abl remains central to disease pathogenesis has stimulated a search for novel Abl kinase inhibitors with activity against mutant Bcr-Abl. Nilotinib, developed from an imatinib backbone, and dasatinib, a dual Abl/Src kinase inhibitor, are currently in phase I/II clinical trials of patients with imatinib-resistant CML, with very encouraging results. While Bcr-Abl is the most attractive target, there are multiple signal transduction pathways downstream that can be intercepted with specific inhibitors, such as blockers of farnesyl transferase and mTOR. Some of these compounds are in clinical trials of imatinib-resistant patients, but results are not yet available. Although imatinib is probably not capable of eradicating CML stem cells, for many patients this agent has turned a life-threatening disease into a chronic disorder that does not significantly affect quality of life.

5.1 Introduction – Drug Targets in Chronic Myeloid Leukemia

Multiple lines of evidence, most importantly animal models, indicate that Bcr-Abl is necessary and probably sufficient to induce the chronic phase of chronic myeloid leukemia (CML) (Daley et al. 1990; Pear et al. 1998). Although there may be some kinase-independent biological effects (Ramaraj et al. 2004), it is undisputed that tyrosine kinase activity is *conditio sine qua non* for Bcr-Abl's ability to transform hematopoietic cells, implicating Bcr-Abl kinase as an attractive therapeutic target (Lugo et al. 1990). Bcr-Abl leads to the activation of multiple signal transduction pathways that confer malignant properties to hematopoietic cells, such as resistance to apoptosis, decreased dependence on growth factors, and perturbed interaction with bone marrow stroma (Deininger et al. 2000; Melo and Deininger 2004). Serine/threonine kinases such as Akt, lipid kinases such as phosphatidyl inositol 3′ kinase (PI3K) and other intermediary proteins including transcription factors and regulators of apoptosis are required for transducing and executing these signals; they constitute an additional set of potential drug targets in cells transformed by Bcr-Abl. It is obvious that pathways downstream of Bcr-Abl, which are essential to Bcr-Abl's capacity to transform hematopoietic cells, are more promising targets than pathways with a high degree of redundancy. While the emphasis of this review will be placed on Bcr-Abl kinase inhibitors, given their dominant role in the clinical management of CML, other potential targets will also be covered.

5.2 ABL Kinase Inhibitors

5.2.1 Preimatinib Inhibitors

In 1989, Gazit and colleagues reported on the synthesis of a novel class of low molecular weight tyrosine kinase inhibitors with selective activity towards epidermal growth factor receptor (EGFR) that they named tyrphostins (Gazit et al. 1989). They suggested that this class of compounds might be useful "as selective antiproliferative agents for proliferative diseases caused by the hyperactivity of protein tyrosine kinases." In 1992, the same investigators reported a tyrphostin that inhibited the tyrosine kinase activity of Bcr-Abl and suggested that it might be possible to design specific compounds for the treatment of Abl-associated human leukemias (Anafi et al. 1992, 1993). Subsequently, the tyrphostins AG568, AG957, and AG1112 were identified as the most specific compounds. Growth inhibition of the CML cell line K562 occurred at micromolar concentrations and was associated with inhibition of Bcr-Abl tyrosine kinase activity (Kaur et al. 1994). Although active in vitro, tyrphostins have not been developed for clinical use. Nonetheless, they provided proof of principle that tyrosine kinases can be selectively inhibited with small molecules.

5.2.2 Imatinib

During the late 1980s protein kinase C (PKC) was ranked highly as a potential drug target in cancer therapy because of its role in cell proliferation. In one medicinal chemistry project performed at Ciba Geigy (now Novartis) with PKC as a target, a 2-phenylaminopyrimidine derivative was identified as the lead compound (Zimmermann et al. 1996, 1997) (Fig. 5.1). This compound, a low potency inhibitor of both serine/threonine and tyrosine kinases, served as the starting point for the synthesis of a series of derivatives. The cellular activity (as opposed to activity in cell-free systems) was enhanced by the addition of a 3′-pyridyl group at the 3′-position of the pyrimidine (Fig. 5.1 A). Activity against tyrosine kinases was enhanced by introduction of a benzamide group at the phenyl ring (Fig. 5.1 B). Analysis

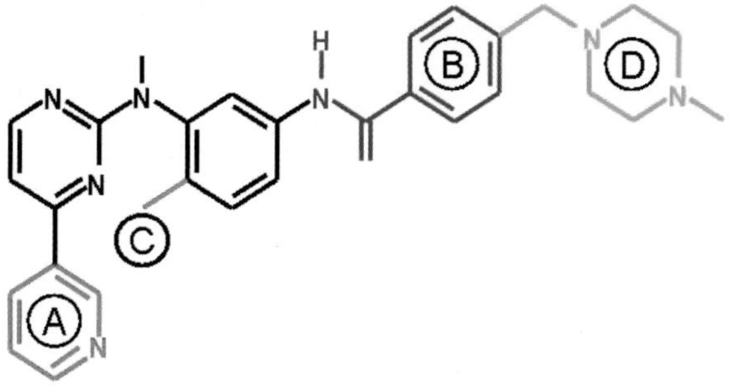

Fig. 5.1. Lead optimization. Development of imatinib from a 2-phenylaminopyrimidine backbone (shown in black). (**A**) Activity in cellular assays was improved by introduction of a 3′ pyridyl group (*red*) at the 3′ position of the pyrimidine. (**B**) Activity against tyrosine kinases was further enhanced by addition of a benzamide group (*blue*) to the phenyl ring. (**C**) Attachment of a "flag-methyl" group (*magenta*) ortho to the diaminophenyl ring strongly reduced activity against PKC. (**D**) Addition of an N-methylpiperazine (*green*) increased water-solubility and oral bioavailability. (Adapted from Deininger et al. 2005)

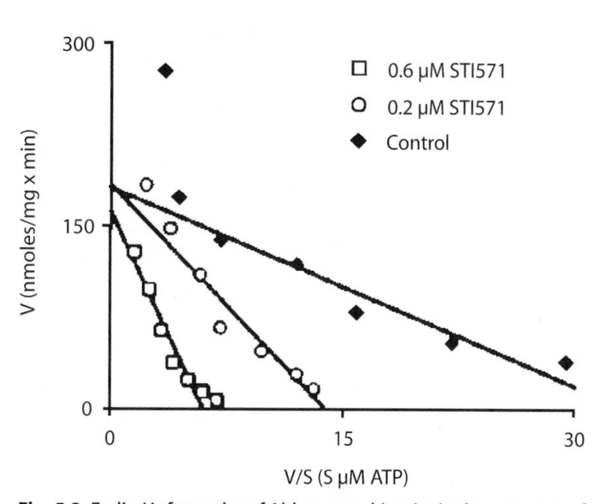

Fig. 5.2. Eadie-Hofstee plot of Abl enzyme kinetics in the presence of imatinib. The concentration of substrate (poly[AlaGluLysTyr]) was kept constant at 50 µg/mL, while ATP concentrations were varied between 1.25 and 100 µM. Vmax (ordinate) remains constant at the various concentrations of imatinib, consistent with competitive inhibition of enzyme activity. (Modified from Cowan-Jacob et al. 2004, with permission)

of structure–activity relationships showed that substitutions at the 6-position of the anilino phenyl ring led to loss of PKC inhibition, while the introduction of a "flag-methyl" group at this position retained or enhanced activity against tyrosine kinases, including Abl (Fig. 5.1 C). The first series of compounds had low water solubility and poor oral bioavailability. The attachment of a highly polar side chain, N-methylpiperazine, markedly improved solubility and oral bioavailability (Fig. 5.1 D). STI571 (formerly CGP57148B, now imatinib mesylate, Gleevec or Glivec) emerged as the most promising compound for clinical development in Philadelphia chromosome (Ph)-positive leukemia, since it had the highest selectivity for growth inhibition of Bcr-Abl-expressing cells.

5.2.2.1 Biochemical Characteristics

The IC_{50} (i.e., the concentration of compound that induces a 50% reduction of a defined activity) for inhibition of substrate phosphorylation by Abl and its oncogenic derivatives Bcr-Abl, Tel-Abl, and *v*-Abl is in the range of 25 nM in biochemical assays (in vitro kinase assays) (Buchdunger et al. 1996; Druker et al. 1996). This is approximately tenfold lower than the IC_{50} for inhibition of cell proliferation of cell lines expressing Bcr-Abl, a difference that may reflect the fact that intracellular ATP concentrations are higher (in the range of 1–2 mM) than the micromolar concentrations commonly used in kinase assays. Alternatively, drug transporters such as p-glycoprotein may actively lower intracellular drug concentrations. Besides Abl, imatinib inhibits the platelet-derived growth factor receptors (PDGFR), the stem cell factor receptor Kit and the gene product of the *ABL*-related gene ARG (also known as Abl2) (Table 5.1) (Heinrich et al. 2000). Kinase assays performed in the presence of graded ATP concentrations showed that imatinib acts as an ATP-competitive inhibitor of substrate phosphorylation (Fig. 5.2) (Cowan-Jacob et al. 2004).

5.2.2.2 Structure – Function Relationships (Fig. 5.3)

The catalytic domains of tyrosine kinases exhibit a universal bilobar structure. The smaller N-terminal lobe consists predominantly of antiparallel beta-sheets, while the C-lobe is largely alpha-helical. The amino acid residues lining the cleft between the two lobes form the catalytic machinery and include the ATP-binding loop (p-loop), the conserved DFG (aspartate-phenylalanine-glycine) motif, and the activation loop (activation loop). In active kinases, the activation loop is stabilized in an open conformation by phosphorylation on key tyrosine or serine/threonine residues within the loop. In this conformation of Abl, a short antiparallel beta-sheet pro-

Table 5.1. Inhibition of protein kinases by imatinib

Enzyme	Substrate phosphorylation IC_{50} [μM]	Cellular tyrosine phosphorylation IC_{50} [μM]
c-ABL	0.2; 0.025*	
v-ABL	0.038	0.1–0.3
$p210^{BCR-ABL}$	0.025*	0.25
$p185^{BCR-ABL}$	0.025*	0.25
TEL-ABL	ND	0.35
PDGF-R α and β	0.38 (PDGF-Rβ)	0.1
Tel-PDGF-R	ND	0.15
c-KIT	0.41	0.1
c-FMS	ND	0.3–1.4
FLT-3	>10	>10
Btk	>10	ND
c-SRC	>100	ND
v-SRC	ND	>10
c-LYN	>100	ND
c-FGR	>100	ND
LCK	9.0	ND
SYK (TPK-IIB)	>100	ND
JAK-2	>100*	>100
EGF-R	>100	>100
Insulin receptor	>10	>100
IGF-IR	>10	>100
FGF-R1	31.2	ND
VEGF-R2 (KDR)	10.7	ND
VEGF-R1 (FLT-1)	19.5	ND
VEGF-R3 (FLT-4)	5.7	ND
TIE-2 (TEK)	>50	ND
c-MET	>100	ND
PKA	>500	ND
PPK	>500	ND
PKCα, β1, β2, γ, δ, ε, ζ, or η	>100	ND
Protein kinase CK-1, CK-2	>100	ND
PKB	>10	ND
p38	>10	ND
PDK1	>10	ND
c-Raf-1	0.97	ND
CDC2/cyclin B	>100	ND

ND, not done

Imatinib concentrations causing a 50% reduction in kinase activity (IC_{50}) are given. *IC_{50} was determined in immunocomplex assays. PDGF-R, platelet-derived growth factor receptor; Btk, Bruton's tyrosine kinase; TPK, tyrosine-protein kinase; EGF-R, epidermal growth factor receptor; IGF-IR, insulin-like growth factor receptor I, FGF-R1, fibroblast growth factor receptor 1; VEGF-R, vascular endothelial growth factor receptor; PKA, cAMP-dependent protein kinase; PPK, phosphorylase kinase; PKC, protein kinase C; CK, casein kinase; PKB, protein kinase B (also known as Akt); PKD1, 3-phosphoinoside-dependent protein kinase 1

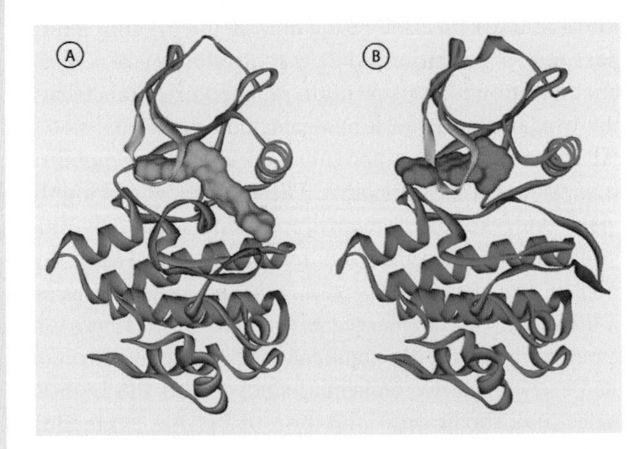

Fig. 5.3. Structure of the Abl KD in complex with kinase inhibitors. Shown is (**A**) the conformation of Abl (*blue*) in complex with imatinib (*orange*), with the Activation loop (*magenta*) in a "closed" conformation, and (**B**) the Abl conformation (*green*) in the PD180970 (*red*) complex with the Activation loop (*magenta*) in an "open" conformation. The p-loop (*yellow*) folds down over the inhibitor in both cases. [Figure prepared by Sandra W. Cowan-Jacob based on reported structures (Nagar et al. 2002; Schindler et al. 2000)]. (From Deininger et al. 2005)

vides a platform for substrate binding. The DFG motif at the N-terminal end of the activation loop is held in a position that allows the binding of metal cations by the aspartate side chain that in turn coordinate the phosphates of ATP bound to the p-loop. In the active state the activation loops of various kinases assume very similar conformations, while the activation loop conformations of inactive kinases are quite distinct. Frequently, the activation loop occludes the "mouth" of the kinase and the DFG motif is displaced outward such that productive nucleotide binding is impossible.

Since it was assumed that imatinib would compete with ATP for binding to the active site, its high selectivity for Abl over closely related kinases such as Src remained unexplained. This discrepancy was reconciled when the crystal structure of the Abl kinase domain (KD) in complex with an imatinib analogue, and subsequently imatinib itself (AblK:imatinib) was solved at high resolution (Nagar et al. 2002; Schindler et al. 2000). Imatinib was found to engage no less than 21 amino acid residues in hydrogen bonds and hydrophobic interactions, affording a very high degree of surface complementarity (Fig. 5.4). Contrary to expectations, Abl was in an inactive conformation in the AblK:imatinib complex, with the activation loop in a closed position, mimicking a substrate bound to the kinase and the regulatory tyrosine 393 in a hydrogen bond with asparagine 363, a highly conserved residue. Since in this conformation the DFG motif is displaced away from the catalytic center, tyrosine 393 cannot be phosphorylated. Given the similarity of the activation loop conformation to a bound substrate, it is very likely that imatinib stabilizes a naturally occurring inactive conformation. The fact that imatinib binds an inactive conformation of Abl explains its exceptional specificity. What is not yet clear is why the activation loops of closely related kinases such as Src are unable to assume this specific conformation (Nagar et al. 2002). The data from the crystal structure analysis were corroborated by biochemical studies. Since phosphorylation of tyrosine 393 (within the activation loop) activates Abl, it was predicted that phosphorylated forms of Abl would be resistant to imatinib. In fact, this was confirmed in in vitro kinase assays using phosphorylated and dephosphorylated proteins (Nagar et al. 2002; Schindler et al. 2000). An additional important observation from the crystal structure analysis was that the p-loop, a glycine-rich flexible structure, undergoes a major downward displacement upon binding of imatinib. This "induced fit" interaction is stabilized by a water-mediated hydrogen bond between Y253 and N322 (Schindler et al. 2000) and the formation of a hydrophobic cage surrounding a portion of imatinib, in which Y253, L370, and F382 make van der Waals interactions with the inhibitor. Knowledge of the AblK:imatinib crystal structure proved to be instrumental for understanding the mechanisms of acquired resistance to imatinib.

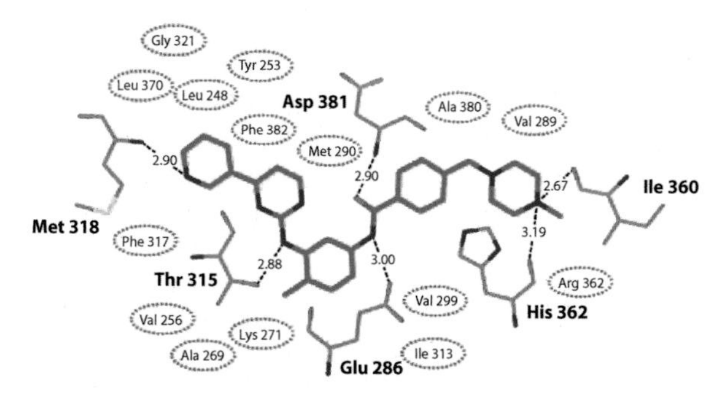

Fig. 5.4. Amino acids residues interacting with Abl in the AblK: imatinib complex. Residues engaged in hydrophobic interactions are indicated by *green dotted lines*. *Dashed lines* indicate hydrogen bonds, with distances in Å. Imatinib carbon atoms are drawn in *green*, nitrogen atoms in *orange* and oxygen atoms in *red*. Amino acid numbering is according to Abl variant containing exon Ia. (From Nagar et al. 2002, with permission)

5.2.2.3 Biological Characteristics

The mesylate salt of imatinib is a white powder with good water solubility. The watery solution has a pH of 5.5 and a yellowish color. Imatinib inhibits the proliferation of Bcr-Abl expressing cell lines with IC_{50}s of 0.1–0.5 μM, and inhibition of proliferation is accompanied by induction of apoptosis, in line with key biological effects of Bcr-Abl (Beran et al. 1998; Deininger et al. 1997). Growth suppression in clonogenic assays of primary CML progenitor cells was observed at similar concentrations, although some *BCR-ABL*-positive colonies survived up to 10 μM of drug (Deininger et al. 1997). Imatinib administered orally at doses ranging from 10 to 50 mg/kg twice daily inhibited tumor formation by 32D cells expressing $P210^{BCR\text{-}ABL}$ injected subcutaneously into Balb/c mice. However, the drug failed to eradicate the disease (Druker et al. 1996). Subsequent studies revealed that the efficacy in the murine model was highly dependent on the drug administration scheme. Thus, in a nude mouse model using the human CML-derived cell line KU812, imatinib administered once or twice daily produced some tumor regression, but only three times daily dosing induced lasting complete remissions (le Coutre et al. 1999). A suboptimal twice-daily dosing scheme may explain why imatinib showed only rather moderate activity in a retroviral transduction-transplantation model of *BCR-ABL*-positive leukemia that resembles CML (Wolff and Ilaria, Jr. 2001). Fortunately, pharmacokinetics in humans proved to be more favorable than in mice. In the phase I study trough levels in patients treated with 400 mg daily averaged 1.46 μM (Druker et al. 2001b), approximately three- to fivefold the IC_{50} in cell proliferation assays (Deininger et al. 1997). Consistent with this, dephosphorylation of CrkL, a specific substrate of the Bcr-Abl kinase, in CML cells was demonstrated in patients. Practically all patients receiving at least 300 mg imatinib daily achieved a complete hematologic response, and this correlated with dephosphorylation of CrkL. As expected, higher trough levels (approximately 5.4 μM) were seen with 400 mg twice daily (Peng et al. 2004). Peak levels at 400 mg once and twice daily were 5.2 and 7.4 μM, respectively. Based on "wash out" experiments and the animal data it is likely that trough rather than peak levels determine efficacy (le Coutre et al. 1999).

In the phase I trials imatinib was generally well tolerated (Druker et al. 2001a, b). Significant (grade 3–4) myelosuppression was common, particularly in patients with advanced disease, likely reflecting antileukemic efficacy in the presence of a limited pool of Ph-negative stem cells capable of restoring nonleukemic hematopoiesis. Nonhematopoietic side effects were also frequent but usually mild and only rarely required permanent discontinuation of therapy. Because of the relative lack of side effects combined with the observation of almost 100% complete hematologic responses at 300 mg daily, no maximum tolerated drug dose was formally established in the phase I trial of CML. Somewhat arbitrarily 400 mg QD was chosen as the dose for the phase II trials. The phase II trials, although not designed to compare 400 vs. 600 mg daily, strongly suggested superiority of the higher dose in patients with accelerated phase or blast crisis (Sawyers et al. 2002; Talpaz et al. 2002). Higher doses of imatinib (400 mg twice daily) may also be more effective in terms of major and complete molecular responses in patients with chronic phase CML (Cortes et al. 2003b; Kantarjian et al. 2004). The maximum tolerated dose (MTD) of imatinib was subsequently established in patients with gastrointestinal stromal tumors (GIST) and is in the range of 1000 mg daily (van Oosterom et al. 2001).

Should the MTD have been used in the phase II studies of imatinib? As this information was unavailable at the time, it would have been necessary to delay the phase II studies. In addition, clinical resistance to imatinib and its mechanisms had neither been investigated in any detail nor was the extent of this problem known at the time. More fundamental is the question whether the MTD or a biomarker such as CrkL phosphorylation should generally guide dosing in clinical trials of targeted agents. At closer view the use of CrkL phosphorylation as a biomarker is quite complex. Firstly, the immunoblots used to measure pCrkL are not very sensitive and only semiquantitative. Secondly, the assays are performed on total white cells or mononuclear cells but these differentiated cells may not represent the critical target population that determines durability of response to treatment. Thirdly, it is not clear whether there is a threshold of Bcr-Abl kinase activity, below which results are optimal and not improved with yet greater levels of kinase inhibition. On the other hand, it could be argued that one of the distinctive features of targeted therapy is to dissect maximal therapeutic effects from the MTD. As yet no randomized trial has shown superiority of 400 mg imatinib twice daily over 400 mg once daily in patients with chronic phase disease, although several single-armed studies strongly suggest this may be the case (Cortes et al. 2003b; Kantarjian et al. 2004). Several large randomized trials are underway in the USA and Europe that will clarify this issue.

5.2.2.4 Resistance and Refractoriness to Imatinib

It is important to distinguish between primary resistance (also referred to as refractoriness) and secondary resistance (also referred to as acquired resistance). Acquired resistance is defined as the loss of a response at any level. Refractoriness is defined as the failure to achieve a certain level of response. The distinction is relevant as the mechanisms underlying refractoriness and acquired resistance may be different (Deininger et al. 2005).

5.2.2.5 Modeling Resistance In Vitro

Before acquired resistance to imatinib was recognized as a significant clinical problem, several groups attempted to model resistance in vitro. *BCR-ABL*-positive cell lines exposed to imatinib at gradually increasing concentrations eventually tolerate up to tenfold higher drug concentrations than the parental lines (le Coutre et al. 2000; Mahon et al. 2000; Weisberg and Griffin

2000). Detailed studies of this in vitro resistance revealed increased expression of Bcr-Abl protein as a result of gene amplification or transcriptional upregulation as the predominant mechanism. In addition, expression of Pgp, the product of the *MDR1* drug resistance gene, was demonstrated in a drug-resistant cell line (Okuda et al. 2001). Several subsequent studies showed that imatinib is indeed a substrate for Pgp (Burger and Nooter 2004; Hegedus et al. 2002; Mahon et al. 2003; Widmer et al. 2003). With both of these mechanisms Bcr-Abl kinase remains active in the resistant cells. In contrast, a Bcr-Abl-independent mechanism of resistance was postulated for imatinib-resistant sublines of KCL22 cells, as comparable inhibition of Bcr-Abl kinase activity by imatinib was demonstrated in resistant and sensitive cell clones (Mahon et al. 2000; Tipping et al. 2003). Mutations in the KD of Bcr-Abl, the dominant mechanism of clinical resistance, have only recently been described in cell lines (Ricci et al. 2002; von Bubnoff et al. 2005).

5.2.2.6 Clinical Resistance

The key observation with respect to acquired resistance in most patients is that phosphorylation of CrkL is restored at the time of relapse, indicating that Bcr-Abl signaling has been re-established (Gorre et al. 2001). It turned out that, in contrast to cell lines, point mutations in the KD of Bcr-Abl that impair drug binding are the predominant mechanism of resistance. In various studies of patients with acquired drug resistance, the rate of such mutations ranged from 50 to 90% (Al Ali et al. 2004; Branford et al. 2002; Gorre et al. 2001; Hofmann et al. 2002; Shah et al. 2002; von Bubnoff et al. 2002). The differences between the various studies may reflect differences in the sensitivity of the assays used for mutation screening as well as patient selection. Mutations have been identified in more than 30 different amino acids within the KD, and several clusters are recognized according to their localization, including the p-loop, theonine 315 (T315), methionine 351 (M351), and the activation loop (Table 5.2) (Deininger et al. 2005). Mutations may confer imatinib resistance by one of three mechanisms. Firstly, they may alter sites directly involved in drug binding. The best example is T315, which makes a hydrogen bond with imatinib. In the T315I mutant, threonine is replaced with the bulky isoleucine, eliminating the hydrogen bond and causing a steric clash with imatinib. Secondly, mutations may prevent the conformational changes required for drug binding. Examples include mutations of the p-loop. Thirdly, mutations may favor the active conformation of the kinase, from which imatinib is sterically excluded. This mechanism probably underlies the resistance of activation loop mutants such as H396P. The rather common M351T mutant may also belong to this category, as it eliminates the site of an inhibitory interaction between the Abl kinase and SH2 domain, which may favor the kinase active conformation. However, since M351T confers resistance also in assays using the isolated Abl KD, other mechanisms must contribute. Definitive clarification of the mechanisms will require solving the crystal structure of these mutants. The degree to which KD mutations reduce sensitivity to imatinib is highly variable. Compared to unmutated Bcr-Abl, the IC_{50} concentrations for highly resistant mutants such as T315I, Y253H, and E255V are more than 200-fold higher in kinase assays and more than 30-fold higher in cell proliferation assays (Corbin et al. 2003). Other mutants, such as M351T or M244V, exhibit only moderately reduced drug sensitivity and some mutants, such as F311L, do not show significant resistance at all (Corbin et al. 2003). This has obvious clinical implications, as dose escalation of imatinib may recapture responses in the case of mutants with a low or moderate degree of resistance, while this would not be effective with highly resistant mutants.

Another well-described though less common mechanism of clinical resistance is *BCR-ABL* gene amplification or increased levels of mRNA. It is thought that both result in increased levels of Bcr-Abl protein, although due to the difficulties of detecting Bcr-Abl protein in lysates of primary CML cells, this has not been formally demonstrated. Similar to KD mutations, increased levels of protein will restore Bcr-Abl signaling, as more active kinase will be present at a given drug concentration. In contrast, Bcr-Abl independent mechanisms of resistance appear to be uncommon. Activation of Src kinases has been shown in cell lines from several patients with clinical resistance but is not a common finding (Donato et al. 2003). Clonal cytogenetic evolution in patients on imatinib is an adverse prognostic factor and frequently seen in patients with drug resistance. However, given that the types of chromosomal abnormalities seen in patients treated with imatinib are identical to those seen in historical controls (Schoch et al. 2003), it is difficult to mechanistically link these chromosomal changes to imatinib resistance. The exception is an additional Ph,

Table 5.2. In vitro sensitivity of clinically isolated BCR-ABL KD mutants to imatinib in various assays

Wild-type ABL		Exchange	N=(177)	%	IC_{50} [µM] – BCR-ABL phosphorylation in cells	IC_{50} [µM] – ABL autophosphorylation (in vitro kinase assay)	IC_{50} [µM] – cell proliferation	Comments
Numbering according to ABL exon Ia	Numbering according to ABL exon Ib							
M244	M263	V	3	1.69	NR*	0.03, 0.64, 1	1, 1.6	
L248	L267	V	1	0.56	NR*			L267R: >33-fold increased resistance in proliferation assays
G250	G269	E	6	3.39	7.4 to >10	1.6	4.5 to >20	
G250	G269	A	1	0.56	NR	NR	NR	
Q252	Q271	H	8	4.52	2.9, 10.4	NR	2.8 to 9.3	
		R	1	0.56	10.4	NR	NR	
Y253	Y272	F	6	3.39	5.9, 21.4	72	3 to 8.9	
		H	12	6.78	21.4	150	17.7, >33	
E255	E274	K	34	19.21	27.9	>200	15 to 33	
		V	4	2.26	7.3	3.5, >200	7.7, >33	
D276	D295	G	1	0.56	NR	NR	NR	D276V: twofold increased resistance in proliferation assays
F311	F330	L	1	0.56	NR*	0.031, 1	0.7 to 2.1	
T315	T334	I	37	20.9	>10	>10	5.2 to >10	
T315	T334	N	1	0.56	NR	NR	NR	
F317	F336	L	7	3.95	0.8 to 11.8	0.25, 0.38, 8.3	1.3 to 13	
M343	M362	T	1	0.56		NR	NR	
M351	M370	T	27	15.25	0.6 to 3.9	0.26, <1	0.9 to 7.3	
E355	E374	G	5	2.82	2.8, 10	0.02, 0.8	2.3, 4	
F359	F378	A	1	0.56	NR	NR	NR	
		V	7	3.95	NR	0.05, 1.8	1.4, 2.8	

Table 5.2 (continued)

Wild-type ABL		Exchange	N=(177)	%	IC_{50} [µM] – BCR-ABL phosphorylation in cells	IC_{50} [µM] – ABL autophosphorylation (in vitro kinase assay)	IC_{50} [µM] – cell proliferation	Comments
Numbering according to ABL exon Ia	Numbering according to ABL exon Ib							
V379	V398	I	1	0.56	NR	0.03, 1.1	1, 2	
F382	F401	L	1	0.56	NR	NR	NR	
L387	L406	M	1	0.56	NR	0.06, 2.1	1.1, 2.2	
H396	H415	P	1	0.56	NR	0.34, 0.87	1.4 to 4.3	
H396	H415	R	6	3.39	NR	0.22, 7.3	5.4, 11	
S417	S436	Y	1	0.56	NR	NR	1.8	
E459	E478	K	1	0.56	NR	NR	NR	
F486	F505	S	1	0.56	1.1	0.67	1.4 , 9.1	

The values are given as fold changes over wildtype. The data are compiled from several studies (Al Ali et al. 2004; Azam et al. 2003; Barthe et al. 2001; Corbin et al. 2002, 2003; Gorre et al. 2001; Hochhaus et al. 2002; Leguay et al. 2003; Shah et al. 2002; von Bubnoff et al. 2002).

* Immunoblots were published but IC_{50} values were not given (Azam et al. 2003).

NR, not reported.

which may be equivalent to gene amplification. Thus, clonal cytogenetic evolution is more likely to represent an epiphenomenon than a causal finding in patients with acquired imatinib resistance.

The possible involvement of leukemia cell-extrinsic mechanisms in imatinib resistance has been a controversial issue. In nude mice injected subcutaneously with the human CML cell line KU812, tumor recurrence was observed after a transient response to imatinib (le Coutre et al. 1999). Unexpectedly, the tumor cells remained sensitive to in vitro treatment with imatinib, suggesting the resistance in this model was mediated by an extrinsic mechanism. Increased levels of alpha-1 acidic glycoprotein were subsequently demonstrated in these mice (Gambacorti-Passerini et al. 2000). As alpha-1 acidic glycoprotein avidly binds imatinib, this could reduce plasma levels of active drug. Although an experimentally well-founded hypothesis, no convincing clinical correlation between alpha-1 acidic glycoprotein levels and drug resistance has been demonstrated thus far (le Coutre et al. 2002).

Active drug levels may also be reduced by drugs that induce Cyp3A4/5, the main imatinib-metabolizing enzyme (Deininger et al. 2003). Of greater clinical significance as an extrinsic mechanism of "resistance" may be noncompliance. A survey by Novartis showed that almost one third of drug doses are missed in patients. In addition, underdosing may not be uncommon in the community setting.

5.2.2.7 Refractoriness and Disease Persistence

The incidence of refractoriness depends on the phase of disease and the level of response that is considered. Thus, hematologic refractoriness is rare in patients with CML in chronic phase but quite common in patients with myeloid blast crisis. On the other hand, molecular refractoriness, i.e., the persistence of residual disease at the molecular level as assessed by RT/PCR, is the rule even in newly diagnosed patients with chronic phase (Fig. 5.5). At least in terms of numbers, this is the most relevant group, given that >90% of patients are diagnosed in chronic phase, at least in developed countries, and that more than 80% of these will achieve a complete cytogenetic response with standard dose imatinib (Guilhot 2004). Anecdotal observations show that discontinuation of imatinib is followed by disease recurrence in the majority of cases, with the exception of patients who previously received an allogeneic stem cell transplant (Cortes et al. 2004; Kim et al. 2004; Mauro et al. 2004; Merante et al. 2005) and possibly of patients who had been treated with interferon-alpha prior to imatinib (Rousselot et al. 2005). This indicates that the residual *BCR-ABL*-positive cells are fully leukemogenic. Nonetheless, a few individuals have remained RT/PCR-negative for up to 15 months after imatinib was discontinued. Longer follow-up is required to see whether these responses will last.

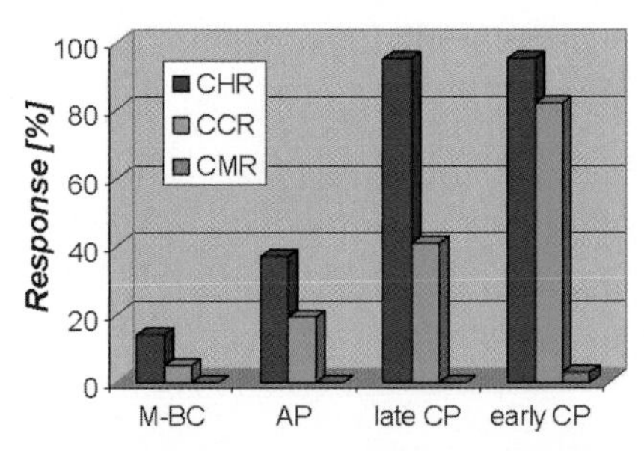

Fig. 5.5. Frequency of complete hematologic, complete cytogenetic and complete molecular responses in CML patients treated with imatinib, according to disease phase (AP, accelerated phase; CP, chronic phase; M-BC, myeloid blast crisis). (From Deininger et al. 2005)

It is currently unknown which specific properties endow persistent cells with the ability to survive in the presence of drug. It has been shown that CML patients harbor an imatinib-resistant quiescent population of cells with the capacity of engrafting SCID-NOD mice (Graham et al. 2002; Holyoake et al. 1999). It is conceivable that these cells represent the persistent population in patients on imatinib but this remains to be formally proven. It is also unknown why quiescent cells are resistant to imatinib. As with acquired resistance, it will be crucial to establish whether or not Bcr-Abl kinase activity is inhibited in the presence of drug. Several mechanisms could explain imatinib's failure to inhibit Bcr-Abl in persistent leukemic progenitor cells, including drug efflux or lack of drug influx, KD mutations, and high levels of Bcr-Abl protein (recently reviewed in Deininger et al. 2005). In one small study, KD mutations were found in 5/13 patients with complete cytogenetic response. An additional four patients tested mutation-positive on follow-up, associated with a rise in *BCR-ABL* mRNA (Chu et al. 2005). Interestingly, the majority of the mutations detected in these patients confer only low level resistance in cell lines, suggesting that in the presence of imatinib they may be sufficient to maintain the clone's viability but insufficient to support its expansion. As the relapse rate in this group was much higher than would be expected from observations in larger studies (Kantarjian et al. 2002; O'Brien et al. 2003), it is doubtful whether the cohort is representative of "typical" patients with complete cytogenetic response. Another possibility is that drug transporters such as Pgp may actively lower intracellular drug levels in the persistent progenitor cells. There is also evidence that imatinib is actively transported into the cell by Oct-1, and thus failure to express this protein could also be relevant (Crossman et al. 2005; Thomas et al. 2004). Lastly, it has been shown that the levels of *BCR-ABL* mRNA are much higher in lineage-negative than in lineage-committed CML progenitor cells (Jiang et al. 2003). It this was reflected in protein levels, then such cells would be innately resistant to much higher drug concentrations than their more differentiated progeny that are assessed with CrkL phosphorylation assays. All these mechanisms have in common the fact that Bcr-Abl remains central to disease pathogenesis, and that they may be overcome with alternative Abl inhibitors which are active against KD mutant Bcr-Abl, have increased potency, or exhibit a different profile of affinity to drug transporters.

Perhaps more disturbing is the possibility that residual leukemic progenitors may be independent of Bcr-Abl kinase activity for their survival. Primary CML progenitor cells are not completely growth-factor-independent, indicating that physiological growth and survival pathways are intact and active. Consistent with this, growth-factor-dependent activation of mitogen-activated protein (MAP) kinase signaling has been demonstrated in CD34-positive cells from CML patients treated ex vivo with imatinib, suggesting that the cells are capable of switching to physiological pathways if forced by inhibition of Bcr-Abl. From a practical point, this would imply that stem-cell-targeted rather than Bcr-Abl-targeted therapy would be required to eradicate residual leukemia (Deininger and Holyoake 2005).

5.2.3 Alternative Abl Kinase Inhibitors

Four classes of alternative Abl inhibitors can be distinguished. The first group consists of structurally diverse compounds with activity against Abl and Src as well as various additional kinases. The most prominent agent is dasatinib (formerly BMS-354825) (Shah et al. 2004). The second class, currently represented only by nilotinib, is based on an imatinib backbone (Weisberg et al. 2005). The third class is substrate rather than ATP competitive and currently includes ON012380 (Gumireddy et al. 2005) and adaphostin (Kaur and Sausville 1996; Mow et al. 2002). Very recently, yet another class of compounds has been described that most likely acts as allosteric inhibitors of Bcr-Abl (Adrian et al. 2006).

5.2.4 Combined Abl/Src Kinase Inhibitors

5.2.4.1 Structural Similarities Between Abl and Src

The N-terminal portions of Abl and Src, excluding the unique N-terminal cap, exhibit a high degree of sequence homology (42% sequence identity), with the three major functional domains (Src homology domains 1–3, SH1-SH3) oriented in an identical fashion (Nagar et al. 2003). The two proteins are different in their C-termini however. The large C-terminus of Abl is unique, containing proline rich sequences, DNA binding motifs, nuclear localization and export signals, and an actin-binding motif at the very C-terminal end (Deininger et al. 2000). Importantly, Abl lacks tyrosine 527, the residue crucial to autoinhibition of Src. Surprisingly, crystal structure analysis has revealed that the inactive (autoinhibited) conformations of the two kinases are similar, although entirely different mechanisms are used for their stabilization (Hantschel et al. 2003; Nagar et al. 2003). In Src, phosphorylated tyrosine 527 binds intramolecularly to the SH2 domain, forming a "clamp" that stabilizes the kinase in an inactive conformation. In Abl, the same is achieved by interaction of the myristoylated N-terminal cap with a hydrophobic pocket in the C-lobe of the KD. It must be stressed that the latter mechanism applies only to the isoform of Abl that contains exon Ib, as only this form contains the N-terminal myristoylation site. Despite these similarities, there are significant differences between the activation loop conformations of inactive Abl and Src that are the basis for imatinib's high level of specificity. Conversely, drugs that bind the active conformation of Abl are expected to bind active Src as well.

5.2.4.2 Classes of Combined Abl/Src Inhibitors

Pyrido[2,3-d]pyrimidine derivatives had been developed as Src kinase inhibitors (Kraker et al. 2000) but were subsequently found to inhibit Abl at nanomolar concentrations and induce apoptosis in Bcr-Abl-expressing leukemia cell lines (Dorsey et al. 2000). The crystal structure of the Abl KD in complex with one derivative, PD173955 was solved and revealed marked differences compared to the AblK:imatinib complex (Nagar et al. 2002). PD173955 was found to engage only 11 amino acids compared to 21 residues contacted by imatinib. As a result, the binding interface is significantly smaller (913 $Å^2$ for PD173955 compared to 1251 $Å^2$ for imatinib). Nonetheless, PD173955 is a more potent inhibitor of Abl, with an IC_{50} in the low nanomolar range. How can this be explained? In contrast to the AblK:imatinib complex, the activation loop in the AblK:PD173955 was found in a conformation similar to that of an active kinase, and modeling of PD173955 into inactive Abl revealed no significant steric clash, suggesting that PD173955 is capable of binding to both active and inactive conformations of the kinase (Fig. 5.3). In contrast, imatinib depends on capturing the kinase in a unique but probably rare inactive conformation. Furthermore, only minor adjustments were required for binding of PD173955 to the p-loop compared to the extensive downward displacement seen in the AblK:imatinib complex. Since the activity of Abl is regulated by phosphorylation of tyrosine 393 within the activation loop, it was predicted that binding of imatinib, but not of PD173955, would be influenced by the phosphorylation state of Abl. Exactly this was seen in kinase assays (Nagar et al. 2002). The Druker lab was the first to show that besides their increased potency, pyrido[2,3-d]pyrimidine derivatives have activity against most Abl KD mutants, except T315I (La Rosee et al. 2002). Unfortunately, although highly active in vitro, the pyrido[2,3-d]pyrimidine derivatives exhibit unfavorable pharmacokinetics, in particular poor oral bioavailability and they were thus not developed clinically. Several other combined Abl/Src inhibitors with diverse chemical backbones have been described (Golas et al. 2003; Huron et al. 2003; O'Hare et al. 2004b; Warmuth et al. 2003; Wisniewski et al. 2002) (Fig. 5.6). These compounds differ mainly in terms of pharmacokinetics. Although for some compounds crystallographic data are not available, it is likely that all these inhibitors bind both the active and inactive conformations of Abl. Compared to imatinib, their key features are increased potency and activity against most Abl KD mutants, with the notable exception of T315I (Table 5.3).

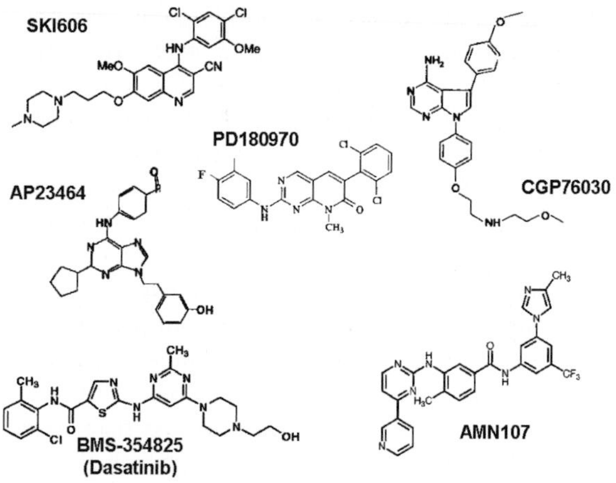

Fig. 5.6. Alternative Abl kinase inhibitors. All compounds shown, except nilotinib, are combined Abl/Src inhibitors, of which only dasatinib is currently in clinical trials. Nilotinib was developed from an imatinib backbone

5.2.4.3 Dasatinib (BMS-354825)

The most promising of the combined Abl/Src inhibitors is dasatinib (BMS-354825), a 2-amino-thiazole-5-carboxamide, has excellent oral bioavailability. The IC_{50} for inhibition of substrate phosphorylation is <1 nM for Abl and most KD mutants except T315I, which is completely resistant (O'Hare et al. 2005). The IC_{50} for inhibition of Src family kinases ranges between 1 and 3 nM. Cell proliferation assays using BaF3 cells expressing the various Bcr-Abl mutants revealed a somewhat more complicated picture (Table 5.4). Most mutants are inhibited at IC_{50}s in the low nanomolar range but slightly higher values were noted for the p-loop mutants Y253 and E255. As expected, BaF3 cells expressing Bcr-Abl T315I were resistant. In a murine model of *BCR-ABL*-positive leukemia, dasatinib was effective against cells expressing unmutated and M351T mutant Bcr-Abl but not against cells expressing T315I (Shah et al. 2004). Dasatinib is currently in phase I/II clinical trials, with encouraging preliminary results (Sawyers et al. 2005) (Table 5.5). As the plasma levels achieved at the MTD (120 mg twice daily) are in the range of 150 nM, all mutants except T315I should be responsive (Sawyers et al. 2005). Based on the phase I/II data dasatinib has been appeared by the FDA for the treatment of imatinib failure.

Table 5.3. ATP-competitive Abl kinase inhibitors with activity against KD mutants. (See also Table 5.4)

Compound	Class	Anti Src activity	IC_{50} (cell proliferation) [nM]					Reference
			Wild-type Bcr-Abl	E255K	M351T	H396P	T315I	
PD180970	Pyridopyrimidine	Yes	25	140	45	15	840	(La Rosee et al. 2002)
SKI DV-M016	Pyridopyrimidine	Yes	~11	~30		~10	>500	(von Bubnoff et al. 2003)
AP23848	Trisubstituted purine	Yes	14	94	24	8	9050	(O'Hare et al. 2004a)
Dasatinib	2-amino-thiazole-5-carboxamide	Yes	0.087–1	5.6	1.1	5.6	>250	(Lee et al. 2004; Shah et al. 2004)
Nilotinib	2-phenylamino-pyrimidine	No	20	150	31	ND	>2000	

Table 5.4. Sensitivity of common Abl kinase domain mutants to imatinib, BMS-453825 and AMN107 in kinase and cell proliferation assays (reproduced from O'Hare et al, Cancer Res (2005) 165(11):4500-4505, with permission)

	Ba/F3 cellular assays								
	Cellular proliferation						Bcr-Abl tyrosine phosphorylation		
	Imatinib		AMN107		BMS-354825		Imatinib	AMN107	BMS-354825*
	IC_{50} (nmol/L)	Fold Change	IC_{50} (nmol/L)	Fold Change	IC_{50} (nmol/L)	Fold Change	IC_{50} (nmol/L)	IC_{50} (nmol/L)	IC_{50} (nmol/L)
WT Bcr-Abl	260	1	13 (28)†	1	0.8 (2.6)†	1	280	10	<10
M244V	2000	8	38 (56)	3	1.3 (1.8)	2	500	8	<10
G250E	1350	5	48 (152)	4	1.8 (3)	2	1000	7	10–100
Q252H	1325	5	70 (156)	5	3.4 (11.2)	4	1500	15	<10
Y253F	3475	13	125 (215)	10	1.4 (3)	2	4200	55	<10
Y253H	>6400	>25	450 (1024)	35	1.3 (3)	2	>5000	155	<10
E255K	5200	20	200 (415)	15	5.6 (12.8)	7	5000	70	10–100
E255V	>6400	>25	430 (2000)	33	11 (27)	14	>5000	250	<10
F311L	480	2	23 (48)	2	1.3 (2.8)	2	600	44	nd
T315I	>6400	>25	>2000	>154	>200	>250	>5000	>5000	>1000
F317L	1050	4	50 (116)	4	7.4 (15)	9	400	47	<10
M351T	880	3	15 (31)	1.2	1.1 (3)	1.4	500	8	<10
F359V	1825	7	175 (385)	13	2.2 (4.8)	3	3100	43	10–100
V379I	1630	6	51 (115)	4	0.8 (1.6)	1	800	15	nd
L387M	1000	4	49 (115)	4	2 (4)	3	2700	33	nd
H396P	850	3	41 (69)	3	0.6 (1.2)	0.8	2700	70	nd
H396R	1750	7	41 (73)	3	1.3 (2.7)	2	1000	22	<10
Parental Ba/F3	>6400	>25	>2000	>154	>200	>250	ns	ns	nd

Note: Fold Change refers to the fold difference in the IC_{50}, relative to WT, which is set to 1.

* Estimated from Shah et al. 2004.

† Values in parentheses are IC_{90} values, given for AMN107 and BMS-354825 only.

Abbreviations: ns, no signal detected, Bcr-Abl not expressed; nd, not determined.

Table 5.5. Early clinical results from phase I studies of dasatinib and nilotinib. Due to slightly different inclusion criteria and shorter follow-up in the nilotinib cohort, the data from the two studies are not directly comparable

Chronic phase CML	Dasatinib (Talpaz et al. 2006)	Nilotinib (Kantarjian et al. 2005)
Complete hematologic response	93%	92%
Complete cytogenetic response	35%	35%
Accelerated phase CML		
Hematologic response	81%	76%
Complete hematologic response	45%	50%
Complete cytogenetic response	18%	14%
Myeloid blast phase CML		
Hematologic response	61%	42%
Complete hematologic response	28%	29%
Major cytogenetic response	35%	17%
Complete cytogenetic response	26%	4%

5.2.5 Nilotinib (AMN107)

In contrast to the combined Abl/Src kinase inhibitors, nilotinib was developed from an imatinib backbone. Compared to imatinib, the N-methylpiperazinyl residue was replaced with a trifluoromethyl/imidazole-substituted phenyl group. This is energetically more favorable, since the need to deprotonate the highly basic N-methylpiperazine "consumes" a significant amount of free binding energy in the AblK:imatinib complex. Thus, although nilotinib still binds the inactive conformation of Abl, this binding is much tighter compared to imatinib, resulting in increased potency. This is reflected by IC_{50} values for inhibition of Abl substrate and autophosphorylation that are at least one order of magnitude lower than for imatinib. As a result of its increased potency, nilotinib is active against many KD mutants, although the differential in drug sensitivity between unmutated and mutated Abl is largely maintained (Table 5.4). Thus, the various mutants can be categorized according to their sensitivity to nilotinib, which implies that plasma levels achieved in patients will determine the breadth of coverage. Emerging data from phase I studies indicate trough levels in the range of 2 μM in patients treated with 400 mg nilotinib twice daily, which is probably the MTD (Kantarjian et al. 2005). Thus, all mutants except for T315I should be inhibited at this dose. Phase I/II clinical trials are underway, with encouraging early results (Kantarjian et al. 2005) (Table 5.5). Another remarkable feature of nilotinib compared to imatinib is that the sensitivity of the three main target kinases Abl, Kit, and PDGFR is reversed. While imatinib is most potent against PDGFR (a fact that explains the response of patients with FIP1L1-PDGFR rearrangements to low doses of imatinib (Gleich et al. 2002)) and least potent against Abl, this is reversed in nilotinib. If some imatinib side effects are indeed mediated by PDGFR inhibition (Deininger et al. 2003), this would be clinically advantageous.

An important question is whether mutations other than those detected in patients with resistance to imatinib may confer resistance to nilotinib or dasatinib. The approach of "saturation mutagenesis" has been taken to predict Bcr-Abl mutations conferring drug resistance to imatinib (Azam et al. 2003). This assay is based on expression of a *BCR-ABL* plasmid in a DNA repair deficient strain of *E. coli*. The mutagenized plasmid is then used to transform BaF3 cells to growth factor independence, followed by selection of cell clones expressing dug resistant mutants in the presence of imatinib. Using this system, a broad range of Bcr-Abl mutants was recovered, including all clinical isolates known at the time. The identical experiment performed with dasatinib in comparison with imatinib revealed that the range of mutants conferring resistance to dasatinib was rather narrow, consistent with less stringent requirements for drug binding and thus fewer "vulnerable" sites. Interestingly however, several mutants were identified that were relatively (i.e., compared to wild type) more resistant to dasatinib compared to imatinib, including F317L/V and

T315A (Burgess et al. 2005). Very few resistant clones were recovered when both agents were combined. These data indicate that combinations of dasatinib with a conformation-sensitive inhibitor such as imatinib may delay the outgrowth of drug resistant clones in patients. It will be interesting to compare and combine dasatinib and nilotinib using this or a recently published cell-line based assay (von Bubnoff et al. 2005). Clearly, any such combination will eventually have to be complemented by an inhibitor with activity against T315I. As a result of threonine 315's function as a gatekeeper of the kinase, the development of such compounds requires entirely different scaffolds, but is not impossible. For example, a novel, crystallography-based approach led to the discovery of a series of molecules with activity against T315I in the nanomolar dose range (Burley 2005).

5.2.6 Non-ATP-Competitive Abl Kinase Inhibitors

Imatinib, nilotinib, and the combined Abl/Src kinase inhibitors described above are all competitive towards ATP. The fact that the T315I mutant is resistant to all these agents has stimulated interest in the development of inhibitors that bind Abl outside the ATP binding pocket. One such compound, termed ON012380 has recently been profiled (Gumireddy et al. 2005). In in vitro kinase assays, ON012380 was found to be competitive vs. recombinant Crk as a substrate of Abl but not vs. ATP (Fig. 5.7). Consistent with binding to different sites in Abl, ON012380 and imatinib appear to be synergistic. The IC_{50} for induction of cell death in 32D cells expressing wild-type Bcr-Abl and a range of KD mutants was between 5.9 nM and 10 nM. Importantly, this included T315I. The compound was also tested in mice injected with 32D cells expressing T315I mutant Bcr-Abl. A reduction of peripheral blood leukemia cells was demonstrated in animals treated with intraperitoneal injections of ON012380, but not imatinib. Unfortunately, no survival data were provided, thus the significance of this murine model remains somewhat elusive. Nonetheless, this study demonstrates the feasibility of generating effective substrate-competitive Abl kinase inhibitors. An intriguing question is whether point mutations may be capable of blocking ON012380 binding, in analogy to ATP-competitive inhibitors. Although the crystal structure of ON012380 in complex with the Abl KD has not been resolved, the prediction is that mutation of residues that make direct contact with this compound will interfere with binding. If kinase activity were preserved in such mutants, this would lead to drug resistance. Another example of a substrate-competitive inhibitor is adaphostin (Kaur et al. 2005). This agent is active against imatinib-resistant cell lines (including lines expressing T315I mutant Bcr-Abl) and primary cells. However, adaphostin effects may be mediated by degradation of Bcr-Abl protein and an increase in intracellular reactive oxygen species rather than by "simple" inhibition of Bcr-Abl kinase activity (Chandra et al. 2005).

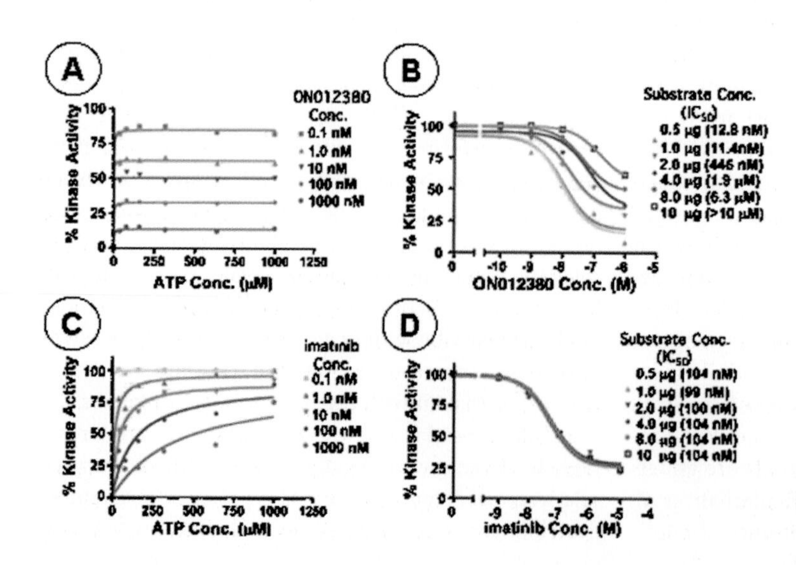

Fig. 5.7. Inhibition of Abl by ON012380 compared to imatinib. (**A, B**) Substrate but not ATP competes with ON012380for inhibition of Abl kinase, consistent with substrate-competitive inhibition. (**C, D**) ATP but not substrate competes with imatinib for inhibition of kinase, consistent with ATP-competitive inhibition (see also Fig. 5.2). (Adapted from Gumireddy et al. 2005, with permission)

5.2.7 Allosteric Inhibitors

Kinase activity can also be influenced through binding of small molecules to allosteric regulatory sites outside the catalytic site, for example the Akt inhibitor Akt-I-1 (Barnett et al. 2005). GNF-2, a recently described compound, probably functions as an allosteric inhibitor of Bcr-Abl by binding to the myristoyl binding pocket in the KD (Adrian et al. 2006). Interestingly, the kinase inhibitory effect was seen only in Bcr-Abl-positive cells (as opposed to cells transformed with Tel-Abl) and only in cells but not in cell-free kinase assays. This, together with the observation that several KD mutants, including T315I and G250E, are resistant to GNF-2, suggests that this compound binds a specific conformation of Bcr-Abl present only in cells. Alternatively, an additional adaptor molecule could be required to allow for binding. It is not yet clear if this class of compounds will have a place in the clinic. One obvious advantage is their high level of selectivity, which would be predicted to minimize side effects.

5.2.8 Selectivity vs. Potency

Preliminary data from phase I/II clinical trials are very encouraging both for nilotinib and dasatinib (Table 5.4). From the standpoint of relative potency, dasatinib is clearly superior, although the clinical relevance of this difference will eventually depend on pharmacokinetics, including achievable plasma levels and plasma protein binding. However, one clear-cut difference is that dasatinib inhibits a broader spectrum of kinases that includes Src in addition to Abl, PDGFR, and Kit. Given the involvement of Src family kinases in multiple cellular signaling processes, one obvious concern is that inhibition of these kinases may lead to significant side effects, especially in view of dasatinib's potency. For example, inhibition of Lck, a Src family kinase required for signal transduction from the T cell receptor, may lead to immunosuppression. Whether this prediction is true remains to be seen in clinical studies. From the efficacy standpoint, it is possible that inhibition of Src may indeed be advantageous. This is based on the notion that activation of Src kinases has been observed in some cases of imatinib resistance (Donato et al. 2003), and that Src kinases may have a role in myeloid blast crisis of CML (Ptasznik et al. 2004) and in Ph-positive acute lymphoblastic leukemia (Hu et al. 2004).

5.2.9 Targeting Bcr-Abl Protein Rather Than Bcr-Abl Kinase Activity

An alternative approach to inhibiting Bcr-Abl function is to target the protein itself rather than its enzymatic activity. In fact, herbimycin A, one of the first Abl kinase inhibitors described, later turned out to induce protein degradation rather than inhibit the kinase (Okabe et al. 1992). Bcr-Abl's stability is dependent on cellular chaperones such as heat shock protein 90 (Hsp90). Consequently, inhibitors of Hsp90, including geldanamycin and its less toxic derivative 17-allylaminogeldanamycin (17-AAG) induce degradation of wild-type and KD mutant Bcr-Abl (Gorre et al. 2002). A phase-I study of 17-AAG in combination with imatinib in patients with resistance to single agent imatinib is currently underway. LAQ824, a histone deacetylase inhibitor, has also been shown to inhibit Hsp90 function by promoting its acetylation. As with 17-AAG, the result is proteasomal degradation of Bcr-Abl. Lastly, arsenic trioxide reduces Bcr-Abl levels by inhibiting its translation (Nimmanapalli et al. 2003a). Synergism between arsenic trioxide and imatinib has been demonstrated in vitro (La Rosee et al. 2004). Moderate activity was seen in a phase I/II study of patients with imatinib-resistant CML (Mauro et al. 2003). Overall, although conceptually appealing, the approach of inducing Bcr-Abl protein degradation has not yet delivered a major clinical breakthrough.

5.3 Inhibitors of Signaling Pathways Downstream of Bcr-Abl

A host of signaling pathways are activated in Bcr-Abl-transformed cells, including MAP kinases, PI3-K, and others (Fig. 5.8). Much effort has been invested into the identification of pathways that are essential for Bcr-Abl's ability to transform cells to malignancy. The emerging picture is that although many pathways contribute to a fully malignant phenotype, few are truly essential, due to the extensive redundancy of the system (Deininger et al. 2000). This may explain why Bcr-Abl is fully leukemogenic in mice with targeted disruption of the STAT5 (Sexl et al. 2000), CBL (Dinulescu et al. 2003), IL-3, or GM-CSF genes (Li et al. 2001), amongst others. The exception to this rule is Gab2, an adaptor molecule that binds to tyrosine 177 of Bcr-Abl via Grb2 (Sattler et al. 2002). Extensive in vitro studies have

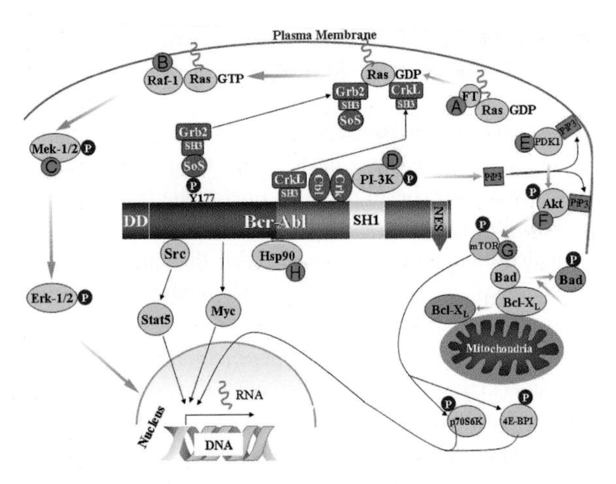

Fig. 5.8. Signal transduction pathways in cells transformed by Bcr-Abl. Potential drug targets other than Abl kinase include (**A**) Farnesyl transferases that prenylate Ras, mediating its binding to the cell membrane; (**B**) Raf, a serine kinase that activates mitogen activated protein (MAP) kinase signaling; (**C**) Mitogen activated protein (MAP) kinases; (**D**) Phosphatidyl inositol 3′ kinase (PI3K) that produces 3,4,5 phosphatidyl inositol (PiP_3), which is required for localization of PDK1 and Akt to the inner leaflet of the cell mebrane; (**E**) PDK1 which activates Akt; (**F**) Akt which activates mammalian target of rapamycin (mTOR); (**G**) mTOR, which phosphorylates and activates p70S6 kinase and 4E-BP1, two major global regulators of gene transcription in response to growth stimuli; (**H**) chaperones like heat shock protein 90 (Hsp90) that stabilize Bcr-Abl protein. (Modified from Deininger and Melo 2004)

tested specific inhibitors of signal transduction pathways downstream of Bcr-Abl alone and in combination with imatinib. In most cases, synergistic or additive effects were demonstrable, in some instances also in imatinib-resistant cell lines. Several of these inhibitors are in clinical testing, alone or in combination with imatinib.

5.3.1 Farnesyl Transferase Inhibitors (FTI)

Bcr-Abl activates Ras, which in turn leads to activation of the MAP kinase-signaling cascade (Cortez et al. 1995; Pendergast et al. 1993; Puil et al. 1994). Since localization of Ras to the cell membrane is required for activation (Marais et al. 1995), and binding of Ras to the membrane is dependent on farnesylation, there is a rationale for FTI inhibitors to suppress Ras signaling. Consistent with predictions, the FTI SCH66336 (Lonafarnib, Sarasar) was shown to inhibit the proliferation of *BCR-ABL*-positive cell lines, although it did not induce apoptosis (Peters et al. 2001). Activity was also seen in imatinib resistant cell lines, but synergism was limited to cell lines with residual sensitivity to imatinib (Hoover et al. 2002). Unexpectedly, the effects of Lonafarnib were more pronounced than those of dominant-negative Ras, suggesting that the drug may modulate additional targets. Candidates include the small GTPases Rheb1, Rheb2 (Basso et al. 2005), and RhoB (Ashar et al. 2001), and the centromere-associated proteins CENP-E and CENP-F (Ashar et al. 2000). Given that the activity of FTIs in *BCR-ABL*-positive cells appears to be predominantly cytostatic, the full potential of these compounds may be realized only in combination with apoptosis-inducing agents. Potentially significant is the fact that FTIs reduced the survival of imatinib-resistant quiescent *BCR-ABL*-positive progenitor cells from CML patients (Jorgensen et al. 2005), a cell population that may be responsible for disease persistence.

5.3.2 Inhibitors of MAP Kinase Signaling

All three groups of MAP kinases have been implicated in Bcr-Abl-induced leukemogenesis. However, the role of the Ras → Raf → Mek1/2 → Erk1/2 axis as a major growth stimulating and antiapoptotic pathway has been established most convincingly (Cortez et al. 1997), while the role of Jnk and p38, the other two pillars of the MAP kinase system, is less well characterized (Parmar et al. 2004; Raitano et al. 1995). In fact, p38 activation may mediate the cytotoxic effects of imatinib rather than promote survival (Parmar et al. 2004). Mek1/2 inhibitors such as PD98059 and U0126 were shown to act synergistically with imatinib (Yu et al. 2002b). Bay 43-9006, a Raf inhibitor (Wilhelm et al. 2004) has in vitro activity against imatinib-resistant cell lines (Choi et al. 2002). This compound was tested in a phase I trial of patients with imatinib-resistant CML. Results have not yet been published. One potentially important application for inhibitors of MAP kinases could arise if MAP kinase activation by Bcr-Abl-independent signals was indeed important for disease persistence, as was suggested by a recent study that showed upregulation of MAP kinase activity in CD34+ progenitor cells from CML patients treated ex vivo with imatinib (Chu et al. 2004). However, the relevance of this finding for persistence in vivo remains to be established. The fact that MAP kinase inhibitors failed to enhance the effects of imatinib on "quiescent" CML progenitor cells does not support this notion (Jorgensen et al. 2005).

5.3.3 Inhibitors of Phosphatidyl-Inositol 3 Kinase (PI3 Kinase) Signaling

PI3K is responsible for the conversion of phosphatidyl inositol-4,5 bisphosphate to phosphatidyl inositol-3,4,5 trisphosphate (PIP_3), a central second messenger in proliferation and survival pathways (Kharas and Fruman 2005). PIP_3 binds to the inner leaflet of the cell membrane, where it facilitates the binding of proteins with pleckstrin homology (PH) domains. PI3K is composed of a catalytic and a regulatory subunit, for both of which there are several isoforms. At least 3 different mechanisms are involved in PI3K activation by Bcr-Abl. The first involves binding of the Grb2 SH2 domain to phosphorylated tyrosine177 of Bcr (Pendergast et al. 1993). Grb2 interacts with Gab2, another adaptor protein that in turn binds one of the SH2 domains of the p85 subunit of PI3K (Sattler et al. 2002). A second mechanism relies on a complex that consists of CrkL bound to the Abl SH3 domain, with tyrosine phosphorylated Cbl mediating between the CrkL and p85 SH2 domains (Gaston et al. 2004). A third option is a Shc-mediated interaction between the SH2 domains of Abl and Grb2 (Tauchi et al. 1994). Current thinking holds that Bcr-Abl and the various adaptor proteins form a multimeric complex that includes and activates PI3K. Various PH domain-containing proteins, including the serine/threonine kinases, PDK-1 and Akt, bind to the cell membrane in a PIP_3-dependent manner (Fig. 5.8). Binding to the cell membrane induces a conformational change in Akt that renders it a substrate for PDK-1, which results in activation (reviewed in Kharas and Fruman 2005). Akt functions as a master switch in PI3K signaling, targeting several major downstream pathways. Probably most important is mammalian target of rapamycin (mTOR), an evolutionary conserved serine threonine kinase. Akt activates mTOR mainly indirectly, via phosphorylation of tuberous sclerosis 2 (TSC2). Unphosphorylated TSC2, in complex with TSC1, inactivates the small GTPase Rheb. This inhibition is released by Akt phosphorylation of TSC2, which leads to mTOR activation by Rheb. mTOR is a master regulator of translation that drives global responses to growth stimuli. Its major downstream mediators are p70S6 kinase and 4E-BP1 (Ly et al. 2003). In addition to mTOR, substrates of Akt include forkhead transcription factors like FOXO3 and glycogen synthetase kinase β (GSKβ). In Bcr-Abl expressing cells, FOXO3 is targeted for degradation by Akt mediated phosphorylation, resulting in downregulation of FOXO3 target genes (Komatsu et al. 2003). GSK, which negatively regulates cyclin D1 and β-catenin by phosphorylation, is kept in an inactive state when phosphorylated by Akt (Kharas and Fruman 2005). Lastly, Akt has also been shown to phosphorylate the proapoptotic protein Bad, resulting in its sequestration and inactivation by 14-3-3 proteins (Zha et al. 1996) as well as Mdm2, which results in enhanced degradation of the p53 tumor suppresser protein (Goetz et al. 2001). Thus, the PI3K network offers multiple targets, including PI3K itself, Akt, and mTOR.

5.3.4 PI3 Kinase Inhibitors

In vitro and in vivo data have implicated PI3K as an important mediator of *BCR-ABL*-induced leukemogenesis (Skorski et al. 1995). Currently available PI3K inhibitors such as wortmannin and LY 294002 do not discriminate between isoforms of PI3K. Although useful in the laboratory, they are too toxic to be used as drugs. The fact that the expression of PI3K isoforms is to some extent tissue specific may offer the opportunity to selectively target malignant cells (Kang et al. 2005). The expectation is that such isoform-specific inhibitors would be less toxic than pan-PI3K inhibitors.

5.3.5 PDK1 Inhibitors

The role of PDK-1 in Bcr-Abl-mediated leukemogenesis has not been studied. However, based on known biochemical pathways, the PDK-1 inhibitor OSU-03012 was recently tested in cell lines expressing the E255K and T315I mutants of Bcr-Abl. The investigators showed this agent to be growth inhibitory with IC_{50} concentrations of 14 and 30 µM, respectively (Tseng et al. 2005). Activity was correlated with inhibition of Akt. Although these concentrations are not achievable in the plasma, synergism was observed at lower doses, and could possibly be exploited in combination therapy regimens.

5.3.6 mTOR Inhibitors

Rapamycin, an antibiotic isolated from a strain of *Streptococcus hygroscopicus* collected on Easter Island (Rapa Nui), is a powerful immunosuppressant. The cellular target of rapamycin is FKBP-12, a 12-kD protein that is also the target for FK506, another immunosuppressive agent. Rapamycin (Sirolimus) is approved for prevention of renal transplant rejection but has also strong antiproliferative properties in many tumors. Rapamycin and its derivative RAD001 inhibit Bcr-Abl-dependent cell growth in vitro and in vivo (Ly et al. 2003; Mohi et al. 2004). Synergism depends on residual sensitivity of the leukemia cells to imatinib (Dengler et al. 2005), a common theme with imatinib combinations (La Rosee et al. 2004). RAD001 is currently in phase I testing in patients with imatinib-resistant leukemia. Results are not yet available.

5.4 Nonkinase Targets Related to Bcr-Abl and Semispecific Agents

5.4.1 Inhibitors of Protein Interaction

Bcr-Abl contains several structural motifs that allow for binding of other proteins involved in signal transduction. In some instances small molecules or peptides that specifically block important interactions have been developed.

5.4.1.1 Dimerization Domain of Bcr

The N-terminus of Bcr contains a coiled-coil motif, which is required for dimerization. Dimerization in turn is critical for transformation (He et al. 2002; McWhirter et al. 1993; Smith et al. 2003). Crystallography revealed a rather specific structure of the dimerization domain (Zhao et al. 2002) that may allow developing specific inhibitors.

5.4.1.2 Tyrosine 177 and Grb2

Phosphorylated tyrosine 177 binds Grb2, an interaction that is crucial for activation of MAP kinase signaling via binding of the SH3 domain of Grb2 to Sos, which stabilizes Ras in its active GTP-bound form (Pendergast et al. 1993). Peptides that disrupt this interaction inhibit the growth of Bcr-Abl-positive cells (Kardinal et al. 2001). A small molecule inhibitor could conceivably be developed to the same effect. More recently it was shown that Grb2 is also required for binding of the Gab2 adaptor protein, which links Bcr-Abl to the PI3 kinase pathway (Sattler et al. 2002). It has not been reported whether the aforementioned peptides disrupt this interaction.

5.4.1.3 Additional Targets in Bcr-Abl

There are additional targets in Bcr-Abl that could potentially be exploited, including the Abl SH3 domain. The SH3 domain appears to have an inhibitory role, as deletion of SH3 activates the kinase. Several proteins are known to bind SH3, and at least one of them, Pag (MSP23) inhibits Abl kinase (Wen and van Etten 1997). This has not been formally exploited for drug development. Lastly, it may be possible to disrupt the multimeric Bcr-Abl signaling complex by interfering with binding of other proteins in the complex, including CrkL and Cbl. As this complex is held together by multiple interactions (Gaston et al. 2004), this task could hardly be accomplished with a single compound.

5.4.2 Intracellular Redistribution

In contrast to Abl, Bcr-Abl is localized almost exclusively in the cytoplasm in association with F-actin. Disruption of the F-actin binding site in the C-terminus of Abl impairs cellular transformation (McWhirter and Wang 1993). Interestingly, keeping kinase active Bcr-Abl in the cytoplasm and out of the nucleus appears to be important. Thus, inhibition of Bcr-Abl kinase with imatinib leads to nuclear accumulation. If such cells are then released from kinase inhibition in the presence of leptomycin B, a drug that inhibits Bcr-Abl's export from the nucleus into the cytoplasm, trapping active kinase in the nucleus, apoptosis is induced (Vigneri and Wang 2001). With nuclear export inhibitors that are less toxic than leptomycin, this could potentially be exploited therapeutically. Obviously, this strategy is dependent on achieving inhibition of Bcr-Abl kinase in the first place and would not be effective in the case of the T315I mutant.

5.4.3 Semispecific Agents

It is obvious that inhibition of targets "farther away" from Bcr-Abl as the disease-initiating protein will be less specific, as they will be downstream of an increasing number of physiological signaling networks. Inhibitors of canonical physiologic processes such as histone deacetylation or cell cycle progression should not be referred to as "targeted" therapeutics as their specificity is strictly biochemical but not biological. One could easily argue that these agents are in principle not different from some conventional anticancer drugs like topoisomerase II inhibitors that target a specific enzyme but not specific cancer cells.

Flavopiridol is a broad spectrum inhibitor of cyclin-dependent kinases (Sausville et al. 1999), a class of serine/threonine kinases that are essential for cell cycle progression. Synergism with imatinib has been demonstrated in *BCR-ABL*-positive cell lines (Yu et al. 2002a) and synergism with the proteasome inhibitor bortezomib in imatinib-resistant lines (Dai et al. 2004). Flavopiridol is currently being tested with imatinib in a phase I study in patients with imatinib-resistant CML. Results are not yet available, but given the overall rather sobering results with this agent in clinical trials of other malignancies, optimism is guarded (Blagosklonny 2004).

Bortezomib (Velcade), a drug with excellent activity in multiple myeloma, has been tested as a single agent in a phase II study. Moderate responses were seen in some patients, such as return from accelerated phase to chronic phase but not cytogenetic responses or lasting remissions (Cortes et al. 2003a). The final results of this trial have not yet been published.

Histone deacetylase inhibitors are another novel class of antileukemic agents. Synergy with imatinib has been shown in vitro, although at least some effects may be mediated via inhibition of Hsp90 (Nimmanapalli et al. 2003b).

Demethylating agents such as decitabine have rather impressive single agent activity in CML (Kantarjian et al. 1997) and are synergistic with imatinib in vitro (La Rosee et al. 2004). A clinical trial in patients with imatinib refractory CML is ongoing but results have not yet been reported.

Oblimersen, a Bcl2 antisense molecule, has shown activity in a nude mouse model of imatinib-resistant Ph-positive leukemia (Tauchi et al. 2003). A clinical trial in combination with imatinib in CML patients with resistance to imatinib is ongoing but results have not yet been published.

5.5 Summary and Perspective

Given its central role in the pathogenesis of CML, Bcr-Abl is undoubtedly the optimal drug target in this disease. The strongest confirmation for this is the clinical success of imatinib. Can we do still better? Alternative Abl inhibitors such as dasatinib and nilotinib show promise in relapsed or refractory disease, raising the question whether they will eventually replace imatinib as the first line therapy in patients with newly diagnosed chronic phase CML. This will depend on efficacy as much as on tolerability. Both agents are not only active against KD mutants but they are also much more potent against unmutated Bcr-Abl. One would suspect that this will translate into better outcomes. However, in view of the high rates of complete cytogenetic response and the excellent progression-free and overall survival with imatinib, long observation times and large cohorts of patients will be required to demonstrate superiority of a novel Abl kinase inhibitor using these endpoints. Molecular endpoints, such as a major (Hughes et al. 2003) or complete molecular response (sustained negativity by RT-PCR) are more likely to show differences within a reasonable period of follow-up that may later translate into improved progression-free and overall survival. A word of caution is warranted. Although very likely, it remains to be formally proven that responses are equally durable regardless of whether they were attained with standard dose imatinib or with a highly potent Abl inhibitor (or high doses of imatinib). A related question is whether more potent Abl inhibitors will be capable of eradicating the leukemic cell clone. Clinical observations and mathematical modeling suggest that imatinib, unlike allografting, is not capable of eliminating residual disease (Cortes et al. 2004; Kim et al. 2004; Lange et al. 2003, 2005; Mauro et al. 2004), as it does not deplete the leukemic stem cell pool (Michor et al. 2005), and lifelong therapy is required. It is not known whether more potent Abl inhibitors will be different. If not, then the side effects of treating a disease that is increasingly perceived as a chronic ailment rather than as a life threatening condition may become the central issue.

One of the most fascinating observations with Bcr-Abl-kinase-targeted therapy of CML is that acquired resistance is, at least in the majority of cases, associated with reactivation of Bcr-Abl. This implies that Bcr-Abl (and perhaps other activating tyrosine kinase mutations) have a high degree of target cell specificity and consequently cannot easily be replaced by other mutations. From the therapeutic standpoint this is good news as there continues to be one uniform drug target at the time of relapse, rather than a diversity of genetic lesions. It also implies that targets other than Bcr-Abl remain second choice, even at the time of disease recurrence. A different scenario would arise if leukemic stem cells were found to shift to physiological signaling pathways to maintain survival in the face of Bcr-Abl inhibition. If such pathways were essential under these conditions, they would be excellent targets for drug combinations.

Acknowledgements. The author is grateful to Chris Koontz, OHSU, for editorial assistance and John M. Goldman, NHLBI, Bethesda, USA, for helpful discussions.

References

Adrian FJ, Ding Q, Sim T, Velentza A, Sloan C, Liu Y, Zhang G, Hur W, Ding S, Manley P, Mestan J, Fabbro D, Gray NS (2006) Allosteric inhibitors of Bcr-abl-dependent cell proliferation. Nat Chem Biol 2:95–102

Al Ali HK, Heinrich MC, Lange T, Krahl R, Mueller M, Muller C, Niederwieser D, Druker BJ, Deininger MW (2004) High incidence of BCR-ABL kinase domain mutations and absence of mutations of the PDGFR and KIT activation loops in CML patients with secondary resistance to imatinib. Hematol J 5:55–60

Anafi M, Gazit A, Gilon C, Ben Neriah Y, Levitzki A (1992) Selective interactions of transforming and normal abl proteins with ATP, tyrosine-copolymer substrates, tyrphostins. J Biol Chem 267:4518–4523

Anafi M, Gazit A, Zehavi A, Ben Neriah Y, Levitzki A (1993) Tyrphostin-induced inhibition of p210bcr-abl tyrosine kinase activity induces K562 to differentiate. Blood 82:3524–3529

Ashar HR, James L, Gray K, Carr D, Black S, Armstrong L, Bishop WR, Kirschmeier P (2000) Farnesyl transferase inhibitors block the farnesylation of CENP-E and CENP-F and alter the association of CENP-E with the microtubules. J Biol Chem 275:30451–30457

Ashar HR, James L, Gray K, Carr D, McGuirk M, Maxwell E, Black S, Armstrong L, Doll RJ, Taveras AG, Bishop WR, Kirschmeier P (2001) The farnesyl transferase inhibitor SCH 66336 induces a G(2) → M or G(1) pause in sensitive human tumor cell lines. Exp Cell Res 262:17–27

Azam M, Latek RR, Daley GQ (2003) Mechanisms of autoinhibition and STI-571/imatinib resistance revealed by mutagenesis of BCR-ABL. Cell 112:831–843

Barnett SF, Defeo-Jones D, Fu S, Hancock PJ, Haskell KM, Jones RE, Kahana JA, Kral AM, Leander K, Lee LL, Malinowski J, McAvoy EM, Nahas DD, Robinson RG, Huber HE (2005) Identification and characterization of pleckstrin-homology-domain-dependent and isoenzyme-specific Akt inhibitors. Biochem J 385:399–408

Barthe C, Cony-Makhoul P, Melo JV, Mahon JR (2001) Roots of clinical resistance to STI-571 cancer therapy. Science 293:2163

Basso AD, Mirza A, Liu G, Long BJ, Bishop WR, Kirschmeier P (2005) The FTI SCH66336 (Lonafarnib) inhibits Rheb farnesylation and mTOR signaling: Role in FTI enhancement of taxane and tamoxifen antitumor activity. J Biol Chem 280:31101–31108

Beran M, Cao X, Estrov Z, Jeha S, Jin G, O'Brien S, Talpaz M, Arlinghaus RB, Lydon NB, Kantarjian H (1998) Selective inhibition of cell proliferation and BCR-ABL phosphorylation in acute lymphoblastic leukemia cells expressing Mr 190,000 BCR-ABL protein by a tyrosine kinase inhibitor (CGP-57148). Clin Cancer Res 4:1661–1672

Blagosklonny MV (2004) Flavopiridol, an inhibitor of transcription: implications, problems and solutions. Cell Cycle 3:1537–1542

Branford S, Rudzki Z, Walsh S, Grigg A, Arthur C, Taylor K, Herrmann R, Lynch KP, Hughes TP (2002) High frequency of point mutations clustered within the adenosine triphosphate-binding region of BCR/ABL in patients with chronic myeloid leukemia or Ph-positive acute lymphoblastic leukemia who develop imatinib (STI571) resistance. Blood 99:3472–3475

Buchdunger E, Zimmermann J, Mett H, Meyer T, Muller M, Druker BJ, Lydon NB (1996) Inhibition of the Abl protein-tyrosine kinase in vitro and in vivo by a 2-phenylaminopyrimidine derivative. Cancer Res 56:100–104

Burger H, Nooter K (2004) Pharmacokinetic resistance to imatinib mesylate: role of the ABC drug pumps ABCG2 (BCRP) and ABCB1 (MDR1) in the oral bioavailability of imatinib. Cell Cycle 3:1502–1505

Burgess MR, Skaggs BJ, Shah NP, Lee FY, Sawyers CL (2005) Comparative analysis of two clinically active BCR-ABL kinase inhibitors reveals the role of conformation-specific binding in resistance. Proc Natl Acad Sci 102:3395–3400

Burley S (2005) Application of FAST™ fragment-based lead discovery and structure-guided design to discovery of small molecule inhibitors of BCR-ABL tyrosine kinase active against the T315I imatinib-resistant mutant. Blood 106:206a

Chandra J, Tracy J, Loegering D, Flatten K, Verstovsek S, Beran M, Gorre M, Estrov Z, Donato N, Talpaz M, Sawyers C, Bhalla K, Karp J, Sausville E, Kaufmann SH (2005) Adaphostin-induced oxidative stress overcomes bcr/abl mutation-dependent and -independent imatinib resistance. Blood 15:2501–2506

Choi YJ, Qing W, White S, Gorre M, Sawyers CL, Bollag G (2002) Imatinib-resistant cell lines are sensitive to the Raf inhibitor BAY 43-9006. Blood 100:369A

Chu S, Holtz M, Gupta M, Bhatia R (2004) BCR/ABL kinase inhibition by imatinib mesylate enhances MAP kinase activity in chronic myelogenous leukemia CD34+ cells. Blood 103:3167–3174

Chu S, Xu H, Shah NP, Snyder DS, Forman SJ, Sawyers CL, Bhatia R (2005) Detection of BCR-ABL kinase mutations in CD34+ cells from chronic myelogenous leukemia patients in complete cytogenetic remission on imatinib mesylate treatment. Blood 105:2093–2098

Corbin AS, Buchdunger E, Pascal F, Druker BJ (2002) Analysis of the structural basis of specificity of inhibition of the Abl kinase by STI571. J Biol Chem 277:32214–32219

Corbin AS, Rosee PL, Stoffregen EP, Druker BJ, Deininger MW (2003) Several Bcr-Abl kinase domain mutants associated with imatinib mesylate resistance remain sensitive to imatinib. Blood 101:4611–4614

Cortes J, Giles F, O'Brien S, Beran M, McConkey D, Wright J, Schenkein D, Patel G, Verstovsek S, Pate O, Talpaz M, Kantarjian H (2003 a) Phase II study of bortezomib (Velcade, formerly PS-341) for patients with imatinib-refractory chronic myeloid leukemia (CML) in chronic (CP) or accelerated phase (AP). Blood 312 ab

Cortes J, Giles F, O'Brien S, Thomas D, Garcia-Manero G, Rios MB, Faderl S, Verstovsek S, Ferrajoli A, Freireich EJ, Talpaz M, Kantarjian H (2003 b) Result of high-dose imatinib mesylate in patients with Philadelphia chromosome – positive chronic myeloid leukemia after failure of interferon-α. Blood 102:83–86

Cortes J, O'Brien S, Kantarjian H (2004) Discontinuation of imatinib therapy after achieving a molecular response. Blood 104:2204–2205

Cortez D, Kadlec L, Pendergast AM (1995) Structural and signaling requirements for BCR-ABL-mediated transformation and inhibition of apoptosis. Mol Cell Biol 15:5531–5541

Cortez D, Reuther GW, Pendergast AM (1997) The BCR-ABL tyrosine kinase activates mitotic signaling pathways and stimulates G1-to-S phase transition in hematopoietic cells. Oncogene 15:2333–2342

Cowan-Jacob SW, Guez V, Fendrich G, Griffin JD, Fabbro D, Furet P, Liebetanz J, Mestan J, Manley PW (2004) Imatinib (STI571) resistance in chronic myelogenous leukemia: molecular basis of the underlying mechanisms and potential strategies for treatment. Mini Rev Med Chem 4:285–299

Crossman LC, Druker BJ, Deininger MW, Pirmohamed M, Wang L, Clark RE (2005) hOCT 1 and resistance to imatinib. Blood 106:1133–1134

Dai Y, Rahmani M, Pei XY, Dent P, Grant S (2004) Bortezomib and flavopiridol interact synergistically to induce apoptosis in chronic myeloid leukemia cells resistant to imatinib mesylate through both Bcr/Abl-dependent and -independent mechanisms. Blood 104:509–518

Daley GQ, Van Etten RA, Baltimore D (1990) Induction of chronic myelogenous leukemia in mice by the P210bcr/abl gene of the Philadelphia chromosome. Science 247:824–830

Deininger M, Goldman JM, Lydon NB, Melo JV (1997) The tyrosine kinase inhibitor CGP57148B selectively inhibits the growth of BCR-ABL positive cells. Blood 90:3691–3698

Deininger M, Buchdunger E, Druker BJ (2005) The development of imatinib as a therapeutic agent for chronic myeloid leukemia. Blood 105:2640–2653

Deininger MW, Holyoake TL (2005) Can we afford to let sleeping dogs lie? Blood 105:1840–1841

Deininger MW, Goldman JM, Melo JV (2000) The molecular biology of chronic myeloid leukemia. Blood 96:3343–3356

Deininger MW, O'Brien SG, Ford JM, Druker BJ (2003) Practical management of patients with chronic myeloid leukemia receiving imatinib. J Clin Oncol 21:1637–1647

Dengler J, von Bubnoff N, Decker T, Peschel C, Duyster J (2005) Combination of imatinib with rapamycin or RAD001 acts synergistically only in Bcr-Abl-positive cells with moderate resistance to imatinib. Leukemia 19:1835–1838

Dinulescu DM, Wood LJ, Shen L, Loriaux M, Corless CL, Gross AW, Ren R, Deininger MW, Druker BJ (2003) c-CBL is not required for leukemia induction by Bcr-Abl in mice. Oncogene 22:8852–8860

Donato NJ, Wu JY, Stapley J, Gallick G, Lin H, Arlinghaus R, Talpaz M (2003) BCR-ABL independence and LYN kinase overexpression in chronic myelogenous leukemia cells selected for resistance to STI571. Blood 101:690–698

Dorsey JF, Jove R, Kraker AJ, Wu J (2000) The pyrido[2,3-d]pyrimidine derivative PD180970 inhibits p210Bcr-Abl tyrosine kinase and induces apoptosis of K562 leukemic cells. Cancer Res 60:3127–3131

Druker BJ, Tamura S, Buchdunger E, Ohno S, Segal GM, Fanning S, Zimmermann J, Lydon NB (1996) Effects of a selective inhibitor of the Abl tyrosine kinase on the growth of Bcr-Abl positive cells. Nat Med 2:561–566

Druker BJ, Sawyers CL, Kantarjian H, Resta DJ, Reese SF, Ford JM, Capdeville R, Talpaz M (2001 a) Activity of a specific inhibitor of the BCR-ABL tyrosine kinase in the blast crisis of chronic myeloid leukemia and acute lymphoblastic leukemia with the Philadelphia chromosome. N Engl J Med 344:1038–1042

Druker BJ, Talpaz M, Resta DJ, Peng B, Buchdunger E, Ford JM, Lydon NB, Kantarjian H, Capdeville R, Ohno-Jones S, Sawyers CL (2001 b) Efficacy and safety of a specific inhibitor of the BCR-ABL tyrosine kinase in chronic myeloid leukemia. N Engl J Med 344:1031–1037

Gambacorti-Passerini C, Barni R, le Coutre P, Zucchetti M, Cabrita G, Cleris L, Rossi F, Gianazza E, Brueggen J, Cozens R, Pioltelli P, Pogliani E, Corneo G, Formelli F, D'Incalci M (2000) Role of alpha1 acid glycoprotein in the in vivo resistance of human BCR-ABL(+) leukemic cells to the abl inhibitor STI571. J Natl Cancer Inst 92:1641–1650

Gaston I, Johnson KJ, Oda T, Bhat A, Reis M, Langdon W, Shen L, Deininger MW, Druker BJ (2004) Coexistence of phosphotyrosine-dependent and -independent interactions between Cbl and Bcr-Abl. Exp Hematol 32:113–121

Gazit A, Yaish P, Gilon C, Levitzki A (1989) Tyrphostins I: synthesis and biological activity of protein tyrosine kinase inhibitors. J Med Chem 32:2344–2352

Gleich GJ, Leiferman KM, Pardanani A, Tefferi A, Butterfield JH (2002) Treatment of hypereosinophilic syndrome with imatinib mesilate. Lancet 359:1577–1578

Goetz AW, van der KH, Maya R, Oren M, Aulitzky WE (2001) Requirement for Mdm2 in the survival effects of Bcr-Abl and interleukin 3 in hematopoietic cells. Cancer Res 61:7635–7641

Golas JM, Arndt K, Etienne C, Lucas J, Nardin D, Gibbons J, Frost P, Ye F, Boschelli DH, Boschelli F (2003) SKI-606, a 4-anilino-3-quinolinecarbonitrile dual inhibitor of Src and Abl kinases, is a potent antiproliferative agent against chronic myelogenous leukemia cells in culture and causes regression of K562 xenografts in nude mice. Cancer Res 63:375–381

Gorre ME, Mohammed M, Ellwood K, Hsu N, Paquette R, Rao PN, Sawyers CL (2001) Clinical resistance to STI-571 cancer therapy caused by BCR-ABL gene mutation or amplification. Science 293:876–880

Gorre ME, Ellwood-Yen K, Chiosis G, Rosen N, Sawyers CL (2002) BCR-ABL point mutants isolated from patients with imatinib mesylate-resistant chronic myeloid leukemia remain sensitive to inhibitors of the BCR-ABL chaperone heat shock protein 90. Blood 100:3041–3044

Graham SM, Jorgensen HG, Allan E, Pearson C, Alcorn MJ, Richmond L, Holyoake TL (2002) Primitive, quiescent, Philadelphia-positive stem cells from patients with chronic myeloid leukemia are insensitive to STI571 in vitro. Blood 99:319–325

Guilhot F (2004) Sustained durability of responses plus high rates of cytogenetic responses result in long-term benefit for newly diagnosed chronic phase chronic myeloid leukemia (CML-CP) treated with imatinib (IM) therapy: update from the IRIS Study. Blood 104:10 a

Gumireddy K, Baker SJ, Cosenza SC, John P, Kang AD, Robell KA, Reddy MV, Reddy EP (2005) A non-ATP-competitive inhibitor of BCR-ABL overrides imatinib resistance. Proc Natl Acad Sci 102(6):1992–1997

Hantschel O, Nagar B, Guettler S, Kretzschmar J, Dorey K, Kuriyan J, Superti-Furga G (2003) A myristoyl/phosphotyrosine switch regulates c-Abl. Cell 112:845–857

He Y, Wertheim JA, Xu L, Miller JP, Karnell FG, Choi JK, Ren R, Pear WS (2002) The coiled-coil domain and Tyr177 of bcr are required to induce a murine chronic myelogenous leukemia-like disease by bcr/abl. Blood 99:2957–2968

Hegedus T, Orfi L, Seprodi A, Varadi A, Sarkadi B, Keri G (2002) Interaction of tyrosine kinase inhibitors with the human multidrug transporter proteins, MDR1 and MRP1. Biochim Biophys Acta 1587:318–325

Heinrich MC, Griffith DJ, Druker BJ, Wait CL, Ott KA, Zigler AJ (2000) Inhibition of c-kit receptor tyrosine kinase activity by STI 571, a selective tyrosine kinase inhibitor. Blood 96:925–932

Hochhaus A, Kreil S, Corbin AS, La Rosee P, Muller MC, Lahaye T, Hanfstein B, Schoch C, Cross NC, Berger U, Gschaidmeier H, Druker BJ, Hehlmann R (2002) Molecular and chromosomal mechanisms of resistance to imatinib (STI571) therapy. Leukemia 16:2190–2196

Hofmann WK, Jones LC, Lemp NA, de Vos S, Gschaidmeier H, Hoelzer D, Ottmann OG, Koeffler HP (2002) Ph(+) acute lymphoblastic leukemia resistant to the tyrosine kinase inhibitor STI571 has a unique BCR-ABL gene mutation. Blood 99:1860–1862

Holyoake T, Jiang X, Eaves C, Eaves A (1999) Isolation of a highly quiescent subpopulation of primitive leukemic cells in chronic myeloid leukemia. Blood 94:2056–2064

Hoover RR, Mahon FX, Melo JV, Daley GQ (2002) Overcoming STI571 resistance with the farnesyl transferase inhibitor SCH66336. Blood 100:1068–1071

Hu Y, Liu Y, Pelletier S, Buchdunger E, Warmuth M, Fabbro D, Hallek M, Van Etten RA, Li S (2004) Requirement of Src kinases Lyn, Hck and Fgr for BCR-ABL1-induced B-lymphoblastic leukemia but not chronic myeloid leukemia. Nat Genet 36:453–461

Hughes TP, Kaeda J, Branford S, Rudzki Z, Hochhaus A, Hensley ML, Gathmann I, Bolton AE, van Hoomissen IC, Goldman JM, Radich JP (2003) Frequency of major molecular responses to imatinib or interferon alfa plus cytarabine in newly diagnosed chronic myeloid leukemia. N Engl J Med 349:1423–1432

Huron DR, Gorre ME, Kraker AJ, Sawyers CL, Rosen N, Moasser MM (2003) A novel pyridopyrimidine inhibitor of Abl kinase is a picomolar inhibitor of Bcr-Abl-driven K562 cells and is effective against STI571-resistant Bcr-Abl mutants. Clin Cancer Res 9:1267–1273

Jiang X, Zhao Y, Chan P, Eaves A, Eaves C (2003) Quantitative real-time RT-PCR analysis shows BCR-ABL expression progressively decreases as primitive leukemic cells from patients with chronic myeloid leukemia (CML) differentiate in vivo. Exp Hematol 31: 228–229

Jorgensen HG, Allan EK, Graham SM, Godden JL, Richmond L, Elliott MA, Mountford JC, Eaves CJ, Holyoake TL (2005) Lonafarnib reduces the resistance of primitive quiescent CML cells to imatinib mesylate in vitro. Leukemia 19:1184–1191

Kang S, Song J, Kang J, Kang H, Lee D, Lee Y, Park D (2005) Suppression of the alpha-isoform of class II phosphoinositide 3-kinase gene expression leads to apoptotic cell death. Biochem Biophys Res Commun 329:6–10

Kantarjian HM, O'Brien SM, Keating M, Beran M, Estey E, Giralt S, Kornblau S, Rios MB, de Vos D, Talpaz M (1997) Results of decitabine therapy in the accelerated and blastic phases of chronic myelogenous leukemia. Leukemia 11:1617–1620

Kantarjian H, Sawyers C, Hochhaus A, Guilhot F, Schiffer C, Gambacorti-Passerini C, Niederwieser D, Resta D, Capdeville R, Zoellner U, Talpaz M, Druker B (2002) Hematologic and cytogenetic responses to imatinib mesylate in chronic myelogenous leukemia. N Engl J Med 346:645–652

Kantarjian H, Talpaz M, O'Brien S, Garcia-Manero G, Verstovsek S, Giles F, Rios MB, Shan J, Letvak L, Thomas D, Faderl S, Ferrajoli A, Cortes J (2004) High-dose imatinib mesylate therapy in newly diagnosed Philadelphia chromosome-positive chronic phase chronic myeloid leukemia. Blood 103:2873–2878

Kantarjian H, Ottmann OG, Cortes J, Wassmann B, Wunderle L, Bhalla K, Jones D, Hochhaus A, Rae P, Alland L, Dugan M, Albitar M, Giles F (2005) AMN107, a novel aminopyrimidine inhibitor of Bcr-Abl, has significant activity in imatinib-resistant chronic myeloid leukemia (CML) or Philadelphia-chromosome positive acute lymphoid leukemia (Ph + ALL). Blood 106:15 a

Kardinal C, Konkol B, Lin H, Eulitz M, Schmidt EK, Estrov Z, Talpaz M, Arlinghaus RB, Feller SM (2001) Chronic myelogenous leukemia blast cell proliferation is inhibited by peptides that disrupt Grb2-SoS complexes. Blood 98:1773–1781

Kaur G, Sausville EA (1996) Altered physical state of p210bcr-abl in tyrphostin AG957-treated K562 cells. Anticancer Drugs 7:815–824

Kaur G, Gazit A, Levitzki A, Stowe E, Cooney DA, Sausville EA (1994) Tyrphostin induced growth inhibition: correlation with effect on p210bcr-abl autokinase activity in K562 chronic myelogenous leukemia. Anticancer Drugs 5:213–222

Kaur G, Narayanan VL, Risbood PA, Hollingshead MG, Stinson SF, Varma RK, Sausville EA (2005) Synthesis, structure-activity relationship, p210(bcr-abl) protein tyrosine kinase activity of novel AG 957 analogs. Bioorg Med Chem 13:1749–1761

Kharas MG, Fruman DA (2005) ABL oncogenes and phosphoinositide 3-kinase: mechanism of activation and downstream effectors. Cancer Res 65:2047–2053

Kim Y-J, Kim D-W, Lee S, Eom K-S, Min C-K, Kim H-J, Lee J-W, Min W-S, Kim C-C (2004) Monitoring of BCR-ABL transcript levels after discontinuation of imatinib therapy in chronic myelogenous leukemia patients achieving complete cytogenetic response. Blood 104:255 b

Komatsu N, Watanabe T, Uchida M, Mori M, Kirito K, Kikuchi S, Liu Q, Tauchi T, Miyazawa K, Endo H, Nagai T, Ozawa K (2003) A member of Forkhead transcription factor FKHRL1 is a downstream effector of STI571-induced cell cycle arrest in BCR-ABL-expressing cells. J Biol Chem 278:6411–6419

Kraker AJ, Hartl BG, Amar AM, Barvian MR, Showalter HD, Moore CW (2000) Biochemical and cellular effects of c-Src kinase-selective pyrido[2,3-d]pyrimidine tyrosine kinase inhibitors. Biochem Pharmacol 60:885–898

La Rosee P, Corbin AS, Stoffregen EP, Deininger MW, Druker BJ (2002) Activity of the Bcr-Abl kinase inhibitor PD180970 against clinically relevant Bcr-Abl isoforms that cause resistance to imatinib mesylate (Gleevec, STI571). Cancer Res 62:7149–7153

La Rosee P, Johnson K, Corbin AS, Stoffregen EP, Moseson EM, Willis S, Mauro MM, Melo JV, Deininger MW, Druker BJ (2004) In vitro efficacy of combined treatment depends on the underlying mechanism of resistance in imatinib-resistant Bcr-Abl-positive cell lines. Blood 103:208–215

Lange T, Niederwieser DW, Deininger MW (2003) Residual disease in chronic myeloid leukemia after induction of molecular remission. N Engl J Med 349:1483–1484

Lange T, Bumm T, Mueller M, Otto S, Al Ali HK, Grommisch L, Musiol S, Franke C, Krahl R, Niederwieser D, Deininger MW (2005) Durability of molecular remission in chronic myeloid leukemia patients treated with imatinib vs allogeneic stem cell transplantation. Leukemia 19:1262–1265

le Coutre P, Mologni L, Cleris L, Marchesi E, Buchdunger E, Giardini R, Formelli F, Gambacorti-Passerini C (1999) In vivo eradication of human BCR/ABL-positive leukemia cells with an ABL kinase inhibitor. J Natl Cancer Inst 91:163–168

le Coutre P, Tassi E, Varella-Garcia M, Barni R, Mologni L, Cabrita G, Marchesi E, Supino R, Gambacorti-Passerini C (2000) Induction of resistance to the Abelson inhibitor STI571 in human leukemic cells through gene amplification. Blood 95:1758–1766

le Coutre P, Kreuzer KA, Na IK, Lupberger J, Holdoff M, Appelt C, Schwarz M, Muller C, Gambacorti-Passerini C, Platzbecker U, Bonnet R, Ehninger G, Schmidt CA (2002) Determination of alpha-1 acid glycoprotein in patients with Ph+ chronic myeloid leukemia during the first 13 weeks of therapy with STI571. Blood Cells Mol Dis 28:75–85

Lee FY, Lombardo L, Borzilleri R, Camuso A, Castaneda S, Donato NJ, Fager K, Flefleh C, Gray H, Inigo I, Kan D, Luo R, Pang S, Wem ML, Wild R, Wong TW, Talpaz M, Kramer R (2004) BMS-354825 – a potent SRC/ABL kinase inhibitor possessing curative efficacy against imatinib sensitive and resistant human CML models in vivo. AACR meeting 2004

Leguay T, Desplat V, Barthe C, Rousselot P, Reiffers J, Marit G, Mahon FX (2003) Study of mutations in the ATP binding domain and the SH2/SH3 domain of BCR-ABL in 43 chronic myeloid leukemia patients treated by imatinib mesylate (STI571). Blood 100:369 a

Li S, Gillessen S, Tomasson MH, Dranoff G, Gilliland DG, Van Etten RA (2001) Interleukin 3 and granulocyte-macrophage colony-stimulating factor are not required for induction of chronic myeloid leukemia-like myeloproliferative disease in mice by BCR/ABL. Blood 97:1442–1450

Lugo TG, Pendergast AM, Muller AJ, Witte ON (1990) Tyrosine kinase activity and transformation potency of bcr-abl oncogene products. Science 247:1079–1082

Ly C, Arechiga AF, Melo JV, Walsh CM, Ong ST (2003) Bcr-Abl kinase modulates the translation regulators ribosomal protein S6 and 4E-BP1 in chronic myelogenous leukemia cells via the mammalian target of rapamycin. Cancer Res 63:5716–5722

Mahon FX, Deininger MW, Schultheis B, Chabrol J, Reiffers J, Goldman JM, Melo JV (2000) Selection and characterization of BCR-ABL positive cell lines with differential sensitivity to the tyrosine kinase inhibitor STI571: diverse mechanisms of resistance. Blood 96: 1070–1079

Mahon FX, Belloc F, Lagarde V, Chollet C, Moreau-Gaudry F, Reiffers J, Goldman JM, Melo JV (2003) MDR1 gene overexpression confers resistance to imatinib mesylate in leukemia cell line models. Blood 101:2368–2373

Marais R, Light Y, Paterson HF, Marshall CJ (1995) Ras recruits Raf-1 to the plasma membrane for activation by tyrosine phosphorylation. EMBO J 14:3136–3145

Mauro MJ, Deininger MWN, O'Dwyer ME, Maziarz RT, Walker T, Kurilik G, Druker BJ (2003) Phase I/II study of arsenic trioxide (trisemox) in combination with imatinib mesylate (Gleevec, STI571) in patients with Gleevec-resistant chronic myelogenous leukemia in chronic phase. Blood 100:781 a

Mauro MJ, Druker BJ, Maziarz RT (2004) Divergent clinical outcome in two CML patients who discontinued imatinib therapy after achieving a molecular remission. Leuk Res 28:S71–S73

McWhirter JR, Wang JY (1993) An actin-binding function contributes to transformation by the Bcr-Abl oncoprotein of Philadelphia chromosome-positive human leukemias. EMBO J 12:1533–1546

McWhirter JR, Galasso DL, Wang JY (1993) A coiled-coil oligomerization domain of Bcr is essential for the transforming function of Bcr-Abl oncoproteins. Mol Cell Biol 13:7587–7595

Melo JV, Deininger MW (2004) Biology of chronic myelogenous leukemia-signaling pathways of initiation and transformation. Hematol Oncol Clin North Am 18:545-viii

Merante S, Orlandi E, Bernasconi P, Calatroni S, Boni M, Lazzarino M (2005) Outcome of four patients with chronic myeloid leukemia after imatinib mesylate discontinuation. Haematologica 90:979–981

Michor F, Hughes TP, Iwasa Y, Branford S, Shah NP, Sawyers CL, Nowak MA (2005) Dynamics of chronic myeloid leukaemia. Nature 435:1267–1270

Mohi MG, Boulton C, Gu TL, Sternberg DW, Neuberg D, Griffin JD, Gilliland DG, Neel BG (2004) Combination of rapamycin and protein tyrosine kinase (PTK) inhibitors for the treatment of leukemias caused by oncogenic PTKs. Proc Natl Acad Sci USA 101:3130–3135

Mow BM, Chandra J, Svingen PA, Hallgren CG, Weisberg E, Kottke TJ, Narayanan VL, Litzow MR, Griffin JD, Sausville EA, Tefferi A, Kaufmann SH (2002) Effects of the Bcr/abl kinase inhibitors STI571 and adaphostin (NSC 680410) on chronic myelogenous leukemia cells in vitro. Blood 99:664–671

Nagar B, Bornmann WG, Pellicena P, Schindler T, Veach DR, Miller WT, Clarkson B, Kuriyan J (2002) Crystal structures of the kinase domain of c-Abl in complex with the small molecule inhibitors PD173955 and imatinib (STI-571). Cancer Res 62:4236–4243

Nagar B, Hantschel O, Young MA, Scheffzek K, Veach D, Bornmann W, Clarkson B, Superti-Furga G, Kuriyan J (2003) Structural basis for the autoinhibition of c-Abl tyrosine kinase. Cell 112:859–871

Nimmanapalli R, Bali P, O'Bryan E, Fuino L, Guo F, Wu J, Houghton P, Bhalla K (2003 a) Arsenic trioxide inhibits translation of mRNA of bcr-abl, resulting in attenuation of Bcr-Abl levels and apoptosis of human leukemia cells. Cancer Res 63:7950–7958

Nimmanapalli R, Fuino L, Bali P, Gasparetto M, Glozak M, Tao J, Moscinski L, Smith C, Wu J, Jove R, Atadja P, Bhalla K (2003 b) Histone deacetylase inhibitor LAQ824 both lowers expression and promotes proteasomal degradation of Bcr-Abl and induces apoptosis of imatinib mesylate-sensitive or -refractory chronic myelogenous leukemia-blast crisis cells. Cancer Res 63:5126–5135

O'Brien SG, Guilhot F, Larson RA, Gathmann I, Baccarani M, Cervantes F, Cornelissen JJ, Fischer T, Hochhaus A, Hughes T, Lechner K, Nielsen JL, Rousselot P, Reiffers J, Saglio G, Shepherd J, Simonsson B, Gratwohl A, Goldman JM, Kantarjian H, Taylor K, Verhoef G, Bolton AE, Capdeville R, Druker BJ (2003) Imatinib compared with interferon and low-dose cytarabine for newly diagnosed chronic phase chronic myeloid leukemia. N Engl J Med 348:994–1004

O'Hare T, Pollock R, Stoffregen EP, Keats JA, Abdullah OM, Moseson EM, Rivera VM, Tang H, Metcalf III CA, Bohacek RS, Wang Y, Sundaramoorthi R, Shakespeare WC, Dalgarno D, Clackson T, Sawyer TK, Deininger MW, Druker BJ (2004 a) Inhibition of wild-type and mutant Bcr-Abl by AP23464, a potent ATP-based oncogenic protein kinase inhibitor: Implications for CML. Blood 104:2532–2539

O'Hare T, Pollock R, Stoffregen EP, Keats JA, Abdullah OM, Moseson EM, Rivera VM, Tang H, Metcalf CA, III, Bohacek RS, Wang Y, Sundaramoorthi R, Shakespeare WC, Dalgarno D, Clackson T, Sawyer TK, Deininger MW, Druker BJ (2004 b) Inhibition of wild-type and mutant Bcr-Abl by AP23464, a potent ATP-based oncogenic protein kinase inhibitor: implications for CML. Blood 104:2532–2539

O'Hare T, Walters DK, Stoffregen EP, Jia T, Manley PW, Mestan J, Cowan-Jacob SW, Lee FY, Heinrich MC, Deininger MW, Druker BJ (2005) In vitro activity of Bcr-Abl inhibitors AMN107 and BMS-354825 against clinically relevant imatinib-resistant Abl kinase domain mutants. Cancer Res 65:4500–4505

Okabe M, Uehara Y, Miyagishima T, Itaya T, Tanaka M, Kuni Eda Y, Kurosawa M, Miyazaki T (1992) Effect of herbimycin A, an antagonist of tyrosine kinase, on bcr/abl oncoprotein-associated cell proliferations: abrogative effect on the transformation of murine hematopoietic cells by transfection of a retroviral vector expressing oncoprotein P210bcr/abl and preferential inhibition on Ph1-positive leukemia cell growth. Blood 80:1330–1338

Okuda K, Weisberg E, Gilliland DG, Griffin JD (2001) ARG tyrosine kinase activity is inhibited by STI571. Blood 97:2440–2448

Parmar S, Katsoulidis E, Verma A, Li Y, Sassano A, Lal L, Majchrzak B, Ravandi F, Tallman MS, Fish EN, Platanias LC (2004) Role of the p38 mitogen-activated protein kinase pathway in the generation of the effects of imatinib mesylate (STI571) in BCR-ABL-expressing cells. J Biol Chem 279:25345–25352

Pear WS, Miller JP, Xu L, Pui JC, Soffer B, Quackenbush RC, Pendergast AM, Bronson R, Aster JC, Scott ML, Baltimore D (1998) Efficient and rapid induction of a chronic myelogenous leukemia-like myeloproliferative disease in mice receiving P210 bcr/abl-transduced bone marrow. Blood 92:3780–3792

Pendergast AM, Quilliam LA, Cripe LD, Bassing CH, Dai Z, Li N, Batzer A, Rabun KM, Der CJ, Schlessinger J et al (1993) BCR-ABL-induced oncogenesis is mediated by direct interaction with the SH2 domain of the GRB-2 adaptor protein. Cell 75:175–185

Peng B, Hayes M, Resta D, Racine-Poon A, Druker BJ, Talpaz M, Sawyers CL, Rosamilia M, Ford J, Lloyd P, Capdeville R (2004) Pharmacokinetics and pharmacodynamics of imatinib in a phase I trial with chronic myeloid leukemia patients. J Clin Oncol 22:935–942

Peters DG, Hoover RR, Gerlach MJ, Koh EY, Zhang H, Choe K, Kirschmeier P, Bishop WR, Daley GQ (2001) Activity of the farnesyl protein transferase inhibitor SCH66336 against BCR/ABL-induced murine leukemia and primary cells from patients with chronic myeloid leukemia. Blood 97:1404–1412

Ptasznik A, Nakata Y, Kalota A, Emerson SG, Gewirtz AM (2004) Short interfering RNA (siRNA) targeting the Lyn kinase induces apoptosis in primary, drug-resistant, BCR-ABL1(+) leukemia cells. Nat Med 10:1187–1189

Puil L, Liu J, Gish G, Mbamalu G, Bowtell D, Pelicci PG, Arlinghaus R, Pawson T (1994) Bcr-Abl oncoproteins bind directly to activators of the Ras signalling pathway. EMBO J 13:764–773

Raitano AB, Halpern JR, Hambuch TM, Sawyers CL (1995) The Bcr-Abl leukemia oncogene activates Jun kinase and requires Jun for transformation. Proc Natl Acad Sci USA 92:11746–11750

Ramaraj P, Singh H, Niu N, Chu S, Holtz M, Yee JK, Bhatia R (2004) Effect of mutational inactivation of tyrosine kinase activity on BCR/ABL-induced abnormalities in cell growth and adhesion in human hematopoietic progenitors. Cancer Res 64:5322–5331

Ricci C, Scappini B, Divoky V, Gatto S, Onida F, Verstovsek S, Kantarjian HM, Beran M (2002) Mutation in the ATP-binding pocket of the ABL kinase domain in an STI571-resistant BCR/ABL-positive cell line. Cancer Res 62:5995–5998

Rousselot P, Huguet F, Cayuela JM, Maarek O, Marit G, Gluckman E, Reiffers J, Mahon FX (2005) Imatinib mesylate discontinuation in patients with chronic myelogenous leukaemia in complete colecular remission for more than two tears. Blood 106:321 a

Sattler M, Mohi MG, Pride YB, Quinnan LR, Malouf NA, Podar K, Gesbert F, Iwasaki H, Li S, Van Etten RA, Gu H, Griffin JD, Neel BG (2002) Critical role for Gab2 in transformation by BCR/ABL. Cancer Cell 1:479–492

Sausville EA, Zaharevitz D, Gussio R, Meijer L, Louarn-Leost M, Kunick C, Schultz R, Lahusen T, Headlee D, Stinson S, Arbuck SG, Senderowicz A (1999) Cyclin-dependent kinases: initial approaches to exploit a novel therapeutic target. Pharmacol Ther 82:285–292

Sawyers CL, Hochhaus A, Feldman E, Goldman JM, Miller CB, Ottmann OG, Schiffer CA, Talpaz M, Guilhot F, Deininger MW, Fischer T, O'Brien SG, Stone RM, Gambacorti-Passerini CB, Russell NH, Reiffers JJ, Shea TC, Chapuis B, Coutre S, Tura S, Morra E, Larson RA, Saven A, Peschel C, Gratwohl A, Mandelli F, Ben Am M, Gathmann I, Capdeville R, Paquette RL, Druker BJ (2002) Imatinib induces hematologic and cytogenetic responses in patients with chronic myelogenous leukemia in myeloid blast crisis: results of a phase II study. Blood 99:3530–3539

Sawyers CL, Kantarjian H, Shah N, Cortes J, Paquette R, Donato NJ, Nicoll J, Bleickard E, Chen T, Talpaz M (2005) Dasatinib (BMS-354825) in patients with chronic myeloid leukemia (CML) and Philadelphia-chromosome positive acute lymphoblastic leukemia (Ph+ALL) who are resistant or intolerant to imatinib: update of a phase I study. Blood 106:16 a

Schindler T, Bornmann W, Pellicena P, Miller WT, Clarkson B, Kuriyan J (2000) Structural mechanism for STI-571 inhibition of abelson tyrosine kinase. Science 289:1938–1942

Schoch C, Haferlach T, Kern W, Schnittger S, Berger U, Hehlmann R, Hiddemann W, Hochhaus A (2003) Occurrence of additional chromosome aberrations in chronic myeloid leukemia patients treated with imatinib mesylate. Leukemia 17:461–463

Sexl V, Piekorz R, Moriggl R, Rohrer J, Brown MP, Bunting KD, Rothammer K, Roussel MF, Ihle JN (2000) Stat5a/b contribute to interleukin 7-induced B-cell precursor expansion, but abl- and bcr/abl-induced transformation are independent of stat5. Blood 96:2277–2283

Shah NP, Nicoll JM, Nagar B, Gorre ME, Paquette RL, Kuriyan J, Sawyers CL (2002) Multiple BCR-ABL kinase domain mutations confer polyclonal resistance to the tyrosine kinase inhibitor imatinib (STI571) in chronic phase and blast crisis chronic myeloid leukemia. Cancer Cell 2:117–125

Shah NP, Tran C, Lee FY, Chen P, Norris D, Sawyers CL (2004) Overriding imatinib resistance with a novel ABL kinase inhibitor. Science 305:399–401

Skorski T, Kanakaraj P, Nieborowska Skorska M, Ratajczak MZ, Wen SC, Zon G, Gewirtz AM, Perussia B, Calabretta B (1995) Phosphatidylinositol-3 kinase activity is regulated by BCR/ABL and is required for the growth of Philadelphia chromosome-positive cells. Blood 86:726–736

Smith KM, Yacobi R, Van Etten RA (2003) Autoinhibition of Bcr-Abl through its SH3 domain. Mol Cell 12:27–37

Talpaz M, Silver RT, Druker BJ, Goldman JM, Gambacorti-Passerini C, Guilhot F, Schiffer CA, Fischer T, Deininger MW, Lennard AL, Hochhaus A, Ottmann OG, Gratwohl A, Baccarani M, Stone R, Tura S, Mahon FX, Fernandes-Reese S, Gathmann I, Capdeville R, Kantarjian HM, Sawyers CL (2002) Imatinib induces durable hematologic and cytogenetic responses in patients with accelerated phase chronic myeloid leukemia: results of a phase 2 study. Blood 99:1928–1937

Talpaz M, Rousselot P, Kim D-W, Guilhot F, Corm S, Bleickard E, Zink R, Rosti G, Coutre S, Sawyers C (2006) A phase II study of dasatinib in patients with chronic myeloid leukemia (CML) in myeloid blast crisis who are resistant or intolerant to imatinib: first results of the CA180006 'START-B' study. Blood 106:16a

Tauchi T, Boswell HS, Leibowitz D, Broxmeyer HE (1994) Coupling between p210bcr-abl and Shc and Grb2 adaptor proteins in hematopoietic cells permits growth factor receptor-independent link to ras activation pathway. J Exp Med 179:167–175

Tauchi T, Sumi M, Nakajima A, Sashida G, Shimamoto T, Ohyashiki K (2003) BCL-2 antisense oligonucleotide genasense is active against imatinib-resistant BCR-ABL-positive cells. Clin Cancer Res 9:4267–4273

Thomas J, Wang L, Clark RE, Pirmohamed M (2004) Active transport of imatinib into and out of cells: implications for drug resistance. Blood 104:3739–3745

Tipping AJ, Deininger MW, Goldman JM, Melo JV (2003) Comparative gene expression profile of chronic myeloid leukemia cells innately resistant to imatinib mesylate. Exp Hematol 31:1073–1080

Tseng PH, Lin HP, Zhu J, Chen KF, Hade EM, Young DC, Byrd JC, Grever M, Johnson K, Druker BJ, Chen CS (2005) Synergistic interactions between imatinib mesylate and the novel phosphoinositide-dependent kinase-1 inhibitor OSU-03012 in overcoming imatinib mesylate resistance. Blood 105:4021–4027

van Oosterom AT, Judson I, Verweij J, Stroobants S, Donato dP, Dimitrijevic S, Martens M, Webb A, Sciot R, Van Glabbeke M, Silberman S, Nielsen OS (2001) Safety and efficacy of imatinib (STI571) in metastatic gastrointestinal stromal tumours: a phase I study. Lancet 358:1421–1423

Vigneri P, Wang JY (2001) Induction of apoptosis in chronic myelogenous leukemia cells through nuclear entrapment of BCR-ABL tyrosine kinase. Nat Med 7:228–234

von Bubnoff N, Schneller F, Peschel C, Duyster J (2002) BCR-ABL gene mutations in relation to clinical resistance of Philadelphia-chromosome-positive leukaemia to STI571: a prospective study. Lancet 359:487–491

von Bubnoff N, Veach DR, Miller WT, Li W, Sanger J, Peschel C, Bornmann WG, Clarkson B, Duyster J (2003) Inhibition of wild-type and mutant Bcr-Abl by pyrido-pyrimidine-type small molecule kinase inhibitors. Cancer Res 63:6395–6404

von Bubnoff N, Veach DR, van der KH, Aulitzky WE, Sanger J, Seipel P, Bornmann WG, Peschel C, Clarkson B, Duyster J (2005) A cell-based screen for resistance of Bcr-Abl-positive leukemia identifies the mutation pattern for PD166326, an alternative Abl kinase inhibitor. Blood 105:1652–1659

Warmuth M, Simon N, Mitina O, Mathes R, Fabbro D, Manley PW, Buchdunger E, Forster K, Moarefi I, Hallek M (2003) Dual-specific Src and Abl kinase inhibitors, PP1 and CGP76030, inhibit growth and survival of cells expressing imatinib mesylate-resistant Bcr-Abl kinases. Blood 101:664–672

Weisberg E, Griffin JD (2000) Mechanism of resistance to the ABL tyrosine kinase inhibitor STI571 in BCR/ABL-transformed hematopoietic cell lines. Blood 95:3498–3505

Weisberg E, Manley PW, Breitenstein W, Bruggen J, Cowan-Jacob SW, Ray A, Huntly B, Fabbro D, Fendrich G, Hall-Meyers E (2005) Characterization of AMN107, a selective inhibitor of native and mutant Bcr-Abl. Cancer Cell 7:129–141

Wen ST, van Etten RA (1997) The PAG gene product, a stress-induced protein with antioxidant properties, is an Abl SH3-binding protein and a physiological inhibitor of c-Abl tyrosine kinase activity. Genes Dev 11:2456–2467

Widmer N, Colombo S, Buclin T, Decosterd LA (2003) Functional consequence of MDR1 expression on imatinib intracellular concentrations. Blood 102:1142

Wilhelm SM, Carter C, Tang L, Wilkie D, McNabola A, Rong H, Chen C, Zhang X, Vincent P, McHugh M, Cao Y, Shujath J, Gawlak S, Eveleigh D, Rowley B, Liu L, Adnane L, Lynch M, Auclair D, Taylor I, Gedrich R, Voznesensky A, Riedl B, Post LE, Bollag G, Trail PA (2004) BAY 43-9006 exhibits broad spectrum oral antitumor activity and targets the RAF/MEK/ERK pathway and receptor tyrosine kinases involved in tumor progression and angiogenesis. Cancer Res 64:7099–7109

Wisniewski D, Lambek CL, Liu C, Strife A, Veach DR, Nagar B, Young MA, Schindler T, Bornmann WG, Bertino JR, Kuriyan J, Clarkson B (2002) Characterization of potent inhibitors of the Bcr-Abl and the c-kit receptor tyrosine kinases. Cancer Res 62:4244–4255

Wolff NC, Ilaria RL Jr (2001) Establishment of a murine model for therapy-treated chronic myelogenous leukemia using the tyrosine kinase inhibitor STI571. Blood 98:2808–2816

Yu C, Krystal G, Dent P, Grant S (2002a) Flavopiridol potentiates STI571-induced mitochondrial damage and apoptosis in BCR-ABL-positive human leukemia cells. Clin Cancer Res 8:2976–2984

Yu C, Krystal G, Varticovksi L, McKinstry R, Rahmani M, Dent P, Grant S (2002b) Pharmacologic mitogen-activated protein/extracellular signal-regulated kinase kinase/mitogen-activated protein kinase inhibitors interact synergistically with STI571 to induce apoptosis in Bcr/Abl-expressing human leukemia cells. Cancer Res 62:188–199

Zha J, Harada H, Yang E, Jockel J, Korsmeyer SJ (1996) Serine phosphorylation of death agonist BAD in response to survival factor results in binding to 14-3-3 not BCL-X(L). Cell 87:619–628

Zhao X, Ghaffari S, Lodish H, Malashkevich VN, Kim PS (2002) Structure of the Bcr-Abl oncoprotein oligomerization domain. Nat Struct Biol 9:117–120

Zimmermann J, Buchdunger E, Mett H, Meyer T, Lydon NB, Taxler P (1996) Phenylamino-Pyrimidine (PAP)-derivatives: a new class of potent and highly selective PDGF-receptor autophosphorylation inhibitors. Bioorg Med Chem Lett 6:1221–1226

Zimmermann J, Buchdunger E, Mett H, Meyer T, Lydon NB (1997) Potent and selective inhibitors of the Abl kinase Phenylamino-pyrimidine (PAP) derivatives. Bioorg Med Chem Lett 7:187–192

Treatment with Tyrosine Kinase Inhibitors

Andreas Hochhaus

Contents

Abstract. Leukemias have traditionally served as model systems for research on neoplasia because of the easy availability of cell material from blood and marrow for diagnosis, monitoring, and studies on pathophysiology. Beyond these more technical aspects, chronic myeloid leukemia (CML) became the first neoplasia in which the elucidation of the genotype led to a rationally designed therapy of the phenotype. Targeting of the pathogenetically relevant Bcr-Abl tyrosine kinase with the inhibitor imatinib has induced remissions with almost complete disappearance of any signs and symptoms of CML. This therapeutic success has triggered an intensive search for suitable targets in other cancers and has led to the development of numerous inhibitors of potential targets now being studied in preclinical and clinical trials worldwide. Imatinib mesylate has been the first selective inhibitor of Bcr-Abl employed in patients. Its routine use has been considered a revolution in the treatment of CML.

6.1 Medical Treatment of CML

The first drug reported to be active in CML was arsenic in 1865. Currently, arsenic has been reintroduced into CML management as second-line treatment in combination with imatinib. Therapy remained palliative during most of the last century and included splenic irradiation, various cytostatic agents, of which busulfan was standard for almost three decades, and intensive combination therapy. The intention of the treatment became curative with the introduction of stem cell transplantation in the 1970s (Goldman and Melo 2003). At the same time, interferon α (IFN) in combination with hydroxyurea or low-dose cytarabine (ara-C) offered the prospect of prolonging survival, particularly in low-risk patients and in patients who achieve a cytogenetic remission (Bonifazi et al. 2001; Hehlmann et al. 1994, 2003).

6.2 Imatinib Mesylate

6.2.1 Clinical Efficacy

In an effort to identify compounds which could selectively inhibit the aberrantly enhanced tyrosine kinase Bcr-Abl, imatinib mesylate, a 2-phenylaminopyrimidine derivative, was identified (see Chap. 1, entitled Chronic Myeloid Leukemia – A Brief History). Imatinib competitively inhibits the ATP binding site of Bcr-Abl tyrosine kinase and, by inhibiting tyrosine phosphorylation blocks the Bcr-Abl signal transduction cascade. It is highly selective for inhibiting Bcr-Abl, ABL, PDGF-R alpha and beta, ARG, and c-kit (Buchdunger et al. 2000) without inhibiting the proliferation of *BCR-ABL*-negative cells (Druker et al. 1996).

Imatinib is well absorbed from the gut. Peak plasma levels are reached after 2–4 h and bioavailability is 98%. A single oral dose of 400 mg/day produces a steady state plasma concentration which exceeds the minimal required concentration for inhibiting cellular phosphorylation and causes lysis of *BCR-ABL*-positive cell lines in vitro. The mean elimination half-time of imatinib is 13–16 h. Excretion is primarily via the feces (Druker et al. 2001b). Imatinib is 95% protein bound, predominantly to albumin and α_1 glycoprotein. Metabolism is mainly through the action of the cytochrome P450 (CYP) isoform CYP3A4. The main metabolite (N-demethylated piperazine derivative) has similar in vitro potency to the parent compound.

In a phase I study 83 IFN refractory patients in chronic phase (CP) were treated with imatinib (Druker et al. 2001b). The median duration of IFN pretreatment was 8.5 months (1 week to 8.5 years) and the median duration of imatinib therapy was 310 days (17–607 days). Complete hematologic response (CHR) was noted in 53 of 54 patients treated with more than 300 mg of imatinib (criteria: leukocytes $<10\times10^9$/l and platelets $<450\times10^9$/l for at least 4 weeks). Hematologic responses were attained generally within the first 4 weeks of imatinib therapy and were durable in 51 of 53 patients with a median follow-up of 265 days (17–468 days). A major cytogenetic remission (MCR, Ph+ metaphases <35%) was noted in 17 (31%), being complete in 7 patients (13%). The median time to best cytogenetic response was 148 days (48–331 days). The side effects (i.e., nausea, diarrhea, myalgias, and periorbital edema) were relatively frequent (25–43%) but mostly mild (WHO grades I and II). In some patients abnormal liver function tests were noted. An initial drop of hemoglobin of 1–2 g/dl, which was dose related, occurred frequently. Leukopenia and thrombocytopenia (WHO grade III) occurred in 14% and 16%, respectively, and was not dose limiting. The highest dose of imatinib administered was 1000 mg daily and the maximum tolerable dose was not defined.

In a second phase I study 58 patients with myeloid (n=38) or lymphoid blast crisis (BC) or Ph-positive acute lymphoblastic leukemia (ALL, n=20) were treated with 300–1000 mg of imatinib daily (Druker et al. 2001a). The median age was 48 years (range, 24 to 76). Additional chromosomal abnormalities were noted in 58% and 65%, respectively. Twenty-one patients with myeloid BC (55%) achieved a hematologic response, which was complete in four patients (11%). In 12 patients (32%) less than 5% blasts were noted in the bone marrow.

In patients with lymphoid BC, hematologic response rate was 70%, which was complete in 20%. In 11 patients (55%) less than 5% blasts were noted in the bone marrow. Seven of 58 patients (12%) attained MCR, which was complete in five patients (3 and 2 patients, respectively from each group). Response rates were not closely related to the administered doses. Of the 21 patients with myeloid BC who had attained a hematologic response, nine patients relapsed after a median of 84 days (42–194 days). All but one of the patients with lymphoid BC relapsed after a median of 58 days. The side-effect profiles were comparable to the aforementioned study in CP CML. Overall, 16 patients died due to disease progression. Phosphorylation of CRK-oncogene-like protein (CRKL), a major substrate of Bcr-Abl kinase, was markedly reduced in leukemic cells, demonstrating the effect of imatinib on its target.

Phase II trials were conducted in BC (n=260), accelerated phase (AP) (n=235), and CP after IFN resistance or intolerance (n=532). According to the original publications, in patients with BC hematologic response rate was 52% (complete in 8%), MCR occurred in 16%, with 7% of the responses being complete (Sawyers et al. 2002). Time to progression and median survival were significantly shorter in pretreated patients. In patients with AP imatinib induced sustained hematologic responses lasting at least 4 weeks in 69% (complete in 34%) (Talpaz et al. 2002). MCR rate was 24%. Estimated 12-month overall survival was 74%. In IFN refractory or intolerant patients in CP CML imatinib induced CHR in 95%, MCR in 60%, with 41% of the responses being complete (Kantarjian et al. 2002). The median time to onset of CHR was 0.7 months, of MCR 2.9 months. Updated results are provided in Table 6.1 (Silver et al. 2004). Phase-II data were confirmed by a large expanded access program with more than 7,000 patients (Hensley et al. 2003).

A subsequent phase III randomized controlled trial (IRIS – International Randomized Study of Interferon and STI571) in 1,106 patients with newly diagnosed CML in CP recruited between June 2000 and January 2001, has shown the superiority of imatinib, 400 mg/

Table 6.1. Rates of hematologic and cytogenetic responses with imatinib (Phase II-studies, update 2004, Kantarjian et al. 2002; Sawyers et al. 2002; Silver et al. 2004; Talpaz et al. 2002)

	Recruited	Complete hematologic response (%)	Major cytogenetic response (≤35% Ph-positive metaphases) (%)	Complete cytogenetic response (%)
Chronic phase	532	96	66	55
Accelerated phase	235	40	28	20
Myeloid blast crisis	260	8.7	16	7.4

day, over the combination of IFN and cytarabine in all relevant endpoints. At 18 months the hematologic and cytogenetic response rates in the imatinib arm were 97% and 87%, respectively, which is much higher than comparable figures for the IFN/cytarabine arm (69% and 22%, respectively); the toxicity with imatinib was lower. Time to progression to blast phase, duration of progression-free survival irrespective of the prognostic-factor score at the time of study entry, and the perceived occurrence of adverse events were advantageous for primary imatinib therapy (O'Brien et al. 2003). Due to the large numbers of crossovers from IFN to imatinib, a long-term comparison of both therapies is impossible.

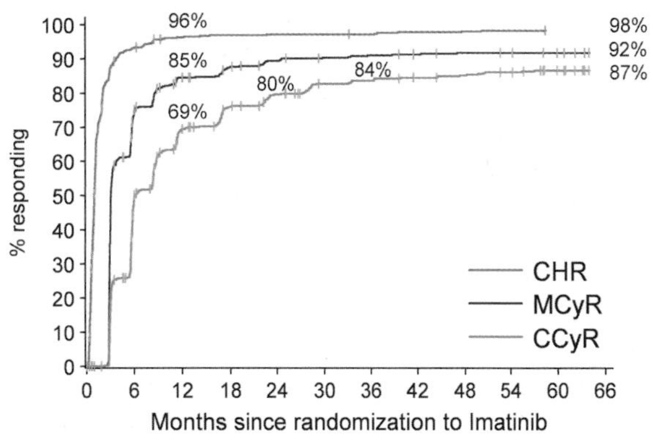

Fig. 6.1. Estimated response to first-line imatinib. CHR, complete hematologic response; MCR, major cytogenetic response (Ph+≤35%); CCR, complete hematologic response (Druker et al. 2006; O'Brien et al. 2003)

A 60-month update of the imatinib group showed complete hematologic remissions in 98%, partial cytogenetic remissions in 92%, and complete cytogenetic remissions in 87% of cases (Druker et al. 2006) (Figs. 6.1, 6.2). Annual rate of relapse was 3.3, 7.5 and 4.8% in the first three years and decreased to 1.5 and 0.9% in the fourth and fifth year after start of treatment. The time to complete hematologic remission was much shorter with imatinib (about 90% after 3 months) than with IFN. Similar to the effects observed with IFN, the achievement of complete cytogenetic remissions was followed in most patients by a continuous decline of *BCR-ABL* transcript levels which continues up to 42 months. Major parameters with favorable prognostic impact were any cytogenetic response after 6 months (Fig. 6.3) and major cytogenetic response (Fig. 6.4) after 12 months of therapy (Druker et al. 2003; Hughes et al. 2003).

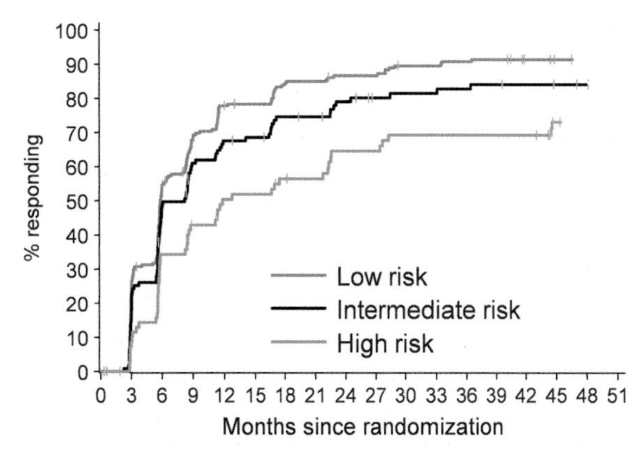

Fig. 6.2. Estimated CCR to first-line Imatinib by Sokal Group (Guilhot 2004; O'Brien et al. 2003)

Quality-of-life analysis has demonstrated advantages of imatinib compared with IFN + cytoarabine as first-line treatment of CP CML. In addition, patients who cross over to imatinib from IFN-based therapies experience a significant improvement in quality of life (Hahn et al. 2003).

There are a number of questions that have been answered definitively by the IRIS study. The study has shown that in terms of hematologic and cytogenetic responses, progression-free survival, and side effects, tolerability, and quality of life, imatinib is superior to IFN plus low-dose cytarabine. However, two important related questions have not definitely been answered by this

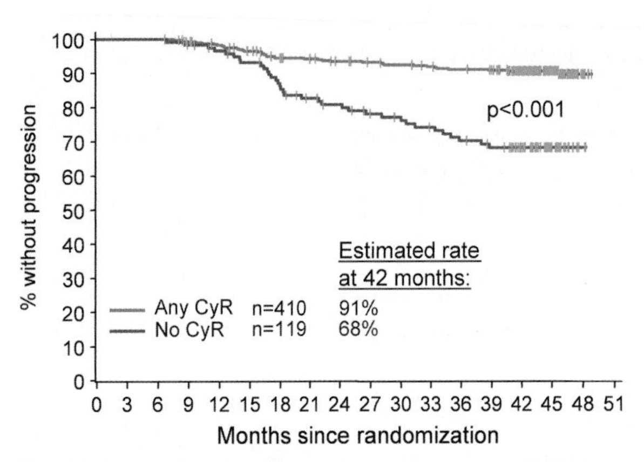

Fig. 6.3. Prognostic value of any cytogenetic response (CyR) at 6 months (Guilhot 2004; O'Brien et al. 2003)

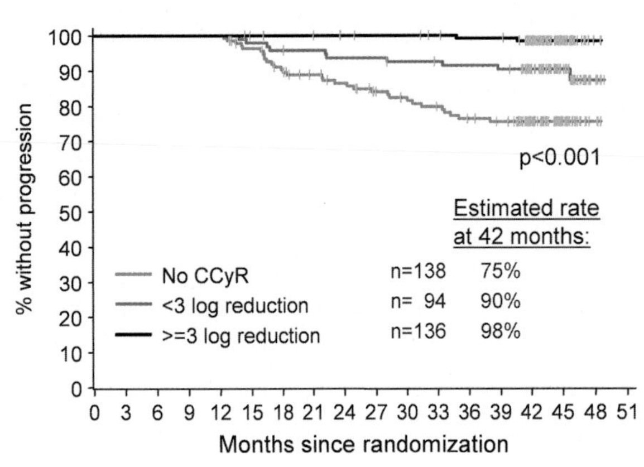

Fig. 6.4. Progression-free survival on first-line imatinib by molecular response (MR) at 12 months (Guilhot 2004; O'Brien et al. 2003)

study, namely (1) is imatinib superior to IFN plus cytarabine in terms of long-term survival? and (2) what will be the outcome of imatinib-treated patients in the longer term? By extrapolation from survival data of IFN-treated CML patients who achieved complete cytogenetic remissions, a 10-year survival rate of at least 51% was estimated for imatinib-treated patients (Hasford et al. 2005). Assuming the relationship between CCR and survival with IFN holds good for imatinib, the much higher CCR rates with imatinib therapy will result in an estimated 6.23 life-years gained compared with treatment with IFN plus low-dose cytarabine (Anstrom et al. 2004).

It can be concluded that imatinib is superior to IFN with regard to response rate, progression-free survival and adverse effects. Comparison with historic data indicates a clear survival advantage of imatinib compared to IFN in patients with early CP CML (Kantarjian et al. 2003).

Another critical issue of course is whether imatinib can cure CML. Current in vitro and in vivo data suggest that dormant or "quiescent" nondividing *BCR-ABL*-positive stem cells are not responsive to imatinib and may produce relapse after withdrawal of imatinib (Druker et al. 2006; Graham et al. 2002).

6.2.2 Side Effects of Imatinib

The majority of imatinib-treated patients experience adverse events at some time. Most events are of mild to moderate grade. The most frequently reported drug-related adverse events are nausea, vomiting, edema, and muscle cramps. Edema is most frequently periorbital or in lower limbs and is manageable with diuretics. The frequency of severe edema in phase I–III trials was 2–5%. Some of the adverse events observed are attributable to local or general fluid retention including pleural effusion, ascites, pulmonary edema, and rapid weight gain with or without superficial edema. The incidence of edema was dose and age related; it was about 20% higher for patients who received imatinib 600 mg/day vs. 400 mg/day and for patients >65 years of age (Table 6.2).

Myelosuppression is common in CML patients treated with imatinib (more common in patients with advanced disease and in the initial phase of therapy). In the phase III randomized trial of newly diagnosed patients in the CP treated with imatinib at 400 mg/day, grade 3 neutropenia (ANC $<1\times10^9$/l) was experienced by 11% of patients, grade 4 neutropenia (ANC $<0.5\times10^9$/l) occurred in 2% of patients, grade 3 thrombocytopenia (platelets $<50\times10^9$/l) occurred in 6.9% of patients, and grade 4 thrombocytopenia (platelets $<10\times10^9$/l) occurred in less than 1% of patients (O'Brien et al. 2003).

Both *in vitro* and *in vivo* data indicate that inhibition of normal hematopoiesis during imatinib treatment is minimal; it is seen primarily as neutropenia and is largely restricted to high doses (Deininger et al. 2003). The much lower rate of infectious complications observed as compared to that expected in patients with a similar level of myelosuppression induced by conventional chemotherapy may be related to the lack of mucous membrane damage in patients on imatinib. Most patients, even patients with advanced phase CML, experience recovery of normal blood counts during continuous therapy with imatinib. Interventions with hematopoietic growth factors are under investigation.

Table 6.2. Management of side effects from imatinib (Garcia-Manero et al. 2003)

Side effect	Management
Nausea and/or emesis	Avoid taking imatinib on an empty stomach
	Antiemetics (e.g., ondansetron at a dose of 8 mg orally or prochlorperazine at a dose of 10 mg orally 30 min prior to intake of imatinib)
	Adequate fluid intake
Diarrhea	Loperamide at a dose of 2 mg orally after each loose bowel movement (up to 16 mg daily) or diphenoxylate atropine at a dose of 20 mg orally daily in 3–4 divided doses
Skin rashes	Avoid sun exposure
	Topical steroids (e.g., 0.1% triamcinolone cream topically as needed)
	Systemic steroids (e.g., prednisone at a dose of 20 mg orally daily for 3–5 days)
Muscle cramps	Electrolyte substitution
	Tonic water (quinine)
	Mg^{2+} replacements
Bone aches	Cox-2 inhibitors (e.g., celecoxib at a dose of 200 mg orally daily or rofecoxib at a dose of 25 mg orally daily)
Liver function abnormalities	Hold imatinib
	Resume within 1–2 weeks
	Consider decreasing the dose (no less than 300 mg orally daily)
Myelosuppression	
Anemia	Erythropoietin as needed
Neutropenia	G-CSF as needed
Thrombocytopenia	Hold if platelets $\leq 40 \times 10^9$/L
	High-dose folic acid
	Interleukin-11 as needed
	Resume at lower dose level (no less than 300 mg orally daily)

6.2.3 Dosage of Imatinib

The recommended dosage of imatinib is 400 mg/day for patients in CP CML and 600 mg/day for patients with AP or BC CML. Consecutive cohorts of patients treated with 400 mg and 600 mg imatinib demonstrated the advantage of 600 mg/day in advanced disease. Retrospective analysis of prognostic factors showed that the 400 mg and 600 mg cohorts were well matched.

Dose increases from 400 mg to 600 mg/day in patients with CP CML or from 600 mg to 800 mg/day in patients with advanced disease may be considered for patients with progressive disease, if a satisfactory hematologic response is not achieved after >3 months of treatment, if cytogenetic remission is not achieved after 6–12 months of treatment or if a previously achieved hematologic or cytogenetic remission is lost (in the absence of severe nonleukemia-related neutropenia or thrombocytopenia).

The increase of imatinib dosage has been previously shown to improve response in patients with accelerated disease. Accelerated disease was found to have higher response rates with 600 mg imatinib than with 400 mg. Kantarjian et al. (2004) have reported in a historical comparison that higher cytogenetic and molecular remission rates can be achieved in shorter time intervals with an imatinib dosage of 800 mg daily as compared to 400 mg in CP CML. The disadvantage of the higher imatinib dose is a higher rate of adverse effects, in particular myelosuppression and fluid retention. It is unknown whether the effect of high-dose imatinib is sustained and provides a survival benefit. The dosage of imatinib should be adjusted or treatment interrupted if severe neutropenia or thrombocytopenia occurs.

Dose increase is suggested in case of suboptimal response, which is defined as:

1. Failure to achieve a complete hematologic response after 3 months,
2. failure to achieve any cytogenetic response after 6 months, or
3. failure to achieve a major cytogenetic response after 12 months of imatinib therapy (Druker et al. 2003; Hughes et al. 2003).

High-dose imatinib therapy was tested in CML patients after IFN failure and in newly diagnosed patients. Cytogenetic and molecular responses were achieved faster with 800 mg imatinib/day (Cortes et al. 2003; Kantarjian et al. 2004). The TIDEL multicenter study in Australia examined the effect of 600 mg/day among newly diagnosed patients with CP CML. Dose escalation to 800 mg/day was allowed if patients did not achieve a CHR at 3 months, an MCR at 6 months, a CCR at 9 months, or became PCR negative at 12 months. Additionally, patients who did not achieve hematologic or cytogenetic responses following dose escalation to imatinib 800 mg/day were allowed to add intermittent ara-C to their regimen. When compared with historical data from the IRIS study, a significantly higher proportion of patients in the TIDEL study achieved an MCR and CCR (Hughes et al. 2004).

6.2.4 Imatinib in Combination

Combinations of imatinib with other drugs have been extensively analyzed in vitro and have shown that a number of drugs are synergistic with imatinib in vitro. Of particular interest were the combinations of imatinib with IFN or low-dose ara-C. The feasibility of the combinations of imatinib with IFN (Pegasys, Peg-Intron) and low-dose cytarabine has been shown in phase I and II studies (Baccarani et al. 2004; Hochhaus et al. 2002).

On the basis of these studies, randomized trials were designed by national study groups in Germany, France, UK, and USA to compare imatinib monotherapy at 400 mg with imatinib in various combinations (IFN, cytarabine) and dosages (600 mg, 800 mg). The first of these studies, the German CML Study IV, started recruitment in July 2002 and compared imatinib 400 mg/d with imatinib + IFN, imatinib + cytarabine and imatinib after IFN failure in newly diagnosed patients with CP CML. By June 2006, 810 patients were randomized. According to the Hasford score, 35% of patients were low risk, 54% intermediate risk, and 11% high risk. Rate of progression was rare, within the first year 13/335 patients (6 low, 3 intermediate, 4 high risk; 4%) progressed to BC, 4 of them revealed clonal evolution (complex aberrant karyotype, n = 3; +8, n = 1), two other *BCR-ABL* mutations. Within the second year 3/232 patients progressed to BC. During the first year of treatment imatinib therapy was stopped due to side effects or resistance in 6% of patients in the imatinib 400 mg arm, in 2% of patients in the imatinib+IFN arm, and in 2% of patients in the imatinib+cytarabine arm. IFN was stopped in 21% and cytarabine in 18% of patients. The interim analysis of a prospective randomized trial with imatinib and imatinib in combination for newly diagnosed patients with CML has proven the feasibility of imatinib combinations in addition to high response and low progression rates (Berger et al. 2004).

In September 2003, the French study was started which compares imatinib monotherapy at 400 mg vs. imatinib at 600 mg vs. imatinib plus IFN (Pegasys) vs. imatinib plus low-dose cytarabine. After an observation period, it is planned to reduce the study to two arms. The UK study compares imatinib monotherapy at 400 mg vs. imatinib at 800 mg vs. imatinib plus IFN (Pegasys). The USA study is focusing on the comparison of 400 mg and 800 mg imatinib therapy only.

The emergence of resistance to imatinib monotherapy has led to a search for downstream targets of the Bcr-Abl kinase that may mediate the altered growth properties of *BCR-ABL*-transformed cells. Identification of signaling pathways downstream of ABL tyrosine kinase may increase our understanding of the pathogenesis of CML and suggest strategies to improve clinical treatment of the disease.

Farnesyl transferase inhibitors enhance the antiproliferative effects of imatinib against *BCR-ABL*-expressing cells, including imatinib-resistant cells. Cells resistant to imatinib because of amplification of *BCR-ABL* remain sensitive to tipifarnib and lonafarnib and cotreatment of these cells with imatinib plus farnesyl transferase inhibitors leads to enhanced antiproliferative or proapoptotic effects even in cells that are resistant to imatinib based on the expression of a Bcr-Abl kinase domain mutation (T315I) that is completely insensitive to imatinib. Although this mutant is sensitive to lonafarnib, the addition of lonafarnib to imatinib yielded no increase in antiproliferative effects. These results raise critically important issues of how and when to molecularly targeted agents should be combined for optimal results. Although the discussion that follows will focus on CML and Bcr-Abl signal transduction, this paradigm could be applied to any agent that targets signaling pathways (Peters et al. 2001).

Early clinical studies using a combination of imatinib and farnesyl transferase inhibitors in advanced phase CML patients demonstrated feasibility but showed only moderate activity, probably due to clonal evolution with novel molecular or cytogenetic aberrations in addition to *BCR-ABL* not responding to farnesyl transferase inhibitors (Cortes et al. 2003).

It is shown that the PI3-kinase/Akt pathway is a critical contributor to survival/proliferation of *BCR-ABL*-transformed cells. The serine/threonine protein kinase mTOR (mammalian target of rapamycin) is a downstream component of the PI3-Kinase/Akt pathway, and plays an important role in controlling cell growth and proliferation. The mTOR pathway is constitutively activated by Bcr-Abl in CML cells. Two of its known substrates, ribosomal protein S6 and 4E-BP1, are constitutively phosphorylated in a Bcr-Abl-dependent manner in *BCR-ABL*-expressing cell lines and CML cell lines. These data suggest that Bcr-Abl may regulate translation of critical targets in CML cells via mTOR.

The effect of rapamycin in three different imatinib-resistant Bcr-Abl mutant cell lines (Ba/F-*BCR-ABL* T315I, G250E, M351T) has been described. Rapamycin alone inhibited proliferation to a degree that would be predicted if mTOR was a critical downstream effector of Bcr-Abl, while the combination of low-dose rapamycin with imatinib markedly enhanced this growth inhibitory effect. The synergy between rapamycin and imatinib, occurring at doses well below typical serum levels obtained during monotherapy with each of these agents represents a strong argument in favor of investigating the clinical activity of the combination (Ly Chi et al. 2003).

6.2.5 Imatinib Resistance

Several questions remain open, notably those concerning the development of imatinib resistance, which is rare in early CP, but increases in frequency along the course of the disease (Hochhaus and La Rosée 2004). Essentially two mechanisms underlie the development of imatinib resistance:

1. Mutations of the ATP-binding site of the Bcr-Abl tyrosine kinase, and
2. clonal evolution with aberrant karyotypes ultimately leading to BC.

Pharmacological mechanisms including activation of multidrug resistance proteins may cause variations in the individual intracellular imatinib concentrations, which may contribute to the development of resistance.

etailed sequence analysis of the Bcr-Abl kinase domain has been performed to elucidate which mutations are responsible for the development of imatinib resistance. More than 30 different mutations have been recognized which are detailed elsewhere (Hochhaus and La Rosée 2004; Shah et al. 2004). The prognostically most-serious mutations concern the so-called P-loop domain of the tyrosine kinase. P-loop mutations have been associated with an especially poor prognosis (Branford et al. 2003), but cessation of imatinib therapy and alternative therapy with other drugs seem to be able to improve prognosis. Novel methods are available to screen for small clones of mutated leukemic cells, e.g., denaturing high-performance liquid chromatography (D-HPLC). The impact of the results of such assays needs to be explored in prospective clinical trials (Soverini et al. 2005).

6.2.6 Prediction of Response

Attempts have been made to develop prognostic models to predict the outcome of CML patients on imatinib therapy. In CP patients after IFN failure, a low neutrophil count and poor cytogenetic response at 3 months were identified as independent factors by investigators of the Hammersmith Hospital in London (Marin et al. 2003), but data are conflicting and were not confirmed by others (Lahaye et al. 2005).

6.3 Novel Bcr-Abl Inhibitors in Clinical Trials

6.3.1 Nilotinib (AMN107)

Nilotinib (AMN107) is a novel aminopyrimidine, available as an oral formulation. It is a competitive inhibitor of the protein tyrosine kinase activity of Bcr-Abl and

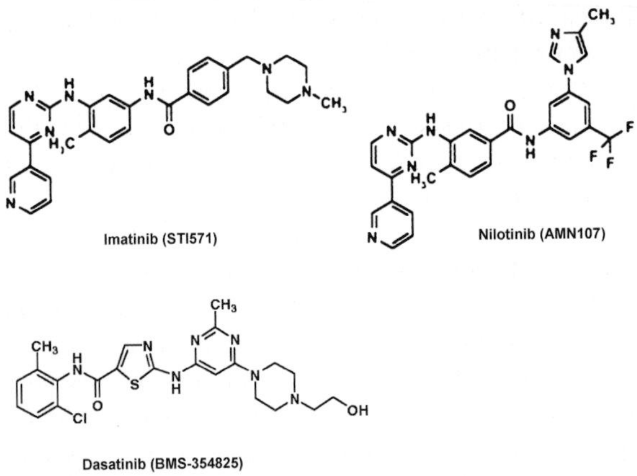

Imatinib (STI571)

Nilotinib (AMN107)

Dasatinib (BMS-354825)

Fig. 6.5. Chemical structure of imatinib, nilotinib, and dasatinib (Shah et al. 2004; Weisberg et al. 2005)

prevents the activation of Bcr-Abl-dependent mitogenic and antiapoptotic pathways (e.g., PI-3 kinase and STAT5), resulting in death of the Bcr-Abl-induced phenotype. In cellular autophosphorylation assays and mediated cell proliferation, nilotinib is a highly potent inhibitor of the Bcr-Abl tyrosine kinase. An important feature of nilotinib is its ability to inhibit most imatinib-resistant mutant forms of BCR-ABL. Based on this activity, nilotinib may provide therapeutic benefit in patients with CML who have developed resistance to imatinib therapy due to mutations within the Bcr-Abl kinase.

The effects of nilotinib on Bcr-Abl autophosphorylation have been evaluated in K562 and KU-812F human leukemia cell lines, which naturally express Bcr-Abl, as well as with p190 or p210-BCR-ABL transfected murine hematopoietic 32D and p210-BCR-ABL transfected Ba/F3 cells. In addition, the compound has been evaluated for effects on autophosphorylation in a panel of Ba/F3 cells, expressing different mutant forms of the Bcr-Abl kinase.

Nilotinib potently inhibits the Bcr-Abl kinase in cell lines derived from human leukemic CML cells and from transfected murine hematopoietic cells, with IC_{50} values in the range of 20 nM to 60 nM. Nilotinib also potently inhibited most of the imatinib-resistant mutant forms of BCR-ABL. Thus, M237I, M244V, L248V, G250A (E, V), Q252H, E255D (K), E275K, E276G, E281K, K285N, E292K, F311V, F317L (C, V), D325N, S348L, M351T, E355 (G), A380S, L387F, M388L, F486S are inhibited with IC_{50} values in the 1–200 nM range, Y253H, E255R (V), and F359C (V), are inhibited with IC_{50} values between 200 nM and 800 nM, leaving only the T315I mutant unaffected by nilotinib at concentrations <8000 nM.

The selectivity of nilotinib as a protein kinase inhibitor has been demonstrated by its lack of appreciable activity (IC_{50} value for inhibition of cell proliferation >3000 nM) against a panel of Ba/F3 cells transfected to express a variety of different kinases (Weisberg et al. 2005). Excellent efficacy in models of myeloproliferative disease was observed. In an acute model in which NOD-SCID mice were injected with murine 32D cells harboring the firefly luciferase gene and transfected to be dependent upon p210 Bcr-Abl, nilotinib (100 mg/kg QD) markedly reduced tumor burden, as assessed by noninvasive imaging. Furthermore, nilotinib (75 mg/kg p.o., QD) prolonged the survival and reduced tumor burden, as assessed by spleen weights, of mice having either p210 or mutant (E255V, M351T) Bcr-Abl myeloproliferative disease. Nilotinib was also evaluated in a disease model using primary hematopoietic cells, in which mice were transplanted with bone-marrow cells transfected to express Bcr-Abl. Treated animals showed reduced morbidity and had spleen weights within the normal range. Similar, although slightly reduced efficacy was observed in mice receiving bone-marrow transplants after infection with either E255V or M351T Bcr-Abl (Weisberg et al. 2005).

A Phase I/II study of nilotinib is currently ongoing in adult patients with imatinib-resistant CML in CP, AP, or BC relapsed/refractory Ph+ acute lymphoblastic leukemia, and other hematological malignancies. The phase I portion of this study has completed its enrollment and the phase-II portion is currently ongoing. During the phase I part of this study, 119 patients were initially treated in dose cohorts from 50 mg to 1200 mg on a once daily schedule with intrapatient dose escalation, and subsequently a twice daily dosing schedule with 400 mg and 600 mg cohorts. For the phase II part of the study, the 400 mg BID dose was selected on the basis of safety and acceptability; this improved serum exposure over once daily dosing in the phase I patients.

In the Phase I study nilotinib was orally administered after a light breakfast and a 2-h fast in sequential cohorts of patients at escalating once daily doses of 50, 100, 200, 400, 600, 800, and 1200 mg. Since a limited increase in serum exposure to nilotinib occurred at higher dose levels, the protocol was amended to add a twice daily dosing schedule of 400 mg (800 mg/day) and 600 mg (1200 mg/day). Nilotinib doses, up to 1200 mg orally once per day or 400 mg orally twice per day, were well tolerated with the majority of adverse events reflecting those commonly seen in patients with advanced leukemia. Overall, 20% of patients experienced thrombocytopenia, 13% experienced neutropenia, 4% developed anemia, and bone marrow aplasia occurred in 2%. There was a higher incidence of neutropenia (22% vs. 9%) in the 600 mg BID cohort compared with the 400-mg BID cohort.

Additional adverse events that were suspected to be study-drug-related included rash and pruritus. Various descriptive terms of rash, including erythema and exanthema, were described in 33% of patients, the majority of which were mild (grades 1 and 2), and 11% at grade 3. Pruritus was reported separately in 15% of patients, 2 (1.6%) of which were grade 3. These cutaneous changes responded to topical corticosteroids in most cases. Nausea (grade 1 or 2) was reported in 7% of patients and emesis in 3%. Fatigue (grades 1–3) has been reported in 5% of patients. Lipase elevations, the majority of which were asymptomatic, have been reported usually during the first cycle of nilotinib therapy. The incidence of clinically recognized pancreatitis was approximately 3%. Transient hyperbilirubinemia occurred early during nilotinib therapy and affected approximately 20% of patients. Most instances of hyperbilirubinemia were due to the unconjugated fraction. These abnormalities generally resolved without further intervention and most patients continued therapy without further recurrence (Kantarjian et al. 2006).

The interim efficacy analysis of the phase-I/II study revealed complete hematologic response in 92% of CP, 51% of AP, and 6% of BC patients. Complete cytogenetic response was achieved in 35%, 14%, and 6% of patients, respectively (Kantarjian et al. 2006).

6.3.2 Dasatinib (BMS 354825)

Dasatinib (BMS-354825) is a potent, orally active inhibitor of the Bcr-Abl, c-KIT, and SRC family kinases. It belongs to the thiazolecarboxamides and is structurally different from imatinib and nilotinib. In preclinical studies, dasatinib has been shown to be a more potent inhibitor of Bcr-Abl (260-fold), c-kit (eightfold), PDGFRβ (60-fold), and SRC (>1000-fold) than imatinib.

Dasatinib inhibits the Bcr-Abl kinase with an *in vitro* IC_{50} of 3 nM. In cellular assays, dasatinib killed or inhibited the proliferation of all Bcr-Abl-dependent leukemic cell lines tested. *In vitro* results suggest that dasatinib is effective in reducing the proliferation or survival of both imatinib sensitive and resistant cells, and its inhibitory activity is not solely dependent on Bcr-Abl. The only imatinib-associated Bcr-Abl mutation resistant to dasatinib is T315I (Shah et al. 2004). Dasatinib is a strong inhibitor of the human CYP3A4 enzyme, so it may reduce clearance of drugs that are significantly metabolized by that enzyme.

A phase-I study with dasatinib in CML patients was initiated in November 2003. Complete hematologic remission was achieved in 92% of CP, 45% of AP, 35% of myeloid BC and 70% of lymphoid BC or Ph+ ALL patients. Complete cytogenetic response was seen in 35%, 18%, 26% and 30% of patients, respectively (Talpaz et al. 2006). Overall hematologic and nonhematologic toxicities have been manageable in the context of the phase-I population. In CP patients, hematologic toxicity consisting mostly of thrombocytopenia was seen at all dose levels. Nonhematologic adverse events usually consisted of grade 1 or 2 events such as pleural effusions, rash, nausea, or fever. They occurred at any dose level without evidence of dose effect.

Pharmacodynamic data (CRKL-phosphorylation assay) suggested a twice-daily schedule. However, the best *in vivo* schedule is being tested in two randomized phase II studies with once-daily and twice-daily schedules at different dose levels (Sawyers et al. 2005).

The advent of selective tyrosine kinase inhibitors has significantly changed CML therapy. However, despite promising results patients should be identified in whom treatment requires optimization, either by dose escalation of imatinib or combination with other drugs. In case of resistance, novel tyrosine kinase inhibitors are available within clinical trials. In addition to hematologic and cytogenetic monitoring, molecular surveillance of response and resistance is essential for therapeutic decisions.

References

Anstrom KJ, Reed SD, Allen AS, Glendenning GA, Schulman KA (2004) Long-term survival estimates for imatinib versus interferon-alpha plus low-dose cytarabine for patients with newly diagnosed chronic-phase chronic myeloid leukemia. Cancer 101:2584–2592

Baccarani M, Martinelli G, Rosti G, Trabacchi E, Testoni N, Bassi S, Amabile M, Soverini S, Castagnetti F, Cilloni D, Izzo B, de Vivo A, Messa E, Bonifazi F, Poerio A, Luatti S, Giugliano E, Alberti D, Fincato G, Russo D, Pane F, Saglio G (2004) GIMEMA Working Party on Chronic Myeloid Leukemia. Imatinib and pegylated human recombinant interferon-α2b in early CP chronic myeloid leukemia. Blood 104:4245–4251

Berger U, Engelich G, Reiter A, Hochhaus A, Hehlmann R and the German CML Study Group (2004) Imatinib and beyond – the new CML-Study IV. A randomised controlled comparison of imatinib vs. imatinib/interferon-alpha vs. imatinib/low-dose AraC vs. interferon-alpha standard therapy in newly diagnosed CP chronic myeloid leukemia. Ann Hematol 83:258–264

Bonifazi F, De Vivo A, Rosti G, Guilhot F, Guilhot J, Trabacchi E, Hehlmann R, Hochhaus A, Shepherd PCA, Steegmann JL, Kluin-Nelemans HC, Thaler J, Simonsson B, Louwagi A, Reiffers J, Mahon FX, Montefusco E, Alimena G, Hasford J, Richards S, Saglio G, Testoni N, Martinelli G, Tura S, Baccarani M for the European Study Group on Interferon in Chronic Myeloid Leukemia (2001) Chronic myeloid leukemia and interferon-alpha: a study of complete cytogenetic responders. Blood 98:3074–3081

Branford S, Rudzki Z, Walsh S, Parkinson I, Grigg A, Szer J, Taylor K, Herrmann R, Seymour JF, Arthur C, Joske D, Lynch K, Hughes T (2003) Detection of BCR-ABL mutations in patients with CML treated with imatinib is virtually always accompanied by clinical resistance, and mutations in the ATP phosphate-binding loop (P-loop) are associated with a poor prognosis. Blood 102:276–283

Buchdunger E, Cioffi CL, Law N, Stover D, Ohno-Jones S, Druker BJ, Lydon NB (2000) Abl protein-tyrosine kinase inhibitor STI571 inhibits in vitro signal transduction mediated by c-kit and platelet-derived growth factor receptors. J Pharmacol Exp Ther 295:139–145

Cortes J, Albitar M, Thomas D et al (2003) Efficacy of the farnesyl transferase inhibitor, Zarnestra (R115777), in chronic myeloid leukemia and other hematologic malignancies. Blood 101:1692–1697

Cortes J, Giles F, O'Brien S, Thomas D, Garcia-Manero G, Rios MB, Faderl S, Verstovsek S, Ferrajoli A, Freireich EJ, Talpaz M, Kantarjian H (2003) Result of high-dose imatinib mesylate in patients with Philadelphia chromosome-positive chronic myeloid leukemia after failure of interferon-alpha. Blood 102:83–86

Deininger MW, O'Brien SG, Ford JM, Druker BJ (2003) Practical management of patients with chronic myeloid leukemia receiving imatinib. J Clin Oncol 21:1637–1647

Druker BJ, Tamura S, Buchdunger E, Ohno S, Segal GM, Fanning S, Zimmermann J, Lydon NB (1996) Effects of a selective inhibitor of the Abl tyrosine kinase on the growth of Bcr-Abl positive cells. Nat Med 2:561–566

Druker BJ, Sawyers CL, Kantarjian H, Resta DJ, Reese SF, Ford JM, Capdeville R, Talpaz M (2001 a) Activity of a specific inhibitor of the Bcr-Abl tyrosine kinase in the BC of chronic myeloid leukemia and acute lymphoblastic leukemia with the Philadelphia chromosome. N Engl J Med 344:1038–1042

Druker BJ, Talpaz M, Resta DJ, Peng B, Buchdunger E, Ford JM, Lydon NB, Kantarjian H, Capdeville R, Ohno-Jones S, Sawyers CL (2001 b) Efficacy and safety of a specific inhibitor of the BCR-ABL tyrosine kinase in chronic myeloid leukemia. N Engl J Med 344:1031–1037

Druker B, Guilhot F, O'Brien S, Larson R (2006) Long-term benefits of imatinib (IM) for patients newly diagnosed with chronic myelogenous leukemia in chronic phase (CML-CP): the 5-year update from the IRIS study. Proc ASCO 24:Abstract 6506

Druker BJ, Gathmann I, Bolton AE, Larson R, on behalf of the IRIS Study Group (2003) Probability and impact of obtaining a cytogenetic response to imatinib as initial therapy for chronic myeloid leukemia (CML) in chronic phase. Blood 102:182 a

Garcia-Manero G, Faderl S, O'Brien S, Cortes J, Talpaz M, Kantarjian HM (2003) Chronic myelogenous leukemia: a review and update of therapeutic strategies. Cancer 98:437–457

Goldman JM, Melo JV (2003) Chronic myeloid leukemia – advances in biology and new approaches to treatment. N Engl J Med 349: 1451–1464

Graham SM, Jorgensen HG, Allan E, Pearson C, Alcorn MJ, Richmond L, Holyoake TL (2002) Primitive, quiescent, Philadelphia-positive stem cells from patients with chronic myeloid leukemia are insensitive to STI571 in vitro. Blood 99:319–325

Guilhot F (2004) Sustained durability of responses plus high rates of cytogenetic responses result in long-term benefit for newly diagnosed chronic-phase chronic myeloid leukemia (CML-CP) treated with imatinib (IM) therapy: update from the IRIS study. Blood 104:11

Hahn EA, Glendenning GA, Sorensen MV, Hudgens SA, Druker BJ, Guilhot F, Larson RA, O'Brien SG, Dobrez DG, Hensley ML, Cella D, IRIS Investigators (2003) Quality of life in patients with newly diagnosed chronic phase chronic myeloid leukemia on imatinib versus interferon alfa plus low-dose cytarabine: results from the IRIS Study. J Clin Oncol 21:2138–2146

Hasford J, Pfirrmann M, Hochhaus A (2005) How long will chronic phase CML pateints treated with imatinib live? Leukemia 19: 497–499

Hehlmann R, Berger U, Pfirrmann M, Hochhaus A, Metzgeroth G, Maywald O, Hasford J, Reiter A, Hossfeld DK, Kolb HJ, Löffler H, Pralle H, Queisser W, Griesshammer M, Nerl C, Kuse R, Tobler A, Eimermacher H, Tichelli A, Aul C, Wilhelm M, Fischer JT, Perker M, Scheid C, Schenk M, Weiss J, Meier CR, Kremers S, Labedzki L, Schmeiser T, Lohrmann HP, Heimpel H, German CML-Study Group (2003) Randomized comparison of interferon alpha and hydroxyurea with hydroxyurea monotherapy in chronic myeloid leukemia (CML-Study II): prolongation of survival by the combination of interferon alpha and hydroxyurea. Leukemia 17:1529–1537

Hehlmann R, Heimpel H, Hasford J, Kolb HJ, Pralle H, Hossfeld DK, Queißer W, Löffler H, Hochhaus A, Heinze B, Georgii A, Bartram CR, Grießhammer M, Bergmann L, Essers U, Falge C, Queißer U, Meyer P, Schmitz N, Eimermacher H, Walther F, Fett W, Kleeberg UR, Käbisch A, Nerl C, Zimmermann R, Meuret G, Tichelli A, Kanz L, Tigges F-J, Schmid L, Brockhaus W, Tobler A, Reiter A, Perker M, Emmerich B, Verpoort K, Zankovich R v. Wussow P, Prümmer O, Thiele J, Buhr T, Ansari H, German CML Study Group (1994) Randomized comparison of interferon-alpha with busulfan and hydroxyurea in chronic myelogenous leukemia. Blood 84:4064–4077

Hensley ML, van Hoomissen IC, Krahnke T, Gathmann I, Thomas E, Ben-Am M, Koehler J, Zoellner U, Schneider A, Capdeville R (2003) Imatinib in chronic myeloid leukemia (CML): outcomes in >7000 patients treated on expanded access program (EAP). Proc Am Soc Clin Oncol 22:579

Hochhaus A, Fischer T, Brümmendorf TH, Schoch C, Müller MC, Merx K, Bostel T, Berger U, Rose MT, Gschaidmeier H, Hehlmann R (2002) Imatinib (Glivec) and pegylated interferon α2a (Pegasys) phase I/II combination study in chronic phase chronic myelogenous leukemia (CML). Blood 1:164 a–165 a

Hochhaus A, La Rosée P (2004) Imatinib therapy in chronic myelogenous leukemia: strategies to avoid and overcome resistance. Leukemia 18:1321–1331

Hughes T, Branford S, Reynolds J, Seymour J, Taylor K, Guzzo-Pernell N, Filshie R, Arthur C, Schwarer A, Hertzberg M, Rudzki Z, Copeman M, Lynch K, Grigg A (2004) Higher-dose imatinib (600 mg/day) with selective intensification in newly diagnosed CML patients in chronic phase: cytogenetic response rates at 12 months are superior to IRIS. Blood 1:286a

Hughes TP, Kaeda J, Branford S, Rudzki Z, Hochhaus A, Hensley ML (2003) Frequency of major molecular responses to imatinib or interferon alfa plus cytarabine in newly diagnosed chronic myeloid leukemia. N Engl J Med 349:1423–1432

Kantarjian H, Sawyers C, Hochhaus A, Guilhot F, Schiffer C, Gambacorti-Passerini C, Niederwieser D, Stone R, Goldman J, Fischer T, Cony-Makhoul P, Miller C, Tallman M, O'Brien S, Brown R, Schuster M, Gratwohl A, Loughran T, Mandelli F, Saglio G, Ottmann O, Lazzarino M, Tura S, Baccarani M, Facon T, Morra E, Russell N, Zoellner U, Resta D, Capdeville R, Talpaz M, Druker B (2002) Hematologic and cytogenetic responses to imatinib mesylate in chronic myelogenous leukemia. N Engl J Med 346:645–652

Kantarjian HM, O'Brien S, Cortes J, Giles FJ, Rios MB, Shan J, Faderl S, Garcia-Manero G, Ferrajoli A, Verstovsek S, Wierda W, Keating M, Talpaz M (2003) Imatinib mesylate therapy improves survival in patients with newly diagnosed Philadelphia chromosome-positive chronic myelogenous leukemia in the chronic phase: comparison with historic data. Cancer 98:2636–2642

Kantarjian H, Talpaz M, O'Brien S, Gracia-Manero G, Verstovsek S, Giles F (2004) High-dose imatinib mesylate therapy in newly diagnosed Philadelphia chromosome-positive chronic phase chronic myeloid leukemia. Blood 103:2873–2878

Kantarjian H, Giles F, Wunderle L, Bhalla K, O'Brien S, Wassmann B, Tanaka C, Manley P, Rae P, Mietlowski W, Bochinski K, Hochhaus A, Griffin JD, Hoelzer D, Albitar M, Dugan M, Cortes J, Alland L, Ottmann OG (2006) Nilotinib in imatinib-resistant CML and Philadelphia chromosome-positive ALL. N Engl J Med 354:2542–2551

Lahaye T, Riehm B, Berger U, Paschka P, Müller MC, Kreil S, Merx K, Schwindel U, Schoch C, Hehlmann R, Hochhaus A (2005) Response and resistance in 300 patients with BCR-ABL-positive leukemias treated with imatinib in a single center: a 4.5-year follow-up. Cancer 103:1659–1669

Ly Chi, Arechiga A, Melo JV et al (2003) Bcr-Abl kinase modulates the translation regulators ribosomal protein S6 and 4E-BP1 in chronic myelogenous leukemia cells via the mammalian target of rapamycin. Cancer Res 63:5716–5722

Marin D, Marktel S, Bua M, Szydlo RM, Franceschino A, Nathan I, Foot N, Crawley C, Nakorn T, Olavarria E, Lennard A, Neylon A, O'Brien SG, Goldman JM, Apperley JF (2003) Prognostic factors for patients with chronic myeloid leukaemia in chronic phase treated with imatinib mesylate after failure of interferon alfa. Leukemia 17:1448–1453

O'Brien S, Guilhot F, Larson R, Gathmann I, Baccarani M, Cervantes F, Cornelissen JJ, Fischer T, Hochhaus A, Hughes T, Lechner K, Nielsen JL, Rousselot P, Reiffers J, Saglio G, Shepherd J, Simonsson B, Gratwohl A, Goldman JM, Kantarjian H, Taylor K, Verhoef G, Bolton AE, Capdeville R, Druker BJ for the IRIS Investigators (2003) The IRIS study: international randomized study of interferon and low-dose ara-C versus STI571 (imatinib) in patients with newly-diagnosed chronic phase chronic myeloid leukemia. N Engl J Med 348:994–1004

Peters DG, Hoover RR, Gerlach MJ et al (2001) Activity of the farnesyl protein transferase inhibitor SCH66336 against BCR/ABL-induced murine leukemia and primary cells from patients with chronic myeloid leukemia. Blood 97:1404–1412

Sawyers CL, Hochhaus A, Feldman E, Goldman JM, Miller C, Ottmann OG, Schiffer CA, Talpaz M, Guilhot F, Deininger MWN, Fischer T, O'Brien SG, Stone R, Gambacorti-Passerini C, Russell N, Reiffers J, Shea T, Chapuis B, Coutre S, Tura S, Morra E, Larson RA, Saven A, Peschel C, Gratwohl A, Mandelli F, Ben-Am M, Gathmann I, Capdeville R, Paquette RL, Druker BJ (2002) Gleevec/Glivec (imatinib mesylate) induces hematologic and cytogenetic responses in patients with chronic myeloid leukemia in myeloid blast crisis: results of a phase II study. Blood 99:3530–3539

Shah NP, Tran C, Lee FY, Chen P, Norris D, Sawyers CL (2004) Overriding imatinib resistance with a novel ABL kinase inhibitor. Science 305:399–401

Silver RT, Talpaz M, Sawyers CL, Druker BJ, Hochhaus A, Schiffer CA, Guilhot F, Goldman JM, Smith BD, Mone M, Krahnke T, Kantarjian HM (2004) Four years of follow-up of 1027 patients with late chronic phase (L-CP), accelerated phase (AP), or blast crisis (BC) chronic myeloid leukemia (CML) treated with imatinib in three large phase ii trials. Blood 104 Suppl 1:11a

Soverini S, Martinelli G, Rosti G, Bassi S, Amabile M, Poerio A, Giannini B, Trabacchi E, Castagnetti F, Testoni N, Luatti S, de Vivo A, Cilloni D, Izzo B, Fava M, Abruzzese E, Alberti D, Pane F, Saglio G, Baccarani M (2005) ABL mutations in late chronic phase chronic myeloid leukemia patients with up-front cytogenetic resistance to imatinib are associated with a greater likelihood of progression to blast crisis and shorter survival: a study by the GIMEMA Working Party on Chronic Myeloid Leukemia. J Clin Oncol 23:4100–4109

Talpaz M, Silver RT, Druker BJ, Goldman JM, Gambacorti-Passerini C, Guilhot F, Schiffer CA, Deininger MWN, Lennard AL, Hochhaus A, Ottmann OG, Gratwohl A, Baccarani M, Stone R, Tura S, Mahon FX, Fernandes-Reese S, Gathmann I, Capdeville R, Kantarjian HM, Sawyers CL (2002) Imatinib induces durable hematologic and cytogenetic responses in patients with accelerated phase chronic myeloid leukemia: results of a phase 2 study. Blood 99:1928–1937

Weisberg E, Manley PW, Breitenstein W, Bruggen J, Cowan-Jacob SW, Ray A, Huntly B, Fabbro D, Fendrich G, Hall-Meyers E, Kung AL, Mestan J, Daley GQ, Callahan L, Catley L, Cavazza C, Azam M, Neuberg D, Wright RD, Gilliland DG, Griffin JD (2005) Characterization of AMN107, a selective inhibitor of native and mutant Bcr-Abl. Cancer Cell 7:129–141

Allogeneic Transplantation for CML

Charles Crawley, Jerald Radich and Jane Apperley

Contents

Abstract. The management of CML has changed dramatically over the past 5–7 years. The development of the specific tyrosine kinase inhibitor, imatinib, has resulted in incidences of cytogenetic and molecular response that far exceed those achieved with interferon. The median duration of survival is predicted to increase and the role of allogeneic transplantation has correspondingly decreased. However, the technology of allografting has also progressed in that developments in molecular typing methodology and in the management of infection have resulted in an improvement in the outcome of unrelated transplants. The imatinib era has coincided with the development of reduced intensity conditioning regimens and early results suggest that this is an effective strategy in CML associated with low transplant-related mortality. This chapter summarizes the data on the prognostic factors for both disease- and transplant-related outcomes and outlines the current indications for allogeneic transplant in CML. These indications for allografting will continue to evolve. Although allogeneic transplant is no longer the initial therapy in the majority of patients, it remains the strategy with the highest probability of achieving a molecular remission and curing the disease. As such it will continue to play a role in the management of CML.

7.1 Introduction

The decision to offer allogeneic hematopoietic stem cell transplantation to a patient with CML in chronic phase (CP) has always been difficult, with a balance to be drawn between the short-term risks of transplantation with the longer-term disease risks of medical therapy. The introduction of the selective tyrosine kinase inhibitor, imatinib (Glivec, Gleevec, STI571) has replaced interferon and cytarabine as primary medical therapy and while survival data remain immature, the data on surrogate markers of cytogenetic and molecular response are impressive. The evidence to date suggests that these responses will be followed by improvements in survival (Hughes et al. 2003). These data have led to a major re-evaluation of the role of allogeneic transplantation for this disease. The algorithms devised in the 1990s are no longer applicable and opinions remain divided as to the role of allogeneic hematopoietic stem cell transplantation in the management of CP disease in particular.

7.2 Changes in Allogeneic Transplant Practice

During the 1990s there was a steady rise in the use of allogeneic transplant for CML, particularly in CP disease. That trend dramatically reversed after 1999 with a reduction in transplant activity reported to the EBMT (European Group for Blood and Marrow Transplantation) of almost 40%. This fall has been restricted to patients transplanted in first CP and has not been matched by a change in the numbers of transplants performed for more advanced disease (Gratwohl et al. 2001b, 2004) (Fig. 7.1). The change in activity reflects the increased use of imatinib and was in anticipation of any demonstrable survival benefit. It has prompted suggestions that there may be little role for allogeneic transplants in the management of CP disease.

Concurrent with the introduction of imatinib, the past 7 years have also witnessed significant changes in allogeneic transplant practice. These include the introduction of reduced intensity conditioning (RIC) regimens or nonmyeloablative transplants with the associated reduction in procedural-related mortality. RIC accounted for less than 1% of transplants performed in Europe in 1998 but had increased to 27% in 2002–2003 (Gratwohl et al. 2004). Other improvements include better supportive care, which is reflected in the

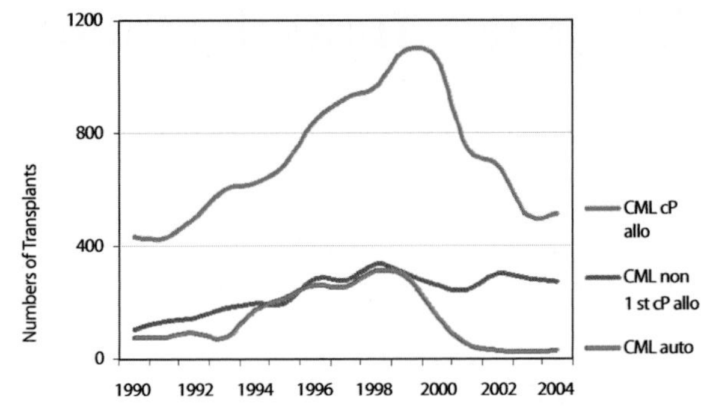

Fig. 7.1. Changes in transplant activity in CML between 1990 and 2003 as reported to EBMT

progressive reduction of infection-related deaths (Gratwohl et al. 2005). Finally, advances in molecular HLA typing methodologies have led to the outcome of unrelated donor transplantation approaching that achieved in HLA matched sibling transplantation (Davies et al. 2001; Hansen et al. 1998; Weisdorf et al. 2002).

The decision to recommend early transplant for patients with CML can only be made after careful consideration of prognostic factors at diagnosis, including those predicting both response to medical therapy and transplantation outcomes. This assessment should be conducted based on current outcome data as outcomes reported in the 1980s and early 1990s do not reflect the result of medical therapy or transplantation in the 21st century. Alternatively, if imatinib is to be offered, there must an attempt to develop criteria for molecular response and imatinib failure that would warrant a reconsideration of treatment strategy.

7.3 Prognostic Features at Diagnosis

There are a number of well-established prognostic models of survival for patients with CML that have been developed based on cohorts of similarly treated patients. These models identify patients who present in CP with high- or lower-risk disease based on the clinical features present at the time of diagnosis. It is important to appreciate that the value of these models varies with different treatments. The best-known score (Sokal et al. 1984) is a model that was based on patients treated predominantly with busulfan and hydroxycarbamide (hydroxyurea) and but is a less useful guide for patients treated with interferon. The Hasford score was developed for patients treated with interferon and confirmed the value of interferon in lower-risk patients (Hasford et al. 1998). Treatment has now changed again and the value of the Hasford score in patients treated with imatinib is uncertain. However, the Sokal score may be of prognostic value in this setting. For patients enrolled in the IRIS study and randomized to imatinib, the probability of achieving cytogenetic remissions were 76% and 49% for Sokal low-risk and high-risk disease, respectively. The Sokal score was also predictive for molecular responses with 66% of the low-risk patients and 45% of high-risk patients achieving a 3 log reduction in BCR-ABL transcript numbers (Hughes et al. 2003).

The applicability of the Sokal and Hasford scores to the outcome of transplantation has been less clear. Recently the International Blood and Marrow Transplant Registry (IBMTR) has analyzed the impact of the two scores on transplant outcome and found that they were entirely nonpredictive for survival (Passweg et al. 2004).

It is likely that prognostic scores based on clinical variables will be surpassed by biological markers as predictors of disease course and response to therapy. Examples include deletions of 9q, which occur in 15–20% of patients and are associated with an inferior outcome (Huntly et al. 2001), although there is some controversy as to whether the prognostic significance of 9q deletions is overcome with imatinib therapy (Huntly et al. 2003; Quintas-Cardama et al. 2005). Recently, gene expression profiling has identified candidate genes such as CD7 and proteinase-3 which may be of greater predictive value (Yong et al. 2006). The next few years may see the incorporation of these or other markers into the treatment algorithms.

7.3.1 Response to First Treatment as an Indicator of Prognosis

Interferon represented a significant advance over hydroxycarbamide and busulfan in that a significant minority (10–15%) of patients with CML achieved a complete cytogenetic remission, albeit after 1–2 years. This group of patients showed the greatest survival advantage. Data from the phase 2 studies suggested and the IRIS study confirmed that the complete cytogenetic remission (CCyR) rate after imatinib is substantially higher (74%) than that achieved with interferon. However, there has been concern over a number of case reports of rapid progression of disease to blast crises despite the achievement of CCyR (Avery et al. 2004; Jabbour et al. 2006; Morimoto et al. 2004). This has led to the question as to whether a CCyR achieved on imatinib carries the same prognostic weight as a remission achieved with interferon. These case reports, however, appear to be the exception and in patients who have achieved a CCyR, the depth of remission as measured by molecular response appears better with imatinib than with interferon. Interferon (or hydroxycarbamide) is now rarely considered as first-line therapy for CML and it is therefore the response to imatinib that is being used to predict outcome in general and progression-free survival in particular. In those patients with a CCyR and a 3 log reduction in BCR-ABL transcript levels as measured by quantitative RT-PCR, the progression-free survival (PFS) at 2 years is 100%. For patients who achieve CCyR but in whom the fall in the BCR-ABL/ABL ratio was less than 3 logs, the PFS is 95% and in those without CCyR the PFS was only 85% (Hughes et al. 2003). At present, the follow-up is too short to demonstrate an overall survival advantage, but given the very low rates of progression, the clear expectation is that this will be seen with time.

7.4 Prognostic Indicators for Transplant Outcome

The most widely used risk assessment score to predict transplant outcome was developed by Gratwohl et al. and is based on five prognostic features (age at transplant, disease stage at transplant, donor type, donor-recipient gender combination, and the interval from diagnosis to transplant) (Table 7.1). Using 3142 patients transplanted for CML from 1984–1994, the score was validated for transplant-related mortality, survival, and disease-free survival (Gratwohl et al. 1998). More recently the IBMTR has confirmed the value of the Gratwohl score using an independent data set comprising 3211 patients (Passweg et al. 2004). The prognostic value of additional factors such as CMV antibody status of patient and donor, donor age, donor/recipient ABO blood group compatibility, and Karnofsky performance score was examined. An initial impression that the Karnofsky score gave useful additional discriminatory power was not confirmed in a validation set of patients and has not been included in subsequent analyses.

Table 7.1 a. BMT transplant risk score

	Original EBMT risk score	
	Criteria	Score
Age	<20 yr	0
	20–40 yr	1
	>40 yr	2
Donor Type	Sibling	0
	Unrelated	1
Disease Phase	Chronic	0
	Accelerated	1
	Blastic	2
Interval Dx-SCT	<1 year	0
	>1 year	1
Sex Match	Female donor – male recipient	0
	All other	1

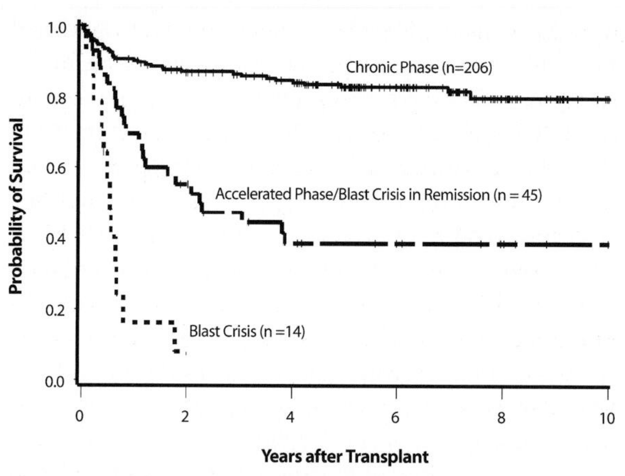

Fig. 7.2. Survival probability of 260 patients transplanted since 1992 according to disease stage at time of transplant (courtesy of Ted Goodey, Fred Hutchinson Cancer Research Center)

7.4.1 Disease Phase

The disease phase at the time of transplant remains the most important determinant of survival (Fig. 7.2) (Clift and Storb 1996; Horowitz et al. 1996). Survival after transplant in CP ranges from 60% to 90% at 5 years (Clift et al. 1999; Gratwohl et al. 1998; Horowitz et al. 1996). The use of chemotherapy preparative regimens, as opposed to total body irradiation (TBI)-based regimens, and improved supportive therapy (including CMV and fungal prophylaxis) may improve survival further. For example, both an initial and a follow-up report of CP CML patients randomized to a preparative regimen of TBI and cyclophosphamide or busulfan and cyclophosphamide (BU/CY) demonstrated similar efficacy of both regimens (Clift and Storb 1996; Clift et al. 1999). Subsequently, a pharmacological assay for blood busulfan levels revealed that patients with levels above 900 ng/ml had better survival and fewer relapses, compared to patients with a level <900 ng/ml (Slattery et al. 1997). This has led to subsequent targeting of busulfan in all patients to a level >900 ng/ml (which also

Table 7.1 b. Survival probabilities according to EBMT score

Risk Score	Number of patients with Score	% of patients with Score	Probability of outcome at 5 years (%)			
			LFS	Survival	TRM	RI
0	65	2	60	72	20	26
1	569	18	60	70	23	23
2	881	28	47	62	31	32
3	867	28	37	48	46	31
4	485	15	35	40	51	28
5	214	7	19	18	71	41
6	57	2	16	22	73	32
7	4	–	–	–	–	–

5-year probability of leukemia-free survival (LFS), survival, transplant-related mortality (TRM), and relapse incidence (RI).

permits correction for patients with a high busulfan level to prevent potential toxicity). This strategy may have contributed to the apparent improvement of survival in CML CP patients transplanted using targeted BU/CY. Indeed, in 131 consecutive CP CML patients treated in Seattle using a preparative regimen of pharmacologically targeted busulfan and cyclophosphamide, the 3-year survival was 85%, with a relapse rate of 8% (Radich et al. 2003). The wide interpatient variation in busulfan pharmacokinetics can also be overcome with the use of intravenous rather than oral busulfan (Kim et al. 2003) . Whether this will allow the Seattle data to be reproduced without the need for pharmacokinetic monitoring is an open question. Unfortunately, advances that may have improved outcomes in CP patients have not been easily translated to accelerated phase (AP) and blast crisis (BC) transplants. Survival rates in these phases have remained relatively static over the last decade, so that survival in AP remains approximately 25–40%, and BC, approximately 10%.

7.4.2 Age at Transplant

Regimen-related toxicity tends to climb with increasing patient age (Gratwohl et al. 1998). However, age limits have gradually increased as the introduction of new preparative regimens and supportive therapies have improved outcomes. For example, CP patients transplanted with matched related donors after TBI-based regimens experience a clear age effect, with superior outcomes in younger patients (<21 years of age), and a steady drop off in survival by increasing decade of age (Clift and Storb 1996). This age effect may be mitigated by the use of non-TBI regimens (e.g., targeted BU/CY), as recent data from the Fred Hutchinson Cancer Research Center in Seattle no longer show an age effect in patients in CP up to 65 years of age (Clift and Storb 1996). Likewise, age does not appear to be an important factor with RIC transplants (Crawley et al. 2005).

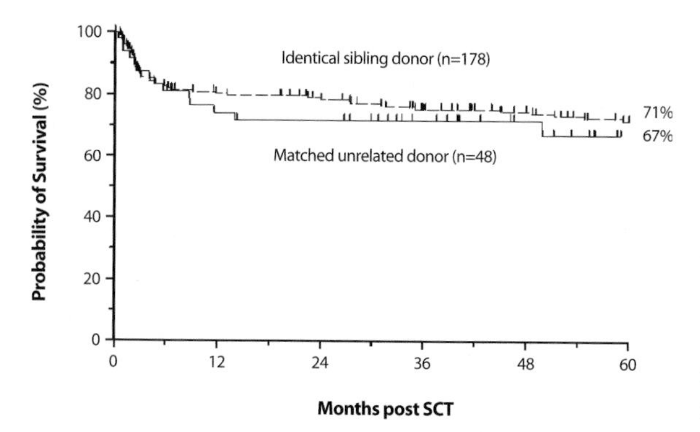

Fig. 7.3. Overall survival of 178 sibling allografts compared to 48 unrelated transplants for CML in first CP (data from Hammersmith Hospital London)

7.4.3 Source of Allograft Donor

For those who lack an HLA-identical sibling donor, the use of unrelated donor transplants is limited by donor availability, and the increased toxicity due to the effects of GVHD its associated infectious complications. Fully matched unrelated donors are now available for over 50% of Caucasian patients, but unfortunately, donors for patients from other ethnic groups are limited.

For "younger" patients (age <40 years), the results in CP CML are similar for fully matched unrelated and related transplants, especially for patients in "good risk" groups. In a series of 226 patients transplanted in first CP at the Hammersmith Hospital in London there were no differences in the transplant outcomes between those patients with unrelated and those with HLA identical sibling donors (Fig. 7.3). In a multicenter analysis of National Marrow Donor Program (NMDP) data, disease-free survival of unrelated and related transplants for CML CP patients aged 30–40 years, transplanted within 1 year of diagnosis, was 67% vs. 57%, respectively (Weisdorf et al. 2002). Two other studies have observed a near-equivalence of disease-free survival for CP CML using either a fully matched unrelated or related donor (Davies et al. 2001; Hansen et al. 1998). Estimates of disease-free survival of more than 70% were found for patients less than 50 years of age transplanted within a year of diagnosis (Hansen et al. 1998). Recent data from the EBMT support this with evidence that the survival after unrelated transplant has more than doubled between 1980–1990 and 2000–2003 from 29% to 63% at 2 years (Gratwohl et al. 2006).

The improved outcomes with unrelated donors are in a large part due to the use of sequence-based typing methodologies for HLA A, B, C, DR, and DQ. Transplant outcomes in CP CML are particularly affected by even a single antigen or allele mismatch (Petersdorf et al. 2004) (Fig. 7.4).

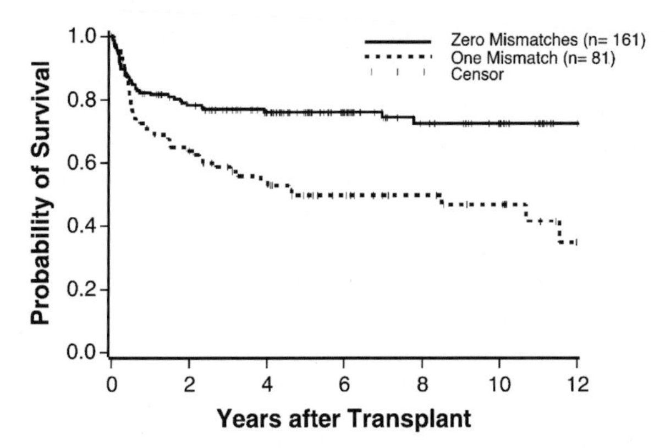

Fig. 7.4. Survival probability after unrelated transplant in CP CML transplanted within 2 years of diagnosis with respect the use a 10 antigen matched donor versus a mismatched donor (courtesy of Effie Petersdorf, Fred Hutchinson Cancer Research Center)

7.4.4 Source of Hematopoietic Stem Cells

Although autologous transplantation now uses almost exclusively peripheral blood-derived stem cells (PBSC) their use in the allogeneic transplant setting has been more controversial. A recent study reported the outcomes of highly purified CD34+PBSC for CP CML (n=49) compared to those of unmanipulated PBSC (n=21) and of BMSC (n=23) in the HLA-compatible sibling donor setting. The estimated probability of grade II –IV acute GVHD was 53% for the PBSC group, 37% for the BMT group, and 20% for the CD34+PBSC group. However, the probabilities for molecular and cytogenetic relapse were 92% and 58% for CD34+PBSCT, and a total of 38 of 49 patients after CD34+ PBSCT required additional T cells on a median of 2 occasions (range 1 to 7). The estimated probability of 3-year survival after transplant was 93% in the CD34+PBSCT compared with 71% in the PBSCT group, and 64% in the BMT group, respectively (Elmaagacli, 2003).

A recent individual patient data meta-analysis combined the data from nine randomized studies of sibling PBSC vs. BMT in a variety of hematological diseases. PBSC were associated as expected with faster engraftment. PBSC did not result in an increase in grades 2–4 acute GvHD but was associated with more grades 3–4 acute GvHD. Chronic GvHD was also more frequent including an increase in extensive chronic GvHD. Despite this, the use of PBSC corresponded to improvements in overall, progression-free survival and a reduction in relapse risk in patients with high-risk disease. An a priori subgroup analysis confirmed that this was true for CML specifically with an advantage for PBSC being seen for patients beyond first CP (Stem Cell Trialists' Collaborative Group 2005).

It is possible that the increased risks of GvHD in the unrelated donor setting may negate any benefit of PBSC. However, two studies from the Essen group evaluating the role of PBSC in the unrelated transplant setting have demonstrated the superiority of PBSC over bone marrow stem cells. The first showed that patients receiving PBSC had the BCR-ABL fusion transcripts detected less often compared to BM patients, suggesting a stronger graft vs. leukemia effect in the PBSC patients (Elmaagacli et al. 1999). The second study compared PBSC with bone marrow in CP CML, and found that the use of PBSC was associated with improved survival (94% vs. 66%), owing largely to a decrease in acute transplant-related mortality (5% vs. 30%). The overall prevalence of acute and chronic GVHD was similar between the two groups (Elmaagacli et al. 2002). Finally, a retrospective study of PBSC transplants compared to a matched set of BM unrelated donor transplants suggested that PBSC and BM transplants had similar rates of GVHD, relapse, and survival (Remberger et al. 2001). The effects appeared similar in all phases of CML.

7.4.5 Therapy Pretransplantation

The time from diagnosis to transplantation is a risk factor for poor outcome, with longer time intervals being associated with decreased survival (Clift and Storb 1996; Goldman 2001; Gratwohl et al. 1998; Sokal et al. 1984). The critical cut-off time is unclear. Data from both the EBMT and IBMTR suggest an outcome advantage for patients transplanted within 1 year from diagnosis in both the related and unrelated setting (Table 7.1); more recent data from Seattle suggests that for matched related donor transplant the cut-off may be at 2 years postdiagnosis (Clift and Storb 1996). The cause of this effect is not clear, but it may be due to both cumulative toxicity of the conventional therapy, leading to an increase in nonleukemic mortality, and from the underlying progression of disease that certainly occurs even during therapy. This is of increasing relevance, as the extensive use of imatinib will result in patients coming to transplant later in the course of their disease.

Prior therapy with busulfan adversely affects transplant outcome, compared with hydroxycarbamide

(Goldman et al. 1993). The effect of prior interferon therapy is controversial. Two studies have shown that prolonged interferon therapy (>6–12 months) was associated with increased nonleukemic mortality and decreased survival (Beelen et al. 1995; Morton et al. 1998). In contrast, no adverse effects of interferon therapy were found on the outcome of allogeneic HLA-identical sibling transplants, provided it was discontinued 90 days before allogeneic bone marrow transplantation (Hehlmann et al. 1999) or only given for a short period of time (median, 2 months) (Giralt et al. 2000).

The effect of pretransplantation therapy with imatinib on transplant morbidity, mortality, and relapse risk is unknown. However, since the introduction of imatinib there have been reports of clonal cytogenetic abnormalities occurring in Ph-chromosome negative cells, a phenomenon previously observed only rarely in patients rendered Ph negative in interferon (Bumm et al. 2003; Medina et al. 2003; O'Dwyer et al. 2003; Terre et al. 2004). These Ph-negative clonal rearrangements may occur in ~5% of patients who obtain a CCyR, and a small subset appears to have MDS/AML. The significance of the majority of these clonal changes in Ph-negative cells is, as yet, unclear. However, these molecular abnormalities may yield important information concerning the stability of the disease and its underlying propensity for transformation.

Relatively few patients have received transplant after prior imatinib therapy and most have been treated by both strategies for advanced phase disease. A recent report from the EBMT looking retrospectively at results of transplant for 70 patients with CML, of whom 44% were in advanced phase, described an estimated transplant-related mortality of 44% and an estimated relapse mortality of 24%. In a multivariate analysis comparing patient outcome with that of historical controls, prior imatinib treatment did not influence overall survival, progression free survival or non-relapse mortality (Deininger et al. 2006). Despite this report, the data are still insufficient to make any categorical statement about the risk and/or benefit of imatinib treatment before any planned transplant procedure.

7.4.6 Patient and Donor Gender

Male patients who receive stem cell products from female donors are known to have poorer survival in the short term largely attributable to an increase in treatment related mortality. This may be entirely due to the allo-recognition of peptides derived from Y chromosome encoded proteins. Although the short-term outcome is inferior in the longer-term, patients who survive such gender mismatch transplants have a corresponding decrease in relapse risk (Gratwohl et al. 2001a; Randolph et al. 2004). Some suggest that male patients at high risk of relapse should be preferentially transplanted from female donors.

7.5 Reduced Intensity Conditioning Transplantation

At the same time as the rapid developments in the tyrosine kinase inhibitors there has been a fundamental rethink of the principles of allogeneic transplantation. Until recently it was assumed that in order to ensure durable engraftment and long-term, disease-free survival, it was necessary to deliver myeloablative doses of chemotherapy and/or radiotherapy. There are a number of studies that suggest that conditioning dose intensity is important in the control of disease (Slattery et al. 1997), however the minimum dose of TBI required to ensure durable engraftment has been defined in the dog studies as 200 cGy, a dose well below that required for myeloablation (Storb et al. 1997). Several groups have taken this approach of immunosuppression rather than myeloablation through into human studies (Giralt et al. 1997; Sandmaier et al. 2000; Slavin et al. 1998). RIC has resulted in a reduction in TRM in most studies and this had enabled the age of patients in whom transplantation can be undertaken at an acceptable risk to be extended by 10–15 years. Over the last 5–7 years there has been a substantial increase in the numbers of RIC transplants and numbers of RIC regimens. Correspondingly, there has been an increase in the terminology, which remains confusing and includes terms such as nonmyeloablative transplants, mini-allografts, and micro-transplants. At present there are no agreed definitions of reduced intensity conditioning.

In comparison to conventional allogeneic hematopoietic stem cell transplantation, the RIC approach relies more on the graft vs. leukemia (GvL) effect than on the antitumor effects of chemotherapy to control disease. CML is a disease where the clinical importance of GvL has been most clearly demonstrated, donor lymphocyte infusions (DLI) being the most tangible example. Response rates to DLI in CML approach 60–70%

Table 7.2. Reported studies of RIC HSCT in CML

Author	N=	Protocol	Disease	Donor	Age	Response	Median Follow-up	NRM	DFS	OS
(Uzunel et al. 2003)	15	Fd/Bu/ATG	15 CP1	10 Sib 5 V'UD	51 yrs	11 BCR-ABL neg (median time 7 months)	20 months	2/15	3 BCR-ABL pos (median 8 months) 1 relapse	13/15
(Weisser et al. 2004)	35	Cy 80–120mg/kg /TBI (8Gy)	26 CP1 9CP2/AP	19 Sib 16 VUD	51 yrs	Cytogenetic 100% Molecular 85%	30 months	Day 100=11% 1 yr 28.5%	49% at 5 years	59% at 2 years
(Sloand et al. 2003)	12	Fd+Cyclo (120 mg/kg)	8 CP1 5 CP2	12 Sib	43 yrs	5 CCR at 6 months 4 mol remission at 1 year 8 mol remission with additional therapy	12 months	Day 100=0%	4 deaths from relapse	8/12
(Or et al. 2003)	24	Fd/Bu/ATG	24 CP1	18 Sib 1 father 5 VUD	35 yrs	100% Molecular remission (3 required DLI)	42 months	Day 100=0% 3 deaths	85% at 5 years	85% at 5 years
(Kerbauy et al. 2005)	24	2 Gy TBI ± Fd	14 CP1 4 CP 2 6 AP	24 Sib	57.5 yrs	15 CCR 13 Molecular remission	36 months	CP1 15% >CP1 12%	Relapse at 2 years CP1 22% >CP1 64%	CP1 70% >CP1 56%
(Das et al. 2003)	17	Fd/Bu/ATG (11) FD/Bu/TBI	16 CP1 1 AP	17 Sib	35	5 molecular remission	30 months	8/17	5/17	6/17
(Bornhauser et al. 2001)	44	Fd/Bu±ATG	26 CP 11 AP 7 BC	19 Sib 15 VUD	52	19/31 molecular remissions 26/31 cytogenetic	14.8 months	15/44	41% at 18 months	24/44

Table 7.2 (continued)

Author	N=	Protocol	Disease	Donor	Age	Response	Median Follow-up	NRM	DFS	OS
(Crawley et al. 2005)	186	Various	118 CP1 26 CP2 30 AP 12BC	113 Sib 20 other related 52 VUD	50 yrs	86.9% Overall	35 months	Day 100 =3.8% 2 yr =18.8%	33% at 3 yrs CP 43% at 3 yrs	54% at 3 yrs CP1 60% at 3yrs
(Ruiz-Arguelles et al. 2005)	24	Bu/Cy/Fd	24 CP	24 Sib	41 yrs	18/24 molecular remissions 5/24 Cytogenetic	15 months	8%	20/24 at 27 months	92% at 27 months

Fd, Fludarabine; Bu, Busulfan; ATG, Antithymocyte globulin; Cy, Cyclophosphamide; Sib, Sibling; VUD, Volunteer unrelated donor; TBI, total body irradiation and even in relapse into AP 30% of patients can be salvaged with DLI alone (Dazzi et al. 2000). As such, CML should be the disease in which RIC allogeneic transplantation is most effective.

Studies of RIC allografts in CML have been limited and the single center experience is summarized in Table 7.2. Data comparing outcomes with conventional conditioning are even more limited and are confounded by differences in patient characteristics and the biases of historical controls. The largest series published to date from the EBMT reported the outcomes on 186 patients. One hundred eighteen were transplanted in first CP, 26 in second CP, and 42 in the accelerated or blastic phases. A variety of different conditioning regimens were employed and the majority (72%) received peripheral blood transplants. Disease phase was the most important factor predicting outcome (RR 3.4) although patients in second CP had a survival only marginally worse than first CP patients (Crawley et al. 2005).

Analysis of outcomes stratified according to the EBMT transplant risk score suggested that disease-free and overall survival were similar if not better than that achieved with conventional conditioning. These conclusions need to be interpreted with caution as the influence of the individual prognostic factors, namely age, female-to-male donors, donor type, and time to transplant have not been established for RIC transplants. Furthermore, the published outcomes based on EBMT risk score are based on data collected between 1989 and 1994. In many diseases, transplant outcomes have improved over the last decade due to improvements in supportive care and better donor identification. There is a real need for comparative studies to determine any potential benefits of RIC compared to conventional transplant.

RIC approaches to allogeneic transplantation are clearly feasible in CML and appear to be associated with a lower nonrelapse mortality than has been seen previously with conventional conditioning (Fig. 7.5). There remain a number of unanswered questions. There are a wide range of different RIC regimens with very variable degrees of myelosuppression and immunosuppression, including some regimens that would previously have been considered to be myeloablative. It is unclear whether the results with different RIC regimens will be equivalent and the relative importance of cytotoxic chemotherapy and immune-mediated GvL in eradicating disease is uncertain. In the EBMT study, the use of fludarabine, busulfan, and antithymocyte globulin (Fd/Bu/ATG) appeared to be associated with improvements in

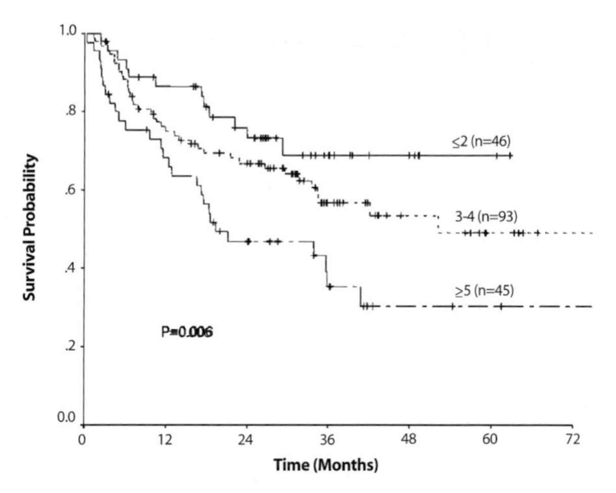

Fig. 7.5. Survival after RIC in 186 patients with CML stratified by EBMT score

disease-free survival (RR 0.7, p = 0.06) and a reduction in treatment-related mortality (RR 0.4, p = 0.02) but did not impact on overall survival. Fd/Bu/ATG is significantly more myelosuppressive with more nonhematological toxicity than the fludarabine and 2 Gy TBI approach pioneered by the Seattle group. Linked to this is the question whether prior cytoreduction with chemotherapy (including imatinib) influences the outcome of RIC transplants by optimizing the GvL effect. It is possible that some of the more myelosuppressive regimens such as Fd/Bu/ATG may be sufficient in their own right, whereas some of the least intensive regimens may benefit from the addition of pretransplant therapy.

A second area of controversy is the use of T cell depletion, most frequently achieved with lymphocyte depleting antibodies such as alemtuzumab and ATG. Their inclusion in the conditioning regimens facilitates engraftment and reduces graft vs. host disease. However, this is at the potential risk of leukemia relapse and delayed immune reconstitution. One strategy adopted to overcome this problem is the pre-emptive use of donor lymphocyte infusions post transplant. The risk of DLI is related to the time post transplant and the T-cell dose (Gilleece and Dazzi 2003). Imatinib is also an option and can be given safely post transplant. In a pilot study of 24 patients receiving RIC transplants at the Hammersmith Hospital, imatinib was given post transplant for 12 months. The imatinib was effective in maintaining molecular remission during administration and allowed the DLI to be delayed to a time where it might be used with a lower risk. Several other groups are exploring related protocols.

7.6 Detection and Management of Residual Disease

The definition of remission of CML has evolved over the last 15 years. It has been recognized for some time that morphological remission of CML is an inadequate endpoint in the control of the disease. In the interferon era cytogenetic remissions were the therapeutic goal and were associated with prolongation in survival. After allogeneic transplant it is now well established that the detection of the chimeric BCR-ABL mRNA transcript by RT-PCR is a powerful predictor of subsequent cytogenetic and hematological relapse. Increasingly molecular responses are being used as a surrogate for remission duration with imatinib therapy (Hughes et al. 2003).

7.6.1 Role of Qualitative RT-PCR for BCR-ABL

Early data relating to the incidence and risk of relapse after allografting were derived from qualitative RT-PCR assays for BCR-ABL transcripts. The highest risk of relapse occurs in patients who were BCR-ABL positive "early" (≤12 months) after transplant (Hughes et al. 1991; Roth et al. 1992; Sawyers et al. 1990). Approximately 25% of patients who appear to be in hematological remission during this time will be qualitatively positive for BCR-ABL (Radich et al. 2001). Minimal residual disease (MRD) can be detected by RT-PCR for years post transplant. BCR-ABL has been detected in 25–50% of patients more than 3 years post transplant, with subsequent relapse rates of approximately 10–20% (Costello et al. 1996; Pichert et al. 1995; Radich et al. 1995, 2001). These data suggest that low levels of BCR-ABL transcripts identified some years after transplant for CML may not be an absolute harbinger of relapse. How patients co-exist with MRD for years while their CML lays "dormant" remains a topic of speculation and research.

7.6.2 Quantitative Studies for *BCR-ABL* in CML

The predictive value of MRD detection is strengthened by BCR-ABL quantification ("Q-PCR") (Lin et al. 1996; Mensink et al. 1998; Mughal et al. 2001; Olavarria et al. 2001; Preudhomme et al. 1995). Several studies have demonstrated that the molecular burden of BCR-ABL mRNA, and the kinetics of increasing BCR-ABL, predict relapse (Lin et al. 1996). Low (or no) residual BCR-ABL was associated with a very low risk of relapse (1%), compared to a 75% relapse rate in patients with increasing or persistently high BCR-ABL levels. Olavarria et al. studied 138 CML patients "early" (3–5 months) post transplant and showed that the BCR-ABL level was highly correlated with relapse (Olavarria et al. 2001). Patients with no evidence of BCR-ABL had a 9% risk of subsequent relapse, whereas patients defined as having a "low" burden of disease (<100 BCR-ABL transcripts/µg RNA) or "high" level of transcripts (>100 copies/µg) had cumulative relapse rates of 30% and 74%, respectively. These results are consistent with a study of 379 CML patients "late" (>18 months) after transplant (Radich et al. 2001). Ninety patients (24%) had at least one assay positive for BCR-ABL, and 13/90 (14%) relapsed whereas 3/289 patients who were persistently BCR-ABL negative relapsed (hazard ratio of relapse=19). Q-PCR for BCR-ABL levels was performed on 344 samples from 85 patients, and a rising BCR-ABL transcript level heralded eventual relapse.

A recent study from the Hammersmith has further attempted to quantify the risk of relapse. This group has previously developed a definition of relapse based on the absolute value of the BCR-ABL/ABL ratio from their laboratory. Patients were considered to have definite evidence of disease recurrence requiring intervention if the BCR-ABL/ABL ratio exceeded 0.02% on three occasions or reached 0.05% on two occasions. They studied 243 patients who had received allogeneic transplants at their institute and had been monitored by quantitative RT-PCR. Four groups of patients could be identified: (1) 36 patients were "durably negative" or had a single low level positive result; (2) 51 patients, "fluctuating positive, low level", had more than one positive result but never more than two consecutive positive results; (3) 27 patients, "persistently positive, low level", had persisting low levels of BCR-ABL transcripts but never more than three consecutive positive results; and (4) 129 patients relapsed. In 107 of these, relapse was based initially only on molecular criteria; in 72 (67.3%) patients the leukemia progressed to cytogenetic or hematologic relapse either prior to or during treatment with donor lymphocyte infusions. The study not only confirmed the value of their definition of relapse, but indicated that the probability of disease recurrence was 20% and 30% in groups 2 and 3, respectively (Kaeda et al. 2006).

7.7 Indications for Allogeneic Transplantation

7.7.1 Primary Therapy

The decision to recommend allogeneic transplantation at presentation is a difficult one. Faced with the relatively low toxicity of imatinib, the risk of allogeneic transplantation is unacceptably high in the majority of patients including those with sibling donors. It should not be forgotten that patients with a low EBMT transplant score have a 5-year survival of 85% after stem cell transplant and with a relapse risk of only 15% they are potentially cured of their leukemia. Despite the impressive imatinib data, durable BCR-ABL molecular negativity rather than molecular response remains an infrequent occurrence. Failure to achieve BCR-ABL negativity is perhaps unsurprising given the data suggesting that there may be inherent resistance to imatinib in leukemic stem cells (Graham et al. 2002). Up-front transplantation remains a treatment option requiring consideration in a minority of patients with low EBMT transplant risk scores, adverse disease characteristics such as a high Sokal score, or adverse biological markers of high-risk disease. Finally, patient preference will remain a fundamental factor in the decision making process.

7.7.2 Allogeneic Transplantation After Imatinib Failure

Allogeneic transplantation should be considered in many patients in the event of failure of imatinib therapy. What is less clear is what constitutes imatinib failure. A working definition is show in Table 7.3. While the thresholds and time cut-offs may be open to debate, the principle of accepting loss of cytogenetic control or the loss of a molecular response is likely to remain. If transplant is to be utilized effectively it is important that it is considered before disease acceleration or blast crises prompts a review of therapeutic strategy.

7.7.3 Management of Persistent or Relapsed Disease Post Transplant

Donor lymphocyte infusions (DLI) have become the treatment of choice for patients who relapse after allo-

Table 7.3. Criteria for imatinib failure (Baccarani et al. 2006)

Time	Failure	Suboptimal response	Warnings
At diagnosis	NA	NA	High risk Del 9q Other chromosome abnormalities in Ph+ cells
3 months	No HR	Less than complete HR	
6 months	Less than complete HR No CyR	Less than partial CyR	
12 months	Less than partial CyR	Less than complete CyR	Less than major molecular response
18 months	Less than complete CyR	Less than major molecular response	
Any time	Loss of complete HR	Other chromosomal abnormalities in Ph+ cells	Any rise in transcript level
	Loss of complete CyR	Loss of major molecular response	Other chromosome abnormalities in Ph– cells
	Mutation (high imatinib insensitivity)	Mutation (low imatinib insensitivity)	

Haematological response (HR)

Cytogenetic response (CyR) complete Ph+ 0, partial Ph+ 1–35%, minor Ph+ 36–65%, minimal Ph+ 66–95%, non Ph+ >95%

Major molecular response as defined by Hughes et al. 2006

geneic SCT and durable molecular remissions are achieved in the majority of patients relapsing into CP (Guglielmi et al. 2002; Kolb et al. 1990, 1995). GVHD and marrow aplasia remain the two most important complications of DLI, but when an escalating dose schedule is used these problems are greatly reduced (Dazzi et al. 2000). In a recent EBMT study, survival after relapse was related to 5 factors: time from diagnosis to transplant, disease phase at transplant and at relapse, time from transplant to relapse, and donor type (Guglielmi et al. 2000). The effects of individual adverse risk factors were cumulative so that patients with two or more adverse features had a significantly reduced survival (35% vs. 65% at 5 years). Furthermore, DLI was less effective in patients who developed GVHD after transplant.

Imatinib is now an alternative to donor lymphocyte infusions with some data to suggest that it is well tolerated after both autologous and allogeneic transplant (Fischer et al. 2002; Kantarjian et al. 2002; Marin et al. 2002; Olavarria et al. 2002). The use of imatinib after allogeneic transplant could potentially be used to achieve remission without GVHD, and could be effective when DLI has failed. It could also be used in combination with lower doses of DLI to maximize responses while minimizing the risk of GVHD.

A number of groups have now used imatinib in the management of patients relapsing after allogeneic transplantation (Olavarria et al. 2003; Wassmann et al. 2001). Most of these patients were treated for relapse into advanced phase disease, as DLI are of limited value in this situation. Other patients were treated for cytogenetic relapse or hematological relapse into CP, often in the presence of on-going immunosuppression for GVHD and/or after failure of DLI. Recently, the Chronic Leukemia Working Party of the EBMT has reported a retrospective analysis of 128 patients treated with imatinib for relapse after allogeneic transplant (Olavarria et al. 2003). At the time of treatment with imatinib, 51 patients were in CP, 31 in AP, and 46 in BC. The median interval between relapse and start of imatinib was 5 months (range, 0 to 65 months). Fifty patients had failed treatment with DLI prior to imatinib. The overall hematological response rate was 84% (98% for patients in CP). The complete cytogenetic response was 58% for patients in CP, 48% for AP and 22% for patients in BC. Complete molecular responses were obtained in 25 patients (26%) of whom 21 were in CP or AP. With a median follow up of 9 months the estimated 2-year survivals for CP, AP, and BC patients were 100%, 86%, and 12% respectively. Of 79 evaluable patients, 45 (57%) achieved full donor and 11 (14%) mixed chimerism after imatinib therapy. Thus, imatinib appeared to have significant activity against relapsed CML after allogeneic transplant. Durable cytogenetic and molecular remissions were obtained in patients in CP, suggesting a certain degree of synergism between imatinib and the graft versus leukemia effect (Savani et al. 2005).

7.8 Summary

The treatment options for the newly diagnosed patient with CML have never been better although the treatment decisions remain difficult and the therapeutic algorithms are complex (Maziarz and Mauro 2003). In the majority of patients, initial therapy will be with imatinib. However, in the absence of long-term outcome data for imatinib, the relative merits of transplantation (with conventional or reduced intensity conditioning) or a tyrosine kinase inhibitor for younger patients will require more detailed consideration. Failure to achieve a CCyR should prompt a re-evaluation of treatment options. As the data mature, molecular responses are likely to become the endpoint of medical as well as transplantation therapies. At present allogeneic transplantation remains the primary alternative therapy although in the future alternative BCR-ABL or downstream signal transduction inhibitors may provide a rescue strategy for those patients in whom the response to imatinib is inadequate.

References

Avery S, Nadal E, Marin D, Olavarria E, Kaeda J, Vulliamy T, Brito Babapulle F, Goldman JM, Apperley JF (2004) Lymphoid transformation in a CML patient in complete cytogenetic remission following treatment with imatinib. Leuk Res 28(Suppl 1):75–77

Baccarani M, Saglio G et al (2006) Evolving concepts in the management of chronic myeloid leukemia. Recommendations from an expert panel on behalf of the European Leukemianet. Blood

Beelen DW, Graeven U, Elmaagacli AH, Niederle N, Kloke O, Opalka B, Schaefer UW (1995) Prolonged administration of interferon-alpha in patients with chronic-phase Philadelphia chromosome-positive chronic myelogenous leukemia before allogeneic bone marrow transplantation may adversely affect transplant outcome. Blood 85:2981–2990

Bornhauser M, Kiehl M, Siegert W, Schetelig J, Hertenstein B, Martin H, Schwerdtfeger R, Sayer HG, Runde V, Kroger N, Theuser C, Ehninger G (2001) Dose-reduced conditioning for allografting in 44 patients with chronic myeloid leukaemia: a retrospective analysis. Br J Haematol 115:119–124

Bumm T, Muller C, Al-Ali HK, Krohn K, Shepherd P, Schmidt E, Leiblein S, Franke C, Hennig E, Friedrich T, Krahl R, Niederwieser D, Deininger MW (2003) Emergence of clonal cytogenetic abnormalities in Ph-cells in some CML patients in cytogenetic remission to imatinib but restoration of polyclonal hematopoiesis in the majority. Blood 101:1941–1949

Clift RA, Storb R (1996) Marrow transplantation for CML: the Seattle experience. Bone Marrow Transplant 17(Suppl 3):1–3

Clift RA, Radich J, Appelbaum FR, Martin P, Flowers ME, Deeg HJ, Storb R, Thomas ED (1999) Long-term follow-up of a randomized study comparing cyclophosphamide and total body irradiation with busulfan and cyclophosphamide for patients receiving allogenic marrow transplants during chronic phase of chronic myeloid leukemia. Blood 94:3960–3962

Costello RT, Kirk J, Gabert J (1996) Value of PCR analysis for long term survivors after allogeneic bone marrow transplant for chronic myelogenous leukemia: a comparative study. Leuk Lymphoma 20:239–243

Crawley C, Szydlo R, Lalancette M, Bacigalupo A, Lange A, Brune M, Juliusson G, Nagler A, Gratwohl A, Passweg J, Komarnicki M, Vitek A, Mayer J, Zander A, Sierra J, Rambaldi A, Ringden O, Niederwieser D, Apperley JF (2005) Outcomes of reduced-intensity transplantation for chronic myeloid leukemia: an analysis of prognostic factors from the Chronic Leukemia Working Party of the EBMT. Blood 106:2969–2976

Das M, Saikia TK, Advani SH, Parikh PM, Tawde S (2003) Use of a reduced-intensity conditioning regimen for allogeneic transplantation in patients with chronic myeloid leukemia. Bone Marrow Transplant 32:125–129

Davies SM, DeFor TE, McGlave PB, Miller JS, Verfaillie CM, Wagner JE, Weisdorf DJ (2001) Equivalent outcomes in patients with chronic myelogenous leukemia after early transplantation of phenotypically matched bone marrow from related or unrelated donors. Am J Med 110:339–346

Dazzi F, Szydlo RM, Cross NC, Craddock C, Kaeda J, Kanfer E, Cwynarski K, Olavarria E, Yong A, Apperley JF, Goldman JM (2000) Durability of responses following donor lymphocyte infusions for patients who relapse after allogeneic stem cell transplantation for chronic myeloid leukemia. Blood 96:2712–2716

Deininger M, Schleuning M, Greinix H, Sayer HG, Fischer T, Martinez J, Maziarz R, Olavarria E, Verdonck L, Schaefer K, Boque C, Faber E, Nagler A, Pogliani E, Russell N, Volin L, Schanz U, Doelken G, Kiehl M, Fauser A, Druker B, Sureda A, Iacobelli S, Brand R, Krahl R, Lange T, Hochhaus A, Gratwohl A, Kolb H, Niederwieser D (2006) The effect of prior exposure to imatinib on transplant-related mortality. Haematologica 91:452–459

Elmaagacli AH, Beelen DW, Opalka B, Seeber S, Schaefer UW (1999) The risk of residual molecular and cytogenetic disease in patients with Philadelphia-chromosome positive first chronic phase chronic myelogenous leukemia is reduced after transplantation of allogeneic peripheral blood stem cells compared with bone marrow. Blood 94:384–389

Elmaagacli AH, Basoglu S, Peceny R, Trenschel R, Ottinger H, Lollert A, Runde V, Grosse-Wilde H, Beelen DW, Schaefer UW (2002) Improved disease-free-survival after transplantation of peripheral blood stem cells as compared with bone marrow from HLA-identical unrelated donors in patients with first chronic phase chronic myeloid leukemia. Blood 99:1130–1135

Elmaagacli AH, Peceny R, Steckel NC, Trenschel R, Ottinger H, Beelen DW (2003) Outcome of transplantation of highly purified peripheral blood CD34+ cells with T cell add-back compared to unmanipulated bone marrow or peripheral blood stem cells from HLA-identical sibling donors in patients with 1st chronic phase CML. Bone Marrow Transplant 31(Abst):O346

Fischer T, Reifenrath C, Hess GR, Corsetti MT, Kreil S, Beck J, Meinhardt P, Beltrami G, Schuch B, Gschaidmeier H, Hehlmann R, Hochhaus A, Carella A, Huber C (2002) Safety and efficacy of STI-571 (imatinib mesylate) in patients with bcr/abl-positive chronic myelogenous leukemia (CML) after autologous peripheral blood stem cell transplantation (PBSCT). Leukemia 16:1220–1228

Gilleece M, Dazzi F (2003) Donor lymphocyte infusions for patients who relapse after allogeneic stem cell transplantation for chronic myeloid leukaemia. Leuk Lymphoma 44:23–28

Giralt S, Estey E, Albitar M, van Besien K, Rondon G, Anderlini P, O'Brien S, Khouri I, Gajewski J, Mehra R, Claxton D, Andersson B, Beran M, Przepiorka D, Koller C, Kornblau S, Korbling M, Keating M, Kantarjian H, Champlin R (1997) Engraftment of allogeneic hematopoietic progenitor cells with purine analog-containing chemotherapy: harnessing graft-versus-leukemia without myeloablative therapy. Blood 89:4531–4536

Giralt S, Szydlo R, Goldman JM, Veum-Stone J, Biggs JC, Herzig RH, Klein JP, McGlave PB, Schiller G, Gale RP, Rowlings PA, Horowitz MM (2000) Effect of short-term interferon therapy on the outcome of subsequent HLA-identical sibling bone marrow transplantation for chronic myelogenous leukemia: an analysis from the international bone marrow transplant registry. Blood 95:410–415

Goldman J (2001) Implications of imatinib mesylate for hematopoietic stem cell transplantation. Semin Hematol 38:28–34

Goldman JM, Szydlo R, Horowitz MM, Gale RP, Ash RC, Atkinson K, Dicke KA, Gluckman E, Herzig RH, Marmont A et al (1993) Choice of pretransplant treatment and timing of transplants for chronic myelogenous leukemia in chronic phase. Blood 82:2235–2238

Graham SM, Jorgensen HG, Allan E, Pearson C, Alcorn MJ, Richmond L, Holyoake TL (2002) Primitive, quiescent, Philadelphia-positive stem cells from patients with chronic myeloid leukemia are insensitive to STI571 in vitro. Blood 99:319–325

Gratwohl A, Hermans J, Goldman JM, Arcese W, Carreras E, Devergie A, Frassoni F, Gahrton G, Kolb HJ, Niederwieser D, Ruutu T, Vernant JP, de Witte T, Apperley J (1998) Risk assessment for patients with chronic myeloid leukaemia before allogeneic blood or marrow transplantation. Chronic Leukemia Working Party of the European Group for Blood and Marrow Transplantation. Lancet 352:1087–1092

Gratwohl A, Hermans J, Niederwieser D, van Biezen A, van Houwelingen HC, Apperley J (2001 a) Female donors influence transplant-related mortality and relapse incidence in male recipients of sibling blood and marrow transplants. Hematol J 2:363–370

Gratwohl A, Passweg J, Baldomero H, Urbano-Ispizua A (2001 b) Hematopoietic stem cell transplantation activity in Europe 1999. Bone Marrow Transplant 27:899–916

Gratwohl A, Schmid O, Baldomero H, Horisberger B, Urbano-Ispizua A (2004) Haematopoietic stem cell transplantation (HSCT) in Europe 2002. Changes in indication and impact of team density. A report of the EBMT activity survey. Bone Marrow Transplant 34:855–875

Gratwohl A, Brand R, Frassoni F, Rocha V, Niederwieser D, Reusser P, Einsele H, Cordonnier C (2005) Cause of death after allogeneic haematopoietic stem cell transplantation (HSCT) in early leukaemias: an EBMT analysis of lethal infectious complications and changes over calendar time. Bone Marrow Transplant 36:757–769

Gratwohl A, Brand R, Apperley JF, Crawley C, Ruutu T, Corradini P, Carreras E, Devergie A, Niederwieser D (2006) Allogeneic hematopoietic stem cell transplantation for chronic myeloid leukemia in Europe 2006: transplant activity, long-term data and current results. An Analysis by the Chronic Leukemia Working Party of the European Group for Blood and Marrow Transplantation (EBMT). Haematologica 99:513–521

Guglielmi C, Arcese W, Hermans J, Bacigalupo A, Bandini G, Bunjes D, Carreras E, Devergie A, Frassoni F, Goldman J, Gratwohl A, Kolb HJ, Iori AP, Niederwieser D, Prentice HG, de Witte T, Apperley J (2000) Risk assessment in patients with Ph+ chronic myelogenous leukemia at first relapse after allogeneic stem cell transplant: an EBMT retrospective analysis. The Chronic Leukemia Working Party of the European Group for Blood and Marrow Transplantation. Blood 95:3328–3334

Guglielmi C, Arcese W, Dazzi F, Brand R, Bunjes D, Verdonck LF, Schattenberg A, Kolb HJ, Ljungman P, Devergie A, Bacigalupo A, Gomez M, Michallet M, Elmaagacli A, Gratwohl A, Apperley J, Niederwieser D (2002) Donor lymphocyte infusion for relapsed chronic myelogenous leukemia: prognostic relevance of the initial cell dose. Blood 100:397–405

Hansen JA, Gooley TA, Martin PJ, Appelbaum F, Chauncey TR, Clift RA, Petersdorf EW, Radich J Sanders JE, Storb RF, Sullivan KM, Anasetti C (1998) Bone marrow transplants from unrelated donors for patients with chronic myeloid leukemia. N Engl J Med 338:962–968

Hasford J, Pfirrmann M, Hehlmann R, Allan NC, Baccarani M, Kluin-Nelemans JC, Alimena G, Steegmann JL, Ansari H (1998) A new prognostic score for survival of patients with chronic myeloid leukemia treated with interferon alfa. Writing Committee for the Collaborative CML Prognostic Factors Project Group. J Natl Cancer Inst 90:850–858

Hehlmann R, Hochhaus A, Kolb HJ, Hasford J, Gratwohl A, Heimpel H, Siegert W, Finke J, Ehninger G, Holler E, Berger U, Pfirrmann M, Muth A, Zander A, Fauser AA, Heyll A, Nerl C, Hossfeld DK, Loffler H, Pralle H, Queisser W, Tobler A (1999) Interferon-alpha before allogeneic bone marrow transplantation in chronic myelogenous leukemia does not affect outcome adversely, provided it is discontinued at least 90 days before the procedure. Blood 94:3668–3677

Horowitz M, Rowlings P, Passweg J (1996) Allogeneic bone marrow transplantation for CML: a report from the International Bone Marrow Transplant Registry. Bone Marrow Transplant Suppl 3: 5–6

Hughes TP, Morgan GJ, Martiat P, Goldman JM (1991) Detection of residual leukemia after bone marrow transplant for chronic myeloid leukemia: role of polymerase chain reaction in predicting relapse. Blood 77:874–878

Hughes TP, Kaeda J, Branford S, Rudzki Z, Hochhaus A, Hensley ML, Gathmann I, Bolton AE, van Hoomissen IC, Goldman JM, Radich JP (2003) Frequency of major molecular responses to imatinib or interferon alfa plus cytarabine in newly diagnosed chronic myeloid leukemia. N Engl J Med, 349:1423–1432

Hughes TP, Deininger M et al (2006) Monitoring CML patients responding to treatment with tyrosine kinase inhibitors: review and recommendations for harmonizing current methodology for detecting BCR-ABL transcripts and kinase domain mutations and for expressing results. Blood 108(1):28–37

Huntly BJ, Guilhot F, Reid AG, Vassiliou G, Hennig E, Franke C, Byrne J, Brizard A, Niederwieser D, Freeman-Edward J, Cuthbert G, Bown N, Clark RE, Nacheva EP, Green AR, Deininger MW (2003) Imatinib improves but may not fully reverse the poor prognosis of patients with CML with derivative chromosome 9 deletions. Blood 102: 2205–2212

Huntly BJ, Reid AG, Bench AJ, Campbell LJ, Telford N, Shepherd P, Szer J, Prince HM, Turner P, Grace C, Nacheva EP, Green AR (2001) Deletions of the derivative chromosome 9 occur at the time of the Philadelphia translocation and provide a powerful and independent prognostic indicator in chronic myeloid leukemia. Blood 98:1732–1738

Jabbour E, Kantarjian H, O'Brien S, Rios MB, Abruzzo L, Verstovsek S, Garcia-Manero G, Cortes J (2006) Sudden blastic transformation in patients with chronic myeloid leukemia treated with imatinib mesylate. Blood 107:480–482

Kaeda J, Szydlo RM, O'Shea D, Olavarria E, Dazzi F, Marin D, Saunders S, Khorashad JS, Cross NCP, Goldman JM, Apperley JF (2006) Serial measurement of BCR-ABL transcripts in the peripheral blood after allogeneic stem cell transplantation for chronic myeloid leukemia: an attempt to define patients who may not require further therapy. Blood 107:4171–4176

Kantarjian HM, O'Brien S, Cortes JE, Giralt SA, Rios MB, Shan J, Giles FJ, Thomas DA, Faderl S, De Lima M, Garcia-Manero G, Champlin R, Arlinghaus R, Talpaz M (2002) Imatinib mesylate therapy for relapse after allogeneic stem cell transplantation for chronic myelogenous leukemia. Blood 100:1590–1595

Kerbauy FR, Storb R, Hegenbart U, Gooley T, Shizuru J, Al-Ali HK, Radich JP, Maloney DG, Agura E, Bruno B, Epner EM, Chauncey TR, Blume KG, Niederwieser D, Sandmaier BM (2005) Hematopoietic cell transplantation from HLA-identical sibling donors after low-dose radiation-based conditioning for treatment of CML. Leukemia 19:990–997

Kim SE, Lee JH, Choi SJ, Kim WK, Lee JS, Sohn HJ, Kang HJ, Park S, Kim K, Kim K, Seol M, Lee YS, Lee KH (2003) Intravenous vs. oral busulfan-based conditioning therapy prior to allogeneic bone marrow transplantation – A case controlled study. Blood 102 (abstract no 2629)

Kolb HJ, Mittermuller J, Clemm C, Holler E, Ledderose G, Brehm G, Heim M, Wilmanns W (1990) Donor leukocyte transfusions for treatment of recurrent chronic myelogenous leukemia in marrow transplant patients. Blood 76:2462–2465

Kolb HJ, Schattenberg A, Goldman JM, Hertenstein B, Jacobsen N, Arcese W, Ljungman P, Ferrant A, Verdonck L, Niederwieser D, van Rhee F, Mittermueller J, de Witte T, Holler E, Ansari H (1995) Graft-versus-leukemia effect of donor lymphocyte transfusions in marrow grafted patients. Blood 86:2041–2050

Lin F, van Rhee F, Goldman JM, Cross NC (1996) Kinetics of increasing BCR-ABL transcript numbers in chronic myeloid leukemia patients who relapse after bone marrow transplantation. Blood 87:4473–4478

Marin D, Marktel S, Bua M, Armstrong L, Goldman JM, Apperley JF, Olavarria E (2002) The use of imatinib (STI571) in chronic myeloid leukemia: some practical considerations. Haematologica 87:979–988

Maziarz RT, Mauro MJ (2003) Transplantation for chronic myelogenous leukemia: yes, no, maybe soAn Oregon perspective. Bone Marrow Transplant 32:459–469

Medina J, Kantarjian H, Talpaz M, O'Brien S, Garcia-Manero G, Giles F, Rios MB, Hayes K, Cortes J (2003) Chromosomal abnormalities in Philadelphia chromosome-negative metaphases appearing during imatinib mesylate therapy in patients with Philadelphia chromosome-positive chronic myelogenous leukemia in chronic phase. Cancer 98:1905–1911

Mensink E, van de Locht A, Schattenberg A, Linders E, Schaap N, Geurts van Kessel A, De Witte T (1998) Quantitation of minimal residual disease in Philadelphia chromosome positive chronic myeloid leukaemia patients using real-time quantitative RT-PCR. Br J Haematol 102:768–774

Morimoto A, Ogami A, Chiyonobu T, Takanashi M, Sugimoto T, Imamura T, Ishida H, Yoshihara T, Imashuku S (2004) Early blastic transformation following complete cytogenetic response in a pediatric chronic myeloid leukemia patient treated with imatinib mesylate. J Pediatr Hematol Oncol 26:320–322

Morton AJ, Gooley T, Hansen JA, Appelbaum FR, Bruemmer B, Bjerke JW, Clift R, Martin PJ, Petersdorf EW, Sanders JE, Storb R, Sullivan KM, Woolfrey A, Anasetti C (1998) Association between pretransplant interferon-alpha and outcome after unrelated donor marrow transplantation for chronic myelogenous leukemia in chronic phase. Blood 92:394–401

Mughal TI, Yong A, Szydlo RM, Dazzi F, Olavarria E, van Rhee F, Kaeda J, Cross NC, Craddock C, Kanfer E, Apperley J, Goldman JM (2001) Molecular studies in patients with chronic myeloid leukaemia in remission 5 years after allogeneic stem cell transplant define the risk of subsequent relapse. Br J Haematol 115:569–574

O'Dwyer ME, Gatter KM, Loriaux M, Druker BJ, Olson SB, Magenis RE, Lawce H, Mauro MJ, Maziarz RT, Braziel RM (2003) Demonstration of Philadelphia chromosome negative abnormal clones in patients with chronic myelogenous leukemia during major cytogenetic responses induced by imatinib mesylate. Leukemia 17:481–487

Olavarria E, Kanfer E, Szydlo R, Kaeda J, Rezvani K, Cwynarski K, Pocock C, Dazzi F, Craddock C, Apperley JF, Cross NC, Goldman JM (2001) Early detection of BCR-ABL transcripts by quantitative reverse transcriptase-polymerase chain reaction predicts outcome after allogeneic stem cell transplantation for chronic myeloid leukemia. Blood 97:1560–1565

Olavarria E, Craddock C, Dazzi F, Marin D, Marktel S, Apperley JF, Goldman JM (2002) Imatinib mesylate (STI571) in the treatment of relapse of chronic myeloid leukemia after allogeneic stem cell transplantation. Blood 99:3861–3862

Olavarria E, Ottmann OG, Deininger M, Clark RE, Bandini G, Byrne J, Lipton J, Vitek A, Michallet M, Siegert W, Ullmann A, Wassmann B, Niederwieser D, Fischer T (2003) Response to imatinib in patients who relapse after allogeneic stem cell transplantation for chronic myeloid leukemia. Leukemia 17:1707–1712

Or R, Shapira MY, Resnick I, Amar A, Ackerstein A, Samuel S, Aker M, Naparstek E, Nagler A, Slavin S (2003) Nonmyeloablative allogeneic stem cell transplantation for the treatment of chronic myeloid leukemia in first chronic phase. Blood 101:441–445

Passweg JR, Walker I, Sobocinski KA, Klein JP, Horowitz MM, Giralt SA (2004) Validation and extension of the EBMT Risk Score for patients with chronic myeloid leukaemia (CML) receiving allogeneic haematopoietic stem cell transplants. Br J Haematol 125:613–620

Petersdorf EW, Anasetti C, Martin PJ, Gooley T, Radich J, Malkki M, Woolfrey A, Smith A, Mickelson E, Hansen JA (2004) Limits of HLA mismatching in unrelated hematopoietic cell transplantation. Blood 104:2976–2980

Pichert G, Roy DC, Gonin R, Alyea EP, Belanger R, Gyger M, Perreault C, Bonny Y, Lerra I, Murray C et al (1995) Distinct patterns of minimal residual disease associated with graft-versus-host disease after allogeneic bone marrow transplantation for chronic myelogenous leukemia. J Clin Oncol 13:1704–1713

Preudhomme C, Wattel E, Lai JL, Henic N, Meyer L, Noel MP, Cosson A, Jouet JP, Fenaux P (1995) Good predictive value of combined cytogenetic and molecular follow up in chronic myelogenous leukemia after non T-cell depleted allogeneic bone marrow transplantation: a report on 38 consecutive cases. Leuk Lymphoma 18:265–271

Quintas-Cardama A, Kantarjian H, Talpaz M, O'Brien S, Garcia-Manero G, Verstovsek S, Rios MB, Hayes K, Glassman A, Bekele BN, Zhou X, Cortes J (2005) Imatinib mesylate therapy may overcome the poor prognostic significance of deletions of derivative chromosome 9 in patients with chronic myelogenous leukemia. Blood 105:2281–2286

Radich JP, Gehly G, Gooley T, Bryant E, Clift RA, Collins S, Edmands S, Kirk J, Lee A, Kessler P et al (1995) Polymerase chain reaction detection of the BCR-ABL fusion transcript after allogeneic marrow transplantation for chronic myeloid leukemia: results and implications in 346 patients. Blood 85:2632–2638

Radich JP, Gooley T, Bryant E, Chauncey T, Clift R, Beppu L, Edmands S, Flowers ME, Kerkof K, Nelson R, Appelbaum FR (2001) The significance of bcr-abl molecular detection in chronic myeloid leukemia patients "late," 18 months or more after transplantation. Blood 98:1701–1707

Radich JP, Gooley T, Bensinger W, Chauncey T, Clift R, Flowers M, Martin P, Slattery J, Sultan D, Appelbaum FR (2003) HLA-matched related hematopoietic cell transplantation for chronic-phase CML using a targeted busulfan and cyclophosphamide preparative regimen. Blood 102:31–35

Randolph SSB, Gooley TA, Warren EH, Appelbaum FR, Riddell SR (2004) Female donors contribute to a selective graft-versus-leukemia effect in male recipients of HLA-matched, related hematopoietic stem cell transplants. Blood 103:347–352

Remberger M, Ringden O, Blau IW, Ottinger H, Kremens B, Kiehl MG, Aschan J, Beelen DW, Basara N, Kumlien G, Fauser AA, Runde V (2001) No difference in graft-versus-host disease, relapse, and survival comparing peripheral stem cells to bone marrow using unrelated donors. Blood 98:1739–1745

Roth MS, Antin JH, Ash R, Terry VH, Gotlieb M, Silver SM, Ginsburg D (1992) Prognostic significance of Philadelphia chromosome-positive cells detected by the polymerase chain reaction after allogeneic bone marrow transplant for chronic myelogenous leukemia. Blood 79:276–282

Ruiz-Arguelles GJ, Gomez-Almaguer D, Morales-Toquero A, Gutierrez-Aguirre CH, Vela-Ojeda J, Garcia-Ruiz-Esparza MA, Manzano C, Karduss A, Sumoza A, de-Souza C, Miranda E, Giralt S (2005) The early referral for reduced-intensity stem cell transplantation in patients with Ph1 (+) chronic myelogenous leukemia in chronic phase in the imatinib era: results of the Latin American Cooperative Oncohematology Group (LACOHG) prospective, multicenter study. Bone Marrow Transplant 36:1043–1047

Sandmaier BM, McSweeney P, Yu C, Storb R (2000) Nonmyeloablative transplants: preclinical and clinical results. Semin Oncol 27:78–81

Savani BN, Montero A, Kurlander R, Childs R, Hensel N, Barrett AJ (2005) Imatinib synergizes with donor lymphocyte infusions to achieve rapid molecular remission of CML relapsing after allogeneic stem cell transplantation. Bone Marrow Transplant 3: 1009–1015

Sawyers CL, Timson L, Kawasaki ES, Clark SS, Witte ON, Champlin R (1990) Molecular relapse in chronic myelogenous leukemia patients after bone marrow transplantation detected by polymerase chain reaction. Proc Natl Acad Sci USA 87:563–567

Slattery JT, Clift RA, Buckner CD, Radich J, Storer B, Bensinger WI, Soll E, Anasetti C, Bowden R, Bryant E, Chauncey T, Deeg HJ, Doney KC, Flowers M, Gooley T, Hansen JA, Martin PJ, McDonald GB, Nash R, Petersdorf EW, Sanders JE, Schoch G, Stewart P, Storb R, Sullivan KM, Thomas ED, Witherspoon RP, Appelbaum FR (1997) Marrow transplantation for chronic myeloid leukemia: The Influence of plasma busulfan levels on the outcome of transplantation. Blood 89:3055–3060

Slavin S, Nagler A, Naparstek E, Kapelushnik Y, Aker M, Cividalli G, Varadi G, Kirschbaum M, Ackerstein A, Samuel S, Amar A, Brautbar C, Ben-Tal O, Eldor A, Or R (1998) Nonmyeloablative stem cell transplantation and cell therapy as an alternative to conventional bone marrow transplantation with lethal cytoreduction for the treatment of malignant and nonmalignant hematologic diseases. Blood 91:756–763

Sloand E, Childs RW, Solomon S, Greene A, Young NS, Barrett AJ (2003) The graft-versus-leukemia effect of nonmyeloablative stem cell allografts may not be sufficient to cure chronic myelogenous leukemia. Bone Marrow Transplant 32:897–901

Sokal J, Cox E, Baccarani M, Tura S, Gomez G, Robertson J, Tso C, Braun T, Clarkson B, Cervantes F (1984) Prognostic discrimination in "good-risk" chronic granulocytic leukemia. Blood 63:789–799

Stem Cell Trialists' Collaborative Group (2005) Allogeneic peripheral blood stem-cell compared with bone marrow transplantation in the management of hematologic malignancies: an individual patient data meta-analysis of nine randomized trials. J Clin Oncol 23:5074–5087

Storb R, Yu C, Wagner JL, Deeg HJ, Nash RA, Kiem HP, Leisenring W, Shulman H (1997) Stable mixed hematopoietic chimerism in DLA-identical littermate dogs given sublethal total body irradiation before and pharmacological immunosuppression after marrow transplantation. Blood 89:3048–3054

Terre C, Eclache V, Rousselot P, Imbert M, Charrin C, Gervais C, Mozziconacci MJ, Maarek O, Mossafa H, Auger N, Dastugue N, Talmant P, Van den Akker J, Leonard C, Khac FN, Mugneret F, Viguie F, Lafage-Pochitaloff M, Bastie JN, Roux GL, Nicolini F, Maloisel F, Vey N, Laurent G, Recher C, Vigier M, Yacouben Y, Giraudier S, Vernant JP, Salles B, Roussi J, Castaigne S, Leymarie V, Flandrin G, Lessard M (2004) Report of 34 patients with clonal chromosomal abnormalities in Philadelphia-negative cells during imatinib treatment of Philadelphia-positive chronic myeloid leukemia. Leukemia 18: 1340–1346

Uzunel M, Mattsson J, Brune M, Johansson JE, Aschan J, Ringden O (2003) Kinetics of minimal residual disease and chimerism in patients with chronic myeloid leukemia after nonmyeloablative conditioning and allogeneic stem cell transplantation. Blood 101:469–472

Wassmann B, Klein SA, Scheuring U, Pfeifer H, Martin H, Gschaidmeier H, Hoelzer D, Ottmann OG (2001) Hematologic and cytogenetic remission by STI571 (Glivec) in a patient relapsing with AP CML after second allogeneic stem cell transplantation. Bone Marrow Transplant 28:721–724

Weisdorf DJ, Anasetti C, Antin JH, Kernan NA, Kollman C, Snyder D, Petersdorf E, Nelson G, McGlave P (2002) Allogeneic bone marrow transplantation for chronic myelogenous leukemia: comparative analysis of unrelated versus matched sibling donor transplantation. Blood 99:1971–1977

Weisser M, Schleuning M, Ledderose G, Rolf B, Schnittger S, Schoch C, Schwerdtfeger R, Kolb HJ (2004) Reduced-intensity conditioning using TBI (8 Gy), fludarabine, cyclophosphamide and ATG in elderly CML patients provides excellent results especially when performed in the early course of the disease. Bone Marrow Transplant 34:1083–1088

Yong AS, Szydlo RM, Goldman JM, Apperley JF, Melo JV (2006) Molecular profiling of CD34+ cells identifies low expression of CD7, along with high expression of proteinase 3 or elastase as predictors of longer survival in patients with CML. Blood 107:205–212

Autografting in Chronic Myeloid Leukemia

Eduardo Olavarria

Contents

Abstract. Autografting was first attempted for patients with chronic myeloid leukemia (CML) in transformation in order to restore a second chronic phase (CP). The principal rationale for autografting in CP resides on the reduction of the tumor burden and the number of leukemic cells at risk of developing blastic transformation, and the possibility of eradicating already mutated cells. In a European Group for Blood and Marrow Transplantation (EBMT) survey, patients with CML in CP, undergoing autologous stem cell transplantation (SCT) for the first time, had an overall survival of 65% at 5 years from transplant with more than 50% of all patients remaining in CP. The main point made by this retrospective study was that in patients refractory to interferon alpha (IFN), 70% achieved a cytogenetic response post autografting, which was complete or major in 31%. Since the advent of imatinib, autografting in CML has experienced a substantial decline. Theoretically, there are several possible ways of using autologous SCT in combination with imatinib: (1) to reverse resistance to imatinib; (2) to eliminate a Ph-positive clone bearing a BCR-ABL kinase domain mutation; and (3) to reduce the level of residual disease after a cytogenetic response to imatinib in patients in whom Ph-negative cells had been harvested.

8.1 Introduction

Autologous stem cell transplantation (auto-SCT) was first attempted for patients with CML in transformation in order to restore a second CP. In 1978, Buckner, et al. used bone marrow harvested during the CP to rescue hematopoiesis after a supralethal myeloablative conditioning regimen including total body irradiation (TBI) (Buckner et al. 1978). Subsequently, Goldman et al. reported that peripheral blood progenitor cells collected at diagnosis could efficiently be used to reconstitute hematopoiesis after similar conditioning (Goldman et al. 1978, 1979). The results of auto-SCT for CML in transformation have been extensively reviewed (Butturini et al. 1990; Haines et al. 1984; Pigneux et al. 1999; Reiffers et al. 1991, 1996 a) and can be summarized as follows. First, hematopoietic recovery is faster after peripheral blood than bone marrow SCT. Second, following auto-SCT, some patients exhibit a "cytogenetic conversion", due to the re-emergence of Ph-negative cells and they seem to have prolonged survival. Third, unsurprisingly, the survival of patients transplanted in accelerated phase is longer than that of those transplanted in blast crisis. Fourth, patients who have received a "double" transplant seem to have a longer survival than those undergoing a single transplant do. Fifth, patients treated with IFN after transplant survive longer than others. Finally, a second CP is obtained in most cases but its duration is usually short, as most patients develop a recurrent blast crisis within 6–9 months, which reflects recrudescence of the clone involved in the first transformation.

Thus, in most patients with advanced disease restoring a prolonged second CP has not proved possible, and so auto-SCT has progressively been abandoned for patients with CML in transformation. However, a double auto-SCT followed by IFN may be beneficial for patients in accelerated phase without a suitable donor. It has been shown by the group in Bordeaux that patients who received a double autograft had a 3-year survival of 47±22% (Pigneux et al. 1999).

8.2 Autografting in Chronic Phase: Rationale

Autografting in CP was increasingly used in Europe in the 1990s as some preliminary results suggested that auto-SCT could increase the proportion of patients with a cytogenetic response, and thus prolong survival (Hehlmann et al. 2000). Although it is well known that the reinfused material contributes to the reappearance of the disease (Deisseroth et al. 1994), the principal rationale for autografting in CP resides on the reduction of the tumor burden and the number of leukemic cells at risk of developing a second genetic event responsible for the blastic transformation (Bhatia et al. 1998; Daley 1996). This, in turn, would delay the emergence of a blastic phase and prolong survival. A second possibility is the "setting back the clock" effect by which the cells that have already mutated will be eradicated and new, fresh, nontransformed cells will replace them after the transplant (Miller 1998). Thirdly, there is the possibility of reversing IFN resistance so that IFN can induce a cytogenetic response when used after autografting in patients previously resistant to IFN. More recently, the group in Genoa has shown the feasibility of collecting Ph negative "stem" cells after in vivo purging with chemotherapy ["mini-ICE" comprising idarubicin, cytarabine and etoposide followed by granulocyte colony-stimulating factor (G-CSF)]. These "normal" Ph-negative cells can be used in an autografting procedure and most patients recover with Ph-negative hemopoiesis (Carella et al. 1996, 1999). This strategy has introduced a new goal in autografting in CML: the possibility of long-term Ph-negative remissions.

8.3 Choice of Progenitor Cells

For many years, auto-SCT was performed using either unmodified bone marrow harvested during CP or peripheral blood cells collected at diagnosis before treatment. In 1978, the group at the Hammersmith Hospital in London (Goldman et al. 1978) first reported that very high numbers of CFU-GM were present in the blood of CML patients at diagnosis and could easily be collected by leukapheresis. Other investigators subsequently confirmed this. For example, in Bordeaux, they performed 1,103 leukapheresis procedures in 212 CML patients, at diagnosis and before any treatment. The median number of nucleated cells and CFU-GM collected per leukapheresis were 2.7 (0.9–12.8)$\times 10^8$/kg and 31.2 (0–1255.2)$\times 10^4$/kg, respectively. The median number of CFU-GM collected in one single leukapheresis was 17.5 ($\times 10^4$/kg) and this was higher than that usually obtained from marrow harvest. Not surprisingly, the cell yield (CFU-GM) was correlated not only with the initial white blood cell count ($r \leq 0.24$; $p < 0.001$) but also with the platelet count ($r = 0.12$; $p = 0.0001$) and the Sokal risk index ($r = 0.2$; $p = 0.005$) (Bouzgarrou et al. 1991). When transplanted, these cells engrafted very quickly in about 15 days, which is more rapidly than observed after autologous bone marrow transplantation for patients with CML (Reiffers 1985). Since peripheral blood and bone marrow in early CP contain Ph-negative progenitors (Coulombel et al. 1983; Jazwieck et al. 1995; Kirk et al. 1995; Petzer et al. 1996), these cells are able to engraft and are probably responsible for the cytogenetic conversions which are regularly seen after auto-SCT, as they have a proliferative advantage (when transplanted), at least in the short term, over Ph-positive progenitor cells (Brito-Babapulle et al. 1989; Haines et al. 1984; Reiffers et al. 1996). Thus, as peripheral blood seems to be at least as effective as bone marrow cells for inducing cytogenetic conversion and to contain more progenitors (leading to quicker engraftment) than bone marrow, most autologous transplants are now performed with Ph-negative peripheral blood stem cells (PBSC).

The advantages of PBSC include more feasibility and easier collection, increased numbers of stem cells collected, the possibility of multiple collections and the option of collecting stem cells after different therapies. The possibility of manipulation of PBSC (either in vitro or in vivo) is discussed in a different chapter. Several attempts have been made to collect stem cells following treatment with IFN in patients with some degree of cytogenetic response (Archimbaud et al. 1997; Olavarria et al. 2000b; Reiffers et al. 1998; Russo et al. 1999). It is now accepted that totally or partially Ph-negative peripheral blood stem cells can be collected after interferon and used for autografting without further manipulation. The use of bone marrow cells has proved technically more difficult (Meloni et al. 1999; The Italian Cooperative Group 1993). Although no survival advantage was seen in early studies (Goldman 1997; Reiffers et al. 1994), it subsequently appeared that bone marrow cells may carry a higher mortality risk and therefore a worse survival after auto-SCT (Olavarria et al. 2002). PBSC have also been collected after auto-SCT, thus allowing for sequential transplants (Spencer et al. 1998).

8.4 Autografting in Chronic Phase: Single Center Results

No prospective study has compared auto-SCT with IFN or other treatment modalities, so it remains unknown whether auto-SCT can prolong survival in CML, and if so which category of patients benefit most. The results of auto-SCT are still very difficult to interpret as most of the studies performed were pilot studies or phase II trials, with only small numbers of patients included and short follow-up (shorter in many cases than the usual median survival of CML!). Moreover, in most series, the indications for auto-SCT were unclear, although most patients seem to have been transplanted for poor prognostic factors such as resistance to IFN treatment. Many single center and multicentric studies have now been published and their principal results are summarized in Table 8.1. They are very difficult to compare given the wide heterogeneity in the characteristics of patients (inclusion criteria) and transplants (e.g., conditioning regimens, source of stem cells, treatment administered after auto-SCT). Despite this heterogeneity, the overall results look similar.

Three main single-center studies have been reported in Europe. First, Meloni, et al. (Meloni et al. 1990) reported 34 patients who were transplanted in CP after Melphalan (60 mg/m^2) and busulfan (4 mg/kg/day, 4 days). Twenty-two treated in the early phase of the disease were transplanted with PBSC within 12 months of diagnosis (group A). Twelve others patients pretreated and responding to IFN had marrow (10 cases) or PBSC collections (2 cases) after a median of 5 months from IFN discontinuation (group B). All patients engrafted and only one patient died early from interstitial pneumonitis. Thirty transplanted patients showing complete hematological reconstitution received low-dose IFN treatment (1×10^6 IU/m^2) as maintenance therapy. At the time of first analysis, 19 patients in group A and

Table 8.1. Summary of results of auto-SCT for CML in chronic phase in Europe using unmanipulated stem cells

Number of patients	Source of stem cells*	Cytogenetic conversion	Outcome**	Reference
34	Unmanipulated PBSC=24 unmanipulated MSC=10	18/32 patients	31/34 A/W (median follow-up of 100 months)	Meloni et al. 1990 (updated 2000)
21	Unmanipulated PBSC	11/17 patients	5-year survival of 56%	Hoyle et al. 1994
20	Unmanipulated PBSC	13/20 patients	5-year survival of 75±42%	Pigneux et al. 1999
120	Unmanipulated PBSC/MSC	Not available	5-year survival of 58±6%	McGlave et al. 1994
316	Unmanipulated PBSC	70/207 patients	5-year survival of 71%	Olavarria et al. 2002

* PBSC, blood stem cells; MSC, marrow stem cells

** A/W: Alive and Well (in chronic phase).

all in group B were in CP after a median time from transplant of respectively 13 and 1.5 months. At 2 months from transplant, 18 of the 32 patients evaluated had a reduction of Ph-positive metaphases greater than 50% (11 among the 22 group A patients and 7 among the 12 group B patients). A recent update of these patients, using the database of the EBMT showed 15 patients still alive after more than 8 years of (median) follow-up. Three of them remain in complete cytogenetic remission. The 8-year probability of survival is just over 50% for the entire group. In London (Hammersmith Hospital), 21 patients were treated with high-dose chemotherapy [Busulfan, 4 mg/kg/day×4 day combined with Melphalan (n=13) or Cyclophosphamide (n=4) or alone (n=1)] or Cyclophosphamide and total body irradiation (TBI) (n=3) followed by the reinfusion of unmanipulated PBSC. One patient failed to engraft and died 4 months posttransplant. Eleven of the 17 patients studied during the first year posttransplant had cytogenetic conversions and seemed to have prolonged survival (Hoyle et al. 1994). The 5-year survival after transplantation was 56%. The survival of these 21 patients was compared to that of 636 age-matched controls in the Medical Research Council's (MRC) database, which had been treated with conventional chemotherapy (without IFN) over the same period. Autografted patients had a significantly longer survival at 5 years than chemotherapy patients (56% vs. 28%). In Bordeaux, 20 patients with poor prognosis CML [initial Sokal index >1.2 (n=6) or no response to IFN (n=14)] were transplanted with PBSC collected at diagnosis before any treatment and without any mobilization, after a conditioning regimen consisting of Busulfan (4 mg/kg/day×4 days) and Melphalan (140 mg/m^2) (Pigneux et al. 1999). All these 20 patients received IFN post auto-SCT. Thirteen patients achieved a cytogenetic response of which five were major and eight minor remissions. For the six patients transplanted with a Sokal index >1.2, one partial and one minor cytogenetic response were observed and for the 14 patients resistant to IFN, four major cytogenetic responses (one complete) and seven minor responses were obtained. No patient died before hematopoietic reconstitution. The 5-year survival was 75±42%, which is similar to those of the London and Rome series. A trend for better survival was observed in patients achieving a major cytogenetic response.

These European results are similar to those reported in USA by the Houston group (Khouri et al. 1996). They transplanted 22 patients who were either resistant to or intolerant of IFN. The preparative regimens used were CBV (cyclophosphamide 1.5 g/m^2/day×4 days, carmustine 300 mg/m^2, etoposide 125 mg/m^2 every 12 h daily×3 days) or Cy/VP16/TBI (cyclophosphamide 60 mg/kg/day×2 days, etoposide 125 mg/m^2 every 12 h×3 days, fractionated TBI of 10.2 Gy). One patient died early and two had graft failure. Eighteen patients achieved a complete hematological response and five of these a partial or complete cytogenetic response. Three of the 18 patients received IFN maintenance therapy after auto-SCT. The median survival of these 22 patients was 34 months (from transplantation).

8.5 Autografting in Chronic Phase: Multicenter Studies

Not surprisingly, results of the retrospective analysis of multicenter studies correspond to those of single center studies. In a recent survey of the EBMT database, 581 patients with CML in CP have been reported to undergo an autologous SCT for the first time (Olavarria et al. 2002). The median follow-up at the time of analysis was 18 months. Median age at SCT was 44 years. The interval between diagnosis and SCT was 20 months. Most patients were transplanted after more than 12 months in CP and the majority had been treated with IFN before SCT. Sixty-seven per cent of IFN-treated patients were refractory at the cytogenetic level and one third were classified as high-risk disease. The transplant procedure was performed using peripheral blood cells alone in more than 70% of cases. Most centers used busulfan alone or in combination with cyclophosphamide or melphalan in the preparative conditioning, although 60 patients received TBI. There was an increase in the numbers of autografts performed with mobilized stem cells in recent years, with nearly 100 cases reported yearly in this survey between 1994 and 1998. The overall transplant mortality was low (4.6%) and seemed to be greater in transplants done with bone marrow stem cells and/or TBI. It was less than 1% for patients transplanted soon after diagnosis. The overall survival was 65% at 5 years from transplant with more than 50% of all patients remaining in CP at 5 years. The use of IFN post autograft was beneficial with more than 80% of patients treated with IFN after SCT surviving at 3 years compared with 55% if they were not given IFN post SCT. Patients transplanted within 6 months from diagnosis and treated with IFN after hematological recovery had an extremely good prognosis with more than 85% alive at 5 years from diagnosis.

Of 207 patients evaluable for cytogenetics within 6 months of auto-SCT, 36 patients (17%) were in complete cytogenetic remission, 34 (16%) in major remission, 74 (36%) in minor remission, and 63 (31%) had no cytogenetic response. Interferon was given post auto-SCT to 267 patients. Results of the cytogenetic analysis within 1–2 years from auto-SCT were available for 117 patients, the majority of whom (n=101) received IFN post SCT: 17 (15%) were in complete cytogenetic response (CCyR), 18 (15%) in major cytogenetic response (MCyR), 24 (20%) in minor cytogenetic response (mCyR), and 58 (50%) had no response (NR). The median survival in this series was 96 months (71–125) from auto-SCT. There was no difference in survival according to cytogenetic status pre- and immediately post auto-SCT. However, patients in CCyR or MCyR at 1–2 years post auto-SCT had a 10-year survival of 66% compared with 36% for patients in mCR or NR (p=0.003). The 5-year survival for patients receiving interferon post auto-SCT was 72% compared with 61% for patients not treated with IFN (p=0.01).

The main point made by this retrospective study was that of 155 patients refractory to IFN pre-auto-SCT (after a median of 18 months of therapy), 70% achieved a cytogenetic response post autograft, which was complete or major in 31%. It is remarkable that only 30% remained 100% Ph positive, indicating that residual Ph-negative (normal) hematopoiesis could be detected in two-thirds of refractory patients after prolonged treatment with IFN. These responses were sustained after 1 or 2 years treatment with IFN in the majority of patients. For the first time we were able to show that autologous SCT can reverse the refractoriness to IFN in a substantial proportion of patients.

McGlave, et al. (1994) reported the results of 200 patients transplanted in eight major transplant centers (4 from Europe). Forty-four of those 200 patients received purged stem cells. One hundred and twenty patients received unmanipulated peripheral blood or bone marrow stem cells while in CP; their 5-year survival was 58% with a median follow-up of 30 months. Transplant-related mortality was influenced by age at the time of transplantation, so that 17% of patients >40 years died during the first year after SCT compared with 1 out of 63 patients <40 years of age. The source of stem cells (blood versus marrow) and the use of ex vivo cell treatment did not influence survival.

In a study from the Scandinavian group (Simonsson et al. 2005) a strategy based on intensive chemotherapy and auto-SCT in newly diagnosed CML patients aged below 56 years, not eligible for allogeneic SCT, resulted in an overall survival of 60% at 10 years, comparable with that of patients in the same study undergoing allogeneic SCT. In this study, after diagnosis, patients received HU and IFN and after 6 months patients with Ph-positive cells still present in the bone marrow received 1–3 courses of intensive AML-like chemotherapy. Those who became Ph-negative after IFN + HU or after 1–3 chemotherapy courses underwent autologous SCT. IFN+HU reduced the percentage of Ph-positive metaphases in 56% of patients, and 1 patient became Ph-negative. After one or two intensive courses of chemotherapy 86% and 88% had a Ph reduction, and 34% and 40% became Ph-negative, respectively. In patients receiving a third intensive chemotherapy course, 92% achieved a Ph reduction and 8% became Ph-negative. The median survival after auto-SCT (n=46) was 7.5 years and the chance of remaining Ph-negative for up to 10 years after autologous SCT was around 20%.

8.6 Autografting in Chronic Phase: Prospective Studies

Unfortunately, by the time that several national groups (Société Française du Greffe de Moelle, SFGM; Grupo Español de Transplante Hemopoyético, GETH; German CML study group, Medical Research Council, MRC; Eastern Cooperative Oncology Group, ECOG) had initiated randomized trials comparing different forms of autografting with IFN, the new tyrosine kinase inhibitors (imatinib) became available in clinical trials. In 1999 the EBMT launched a multicenter, multinational study comparing autografting with IFN in newly diagnosed patients. This trial together with the previous ones, closed prematurely due to poor accrual as a result of the advent of imatinib in clinical practice. A consortium of representatives of all these trials (CML autografting trialists collaboration) is currently working on a meta-analysis: it includes a total of 416 patients randomized between auto-SCT and IFN from six different trials. Notably, there was significant heterogeneity in the design of the different trials and all patients were censored at the time of starting imatinib. Preliminary results suggest that overall survival was identical in both arms but there was an increase in complete cytogenetic remission rates in patients who received an auto-SCT, although this did not reach statistical significance (Apperley et al. 2004).

8.7 Toxicity and Post-SCT Therapy

Auto-SCT performed during CP has a low toxicity (as the transplant-related mortality does not exceed 5% in most series). The mortality seems higher in patients transplanted with bone marrow cells and receiving TBI (Olavarria et al. 2002). Most centers now use chemotherapy only (such as BuCy or BuMel) or even busulfan alone with similar results and a reduced toxicity (Olavarria et al. 2000 a). Hematopoietic reconstitution using peripheral blood stem cells is usually rapid (less than 15 days), and the 5-year survival from transplantation varies between 50% and 70%. These results compare favorably with results after allogeneic SCT. However, unlike the latter, almost all patients have persistent disease after auto-SCT.

Thus, auto-SCT is not a curative treatment for CML but could restore IFN sensitivity and prolong survival. In the EBMT survey, for the first time there is a suggestion that patients previously resistant or refractory to IFN could obtain a cytogenetic remission after autograft and more importantly maintain the cytogenetic response when IFN is used after SCT. Fifteen per cent of IFN refractory patients could expect to achieve a CCyR and 20% a MCyR (Olavarria et al. 2002). In Bordeaux, one third of 41 IFN-resistant patients achieved CCR after auto-SCT and IFN after a median of 2 years of treatment of IFN (Boiron et al. 1999). In the report from Bordeaux referred to above, the investigators showed encouraging results for 14 IFN-resistant patients: they observed no toxic deaths, the 5-year survival was 100%, and 11 patients obtained a cytogenetic response, of whom four had a major cytogenetic response (Pigneux et al. 1999).

While auto-SCT might be able to prolong survival, it is important to know which category of patients with CML in CP could benefit from auto-SCT. For patients responding to IFN (Kantarjian et al. 1995; Mahon et al. 1998; The Italian Study Group on Chronic Myeloid Leukemia 1994) and especially for those who achieve a major (≥65% Ph-negative cells) or CCyR, the probability of surviving at 10 years is 80%. For these patients, it would be very difficult to demonstrate a survival advantage for auto-SCT. As most of these IFN-responding patients do not have a high Sokal index, it could be that auto-SCT is indicated only for patients with high-risk CML. In France they have performed such auto-SCT in 20 CML patients with a Sokal index >1.2 (Reiffers et al. 1993). These patients were given busulfan and melphalan, and then were reinfused with blood stem cells. Fifteen of them received IFN after auto-SCT and three achieved a MCyR. Fifteen of the 20 patients were still alive 1–61 months after transplant. In the EBMT survey, 52 such patients (high-risk disease) were autografted early after diagnosis (27 patients) or in late CP (25 patients) with a trend to a better survival for patients autografted early (72% vs. 39% survival at 5 years).

The use of immunomodulatory agents after auto-SCT has been explored with limited success. Growth factors such as GM-CSF may selectively favor the proliferation of Ph-negative cells and this has been used in combination with hydroxyurea after autografting with unmanipulated PBSC (Carlo-Stella et al. 1997) or with PBSC incubated in vitro with GM-CSF (Gladstone et al. 1999). A small group of seventeen patients received the immunomodulator Roquinimex (linomide) following auto-SCT and cytogenetic responses were seen in all patients, occasionally developing over time, suggesting an immune-mediated and not a post-SCT transient effect (Rowe et al. 1999). Most of the current evidence suggests that IFN post SCT is beneficial. In one case report, a case of post-autograft graft-versus-host disease was described after retreatment with interferon (Rainey et al. 1996).

8.8 Tyrosine Kinase Inhibitors

Since the advent of targeted therapy for BCR-ABL tyrosine kinase activity with imatinib, the use of any modality of SCT in patients with CML has experienced a substantial decline (Fig. 8.1). This is even more so in the case of autologous SCT. In the EBMT database, the number of autologous SCT in the late 1990s was greater than 250 procedures per year. This number has now been reduced to less than 20 in the year 2004. It is evident that, with the advent of imatinib and other tyrosine kinase inhibitors, the role of autografting in the management of CML will have to be redefined.

Theoretically, there are several possible ways of using autologous SCT in combination with imatinib: (1) to reverse primary resistance to imatinib; (2) to eliminate a Ph-positive clone bearing a BCR-ABL kinase do-

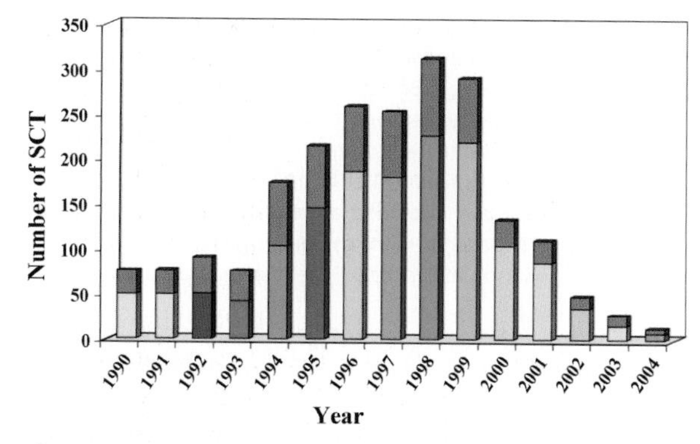

Fig. 8.1. Autologous SCT in Europe since 1990. Data from the EBMT Chronic Leukaemia Working Party registry. *Color bars* show patients with chronic phase CML and *grey bars* show patients with advanced phase CML

main mutation, which confers resistance to imatinib; (3) to reduce the level of residual disease after a cytogenetic response to imatinib in patients in whom Ph-negative cells had been harvested; and (4) to tumor debulk before imatinib.

A number of patients achieving a CCyR to imatinib have had attempts made at stem cell harvesting. Most centers have used mobilization protocols based on G-CSF only. The UK CML Working Party (Drummond et al. 2003) reported on 58 patients in CCyR using recombinant human G-CSF (10 mg/kg/d subcutaneously for at least 4 days), while continuing imatinib treatment. The median number of apheresis procedures was 2 (range 1 to 3) and a median dose of 2.1×10^6/kg CD34+ cells (range 0.1 to 6.5×10(6)/kg) was collected. Some 84% of the 31 collections analyzed were negative for the Ph chromosome by cytogenetics or fluorescence in situ hybridization (FISH), respectively. No toxicity was reported with the regimen. Overall, the target CD34+ dose was attained in 40% of the patients. The German group (Kreuzer et al. 2004) confirmed these observations and performed molecular analysis on the harvested material using nested primer RT-PCR. They showed that 28% of the collections were negative for the presence of *BCR-ABL* transcripts. An Italian group in Monza (Perseghin et al. 2005) has recently reported that a 64% success rate with identical strategy (G-CSF mobilization while continuing on imatinib) could be improved to 80% if imatinib were discontinued temporarily (for 2–4 weeks) prior to the mobilization. Thus, the majority of imatinib responders could have a Ph-negative stem cell collection, which could be reserved for the future. So far, only anecdotal reports exist of patients undergoing auto-SCT with stem cells collected after imatinib therapy, although one patient has been shown to regain CCyR after a cytogenetic relapse on imatinib (Kreuzer et al. 2004).

8.9 Final Considerations

In summary, retrospective and single center trials have shown that auto-SCT in CML could prolong survival if performed in CP. Autografting has been performed in Europe for more than 20 years and we still do not know the exact role that it should play in the management of CML. Many questions remain unanswered: What is the best way of doing an autograft? Is mobilization necessary? Does the use of mainly Ph-negative stem cells influence outcome? But at least we will be ready to ask these and other relevant questions regarding the use of autografting in combination with the newly developed tyrosine kinase inhibitors in the near future.

References

Apperley JF, Boque C, Carella A et al (2004) Autografting in chronic myeloid leukaemia: a meta-analysis of six randomised trials. Bone Marrow Transplant 33:S28

Archimbaud E, Michallet M, Philip I et al (1997) Granulocyte colony-stimulating factor given in addition to interferon-alpha to mobilize peripheral blood stem cells for autologous transplantation in chronic myeloid leukaemia. Br J Haematol 99:678–684

Bhatia R, Forman SJ (1998) Autologous transplantation for the treatment of chronic myelogenous leukemia. Hematol Oncol Clin North Am 12 (1):151–172

Boiron JM, Cahn JY, Meloni G et al (1999) Chronic myeloid leukaemia in first chronic phase not responding to α-interferon: outcome and prognostic factors after autologous transplantation. Bone Marrow Transplant 24:259–264

Bouzgarrou R, Reiffers J (1991) Cellules souches circulantes et LMC: modalités de prélèvement, congélation, décongélation, reconstitution hématologique après greffe. Presented at the Réunion du groupe Hémobiologie du FAG, 22 Octobre 1991

Brito-Babapulle F, Bowcock SJ, Marcus RE et al (1989) Autografting for patients with chronic myeloid leukaemia in chronic phase: peripheral blood stem cells may have a finite capacity for maintaining haematopoiesis. Br J Haematol 73:76–81

Buckner CD, Stewart P, Clift RA et al (1978) Treatment of blastic transformation of chronic granulocytic leukaemia by chemotherapy, total body irradiation and infusion of cryopreserved autologous marrow. Exp Hematol 6:96–109

Butturini A, Keating A, Goldman J, Gale RP (1990) Autotransplants in chronic myelogenous leukaemia: strategies and results. Lancet 335:1255–1258

Carella AM, Frassoni F (1996) ICE, mini-ICE or high-dose hydroxyurea to mobilize Philadelphia [Ph]-negative PBPC in chronic myelogenous leukaemia. Br J Haematol 95:213–214

Carella AM, Frassoni F, Negrin RS (1995) Autografting in chronic myelogenous leukemia: new questions. Leukemia 9:365–369

Carella AM, Lerma E, Corsetti MT et al (1999) Autografting with Philadelphia chromosome negative mobilized hematopoietic progenitor cells in chronic myelogenous leukemia. Blood 83:1534–1539

Carlo-Stella C, Regazzi E, Andrizzi C et al (1997) Use of granulocyte-macrophage colony-stimulating factor (GM-CSF) in combination with hydroxyurea as post-transplant therapy in chronic myelogenous leukemia patients autografted with unmanipulated hematopoietic cells. Haematologica 82(3):291–296

Coulombel L, Kalousek DK, Eaves CJ, Gupta CM, Eaves AC (1983) Long-term marrow culture reveals chromosomally normal hematopoietic progenitor cells in patients with Philadelphia chromosome positive chronic myelogenous leukemia. N Engl J Med 308:1493–1498

Daley GQ (1996) Rationalizing autotransplant strategies for chronic myeloid leukemia. Leuk Lymphoma 21(5–6):353–358

Deisseroth AB, Zu Z, Claxton D et al (1994) Genetic marking shows that Ph+ cells present in autologous transplants of chronic myelogenous leukemia (CML) contribute to relapse after autologous bone marrow in CML. Blood 83:3068–3076

Drummond MW, Marin D, Clark RE et al (2003) Mobilization of Ph chromosome-negative peripheral blood stem cells in chronic myeloid leukaemia patients with imatinib mesylate-induced complete cytogenetic remission. Br J Haematol 123:479–483

Enright H, McGlave P (1998) Bone marrow transplantation for chronic myelogenous leukemia. Curr Opin Oncol 10:100–107

Gladstone DE, Bedi A, Miller CB et al (1999) Philadelphia chromosome-negative engraftment after autologous transplantation with granulocyte-macrophage colony-stimulating factor for chronic myeloid leukemia. Biol Blood Marrow Transplant 5(6): 394–399

Goldman JM (1997) Treatment of chronic myeloid leukaemia: some topical questions. Baillieres Clin Haematol 10(2):405–421

Goldman JM, Th'ng KH, Park DS et al (1978) Collection, cryopreservation and subsequent viability of haemopoietic stem cells intended for treatment of chronic granulocytic leukemia in blast-cell transformation. Br J Haematol 40:185–195

Goldman JM, Catovsky D, Hows J, Spiers ASD, Galton DAG (1979) Cryopreserved peripheral blood cells functioning as autografts in patients with chronic granulocytic leukaemia in transformation. Br Med J 1:1310–1313

Haines ME, Goldman JM, Worsley et al (1984) Chemotherapy and autografting for chronic granulocytic leukaemia in transformation: probable prolongation of survival in some patients. Br J Haematol 58:711–721

Hehlmann R, Hochhaus A, Berger U, Reiter A (2000) Current trends in the management of chronic myelogenous leukemia. Ann Hematol 79:345–54

Hoyle C, Gray R, Goldman J (1994) Autografting for patients with CML in chronic phase: an update. Br J Haematol 86:76–81

Jazwieck B, Mahon FX, Pigneux A et al (1995) 5-Fluorouracil-resistant CD34+ cell population from peripheral blood of chronic myelogenous leukemia patients contains BCR-ABL negative progenitor cells. Exp Hematol 23:1509–1514

Kantarjian HM, Smith TL, O'Brien S et al (1995) Prolonged survival in chronic myelogenous leukemia following cytogenetic response to alpha interferon therapy. Ann Intern Med 122:254–261

Khouri IF, Kantarjian H, Talpaz M et al (1996) Results with high-dose chemotherapy and unpurged autologous stem cell transplantation in 73 patients with chronic myelogenous leukaemia: the MD Anderson experience. Bone Marrow Transplant 17:775–779

Kirk JA, Reems JA, Roecklein BA et al (1995) Benign marrow progenitors are enriched in CD34+/HLA – DR^{lo} population but not in the CD34+/38^{lo} population in chronic myeloid leukemia: an analysis using interphase fluorescence in situ hybridization. Blood 86:737–743

Kreuzer KA, Kluhs C, Baskaynak G et al (2004) Filgrastim-induced stem cell mobilization in chronic myeloid leukaemia patients during imatinib therapy: safety, feasibility and evidence for an efficient in vivo purging. Br J Haematol 124(2):195–199

Mahon FX, Faberes C, Pueyo S et al (1998) Response at three months is a good predictive factor for newly diagnosed chronic myeloid leukemia patients treated by recombinant alpha interferon. Blood 92:4059–4065

McGlave PB, De Fabritiis P, Deisseroth J et al (1994) Autologous transplants for chronic myelogenous leukaemia: results from eight transplant groups. Lancet 343:1486–1488

Meloni G, De Fabritiis P, Alimena F et al (1990) Autologous bone marrow transplantation or peripheral blood stem cell transplantation for patients with chronic myelogenous leukaemia in chronic phase. Bone Marrow Transplant 4(Suppl. 4):92–94

Meloni G, Russo D, Baccarani M et al (1999) A prospective study of alpha-interferon and autologous bone marrow transplantation in chronic myeloid leukemia. The Italian Co-operative Study Group on Chronic Myeloid Leukemia. Haematologica 84:707–715

Miller JS (1998) Innovative therapy for chronic myelogenous leukemia. Hematol Oncol Clin North Am 12(1):173–206

O'Brien SG (1997) Autografting for chronic myeloid leukaemia. Baillieres Clin Haematol 10(2):369–388

Olavarria E, Kanfer E, Szydlo R et al (2000 a) High-dose busulphan alone as cytoreduction before allogeneic or autologous stem cell transplantation for chronic myeloid leukaemia: a single-centre experience. Br J Haematol 108:769–777

Olavarria E, Parker S, Craddock C et al (2000 b) Collection of Ph-negative progenitor cells from interferon responsive patients with chronic myeloid leukemia: effect of granulocyte-colony-stimulating factor mobilization. Haematologica 85(6):647–652

Olavarria E, Reiffers J , Boque C et al (2002) The post-transplant cytogenetic response to interferon is a major determinant of survival after autologous stem cell transplantation for chronic myeloid leukaemia in chronic phase. Br J Haematol 118:762–770

Perseghin P, Gambacorti-Passerini C, Tornaghi L et al (2005) Peripheral blood progenitor cell collection in chronic myeloid leukemia patients with complete cytogenetic response after treatment with imatinib mesylate. Transfusion 45(7):1214–1220

Petzer AL, Eaves CJ, Lansdorp PM et al (1996) Characterization of primitive subpopulation of normal and leukemic cells in the blood of patients with newly diagnosed as well as established chronic myeloid leukemia. Blood 88:2162–2171

Pigneux A, Faberes C, Boiron JM et al (1999) Autologous stem cell transplantation in chronic myeloid leukemia: a single center experience. Bone Marrow Transplant 24:265–270

Rainey MG, Harrison P, Hows JM et al (1996) Spontaneous graft-versus-host disease following autologous peripheral blood progenitor cell transplantation in chronic myeloid leukaemia. Bone Marrow Transplant 17(6):1077–1079

Reiffers J (1985) Autologous transplantation in chronic myelogenous leukemia. Blood Transfusion Immunohematol 28:509–520

Reiffers J, Trouette R, Marit G et al (1991) Autologous blood stem cell transplantation for chronic granulocytic leukaemia in transformation: a report of 47 cases. Br J Haematol 77:339–345

Reiffers J, Cahn JY, Montastruc M et al (1993) Peripheral blood stem cell transplantation followed by recombinant alpha interferon for chronic myelogenous leukemia in chronic phase: preliminary results. Stem Cells 11:23–24

Reiffers J, Goldman J, Meloni G, Cahn JY, Gratwohl A on behalf of the Chronic Leukaemia Working Party of the EBMT (1994) Autologous stem cell transplantation in chronic myelogenous leukaemia: a retrospective analysis of the European Group for Bone Marrow Transplant. Bone Marrow Transplant 14:407–410

Reiffers J, Mahon FX, Boiron JM et al (1996a) Autografting in chronic myeloid leukaemia: an overview. Leukemia 10:385–388

Reiffers J, Goldman JM, Meloni G, Cahn JY, Apperley J (1996b) Autologous stem cell transplantation (Auto-SCT) for chronic myeloid leukemia (CML) in chronic phase: a report of the European Blood and Marrow Transplant (EBMT) Group. 22nd Annual Meeting of the EBMT, Vienna (Austria) Bone Marrow Transplant 17(Suppl.1), S3, abstract no. 56

Reiffers J, Taylor K, Gluckman E et al (1998) Collection of Ph-negative progenitor cells with granulocyte-colony stimulating factor in patients with chronic myeloid leukaemia who respond to recombinant alpha-interferon. Br J Haematol 102:639–646

Rowe JM, Rapoport AP, Ryan DH et al (1999) Treatment of chronic myelogenous leukemia with autologous bone marrow transplantation followed by roquinimex. Bone Marrow Transplant 24(10): 1057–1063

Russo D, Martinelli G, Montefusco V et al (1999) Collection of Ph-negative progenitor cells from Ph+ CML patients in complete cytogenetic remission after long-term interferon-alpha therapy. Haematologica 84(10):953–955

Silver RT, Woolf SH, Helhmann R et al (1999) An evidence-based analysis of the effect of busulfan, hydroxyurea, interferon, and allogeneic bone marrow transplantation in treating the chronic phase of chronic myeloid leukemia: developed for the American Society of Hematology. Blood 94:1517–1536

Simonsson B, Oberg G, Bjoreman M et al (2005) Intensive treatment and stem cell transplantation in chronic myelogenous leukemia: long-term follow-up. Acta Haematol 113(3):155–162

Spencer A, Granter N, Fagan K et al (1998) Collection and analysis of peripheral blood mononuclear cells during haemopoietic recovery following PBSCT for CML: autografting as an in vivo purging manoeuvre? Bone Marrow Transplant 21(1):101–103

The Italian Cooperative Study Group on Chronic Myeloid Leukaemia (1993) Karyotype conversion by interferon as preparative treatment for autologous BMT in Ph positive CML. Leuk Lymphoma 11(Suppl 1):277–280

The Italian Cooperative Study Group on chronic myeloid leukemia (1994) Interferon alpha – 2a as compared with conventional chemotherapy for the treatment of Chronic Myeloid Leukemia. N Engl J Med 330:820–825

Monitoring Disease Response

Timothy Hughes and Susan Branford

Contents

Abstract. Most CML patients will receive imatinib as first-line therapy. For these patients serial analysis of BCR-ABL blood levels by real time quantitative PCR (RQ-PCR) provides the most accurate and clinically relevant monitoring strategy. The major advantage of RQ-PCR is the ability to accurately and frequently monitor the decline in transcript level over a 4–5 log range using peripheral blood. This provides an early indication in most cases that response has been adequate to minimize the risk of disease progression. In suboptimal responders, the RQ-PCR assay provides early warning of imatinib resistance. Frequent RQ-PCR on blood should form the basis of clinical monitoring. Marrow cytogenetics can provide additional information in some cases but its value is quite limited in patients who achieve and maintain a major molecular response. The clinical development of second-generation kinase inhibitors has increased the importance of identifying the cause of imatinib resistance. Many, but not all, of the *BCR-ABL* kinase domain mutations are sensitive to the new inhibitors. Precise molecular monitoring of *BCR-ABL* levels can be used as a sensitive trigger to test for mutations. High-quality molecular monitoring of imatinib-treated CML patients is essential to maximize the clinical benefits.

9.1 Introduction

There have been major changes in the management of patients with chronic myeloid leukaemia (CML) over the past 5–10 years. This includes the range of therapeutic options available and the tests being used to monitor response to therapy. Imatinib, the first Abl kinase inhibitor developed for clinical therapy, is now the most common first-line therapy in most developed countries, (Druker et al. 2001; Kantarjian et al. 2002b; Sawyers et al. 2002; Talpaz et al. 2002), with allogeneic transplant usually being reserved for second-line therapy in selected young patients who have resistance to imatinib. The excellent response rates and good tolerability observed in patients treated with imatinib in chronic phase have driven the rapid change in medical practice. However, the optimal management of CML relies on accurate long-term monitoring of treatment response because not all patients are responsive to imatinib (primary resistance), and some patients lose response (secondary or acquired resistance). The cause of primary resistance is unknown but secondary resistance is due to mutations in the kinase domain of *BCR-ABL* in most cases. Given the recent development of second-generation Abl kinase inhibitors, which may be active in imatinib-resistant patients, and the potential value of allogeneic transplantation in this setting, early detection of suboptimal response or relapse on imatinib therapy assumes increasing importance.

9.2 Methods for Measuring Treatment Response

Monitoring response to therapy has until recently involved following the blood count and aspirating the marrow at regular intervals to determine the percentage of Philadelphia chromosome-(Ph) positive metaphases. The need for a bone marrow aspirate and the limited sensitivity of conventional cytogenetics limits the clinical value of marrow cytogenetics as a regular monitoring test for minimal residual disease.

9.2.1 Cytogenetic Analysis

Cytogenetic analysis is the standard technique for the diagnosis of CML and is particularly useful for the demonstration of karyotypic abnormalities that are additional to the Ph chromosome (clonal evolution). This may be an indicator of advanced disease. The majority of patients have a detectable Ph chromosome; however, about half of the patients without a detectable Ph chromosome have a demonstrable *BCR-ABL* gene. This indicates a submicroscopic insertion of *ABL* into *BCR* on chromosome 22, or *BCR* into *ABL* on chromosome 9 and these patients cannot be monitored by cytogenetic analysis. Traditionally, treatment response has been assessed using cytogenetic determination of the number of cells containing the Ph chromosome. The presence of the Ph chromosome in greater than 95% of cells indicates a lack of cytogenetic response, between 35 and 95% indicates a minor cytogenetic response, 1 to 35% indicates a partial cytogenetic response and 0% indicates a complete cytogenetic response (CCR). A major cytogenetic response (MCR) includes complete and partial responses.

The technique is insensitive as only 20–50 cells in metaphase are usually examined per sample. Therefore, a cytogenetic abnormality may not be detected unless it is present in at least 2–5% of cells. Bone marrow aspirates are required since the method relies on the analysis of dividing cells and peripheral blood contains very few cycling myeloid cells in patients in hematological remission. Consequently, the sample collection is invasive for the patient, which limits the frequency of monitoring. Cells from patients treated with interferon-α or collected early after transplantation often fail to grow well in culture or the cell counts are low resulting in a significant failure rate of cytogenetic analysis. The insensitivity of the technique means that patients with a CCR may still have a considerable leukemic load (Morley, 1998). By the time disease is detectable by cytogenetic analysis in these patients, clinical relapse may be inevitable.

9.2.2 Fluorescent In Situ Hybridization

Fluorescent in situ hybridization (FISH) analysis for *BCR-ABL* allows the examination of dividing cells in metaphase and nondividing cells in interphase. The technique utilizes differently labelled fluorescent DNA probes to give different colored signals. Peripheral blood can be examined by interphase FISH, which averts the need for bone marrow aspirate. The technique is rapid, allows the analysis of more cells than cytogenetic methods (200–500 cells compared to 20–50 cells), and is reasonably reliable in assessing treatment responses (Muhlmann et al. 1998). The method allows the detection of the *BCR-ABL* gene in approximately half of the patients without a detectable Ph chromosome at diagnosis. However, depending on the fluorescent probes used for the detection of the *BCR* and *ABL* signals, the method may be limited by a high false-positive rate of up to 10–15% as well as a high false-negative rate (Chase et al. 1997). Newer probe systems have overcome these problems and the false-positive rate is reduced to approximately 0.2% (Dewald et al. 1998; Grand et al. 1998). Nevertheless, result interpretation is compounded by a number of factors; peripheral blood may have a higher proportion of Ph-negative myeloid progenitors (Sick et al. 2001), which may produce lower Ph-positive signals by FISH analysis as compared to bone marrow in some patients (Seong et al. 1998; Sinclair et al. 1997). Furthermore, in a minority of patients treated with interferon-α or imatinib, bone marrow FISH analysis may give lower Ph-positive values than cytogenetic analysis (Itoh et al. 1999; Kaeda et al. 2002). The false positive rate for the 10–15% of patients with large deletions on the derivative chromosome 9 is significantly increased (Dewald et al. 1999), and the interpretation of signal patterns requires expertise to avoid false-positive results.

9.2.3 Qualitative PCR

The reverse transcription polymerase chain reaction (RT-PCR) technique has significantly enhanced the sensitivity of detection of minimal residual leukemic cells in CML patients. The breakpoints within the DNA sequence of *BCR-ABL* occur over a range spanning many kilobases of sequence and DNA is therefore impractical to use for *BCR-ABL* detection by PCR. However, cDNA is an ideal template following reverse transcription of RNA since the breakpoints in the vast majority of patients result in only two major transcripts that differ by the inclusion of the 75 base pair *BCR* exon 14 (b3). The sensitivity of analysis is improved by performing a nested PCR.

The original RT-PCR analyses of minimal residual disease in CML involved qualitative analysis of *BCR-ABL* in patients following allogeneic transplantation (Cross et al. 1993b; Hughes et al. 1991; Morgan et al. 1989; Radich et al. 1995; Roth et al. 1992). A number of important issues for the reliability of RT-PCR results were recognized by these pioneer studies. Of utmost importance was the stringent control of contamination that will readily produce false positive results (Hughes et al. 1990). Ideally, *BCR-ABL* negative cells should be included in all RNA extraction procedures to assess cross contamination between RNA samples. Additionally, a no template reverse transcription control including all reagents except for RNA will monitor for cross contamination between tubes (Cross et al. 1993b; Hughes et al. 1991). The adoption of other procedures to minimize the risk of contamination were highly recommended (Kwok et al. 1989).

A second issue was the use of appropriate controls. Ubiquitously expressed control genes are regularly included in RT-PCR analysis to control for RNA degradation by providing evidence that the cDNA template is of good quality. Their use is essential for the correct interpretation of samples that are negative for *BCR-ABL*. However, inappropriate control genes such as *β-actin* were frequently used. This gene is highly expressed and is inadequate to detect the minimal RNA degradation that may lead to a false-negative *BCR-ABL*. Additionally, the *β-actin*-amplified products may in fact be derived from contaminating genomic DNA due to the presence of processed pseudogenes, which again can lead to false-negative results (Cross et al. 1994). Furthermore, if PCR primers are used that hybridize within one exon of a control gene rather than across an exon or across exon junctions, then the possibility exists that contaminating genomic DNA will be amplified in the absence of intact RNA. This may lead to the false impression that the reverse transcription of adequate quality RNA has been successful. In this situation the absence of *BCR-ABL* amplification may lead to a false negative interpretation (Melo et al. 1994). Ideally, an appropriate control should be expressed at a constant level at all stages of development; it should not be affected by treatment and should be expressed at a similar level to the target (Bustin 2000). The recommendation for an appropriate control for *BCR-ABL* was a sequence of the normal *ABL* or *BCR* gene that is disrupted in the formation of *BCR-ABL* and that is not amplified in the presence of contaminating DNA. The recommendations for contamination control and the question of the use of appropriate control genes are highly relevant issues for any application of the PCR technique and for the quality and reliability of the results.

The interpretation of qualitative RT-PCR analysis in CML patients post transplantation was not straightforward. Many patients in a CCR remained *BCR-ABL* positive for a number of months without relapsing (Costello et al. 1996; Cross et al. 1993b; Guerrasio et al. 1992; Morgan et al. 1989; Roth et al. 1992). The detection of a positive result in long-term patients did not necessarily correlate with relapse (Miyamura et al. 1993). However, in a large cohort of patients, the detection of a positive result between 6 and 12 months after transplantation was an independent predictor of subsequent relapse (Radich et al. 1995). Therefore, a positive PCR result could be used to identify groups of individuals with an increased risk of relapse but was not predictive for a specific individual. Early PCR positivity by qualitative analysis provided no information on whether the transcripts were decreasing, which may indicate impending molecular remission, or increasing, which may identify early relapse. The realization that qualitative PCR was of limited prognostic value in the monitoring of residual leukemia in CML provided the impetus for the development of quantitative PCR techniques for the assessment of disease activity.

9.2.4 Quantitative PCR

Quantitative RT-PCR assays enable the dynamics of residual disease to be monitored over time. In the late 1990s, real-time quantitative PCR (RQ-PCR) was introduced. The real-time technique is performed on an analyzer that incorporates a thermal cycler, fluorescence detection, and result calculation, which greatly simplifies quantitative PCR. RQ-PCR has largely replaced the more complex competitive quantitative procedures. Nevertheless, the successful application of real-time technology for reliable quantitation requires careful assay design and validation of all aspects of the procedure.

The real-time technology involves two main chemistries; one requires the use of a fluorescent hydrolysis probe (TaqMan probe), and the other uses two fluorescent hybridization probes. Both methods involve fluorescence resonance energy transfer (FRET) to measure accumulated fluorescence during the PCR amplification.

In the TaqMan platform, (Applied Biosystems) the probe has a fluorescent reporter dye on the 5′ end, the emission spectrum of which is quenched by a dye on the 3′ end. During the PCR the probe specifically hybridizes between the forward and reverse primers. The assay utilizes the 5′-nuclease activity of Taq DNA polymerase to hydrolyze the probe. The Taq-mediated primer extension results in the dissociation of the reporter dye from the quencher with a consequent increase in fluorescence that accumulates at every cycle. The intensity of the fluorescence is proportional to the amount of accumulated amplicons.

The hybridization probe system utilizes a probe with a donor fluorescent dye at the 3′ end and a second probe with an acceptor fluorescent dye at the 5′ end. The probes hybridize to the target sequence in very close proximity during the PCR. Excitation of the donor dye results in FRET to the acceptor dye and fluorescence emission. The intensity of the light emitted by the acceptor dye is measured and increasing amounts are proportional to the amount of synthesized DNA. The Lightcycler (Roche Diagnostics) instrument uses this technology.

For both probe systems the point during cycling when amplification of the PCR product is first detected is related to the starting copy number. The higher the starting copy number, the sooner the increase in fluorescence occurs. Analysis is performed by one of two procedures. Relative quantitation involves the comparison of threshold cycles, or C_t, between a control gene and the gene of interest. A requirement for reliable results is that the amplification efficiencies between the control and target are similar. The standard curve method uses serial dilutions of a DNA plasmid or RNA of known quantity.

9.3 Optimization Requirements for RQ-PCR Measurement

Quantitative PCR remains a technically challenging procedure. In order to achieve a high level of reproducibility and the reporting of data in a biologically relevant manner, every aspect of the RQ-PCR technique requires thorough validation and optimization (Bustin 2002; Bustin et al. 2004; Ginzinger 2002). The most important factors for reliable data are: the use of good quality RNA; careful assay design to exclude the amplification of pseudogenes, contaminating DNA, and polymorphisms in primer or probe binding sites; equal amplification efficiency of DNA plasmid standards and cDNA; selection of an appropriate control gene to compensate for variations in the RNA quality and the efficiency of reverse transcription; and the inclusion and appropriate monitoring of quality control samples to detect unreliable results (Hughes et al. 2003; van der Velden et al. 2003).

9.3.1 PCR Amplification Efficiency

When using a DNA standard curve to quantitate cDNA it is essential that the amplification efficiency of both the plasmid and the cDNA is equivalent for accurate results over the whole dynamic range (Hughes et al. 2003). Design factors can influence the amplification efficiency of a PCR reaction such as the amplicon length, the G/C content, and sequence secondary structure. Reaction dynamics can also influence the efficiency such as the enzyme, nonoptimal reagent concentrations, sample impurities, and inhibitors. The advantage of using DNA standards is the superior stability compared to RNA standards. However, the plasmid standard may have a different secondary structure to the patient cDNA. The secondary structure can influence primer hybridization and affect the amplification efficiency. Therefore, it is possible that different templates may have different efficiencies when using the same PCR reaction conditions. These differences should be recognized and corrected by optimization of the reaction conditions for accurate quantitative PCR analysis.

Equal amplification efficiency of the cDNA template and the DNA plasmid standard can be confirmed by demonstrating that when patient cDNA is diluted in a tenfold series, the cDNA values are not significantly different from the expected 1-log reduction at each dilution step. This is illustrated in Table 9.1 for *BCR-ABL* using a RQ-PCR technique with TaqMan probes (Branford et al. 1999). If the DNA standards amplified with a different efficiency, the quantitative value of the diluted samples would be significantly different from a 1-log reduction. Table 9.2 illustrates a quantitative procedure where there was indeed a difference in the amplification efficiency between the DNA plasmid standards and the cDNA target. In this case optimization of the method was required to correct the difference in amplification efficiency.

Table 9.1. Equal amplification efficiency of the DNA plasmid standard and the cDNA target. Patient cDNA was diluted in a tenfold series and the *BCR-ABL* transcript values were not significantly different from the expected 1-log reduction at each dilution step, P=0.78 (Mann-Whitney test)

	Dilution	*BCR-ABL* transcripts	Log decrease at each dilution
Patient 1	0	1.03×10^5	
	1 in 10	1.08×10^4	0.98
	1 in 100	1.10×10^3	0.99
	1 in 1000	1.07×10^2	1.01
Patient 2	0	1.14×10^5	
	1 in 10	1.00×10^4	1.06
	1 in 100	0.90×10^3	1.05
	1 in 1000	1.15×10^2	0.90
Patient 3	0	4.52×10^4	
	1 in 10	4.93×10^3	0.96
	1 in 100	4.24×10^2	1.07
	1 in 1000	4.76×10	0.95

Table 9.2. Unequal amplification efficiency of a DNA plasmid standard and the cDNA target. Patient cDNA was diluted in a tenfold series and Von Willebrand Factor transcript values were significantly different from the expected 1-log reduction at each dilution step, P = 0.006 (Mann-Whitney test). Optimization of the reaction conditions improved the results

	Dilution	Von Willebrands Factor	Log decrease at each dilution
Patient 1	0	2.77×10^{4}	
	1 in 10	3.44×10^{3}	0.91
	1 in 100	7.35×10^{2}	0.67
	1 in 1000	8.01×10^{1}	0.90
Patient 2	0	2.17×10^{5}	
	1 in 10	2.72×10^{4}	0.90
	1 in 100	3.38×10^{3}	0.91
	1 in 1000	3.94×10^{2}	0.93
Patient 3	0	0.96×10^{5}	
	1 in 10	1.23×10^{4}	0.89
	1 in 100	1.62×10^{3}	0.88
	1 in 1000	1.55×10^{2}	1.01

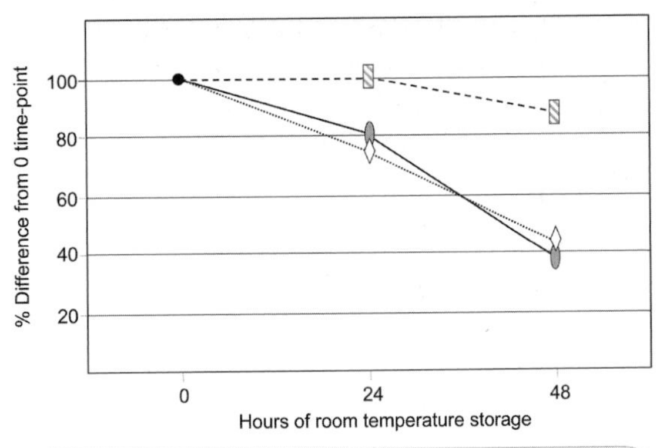

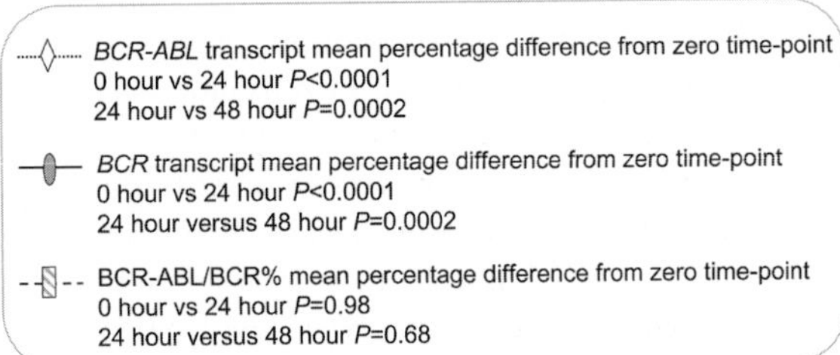

Fig. 9.1. Demonstration that the *BCR* gene is a suitable control to compensate for transcript degradation of the *BCR-ABL* gene. Blood samples from 14 patients were stored at room temperature for 0, 24, and 48 h. The *BCR-ABL* and *BCR* transcript values of each sample and the BCR-ABL/BCR% values were compared to that of their corresponding freshly processed sample (zero time-point). The percent difference from the zero time-point (expressed as 100%) was calculated for each sample. The graph plots the mean percentage difference from the zero time-point for the 14 patients. The degradation was significant for both transcripts over time; however, the rate of degradation was not statistically different between *BCR-ABL* and *BCR* at each time-point (P = 0.68 and P = 0.55 for 24 and 48 h of room temperature storage respectively). Normalizing *BCR-ABL* to *BCR* corrects for the degradation over time

9.3.2 Appropriate Control Gene

Choosing an appropriate control gene constitutes one of the most important aspects for a reliable and reproducible quantitative assay. The control gene can be used to identify RNA samples of unacceptable quality; in samples deemed of acceptable RNA quality the control gene compensates for variations due to the degree of degradation. The control gene adjusts for differences in the efficiency of the reverse transcription reaction, and can determine the sensitivity of each sample measurement (Beillard et al. 2003; Gabert et al. 2003; van der Velden et al. 2003). The control and target should have a similar expression level and stability. Similar RNA stability is important since delays in sample processing may occur.

The two control genes that have been widely assessed for their suitability for *BCR-ABL* quantitation are *BCR* and *ABL*. *BCR* was initially investigated for use as a suitable control in our laboratory since it was reported to have a similar expression level and stability to that of *BCR-ABL* (Collins et al. 1987). Figure 9.1 demonstrates that *BCR* does indeed degrade at the same rate as *BCR-ABL*. To allow RNA degradation, blood samples from 14 patients were stored at room temperature for 24 and 48 h before RNA processing. The quantitative PCR results were compared to the corresponding blood sample that was processed without storage. Significant degradation of both *BCR-ABL* and *BCR* transcripts occurred after 24 and 48 h of room temperature storage [P < 0.0001 and P = 0.0002, respectively (t-test)]. By normalizing the *BCR-ABL* value to *BCR*, the BCR-ABL/BCR% values were not significantly different after 24 and 48 h of room temperature storage (P = 0.68 and P = 0.39, respectively). The data indicate that the *BCR* gene is a suitable control for the quantitation of *BCR-*

ABL as it compensates for the significant degradation of transcripts over time. The EAC recommend *ABL* as the control for RQ-PCR based diagnostics and MRD detection in leukemic patients (Beillard et al. 2003; Gabert et al. 2003). The mean stability of *ABL* and *BCR-ABL* seemed to be comparable, but substantial differences between individual samples were observed upon storage. Either *ABL* or *BCR* are suitable control genes for *BCR-ABL* quantitation. Other genes may also be suitable if the criteria for acceptability are achieved.

9.3.3 Measurement Reliability of the RQ-PCR Assay

The estimation of measurement reliability (also known as uncertainty of measurement) is an important aspect of the development of any quantitative method that is used to monitor treatment response. This is because the ability of any assay to reliably detect a change in values depends on its reproducibility, i.e., the ability of the assay to obtain the same answer for the same sample each time. Reproducibility is normally expressed as the coefficient of variation (CV) of an assay. An assay with a high CV suffers from poor reproducibility. Maximization of the reproducibility of the assay reduces the CV and improves the level of confidence of the results. A number of measures can be implemented to optimize the reproducibility of the quantitative PCR assay (Branford et al. 2004c).

To determine the reproducibility of the *BCR-ABL* quantitative assay it is necessary to measure all aspects of the procedure. The reverse transcription step is the source of most of the variation in a quantitative PCR assay (Freeman et al. 1999), therefore it is particularly important to include this procedure when determining the reproducibility. The interassay variability of the quantitative assay should therefore be based on the *BCR-ABL*/control gene ratio determined using repeated reverse transcription and quantitative PCR analysis of an RNA sample. This approach is an accurate reflection of the variability of the patient results. Many reports of the reproducibility of real-time quantitative PCR assays have been based on the intra- or interassay CV of the threshold cycle (C_t) values. The C_t is defined as the cycle when sample fluorescence exceeds a chosen threshold above calculated background fluorescence. However, it is inappropriate to use these values to determine the assay variability as C_t values are logarithmic units and as such result in a misleading representation of reproducibility (Gabert et al. 2003; Schmittgen et al. 2000).

We and others have found that one of the most significant factors for maximizing the reproducibility is performing the reverse transcription reaction in duplicate with separate quantitative reactions for each cDNA replicate (Branford et al. 1999, 2004c; Stahlberg et al. 2004). It is also essential to ensure that the performance of the assay is consistent. This can be achieved by including at least two quality control samples of different quantitative levels with every reaction. In our laboratory the quality control samples were prepared by mixing *BCR-ABL* expressing cell lines in a negative cell line at different dilution ratios to produce low and high levels (Cross et al. 1993a; Hughes et al. 2003). The diluted cells

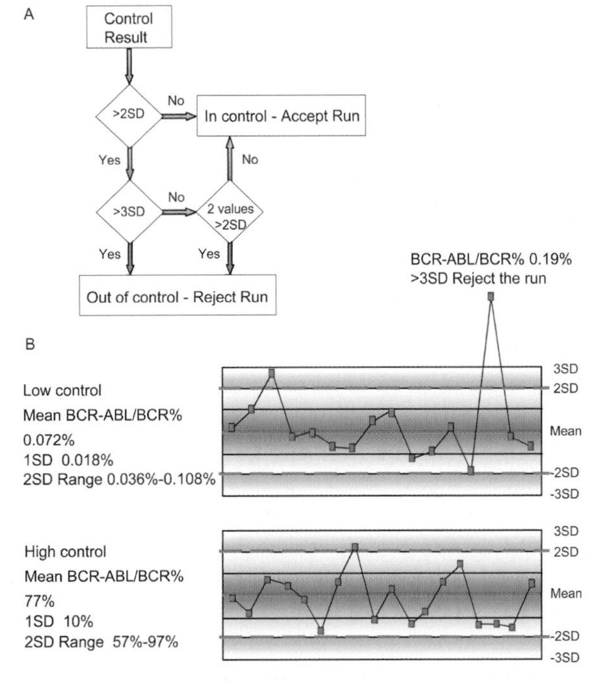

Fig. 9.2. Westgard quality control rules are applied to the quality control results to determine the acceptability of the quantitative PCR assay. **(A)** If the control value is outside the 2 standard deviation range (SD), then the run is only acceptable if the value was within the 3SD range and providing the previous result was within 2SD. Statistically, 5% of results fall between the 2 and 3SD range and are within acceptable limits. The run is rejected if the control value is greater than 3SD. **(B)** Levey-Jennings plot of a series of quality control results for the b3a2 *BCR-ABL* low and high control. The run was rejected when the low control result was outside 3SD from the mean

in each quality control dilution mix were stored in frozen aliquots in an RNA stabilization solution and included in every assay. The mean and standard deviation of the quality control BCR-ABL/BCR% results were determined in separate reverse transcription and quantitative assays measured in several assays. These values determine the acceptability of each assay by applying Westgard Quality Control rules (Westgard et al. 1981) as illustrated in Fig. 9.2. Each result is plotted using a QC Reporter software program (Chiron Healthcare), with automatic acceptance or rejection of the assay using predetermined limits and rules. The assay is rejected if the control value is outside of the acceptable limits. The dilution ratio of each control produces BCR-ABL/BCR% values that differ by approximately 3 logs. Therefore, acceptable quality control results also ensure the maintenance of a linear reaction in every RQ-PCR. In our assay these quality control samples were used to calculate the reproducibility of the assay. The coefficient of variation at high levels of *BCR-ABL* is 13% and at low levels is 25% (Branford et al. 2004c).

In addition to the positive quality control samples a *BCR-ABL* negative control, which is included in each batch of RNA extractions, can monitor for contamination that may be introduced during the extraction procedure (Cross et al. 1993b). Rigorous precautions should be undertaken at every step of the RQ-PCR procedure to prevent cross contamination of plasmid or patient samples as well as contamination with PCR product (Branford et al. 2005b).

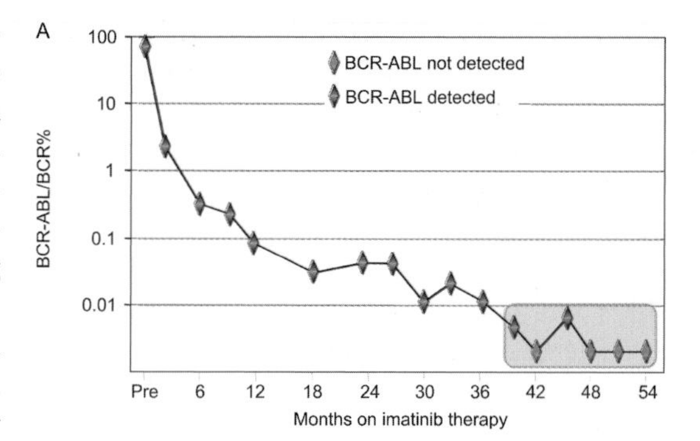

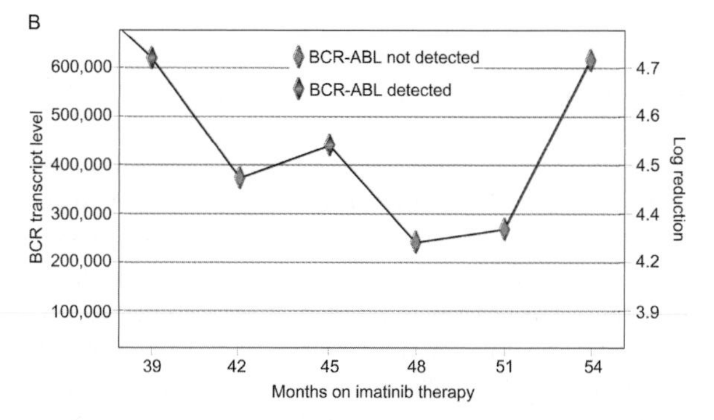

Fig. 9.3. ***BCR-ABL*** **sensitivity reflects the control gene transcript level (in this case the** ***BCR*** **gene), which is an indication of the RNA quality and the efficiency of the reverse transcription and quantitative PCR assays. The higher the control gene level, the better the sensitivity of the assay. (A) represents the** ***BCR-ABL*** **values of a patient plotted against the months of imatinib therapy. The shaded region illustrates that the** ***BCR-ABL*** **value fluctuated between detectable and undetectable. This region is expanded in (B) where the control gene transcript raw data is plotted. The** ***left axis*** **represents the** ***BCR*** **value whereas the** ***right axis*** **represents the corresponding log reduction from the standardized baseline level (Hughes et al., 2003) At month 42 the** ***BCR-ABL*** **transcript was undetectable. However, at month 45 the** ***BCR-ABL*** **transcript was detectable and the** ***BCR*** **value was higher. This indicates an improved assay sensitivity at this time-point compared to month 42. The fact that** ***BCR-ABL*** **was detectable at 39 months with a high** ***BCR*** **value and undetectable at this level of sensitivity at 54 months suggests that there had been a genuine decrease in transcript level over that time**

9.3.4 Undetectable *BCR-ABL* Levels

One of the major reasons for performing RQ-PCR analysis of *BCR-ABL* is to determine the incidence and significance of a complete molecular remission; i.e., an absence of measurable *BCR-ABL*. However, substantial leukemia can still be present without being detectable using current technology (Morley 1998). Furthermore, the validity of a PCR-negative result is highly dependent on a number of factors including the quality of the RNA, the efficiency of the reverse transcription reaction and the sensitivity of the quantitative assay. For this reason we prefer to use the expression "undetectable *BCR-ABL*" at a certain sensitivity level rather than the term "complete molecular remission" since this can be misleading (Hughes et al. 2003). In addition, with technological advances, there will be further improvements in our ability to detect low numbers of *BCR-ABL* transcripts so that "PCR negative" will have different significance as technology advances. Under ideal conditions, where blood samples are processed without delay, a sensitivity of >4.5 logs below baseline is achievable.

The *BCR-ABL* levels for some patients who achieve very low levels may fluctuate between detectable and undetectable depending on the RNA quality and the reaction efficiencies. Figure 9.3 is an example of one such patient and illustrates the varying sensitivity between analyses and between samples, which can influence the detection of *BCR-ABL*. To minimize the possibility of reporting a false-negative result, a control gene transcript level can be determined below which samples are rejected as having inadequate quality RNA.

9.4 The Use of RQ-PCR for Monitoring Treatment Response

At the end of the 1990s, following almost a decade of qualitative and quantitative PCR assessment of *BCR-ABL*, its usefulness in clinical decision making was questioned (Faderl et al. 1999). The studies using these procedures employed different techniques with varying sensitivity. Some had used inappropriate controls, which raised the possibility of both false-positive and false-negative values. The patient numbers were small in some studies and the follow-up was of short duration. The discordance among the studies made interpretation of the results difficult. It was not clear whether persistence of *BCR-ABL* post allogeneic transplant was indeed predictive of relapse. It was suggested that if quantitative data was to be informative, a threshold of residual disease above which a patient is likely to relapse should be defined. This was particularly important in patients in clinical and cytogenetic remission, since aggressive therapeutic intervention using chemotherapy or transplant needs sufficient justification to warrant the associated morbidity and mortality.

It was suggested that guidelines for using PCR techniques to direct treatment of CML were premature and should be viewed critically (Faderl et al. 1999). A quantitative threshold that defined a positive prognosis during drug therapy had also not been established. The methods had not been standardized across laboratories and the reproducibility, specificity and sensitivity had not been acceptably proven.

In response to the question of the validity of quantitative PCR of *BCR-ABL* in decision making, a number of researchers highlighted the relevance of serial quantitative analysis (Goldman et al. 1999; Lion 1999; Moravcova et al. 1999). These researchers considered that quantitative PCR was a very important tool for monitoring minimal residual disease. For some patients who remain PCR negative after transplant a bone marrow examination may never again be necessary. However, it was conceded that variation in the sensitivity of each specimen due to different degrees of RNA quality might account for some of the discrepant results of the PCR studies.

It was clear that further studies were required to clarify a number of questions concerning the use of quantitative PCR of *BCR-ABL* levels in clinical decision making. The introduction of real-time PCR techniques has simplified the cumbersome competitive quantitative procedures. However, the inherent technical complexities of quantitative PCR should not be overlooked. Additionally, certified international reference and control materials are currently not available, although standardization between methods and the development of guidelines for data analysis and for the reporting of minimal residual disease are in progress (Gabert et al. 2003; Hughes et al. 2003, 2006; van der Velden et al. 2003).

Despite the current lack of standardization of RQ-PCR methods, a number of recent studies have demonstrated that *BCR-ABL* mRNA levels accurately reflect the level of leukemic suppression induced by therapy. With the introduction of imatinib mesylate for the treatment of CML, precise and accurate minimal residual disease monitoring using RQ-PCR has become particularly relevant.

9.4.1 Correlation Between the *BCR-ABL* Level and Cytogenetic Response

The *BCR-ABL* levels measured in peripheral blood have been shown to be a reliable alternative to bone marrow cytogenetic analysis (Branford et al. 1999; Hughes et al. 2003; Kantarjian et al. 2003b; Lange et al. 2004; Merx et al. 2002; Muller et al. 2003; Wang et al. 2002). When the RQ-PCR values of imatinib-treated patients were grouped according to the cytogenetic response categories, very little overlap was observed in the *BCR-ABL* levels within the cytogenetic categories amongst 76 patients who had simultaneous blood RQ-PCR and marrow cytogenetics (Hughes et al. 2003). Two studies (Kantarjian et al. 2003b; Merx et al. 2002) have concluded that the BCR-ABL/ABL ratios of patients achieving complete, partial, and minor cytogenetic responses differed significantly, but the range of *BCR-ABL* values for patients in a CCR appeared to be less tightly clustered.

The levels of *BCR-ABL* measured by RQ-PCR analysis in corresponding blood and bone marrow samples display a good correlation (Branford et al. 2003a; Kantarjian et al. 2003b). This allows patients to have more frequent monitoring by molecular analysis using the less invasive procedure of peripheral blood collection.

9.4.2 RQ-PCR Analysis Post Allogeneic Transplant

The main strength of the RQ-PCR assay is in serial measurements, rather than one-off analyses. In patients monitored post allogeneic transplant the sensitivity of the molecular method is considerably higher than that of cytogenetic analysis and can distinguish between rising levels of *BCR-ABL* that may indicate pending relapse and decreasing levels that indicate remission (Branford et al. 1999; Elmaagacli et al. 2001). Persistently undetectable levels of *BCR-ABL* may indicate remission and defines the risk of subsequent relapse (Mughal et al. 2001). In these patients bone marrow analysis is rarely indicated (Goldman et al. 1999; Kaeda et al. 2002).

9.4.3 Predictive Value of Early Molecular Analysis

The early reduction of *BCR-ABL* transcript levels is predictive of the subsequent cytogenetic or molecular response in patients treated with imatinib (Hughes et al. 2003; Lange et al. 2004; Merx et al. 2002; Wang et al. 2002). Merx et al. analyzed 364 blood samples in 106 patients and found that the *BCR-ABL* level at 2 months was predictive for a MCR at 6 months (P = 0.006). This finding was supported in a separate study where patients who achieved a CCR had significant reductions in the *BCR-ABL* level at 3 months of imatinib therapy (Hughes et al. 2003). The early molecular analysis also indicated the risk of subsequent disease progression where patients who failed to achieve at least a 1-log reduction of *BCR-ABL* by 3 months of imatinib therapy had the highest risk (Branford et al. 2003a). In a study of 117 imatinib-treated patients, low quantitative *BCR-ABL* values after 3 months of therapy were correlated with a MCR at 6 months and with progression-free survival (PFS) at 2 years (Lange et al. 2004). The data indicate that valuable predictive information can be gained by molecular analysis very early in the course of therapy.

9.4.4 Relevance of Minimal Residual Disease Monitoring in Imatinib-Treated Patients

In the era of imatinib therapy the residual levels of leukemia fall below the level of detection by bone marrow cytogenetic analysis in most chronic phase patients, i.e., most patients achieve a CCR. The definitive study of imatinib therapy was the Phase III IRIS (International Randomized study of Interferon versus STI571) trial of newly diagnosed patients with chronic phase CML who were randomized to receive either interferon-α (IFN) plus low-dose cytarabine (n = 553) or imatinib at 400 mg/day (n = 553) (O'Brien et al. 2003). By 18 months of imatinib therapy 76% of patients had achieved a CCR compared to 14.5% of patients treated with IFN-AraC. By 42 months of imatinib therapy the percentage of patients achieving a CCR increased to 85% (Guilhot 2004). To further analyze the level of leukemic reduction in patients who had achieved a CCR it was necessary to measure the *BCR-ABL* levels by RQ-PCR.

The IRIS trial molecular study established for the first time a level of *BCR-ABL* that correlated with PFS (Hughes et al. 2003). The definition of progression included loss of a MCR, loss of a complete hematologic response, progression to accelerated phase or blast crisis, and death from other causes while on imatinib. The term "major molecular response" was defined as a ≥3-log reduction in the percentage of BCR-ABL/BCR when compared to the median pretreatment level. For patients in a CCR, 58% achieved a major molecular response by 12 months of first-line imatinib, and these patients had a 100% PFS in the subsequent 12 months (Hughes et al. 2003). This was significantly higher ($p < 0.001$) than the 95% figure for patients in a CCR who did not achieve a major molecular response by 12 months. The early molecular response also predicted the subsequent molecular response. In the IRIS study, 79 of 83 (95%) imatinib-treated patients who achieved a major molecular response maintained or improved the response on subsequent testing 3–12 months later (Hughes et al. 2002). The PFS rate in patients achieving a major molecular response has essentially been maintained at 98% after 42 months of imatinib therapy while those with a CCR but without a major molecular response had an estimated 90% PFS (Guilhot 2004).

In the IRIS trial the median pretreatment *BCR-ABL* level (also called the standardized baseline) was calculated by measuring the level of BCR-ABL/BCR in 30 patients from blood collected just prior to commencement of the study drug (Hughes et al. 2003). A major molecular response in each of the three participating laboratories was defined as a reduction of *BCR-ABL* of ≥3 logs from this standardized baseline level. Each laboratory had a different BCR-ABL/BCR% value for the standardized baseline. This method of determining the molecular response was necessary since many patients did not have samples collected at baseline and it also allowed a comparison of results derived from different molecular methods. Therefore the log reduction from the actual baseline value was not used. The advantage of defining the molecular response according to the reduction from a median pretreatment level is that once a laboratory has established the *BCR-ABL* level that is equivalent to a major molecular response as determined in the IRIS trial, results can be expressed on a common scale internationally. Paschka and colleagues have recently demonstrated that a BCR-ABL/ABL% value of 0.12% in their laboratory is equivalent to a major molecular response as defined in the IRIS trial (Paschka et al. 2004).

In the IRIS study, a *BCR-ABL* level of 4.5 logs below the standardized baseline was defined as the maximum measurable response. We have called this a "4.5-log response" so that it can be differentiated from much more substantial molecular responses that may be verifiable in future studies using improved technology. For the IRIS study, a reduction in *BCR-ABL* level of ≥4.5 logs was detected and verified on at least one occasion in 4% of patients who were in CCR (follow-up 18 months). Similar percentages of patients who have undetectable *BCR-ABL* have been reported in smaller studies (Lin et al. 2003; Merx et al. 2002). At the MD Anderson Cancer Center, Houston, undetectable *BCR-ABL* was reported in 28% of CML patients treated with imatinib 800 mg/day for 18 months compared to 7% in a similar cohort who had received imatinib at a dose of 400 mg/day (Kantarjian et al. 2004).

A subset of patients enrolled in the IRIS trial has been followed in Australia every 3 months for 42 months of first-line imatinib. The median levels of *BCR-ABL* have continued to decline; however, the majority still retained detectable levels of leukemia suggesting that imatinib monotherapy may rarely offer the possibility of a cure (Branford et al. 2004b). Given the steady downward trend in median *BCR-ABL* levels for patients in CCR the number achieving a 4.5-log response will probably increase significantly with longer follow-up.

9.4.5 The Value of Continued and Frequent Molecular Analysis

The IRIS trial and other results showing generally excellent and stable responses (Braziel et al. 2002; Goldman et al. 2003; Kantarjian et al. 2003a, 2004) have led to the widespread acceptance of imatinib as first-line therapy in chronic phase CML. However, there remain concerns regarding imatinib monotherapy in the management of CML, namely suboptimal responders and secondary resistance. These concerns justify a policy of frequent accurate molecular monitoring. Primary and secondary resistance are each seen in 5 to 10% of newly diagnosed CML patients on imatinib (O'Brien et al. 2003). These patients should be identified early in their disease course when intervention may still be effective.

9.5 Are Regular Marrow Cytogenetic Studies Still Needed?

Additional chromosomal abnormalities either in the Ph-positive or (less often) in the Ph-negative cells (Andersen et al. 2002; Bumm et al. 2003; O'Dwyer et al. 2003) can sometimes be observed in patients on imatinib therapy. Whether these additional chromosomal abnormalities are always clinically significant remains uncertain but in some cases they herald disease progression. They may not necessarily be accompanied by significant simultaneous changes in the blood *BCR-ABL* level. Thus there may still be a role for conventional cytogenetics in routine monitoring. In terms of long-term follow-up, the probability of detecting a clinically significant cytogenetic abnormality in the presence of ongoing low *BCR-ABL* levels appears to be quite low Ross et al. Leukemia, in press). Based on these observations, it may be reasonable to reduce the frequency of cytogenetic assessments in patients with substantial molecular responses, as long as *BCR-ABL* levels are falling or stable on regular testing.

9.6 Resistance to Imatinib Due to *BCR-ABL* Kinase Domain Mutations

Primary or acquired imatinib resistance occurs in all phases of the disease. After an initial response to imatinib, relapse occurs in almost all patients treated in blast crisis, in approximately 50% of accelerated phase, and in

15 to 20% of chronic phase patients. Primary resistance is a lack of a response within a defined time frame, and the response criteria vary depending on the disease phase at the start of imatinib. Primary hematologic resistance can be defined as the lack of a complete hematologic response by 3 months in chronic phase patients, and failure to return to chronic phase for at least 4 weeks for patients treated in the accelerated phase or blast crisis. Primary cytogenetic resistance can be defined as failure to achieve a MCR by 6–12 months of imatinib therapy. The definition of acquired resistance is complex and not easily defined but can include loss of a MCR, increase in the percentage of Ph-positive cells by at least 30% at an interval of 3 months or longer, loss of a complete hematologic response, and progression to accelerated phase or blast crisis. Loss of a CCR and an increase in the *BCR-ABL* level of 1 log or more has also been included in the definition of acquired resistance (Goldman 2004). It is important to define the mechanism of resistance in imatinib-treated patients, as it may provide insight into the appropriate therapeutic intervention.

In 2001, Gorre et al (Gorre et al. 2001) published the first study of imatinib resistance in CML patient cells at the time of relapse and identified mutation within the *BCR-ABL* kinase domain as the main mechanism. Further reports confirmed the association of mutations with resistance. These mutations are numerous, with over 40 different amino-acid substitutions now described that confer varying degrees of resistance (Al-Ali et al. 2004; Branford et al. 2002a, 2003b, c; Chu et al. 2005; Corbin et al. 2002, 2003; Deininger et al. 2004; Hochhaus et al. 2002; Kreil et al. 2003; Roche-Lestienne et al. 2002; Shah et al. 2002; Sorel et al. 2004; Soverini et al. 2005; von Bubnoff et al. 2002). The incidence of mutations has been varied and range from 35 to 91% of resistant patients. Mutations have been detected prior to relapse (Branford et al. 2002a, 2003c; Shah et al. 2002) and in some cases prior to commencing imatinib (Kreuzer et al. 2003; Roche-Lestienne et al. 2002, 2003; Shah et al. 2002).

9.7 Strategies for the Detection of *BCR-ABL* Kinase Domain Mutations

Imatinib interacts with 21 amino acids within the kinase domain through hydrogen bonds or van der Waals interaction (Nagar et al. 2002; Schindler et al. 2000). Most of the early studies of *BCR-ABL* mutations examined a region of the kinase domain that included the ATP binding site and the activation loop. This was reasonable considering that imatinib occupies part of the ATP binding site and makes contact with three amino acids in the activation loop. Imatinib does not make direct contact with any residue in the region of the kinase domain carboxy lobe that lies beyond the activation loop and this region was not examined in most studies. Amino acids in this region form hydrophobic interactions that stabilize the conformation of the Bcr-Abl protein. However, an examination of this region in imatinib-resistant patients did indeed reveal that mutations also occurred within this region (Branford et al. 2003c). These mutations were believed to alter the conformation of the Bcr-Abl protein in favor of the active conformation to which imatinib does not bind (Gambacorti-Passerini et al. 2003). This finding was suggested by the crystal structure examination of the Abl kinase domain in complex with an imatinib variant where the snug fit of imatinib hardly allowed for any modification in the kinase domain without compromising binding affinity (Schindler et al. 2000). Of the patients with mutations, approximately 16% have mutations in the region of the kinase domain that is located beyond the activation loop (unpublished observation of the authors).

The initial methods for detecting *BCR-ABL* mutations included subcloning and sequencing ten independent clones, and direct sequencing of the PCR product. The direct sequencing technique was as sensitive as subcloning, where the sensitivity was 20% (Branford et al. 2003c, 2005a; Shah et al. 2002). Furthermore, polyclonal resistance, as indicated by multiple *BCR-ABL* mutations in one patient, can be detected using both methods (Branford et al. 2002a, 2003c; Kreil et al. 2003; Shah et al. 2002).

9.8 Requirements for Accurate Mutation Analysis

The direct sequencing technique is a less complex and cumbersome procedure compared to subcloning multiple independent clones. However, it should be appreciated that the procedure may be prone to inaccuracies and inconsistencies. Just as the RQ-PCR technique requires attention to detail and optimization of all aspects of the procedure to produce reliable and reproducible data, so too does the mutation detection technique. False-positive or negative results, caused by method-

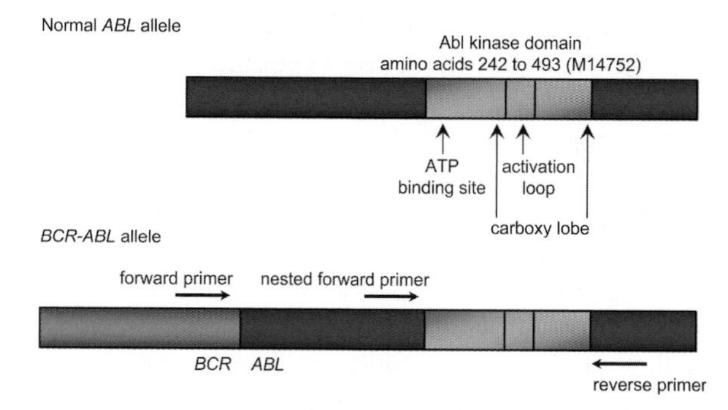

Fig. 9.4. PCR strategy to isolate the kinase domain of the *BCR-ABL* allele for mutation detection by direct sequencing (Branford et al. 2002 a). The diagrams are linear representations of the *ABL* and *BCR-ABL* genes. The forward primer specifically hybridized in *BCR* exon 13 (b2), which therefore excluded the amplification of the kinase domain of the normal *ABL* allele. This strategy increased the sensitivity of mutation detection. A seminested PCR was required for samples with low levels of *BCR-ABL*. The nested forward primer and the reverse primer were used to sequence an 863 base pair fragment that included the *BCR-ABL* kinase domain (GenBank sequence M14752)

ological errors, could lead to inappropriate clinical decisions.

We have implemented a number of procedures to ensure accurate mutation analysis using the direct sequencing technique, particularly for patients with very low levels of *BCR-ABL*. A seminested PCR is used for these patients for sensitive PCR amplification. Amplification products are column purified before the direct sequencing PCR proceeds. This strategy allows the examination of patients with a good response to imatinib, which is essential since it has been found that these patients can harbor *BCR-ABL* mutations that lead to resistance (Branford et al. 2004 a; Chu et al. 2005). Isolation of the *BCR-ABL* allele by careful selection of the PCR primers improves the sensitivity of detection by excluding the amplification of the normal *ABL* allele as illustrated in Fig. 9.4. The enzyme mix that we use for the PCR incorporates two enzymes. One is a proofreading enzyme to optimize the accuracy of sequencing data and the other increases the yield of product (Branford et al. 2002 a, 2003 c). The use of Taq polymerase, which is a standard enzyme for PCR amplification, is avoided since it lacks proofreading capability and therefore has a higher nucleotide misincorporation rate.

9.8.1 The Use of Good Quality RNA

One of the most important aspects for accurate mutation analysis is the use of good quality RNA. Inconsistent and unreliable mutation results occurred when poor quality samples were used (Branford et al. 2003 c; Hughes et al. 2006). The quality of each RNA sample was confirmed before mutation analysis by determining adequate transcript levels of a control gene using quantitative PCR. The control gene was the normal *BCR*, which was also used for the *BCR-ABL* quantitative PCR technique. A *BCR* transcript cut-off value was assigned below which mutation analysis was not performed. Different cut-off levels were used depending on the *BCR-ABL* transcript level. For samples with low levels of *BCR-ABL*, the RNA quality and the *BCR* transcript level had to be particularly high to ensure PCR amplification. The amount of cDNA added to the PCR was also increased for these samples. These measures allowed high-fidelity amplification of the *BCR-ABL* allele for almost all samples of adequate quality. The only exceptions were those with very low *BCR-ABL* levels that corresponded to a >3.5-log reduction from the standardized baseline.

It is important to optimize the PCR template amount for the amplification of samples with low *BCR-ABL* transcript levels. Inadequate input of template amount for low copy number samples has been demonstrated to cause PCR-introduced sequence alterations, even when a proofreading enzyme was used (Akbari et al. 2005; Jacobs et al. 1999; Odeberg et al. 1999). Inconsistencies in mutation analysis have also been reported when using poor quality or low copy number DNA derived from formalin-fixed, paraffin-embedded tumor tissues. In this situation real-time quantitative PCR has also been used to identify samples that would fail analysis and those that required optimization of template input for accuracy of mutation analysis (Farrand et al. 2002).

9.8.2 Adequate PCR Amplification Efficiency for Accurate Mutation Analysis

The accuracy of mutation detection is also dependent on the efficiency of the PCR reaction (Branford et al. 2005 a). On several occasions we have observed that mutations that were present in patients at previous analysis time-points were not detectable. This occurred when the first-round PCR failed to produce an amplification product in samples with *BCR-ABL* levels of sufficient amount that usually produced a product after one round of PCR. Failure of amplification indicated reduced PCR efficiency. These samples required a repeat of the first-round PCR to allow detection of the known mutations.

The results suggested that PCR efficiency impacted on the fidelity of amplification. For this reason a quality control sample that represents a low- to mid-range *BCR-ABL* level is included to monitor for adequate PCR efficiency (Branford et al. 2005 a). If the analysis proceeded despite failure of control amplification, then false-negative mutation results could occur for low abundance mutations. This phenomenon has been reported in other mutation detection systems (Jacobs et al. 1999). To avoid inaccurate results, the PCR is repeated when the positive control fails to amplify.

9.8.3 Confirmation of a Mutation by Repeat of the Whole Procedure

Despite the procedures that we have introduced to optimize the mutation detection system and to exclude inaccurate results, artefact nucleotide substitutions are still occasionally detected. This particularly occurs in patients with low *BCR-ABL* transcript levels. Upon repeat of the samples the nucleotide substitutions may no longer be present. For this reason, the complete mutation analysis procedure is repeated when a mutation is detected in a patient for the first time. The repeat analysis includes repeat of the reverse transcription PCR on a second RNA that was collected at the same sampling time-point or the same RNA if a second sample is unavailable. The second cDNA is used in the repeated mutation detection PCR and sequencing reaction. This procedure was implemented to confirm the mutation or to exclude a PCR-introduced artefact. The mutation is only considered confirmed if it is present upon repeat.

Our decision to repeat the sequencing analysis to confirm mutations and to exclude artefacts has been corroborated by other researchers studying mutations. Mathematical modeling demonstrated that the overall error rate of false-positive results of mutation detection could be reduced if repeated amplifications of the same DNA specimen show an identical result (Jacobs et al. 1999).

9.8.4 Possible Explanation for the Variation in Reported Mutation Frequency

The reported frequency of mutations in patients with imatinib resistance has been variable. The incidence for some studies was less than 50% (Al-Ali et al. 2002; Hochhaus et al. 2002). This is in contrast to the approximately 90% incidence reported in a number of studies of patients with acquired imatinib resistance (Branford et al. 2003 c; Shah et al. 2002; von Bubnoff et al. 2002). Some studies used PCR primers that did not exclude the amplification of the normal *ABL* sequence and thereby reduced the sensitivity of mutation detection. In this situation only about half of the sequences represented in a chromatogram would be derived from the *BCR-ABL* allele. Early studies did not examine the complete kinase domain but restricted the analysis to the ATP binding site and the activation loop. The use of good quality RNA is of paramount importance for accurate mutation detection. Patients with primary imatinib resistance have been reported to have a lower incidence of mutations (Al-Ali et al. 2002; Branford et al. 2002 a). In a minority of cases we have also observed that the mutant *BCR-ABL* clone becomes undetectable at the time of progression to blast crisis (Branford et al. 2003 c). This occurred in three of 14 patients whom we had monitored during imatinib therapy and at the time of blast crisis. These three patients had *BCR-ABL* amplification at the time of blast crisis. This finding serves as a caution that an isolated analysis of a patient at the time of blast crisis may not be reliable when assessing for the presence of a mutation during the course of imatinib therapy. Therefore, a number of factors could account for the variable mutation frequencies, including differences in the patient selection, the mutation detection sensitivity, RNA quality, the timing of mutation analysis, and failure to detect mutations that are located in the kinase domain beyond the activation loop.

9.9 Factors Associated with the Detection of Mutations

To identify the factors that are associated with the detection of mutations, a cohort of 144 patients in accelerated or chronic phase was examined (Branford et al. 2002 b, 2003 c). The analysis was not restricted to patients with resistance but included all patients treated with imatinib who had available RNA for analysis. In all cases mutation screening using a direct sequencing strategy was performed at least every 6 months or more often when resistance was indicated. The aims of the study were to determine if mutations were present in patients without resistance, to determine the frequency of mutations in the different disease phases, and to examine the factors that were associated with the detection of mutations. The phase of disease at the commencement of imatinib therapy, the duration of CML prior to imatinib therapy, and the initial response to imatinib provide the best indication of the risk of mutation development.

Patients who commenced imatinib in accelerated phase had the highest probability of having a detectable mutation and those who commenced in early chronic phase had the lowest (Branford et al. 2002b, 2003c). Those who commenced imatinib more than 4 years since diagnosis had the highest incidence of mutations. The data support the concept that the leukemic clone accumulates sequence errors during DNA replication over the course of the disease. Gradually, a pool of *BCR-ABL* mutants would be generated which, if they have a lower affinity for imatinib, would selectively expand in the presence of imatinib. The data provided the first epidemiological support for a clonal expansion model of imatinib resistance arising from mutant subclones that were present prior to imatinib therapy (Sawyers 2003; Shah et al. 2002).

Studies have suggested a significant association of failure to achieve a MCR with the detection of mutations. In accelerated phase and late chronic phase patients, failure to achieve a MCR by 6 months of imatinib therapy was associated with a higher incidence of mutations (Branford et al. 2003c). In a separate study, Soverini and colleagues found mutations in 48% of late chronic phase patients who failed to achieve a MCR by 12 months of imatinib therapy (Soverini et al. 2005). Failure to achieve a MCR has consistently been shown to predict for the poorest prognosis for imatinib-treated patients (Kantarjian et al. 2002a, b; O'Brien et al. 2003; O'Dwyer et al. 2004; Talpaz et al. 2002). However, these studies did not assess patients for mutations. The data suggest that commencing imatinib therapy early in the disease course and targeting a MCR or better may limit the probability of developing a detectable mutation.

9.10 Clinical Outcome for Patients with Mutations

Several groups determined the in vitro sensitivity of mutations to the antiproliferative and kinase inhibitory effects of imatinib (Corbin et al. 2002, 2003; Gorre et al. 2001; Roumiantsev et al. 2002; Shah et al. 2002). Using biochemical and cellular assays, varying degrees of imatinib resistance were conferred by distinct mutations. Some mutations were highly resistant while others remained inhibited by imatinib and therefore may respond to increased dose. We examined the outcome of the patients with mutations and found that resistance developed rapidly in some patients, leading to a complete loss of the effect of imatinib. In others the mutant clone was still responsive to imatinib and the use of higher doses re-established full or partial disease control (Branford et al. 2003c).

The T315I mutation completely disrupts imatinib binding and confers full resistance. The M351T mutation confers moderate resistance and patients with this mutation in our patient cohort generally responded to an increased imatinib dose. In contrast, a number of chronic phase and accelerated phase patients rapidly progressed to blast crisis after a mutation was detected. An association was found between the location of the mutation and the pattern of loss of response (Branford et al. 2003b, c). Patients with mutations in the region of the kinase domain known as the Phosphate binding loop (P-loop) had a high incidence of blast crisis and a low probability of survival. The association of P-loop mutations with an aggressive clinical course has been reported in a number of other studies (Corm et al. 2004; Kreil et al. 2003; Soverini et al. 2005), whereas one study did not find an association (Jabbour et al. 2004). The T315I mutation has also been associated with an aggressive clinical course (Corm et al. 2004; Gorre et al. 2001).

9.10.1 P-Loop Mutations

Protein kinases share a highly conserved region in the kinase domain known as the phosphate binding loop (P-loop), which is the site of ATP binding. The consensus amino acid sequence is Y-Gly-X-Gly-X-(Phe/Tyr)-Gly-X-Val, where Y is hydrophobic and X is variable (Bossemeyer 1994). The sequence is a critical structure of protein kinases and participates in nucleotide binding, substrate recognition, enzyme catalysis, and the regulation of activity (Bossemeyer 1994; Saraste et al. 1990). The glycines bind the α, β, and γ phosphates of ATP. A catalogue of peptide motifs and protein modules in cell signaling lists the P-loop sequence of several protein kinases including PKA, PKC, Src, and InR that all share the conserved sequence Leu-Gly-X-Gly-X-Phe-Gly-X-Val (http://www.qub.ac.uk/bb/jnpage/modules.html). A characteristic motif of protein kinases is the Rossmann motif consisting of the P-loop plus a lysine. Data by Fainstein et al. indicate that the tyrosine phosphorylating region of *ABL* and *BCR-ABL* includes the ATP binding site composed of the conserved nine amino acid peptide and lysine (Rossmann motif) at positions 248–256 and 271, respectively (Fainstein et al. 1989). These data suggest that the P-loop of *BCR-ABL* consists of the sequence Leu-Gly-Gly-Gly-Gln-Tyr-Gly-Glu-Val spanning amino acid 248–256 (Genbank M14752).

In imatinib-treated patients, the P-loop is a frequent site of mutations. In our study 38% of patients had mutations located in this region. In chronic phase patients, 8 of 13 with P-loop mutations progressed to blast crisis, which was a significantly higher frequency than in those with mutations located outside of this region (4 of 23 patients), P = 0.008 (Branford et al. 2003b).

These observations raise the question of whether some mutations actually confer an enhanced transforming capacity and contribute to disease progression, independent of their resistance to imatinib. In support of this theory, the Y253F P-loop mutation has been shown to activate the leukemogenic potential of the *ABL* proto-oncogene after site-directed mutagenesis (Allen et al. 1996). However the mutation confers only moderate imatinib resistance in vitro and in vivo (Roumiantsev et al. 2002). Furthermore, a recent study demonstrated increased kinase activity in relation to wild-type Bcr-Abl for the E255K P-loop mutation and the T315I mutation (Yamamoto et al. 2004).

It is clear that additional evaluation of imatinib-treated patients is required to confirm the association of P-loop mutations and an aggressive clinical course in CML. Biological studies may reveal that some amino acid substitutions in this region confer a gain of function.

9.11 Screening for *BCR-ABL* Mutations

Monitoring for *BCR-ABL* mutations provides an essential guide for clinical management. Resistance can be predicted early in some patients, which allows timely therapeutic intervention. However, sequencing all patient samples at regular time-points is not feasible in most centers. Undoubtedly, there is a need for a reliable method for identifying the patients likely to harbor mutations.

9.11.1 Denaturing High Performance Liquid Chromatography

Denaturing high performance liquid chromatography (D-HPLC) techniques have recently been developed to identify *BCR-ABL* mutations (Deininger et al. 2004; Irving et al. 2004; Soverini et al. 2004). The technique is dependent on the formation of heteroduplexes between mutant and wild-type sequence strands. An abnormal elution profile suggests the presence of a nucleotide change, which is confirmed by sequencing. Validation experiments using mixtures of wild-type and mutant amplicons showed that the D-HPLC technique was at least as sensitive as direct sequencing and provides a rapid semiautomated system for mutational screening. A disadvantage is that all samples need to be tested to determine when a mutation has developed. Additionally, a mutation may not be apparent when the mutant amplicon comprises >85% of the total amplicons (Deininger et al. 2004). In this situation the D-HPLC will display a homozygote profile, which is similar to the pattern seen when the amplicons are wild type. Therefore all samples with a normal elution pattern require mixture with an equal amount of wild-type amplicon to distinguish an abnormality.

9.11.2 Mutations Are Associated with a Rise in the *BCR-ABL* Level

Serial monitoring of *BCR-ABL* levels by RQ-PCR can identify the patients who harbor mutations (Branford et al. 2004c). In a study of 214 patients, the emergence of mutations was highly associated with a rise in the *BCR-ABL* level. Small increases of *BCR-ABL* on consecutive analysis of just over twofold had biological significance in terms of indicating the patients with mutations. The outcome of this research is that regular mutation screening may not be necessary for patients with stable or decreasing *BCR-ABL* levels.

The ability to reliably detect small increases in the *BCR-ABL* level is highly dependent on the reproducibility of the RQ-PCR assay. Our assay was optimized to limit the variability of results between assays. Quality control samples were included in every run to monitor the performance of the assay and tests were repeated if indicated by control values that fell outside of the acceptable range. These measures resulted in a reproducibility such that a twofold change in consecutive samples could be reliably detected at the level of a 3-log reduction of *BCR-ABL* from a standardized baseline. It is important that each laboratory establish the reproducibility of their quantitative assay. The detection of a twofold change may not be achievable with current practice at each center for various reasons. However, we believe that this level of reliability should be the goal of analysis, since small changes in the *BCR-ABL* level may have biological significance in terms of the detection of mutations.

9.12 Conclusions

In most CML patients serial analysis by RQ-PCR provides the best monitoring strategy. The major clinical advantage of RQ-PCR is the ability to accurately and frequently monitor the decline in transcript level over a 4- to 5-log range using peripheral blood. This provides an early indication in most cases that response has been adequate to minimize the risk of disease progression. However, in suboptimal responders, the RQ-PCR assay provides early warning of imatinib resistance. Frequent RQ-PCR on blood should form the basis of clinical monitoring. Marrow cytogenetics can provide additional information in some cases but is of limited value for patients who achieve and maintain major molecular response. The importance of identifying the underlying mechanism of imatinib resistance has been emphasized by the recent development of second-generation kinase inhibitors (Giles et al. 2004; Sawyers et al. 2004; Shah et al. 2004) and by the evaluation of novel antileukemic agents for their potential for overcoming resistance (La Rosee et al. 2004). Many, but not all of the *BCR-ABL* kinase domain mutations remain sensitive to the new inhibitors. Testing patients for resistant mutations in a timely and cost-effective manner is an essential component of successful patient monitoring. Precise molecular monitoring of *BCR-ABL* levels can be used as a sensitive trigger to test for mutations. We can conclude that treating with imatinib early in the disease course and targeting at least a MCR will minimize the risk of mutation selection and the associated imatinib resistance. However, mutations have also been detected in patients with very low levels of *BCR-ABL* and a good response to imatinib therapy, albeit at a lower frequency. Therefore, the potential exists for the outgrowth of mutations irrespective of the imatinib response and diligent molecular monitoring may facilitate the early detection of mutations in these patients.

References

Akbari M, Dore Hansen M, Halgunset J, Skorpen F, Krokan HE (2005) Low copy number DNA template can render polymerase chain reaction error prone in a sequence-dependent manner. J Mol Diagn 7:36–39

Al-Ali HK, Heinrich MC, Lange T, Krahl R, Mueller M, Muller C, Niederwieser D, Druker BJ, Deininger MW (2004) High incidence of BCR-ABL kinase domain mutations and absence of mutations of the PDGFR and KIT activation loops in CML patients with secondary resistance to imatinib. Hematol J 5:55–60

Al-Ali HK, Leiblein S, Kovacs I, Hennig E, Niederwieser D, Deininger MW (2002) CML with an e1a3 BCR-ABL fusion: rare, benign, and a potential diagnostic pitfall. Blood 100:1092–1093

Allen PB, Wiedemann LM (1996) An activating mutation in the ATP binding site of the ABL kinase domain. J Biol Chem 271:19585–19591

Andersen MK, Pedersen-Bjergaard J, Kjeldsen L, Dufva IH, Brondum-Nielsen K (2002) Clonal Ph-negative hematopoiesis in CML after therapy with imatinib mesylate is frequently characterized by trisomy 8. Leukemia 16:1390–1393

Beillard E, Pallisgaard N, Van Der Velden VH, Bi W, Dee R, Van Der Schoot E, Delabesse E, Macintyre E, Gottardi E, Saglio G, Watzinger F, Lion T, Van Dongen JJ, Hokland P, Gabert J (2003) Evaluation of candidate control genes for diagnosis and residual disease detection in leukemic patients using 'real-time' quantitative reverse-transcriptase polymerase chain reaction (RQ-PCR) – a Europe against cancer program. Leukemia 17:2474–2486

Bossemeyer D (1994) The glycine-rich sequence of protein kinases: a multifunctional element. Trends in Biochemical Sciences 19:201–205

Branford S, Hughes TP, Rudzki Z (1999) Monitoring chronic myeloid leukaemia therapy by real-time quantitative PCR in blood is a reliable alternative to bone marrow cytogenetics. Br J Haematol 107:587–599

Branford S, Hughes TP (2005 a) Detection of BCR-ABL mutations and resistance to imatinib mesylate. In: Iland HJ, Hertzberg M, Marlton P (eds) Myeloid leukemia: methods and protocols, methods in molecular medicine. Humana, Totowa, NJ

Branford S, Hughes TP (2005 b) Diagnosis and monitoring of chronic myeloid leukemia by qualitative and quantitative RT-PCR. In: Iland HJ, Hertzberg M, Marlton P (eds) Myeloid Leukemia: Methods and Protocols, Methods in Molecular Medicine. Humana, Totawa, NJ

Branford S, Rudzki Z, Walsh S, Grigg A, Arthur C, Taylor K, Herrmann R, Lynch KP, Hughes TP (2002a) High frequency of point mutations clustered within the adenosine triphosphate-binding region of BCR/ABL in patients with chronic myeloid leukemia or Ph-positive acute lymphoblastic leukemia who develop imatinib (STI571) resistance. Blood 99:3472–3475

Branford S, Walsh S, Rudzki Z, Grigg A, Taylor K, Herrmann R, Szer J, Seymour J, Arthur C, Lynch K, Hughes T (2002b) The most common cause of Imatinib resistance in late chronic phase and accelerated phase CML is BCR-ABL kinase domain mutations and the incidence is associated with the duration of CML and 6 month cytogenetic response. Blood 100 (abstract):367a

Branford S, Rudzki Z, Harper A, Grigg A, Taylor K, Durrant S, Arthur C, Browett P, Schwarer AP, Ma D, Seymour JF, Bradstock K, Joske D, Lynch K, Gathmann I, Hughes T P (2003a) Imatinib produces significantly superior molecular responses compared to interferon alfa plus cytarabine in patients with newly diagnosed chronic myeloid leukemia in chronic phase. Leukemia 17:2401–2409

Branford S, Rudzki Z, Miller B, Grigg A, Seymour J, Taylor K, Herrmann R, Arthur C, Szer J, Lynch K, Hughes T (2003b) Mutations in the catalytic core (P-loop) of the BCR-ABL kinase domain of imatinib-treated chronic myeloid leukemia patients in chronic phase are strongly associated with imminent progression to blast crisis. Blood 102 (abstract):71a

Branford S, Rudzki Z, Walsh S, Parkinson I, Grigg A, Szer J, Taylor K, Herrmann R, Seymour JF, Arthur C, Joske D, Lynch K, Hughes T (2003c) Detection of BCR-ABL mutations in patients with CML treated with imatinib is virtually always accompanied by clinical resistance, and mutations in the ATP phosphate-binding loop (P-loop) are associated with a poor prognosis. Blood 102:276–283

Branford S, Rudzki Z, Grigg A, Seymour J, Browett P, Taylor K, Herrmann R, Schwarer A, Arthur C, Lynch K, Hughes T (2004a) The frequency of detection of BCR-ABL mutations in imatinib-treated patients with chronic phase CML who attain a complete cytogenetic response (CCR) does not diminish with increasing duration of CCR but the associated loss of response is usually gradual. Blood 104 (abstract):81a

Branford S, Rudzki Z, Grigg A, Seymour J, Taylor K, Browett P, Schwarer A, Bradstock K, Arthur C, Durrant S, Ma D, Joske D, Lynch K, Hughes T (2004b) BCR-ABL levels continue to decrease up to 42 months after commencement of standard dose imatinib in patients with newly diagnosed chronic phase CML who achieve a major molecular response. Blood 104 (abstract):82a

Branford S, Rudzki Z, Parkinson I, Grigg A, Taylor K, Seymour JF, Durrant S, Browett P, Schwarer AP, Arthur C, Catalano J, Leahy MF, Filshie R, Bradstock K, Herrmann R, Joske D, Lynch K, Hughes T (2004c) Real-time quantitative PCR analysis can be used as a primary screen to identify patients with CML treated with imatinib who have BCR-ABL kinase domain mutations. Blood 104:2926–2932

Braziel RM, Launder TM, Druker BJ, Olson SB, Magenis RE, Mauro MJ, Sawyers CL, Paquette RL, O'dwyer ME (2002) Hematopathologic and cytogenetic findings in imatinib mesylate-treated chronic myelogenous leukemia patients: 14 months' experience. Blood 100:435–441

Bumm T, Muller C, Al-Ali HK, Krohn K, Shepherd P, Schmidt E, Leiblein S, Franke C, Hennig E, Friedrich T, Krahl R, Niederwieser D, Deininger MW (2003) Emergence of clonal cytogenetic abnormalities in Ph-cells in some CML patients in cytogenetic remission to imatinib but restoration of polyclonal hematopoiesis in the majority. Blood 101:1941–1949

Bustin SA (2000) Absolute quantification of mRNA using real-time reverse transcription polymerase chain reaction assays. J Mol Endocrinol 25:169–193

Bustin SA (2002) Quantification of mRNA using real-time reverse transcription PCR (RT-PCR): trends and problems. J Mol Endocrinol 29:23–39

Bustin SA, Nolan T (2004) Pitfalls of Quantitative Real-Time Reverse-Transcription Polymerase Chain Reaction. J Biomol Tech 15: 155–166

Chase A, Grand F, Zhang JG, Blackett N, Goldman J, Gordon M (1997) Factors influencing the false positive and negative rates of BCR-ABL fluorescence in situ hybridization. Genes Chromosomes Cancer 18:246–253

Chu S, Xu H, Shah NP, Snyder DS, Forman SJ, Sawyers CL, Bhatia R (2005) Detection of BCR-ABL kinase mutations in CD34+ cells from chronic myelogenous leukemia patients in complete cytogenetic remission on imatinib mesylate treatment. Blood 105:2093–2098

Collins S, Coleman H, Groudine M (1987) Expression of bcr and bcr-abl fusion transcripts in normal and leukaemic cells. Mol Cell Biol 7:2870

Corbin AS, Buchdunger E, Pascal F, Druker BJ (2002) Analysis of the structural basis of specificity of inhibition of the Abl kinase by STI571. J Biol Chem 277:32214–32219

Corbin AS, La Rosee P, Stoffregen EP, Druker BJ, Deininger MW (2003) Several Bcr-Abl kinase domain mutants associated with imatinib mesylate resistance remain sensitive to imatinib. Blood 101:4611–4614

Corm S, Nicollini F, Borie D, Sorel N, Leguay T, Hayette S, Facon T, Roy L, Giraudier S, Marit G, Preudhomme C, Michalet M, Mahon F, Thuilliez M, Guilhot F, Roche-Lestienne C (2004) Mutation status of imatinib mesylate-resistants CML patients and clinical outcomes: A French multicenter retrospective study for the FILMC Group. Blood 104 (abstract):82a

Costello RT, Kirk J, Gabert J (1996) Value of PCR analysis for long term survivors after allogeneic bone marrow transplant for chronic myelogenous leukemia: a comparative study. Leukemia Lymphoma 20:239–243

Cross NC, Feng L, Chase A, Bungey J, Hughes TP, Goldman JM (1993a) Competitive polymerase chain reaction to estimate the number of BCR-ABL transcripts in chronic myeloid leukemia patients after bone marrow transplantation. Blood 82:1929–1936

Cross NC, Hughes TP, Feng L, O'Shea P, Bungey J, Marks DI, Ferrant A, Martiat P, Goldman JM (1993b) Minimal residual disease after allogeneic bone marrow transplantation for chronic myeloid leukaemia in first chronic phase: correlations with acute graft-versus-host disease and relapse. Br J Haematol 84:67–74

Cross NC, Lin F, Goldman JM (1994) Appropriate controls for reverse transcription polymerase chain reaction (RT-PCR). Br J Haematol 87:218

Deininger MW, Mcgreevey L, Willis S, Bainbridge TM, Druker BJ, Heinrich MC (2004) Detection of ABL kinase domain mutations with denaturing high-performance liquid chromatography. Leukemia 18:864–871

Dewald GW, Wyatt WA, Juneau AL, Carlson RO, Zinsmeister AR, Jalal SM, Spurbeck JL, Silver RT (1998) Highly sensitive fluorescence in situ hybridization method to detect double BCR/ABL fusion and monitor response to therapy in chronic myeloid leukemia. Blood 91:3357–3365

Dewald GW, Wyatt WA, Silver RT (1999) Atypical BCR and ABL D-FISH patterns in chronic myeloid leukemia and their possible role in therapy. Leukemia Lymphoma 34:481–491

Druker BJ, Talpaz M, Resta DJ, Peng B, Buchdunger E, Ford JM, Lydon NB, Kantarjian H, Capdeville R, Ohno-Jones S, Sawyers CL (2001) Efficacy and safety of a specific inhibitor of the BCR-ABL tyrosine kinase in chronic myeloid leukemia. N Engl J Med 344:1031–1037

Elmaagacli AH, Freist A, Hahn M, Opalka B, Seeber S, Schaefer UW, Beelen DW (2001) Estimating the relapse stage in chronic myeloid leukaemia patients after allogeneic stem cell transplantation by the amount of BCR-ABL fusion transcripts detected using a new real-time polymerase chain reaction method. Br J Haematol 113:1072–1075

Faderl S, Talpaz M, Kantarjian HM, Estrov Z (1999) Should polymerase chain reaction analysis to detect minimal residual disease in patients with chronic myelogenous leukemia be used in clinical decision making? Blood 93:2755–2759

Fainstein E, Einat M, Gokkel E, Marcelle C, Croce CM, Gale RP, Canaani E (1989) Nucleotide sequence analysis of human abl and bcr-abl cDNAs. Oncogene 4:1477–1481

Farrand K, Jovanovic L, Delahunt B, Mciver B, Hay ID, Eberhardt NL, Grebe SKG (2002) Loss of Heterozygosity studies revisited: prior quantification of the amplifiable DNA content of archival samples improves efficiency and reliability. J Mol Diagn 4:150–158

Freeman WM, Walker SJ, Vrana KE (1999) Quantitative RT-PCR: pitfalls and potential. Biotechniques 26:112–122, 124–125

Gabert J, Beillard E, Van Der Velden VH, Bi W, Grimwade D, Pallisgaard N, Barbany G, Cazzaniga G, Cayuela JM, Cave H, Pane F, Aerts JL, De Micheli D, Thirion X, Pradel V, Gonzalez M, Viehmann S, Malec M, Saglio G, Van Dongen JJ (2003) Standardization and quality control studies of 'real-time' quantitative reverse transcriptase polymerase chain reaction of fusion gene transcripts for residual disease detection in leukemia – a Europe Against Cancer program. Leukemia 17:2318–2357

Gambacorti-Passerini CB, Gunby RH, Piazza R, Galietta A, Rostagno R, Scapozza L (2003) Molecular mechanisms of resistance to imatinib in Philadelphia-chromosome-positive leukaemias. Lancet Oncolol 4:75–85

Giles F, Kantarjian H, Wassmann B, Cortes J, O'Brien S, Tanaka P, Rae W, Mietlowski W, Romano A, Alland L, Dugan M, Albitar, Ottmann O (2004) A Phase I/II study of AMN107, a novel aminopyrimidine inhibitor of Bcr-Abl, on a continuous daily dosing schedule in adult patients (pts) with imatinib-resistant advanced phase chronic myeloid leukemia (CML) or relapsed/refractory Philadelphia chromosome (Ph+) acute lymphocytic leukemia (ALL). Blood 104(abstract):10a

Ginzinger DG (2002) Gene quantification using real-time quantitative PCR: An emerging technology hits the mainstream. Exp Hematol 30:503–512

Goldman JM (2004) Chronic myeloid leukemia-still a few questions. Exp Hematol 32:2–10

Goldman JM, Melo JV (2003) Chronic myeloid leukemia – advances in biology and new approaches to treatment. N Engl J Med 349: 1451–1464

Goldman JM, Kaeda JS, Cross NC, Hochhaus A, Hehlmann R (1999) Clinical decision making in chronic myeloid leukemia based on polymerase chain reaction analysis of minimal residual disease. Blood 94:1484–1486

Gorre ME, Mohammed M, Ellwood K, Hsu N, Paquette R, Rao PN, Sawyers CL (2001) Clinical resistance to STI-571 cancer therapy caused by BCR-ABL gene mutation or amplification. Science 293:876–880

Grand FH, Chase A, Iqbal S, Nguyen DX, Lewis JL, Marley SB, Davidson RJ, Goldman JM, Gordon MY (1998) A two-color BCR-ABL probe that greatly reduces the false positive and false negative rates for fluorescence in situ hybridization in chronic myeloid leukemia. Genes Chromosomes Cancer 23:109–115

Guerrasio A, Martinelli G, Saglio G, Rosso C, Zaccaria A, Rosti G, Testoni N, Ambrosetti A, Izzi T, Sessarego M et al (1992) Minimal residual disease status in transplanted chronic myelogenous leukemia patients: low incidence of polymerase chain reaction positive cases among 48 long disease-free subjects who received unmanipulated allogeneic bone marrow transplants. Leukemia 6:507–512

Guilhot F (2004) On behalf of the IRIS Study Group. Sustained durability of responses plus high rates of cytogenetic responses result in long-term benefit for newly diagnosed chronic-phase chronic myeloid leukemia (CML-CP) treated with imatinib (IM) therapy. Blood 104(abstract):10a

Hochhaus A, Kreil S, Corbin AS, La Rosee P, Muller MC, Lahaye T, Hanfstein B, Schoch C, Cross NC, Berger U, Gschaidmeier H, Druker BJ, Hehlmann R (2002) Molecular and chromosomal mechanisms of resistance to imatinib (STI571) therapy. Leukemia 16:2190–2196

Hughes T, Branford S (2003) Molecular monitoring of chronic myeloid leukemia. Sem Hematol 40:62–68

Hughes T, Branford S (2006) Molecular monitoring of BCR-ABL as a guide to clinical management in chronic myeloid leukaemia. Blood Rev 20:29

Hughes T, Janssen JW, Morgan G, Martiat P, Saglio G, Pignon JM, Pignatti FP, Mills K, Keating A, Gluckman E et al (1990) False-positive results with PCR to detect leukaemia-specific transcript. Lancet 335:1037–1038

Hughes TP, Morgan GJ, Martiat P, Goldman JM (1991) Detection of residual leukemia after bone marrow transplant for chronic myeloid leukemia: role of polymerase chain reaction in predicting relapse. Blood 77:874–878

Hughes T, Kaeda J, Branford S, Rudzki Z, Capdeville R, Gathmann I, Bolton A, Goldman J, Radich J (2002) Molecular responses to imatinib (STI571) as initial therapy for CML; results in the IRIS randomized study versus interferon and cytarabine. Blood 100(abstract):45a

Hughes TP, Kaeda J, Branford S, Rudzki Z, Hochhaus A, Hensley ML, Gathmann I, Bolton AE, Van Hoomissen IC, Goldman JM, Radich JP (2003) Frequency of major molecular responses to imatinib or interferon alfa plus cytarabine in newly diagnosed chronic myeloid leukemia. N Engl J Med 349:1423–1432

Hughes TP, Deininger M, Hochhaus A, Branford S, Radich J, Kaeda J, Baccarani M, Cortes J, Cross NCP, Druker BJ, Gabert J, Grimwade D, Hehlmann R, Kamel-Reid S, Lipton JH, Longtine J, Martinelli G, Saglio G, Soverini S, Stock W, Goldman JM (2006) Monitoring CML patients responding to treatment with tyrosine kinase inhibitors – recommendations for 'harmonizing' current methodology for detecting BCR-ABL transcripts and kinase domain mutations and for expressing results. Blood 108:28–37

Irving JA, O'Brien S, Lennard AL, Minto L, Lin F, Hall AG (2004) Use of denaturing HPLC for detection of mutations in the BCR-ABL kinase domain in patients resistant to Imatinib. Clin Chem 50:1233–1237

Itoh T, Tamura S, Takemoto Y, Kakishita E (1999) A cytogenetic and fluorescence in situ hybridization evaluation of interferon-alpha in the treatment of chronic myeloid leukemia. Intl J Mol Med 4:659–663

Jabbour E, Kantarjian H, Jones D, O'Brien S, Luthra R, Garcia-Manero R, Giles F, Rios M, Verstovsek S, Cortes J (2004) Long-term incidence and outcome of BCR-ABL mutations in patients (pts) with chronic myeloid leukemia (CML) treated with imatinib mesylate – P-Loop mutations are not associated with worse outcome. Blood 104 (abstract):288 a

Jacobs G, Tscholl E, Sek A, Pfreundschuh M, Daus H, Trumper L (1999) Enrichment polymerase chain reaction for the detection of Ki-ras mutations: relevance of Taq polymerase error rate, initial DNA copy number, and reaction conditions on the emergence of false-positive mutant bands. J Cancer Res Clin Oncol 125:395–401

Kaeda J, Chase A, Goldman JM (2002) Cytogenetic and molecular monitoring of residual disease in chronic myeloid leukaemia. Acta Haematol 107:64–75

Kantarjian H, Talpaz M, O'Brien S, Garcia-Manero G, Verstovsek S, Giles F, Rios MB, Shan J, Letvak L, Thomas D, Faderl S, Ferrajoli A, Cortes J (2004) High-dose imatinib mesylate therapy in newly diagnosed Philadelphia chromosome-positive chronic phase chronic myeloid leukemia. Blood 103:2873–2878

Kantarjian HM, O'Brien S, Cortes JE, Smith TL, Rios MB, Shan J, Yang Y, Giles FJ, Thomas DA, Faderl S, Garcia-Manero G, Jeha S, Wierda W, Issa JP, Kornblau SM, Keating M, Resta D, Capdeville R, Talpaz M (2002 a) Treatment of philadelphia chromosome-positive, accelerated-phase chronic myelogenous leukemia with imatinib mesylate. Clin Cancer Res 8:2167–2176

Kantarjian HM, Sawyers C, Hochhaus A, Guilhot F, Schiffer C, Gambacorti-Passerini C, Niederwieser D, Resta D, Capdeville R, Zoellner U, Talpaz M, Druker B, Goldman J, O'Brien SG, Russell N, Fischer T, Ottmann O, Cony-Makhoul P, Facon T, Stone R, Miller C, Tallman M, Brown R, Schuster M, Loughran T, Gratwohl A, Mandelli F, Saglio G, Lazzarino M, Russo D, Baccarani M, Morra E (2002 b) Hematologic and cytogenetic responses to imatinib mesylate in chronic myelogenous leukemia. N Engl J Med 346:645–652

Kantarjian HM, Cortes J E, O'Brien S, Giles F, Garcia-Manero G, Faderl S, Thomas D, Jeha S, Rios MB, Letvak L, Bochinski K, Arlinghaus R, Talpaz M (2003 a) Imatinib mesylate therapy in newly diagnosed patients with Philadelphia chromosome-positive chronic myelogenous leukemia: high incidence of early complete and major cytogenetic responses. Blood 101:97–100

Kantarjian HM, Talpaz M, Cortes J, O'Brien S, Faderl S, Thomas D, Giles F, Rios MB, Shan J, Arlinghaus R (2003 b) Quantitative polymerase chain reaction monitoring of BCR-ABL during therapy with imatinib mesylate (STI571; gleevec) in chronic-phase chronic myelogenous leukemia. Clin Cancer Res 9:160–166

Kantarjian HM, Cortes JE, O'Brien S, Luthra R, Giles F, Verstovsek S, Faderl S, Thomas D, Garcia-Manero G, Rios MB, Shan J, Jones D, Talpaz M (2004) Long-term survival benefit and improved complete cytogenetic and molecular response rates with imatinib mesylate in Philadelphia chromosome-positive chronic-phase chronic myeloid leukemia after failure of interferon-{alpha}. Blood 104:1979–1988

Kreil S, Mueller M, Hanfstein B, La Rosee P, Lahaye T, Helmann R, Hochhaus A (2003) Management and clinical outcome of CML patients after imatinib resistance associated with ABL kinase domain mutations. Blood 102 (abstract):71a

Kreuzer KA, Le Coutre P, Landt O, Na IK, Schwarz M, Schultheis K, Hochhaus A, Dorken B (2003) Preexistence and evolution of imatinib mesylate-resistant clones in chronic myelogenous leukemia detected by a PNA-based PCR clamping technique. Ann Hematol 82:284–289

Kwok S, Higuchi R (1989) Avoiding false positives with PCR. Nature 339:237–238

La Rosee P, Johnson K, Corbin AS, Stoffregen EP, Moseson EM, Willis S, Mauro MM, Melo JV, Deininger MW, Druker BJ (2004) In vitro efficacy of combined treatment depends on the underlying mechanism of resistance in imatinib-resistant Bcr-Abl-positive cell lines. Blood 103:208–215

Lange T, Bumm T, Otto S, Al-Ali HK, Kovacs I, Krug D, Kohler T, Krahl R, Niederwieser D, Deininger MW (2004) Quantitative reverse transcription polymerase chain reaction should not replace conventional cytogenetics for monitoring patients with chronic myeloid leukemia during early phase of imatinib therapy. Haematologica 89:49–57

Lin F, Drummond M, O'Brien S, Cervantes F, Goldman J, Kaeda J (2003) Molecular monitoring in chronic myeloid leukemia patients who achieve complete cytogenetic remission on imatinib. Blood 102:1143

Lion T (1999) Monitoring of residual disease in chronic myelogenous leukemia by quantitative polymerase chain reaction and clinical decision making. Blood 94:1486–1488

Melo JV, Kent NS, Yan XH, Goldman JM (1994) Controls for reverse transcriptase-polymerase chain reaction amplification of BCR-ABL transcripts. Blood 84:3984–3986

Merx K, Muller MC, Kreil S, Lahaye T, Paschka P, Schoch C, Weisser A, Kuhn C, Berger U, Gschaidmeier H, Hehlmann R, Hochhaus A (2002) Early reduction of BCR-ABL mRNA transcript levels predicts cytogenetic response in chronic phase CML patients treated with imatinib after failure of interferon alpha. Leukemia 16:1579–1583

Miyamura K, Tahara T, Tanimoto M, Morishita Y, Kawashima K, Morishima Y, Saito H, Tsuzuki S, Takeyama K, Kodera Y et al (1993) Long persistent bcr-abl positive transcript detected by polymerase chain reaction after marrow transplant for chronic myelogenous leukemia without clinical relapse: a study of 64 patients. Blood 81:1089–1093

Moravcova J, Nadvornikova S, Lukasova M, Klamova H (1999) Polymerase chain reaction analyses should be used as a basis for clinical decision making in patients with chronic myelogenous leukemia. Blood 94:3609–3611

Morgan GJ, Hughes T, Janssen JW, Gow J, Guo AP, Goldman JM, Wiedemann LM, Bartram C R (1989) Polymerase chain reaction for detection of residual leukaemia. Lancet 1:928–929

Morley A (1998) Quantifying leukemia. N Engl J Med 339:627–629

Mughal TI, Yong A, Szydlo RM, Dazzi F, Olavarria E, Van Rhee F, Kaeda J, Cross NC, Craddock C, Kanfer E, Apperley J, Goldman JM (2001) Molecular studies in patients with chronic myeloid leukaemia in remission 5 years after allogeneic stem cell transplant define the risk of subsequent relapse. Br J Haematol 115:569–574

Muhlmann J, Thaler J, Hilbe W, Bechter O, Erdel M, Utermann G, Duba HC (1998) Fluorescence in situ hybridization (FISH) on peripheral blood smears for monitoring Philadelphia chromosome-positive chronic myeloid leukemia (CML) during interferon treatment: a new strategy for remission assessment. Genes Chromosomes Cancer 21:90–100

Muller MC, Gattermann N, Lahaye T, Deininger MW, Berndt A, Fruehauf S, Neubauer A, Fischer T, Hossfeld DK, Schneller F, Krause SW, Nerl C, Sayer HG, Ottmann OG, Waller C, Aulitzky W, Coutre P, Freund M, Merx K, Paschka P, Konig H, Kreil S, Berger U, Gschaidmeier H, Hehlmann R, Hochhaus A (2003) Dynamics of BCR-ABL mRNA expression in first-line therapy of chronic myelogenous leukemia patients with imatinib or interferon alpha/ara-C. Leukemia 17:2392–2400

Nagar B, Bornmann WG, Pellicena P, Schindler T, Veach DR, Miller WT, Clarkson B, Kuriyan J (2002) Crystal structures of the kinase domain of c-Abl in complex with the small molecule inhibitors PD173955 and imatinib (STI-571). Cancer Res 62:4236–4243

O'Brien SG, Guilhot F, Larson RA, Gathmann I, Baccarani M, Cervantes F, Cornelissen JJ, Fischer T, Hochhaus A, Hughes T, Lechner K, Nielsen JL, Rousselot P, Reiffers J, Saglio G, Shepherd J, Simonsson B, Gratwohl A, Goldman JM, Kantarjian H, Taylor K, Verhoef G, Bolton AE, Capdeville R, Druker BJ (2003) Imatinib compared with interferon and low-dose cytarabine for newly diagnosed chronic-phase chronic myeloid leukemia. N Engl J Med 348: 994–1004

O'Dwyer ME, Gatter KM, Loriaux M, Druker BJ, Olson SB, Magenis RE, Lawce H, Mauro MJ, Maziarz RT, Braziel RM (2003) Demonstration of Philadelphia chromosome negative abnormal clones in patients with chronic myelogenous leukemia during major cytogenetic responses induced by imatinib mesylate. Leukemia 17:481–487

O'Dwyer ME, Mauro MJ, Blasdel C, Farnsworth M, Kurilik G, Hsieh YC, Mori M, Druker BJ (2004) Clonal evolution and lack of cytogenetic response are adverse prognostic factors for hematologic relapse of chronic phase CML patients treated with imatinib mesylate. Blood 103:451–455

Odeberg J, Ahmadian A, Williams C, Uhlen M, Ponten F, Lundeberg J (1999) Context-dependent Taq-polymerase-mediated nucleotide alterations, as revealed by direct sequencing of the ZNF189 gene: implications for mutation detection. Gene 235:103–109

Paschka P, Branford S, Lorentz C, Hehlmann R, Hughes T, Hochhaus A (2004) Comparison of "log reduction from median pretherapeutic value" vs ratio Bcr-Abl/Abl to express the therapeutic response in CML. Blood 104(abstract):287a

Radich JP, Gehly G, Gooley T, Bryant E, Clift RA, Collins S, Edmands S, Kirk J, Lee A, Kessler P et al. (1995) Polymerase chain reaction detection of the BCR-ABL fusion transcript after allogeneic marrow transplantation for chronic myeloid leukemia: results and implications in 346 patients. Blood 85:2632–2638

Roche-Lestienne C, Soenen-Cornu V, Grardel-Duflos N, Lai JL, Philippe N, Facon T, Fenaux P, Preudhomme C (2002) Several types of mutations of the Abl gene can be found in chronic myeloid leukemia patients resistant to STI571, and they can pre-exist to the onset of treatment. Blood 100:1014–1018

Roche-Lestienne C, Lai JL, Darre S, Facon T, Preudhomme C (2003) A mutation conferring resistance to imatinib at the time of diagnosis of chronic myelogenous leukemia. N Engl J Med 348:2265–2266

Roth MS, Antin JH, Ash R, Terry VH, Gotlieb M, Silver SM, Ginsburg D (1992) Prognostic significance of Philadelphia chromosome-positive cells detected by the polymerase chain reaction after allogeneic bone marrow transplant for chronic myelogenous leukemia. Blood 79:276–282

Roumiantsev S, Shah NP, Gorre ME, Nicoll J, Brasher BB, Sawyers CL, Van Etten RA (2002) Clinical resistance to the kinase inhibitor STI-571 in chronic myeloid leukemia by mutation of Tyr-253 in the Abl kinase domain P-loop. Proc Nat Acad Sci U S A 99:10700–10705

Saraste M, Sibbald PR, Wittinghofer A (1990) The P-loop – a common motif in ATP- and GTP-binding proteins. Trends Biochem Sci 15:430–434

Sawyers C, Shah N, Kantarjian H, Donato N, Nicoll J, Bai S, Huang F, Clark E, Decillis A, Talpaz M (2004) Hematologic and cytogenetic responses in imatinib-resistant chronic phase chronic myeloid leukemia patients treated with the dual SRC/ABL kinase inhibitor BMS-354825: Results from a Phase I dose escalation study. Blood 104(abstract):4 a

Sawyers CL (2003) Resistance to imatinib: more and more mutations. Blood 102:4–5

Sawyers CL, Hochhaus A, Feldman E, Goldman JM, Miller C , Ottmann O G, Schiffer CA, Talpaz M, Guilhot F, Deininger MW, Fischer T, O'Brien SG, Stone RM, Gambacorti-Passerini CB, Russell NH, Reiffers JJ, Shea TC, Chapuis B, Coutre S, Tura S, Morra E, Larson RA, Saven A, Peschel C, Gratwohl A, Mandelli F, Ben-Am M, Gathmann I, Capdeville R, Paquette RL, Druker BJ (2002) Imatinib induces hematologic and cytogenetic responses in patients with chronic myelogenous leukemia in myeloid blast crisis: results of a phase II study. Blood 99:3530–3539

Schindler T, Bornmann W, Pellicena P, Miller WT, Clarkson B, Kuriyan J (2000) Structural mechanism for STI-571 inhibition of abelson tyrosine kinase. Science 289:1938–1942

Schmittgen TD, Zakrajsek BA, Mills AG, Gorn V, Singer MJ, Reed MW (2000) Quantitative reverse transcription-polymerase chain reaction to study mRNA decay: comparison of endpoint and real-time methods. Anal Biochem 285:194–204

Seong D, Thall P, Kantarjian HM, Talpaz M, Swantkowski J, Xu J, Shen Y, Glassman A, Ramagli L, Siciliano MJ (1998) Philadelphia chromosome-positive myeloid cells in the peripheral blood of chronic myelogenous leukemia patients: comparison with the frequency detected in cycling cells of the bone marrow. Clin Cancer Res 4:861–867

Shah NP, Nicoll JM, Nagar B, Gorre ME, Paquette RL, Kuriyan J, Sawyers CL (2002) Multiple BCR-ABL kinase domain mutations confer polyclonal resistance to the tyrosine kinase inhibitor imatinib (STI571) in chronic phase and blast crisis chronic myeloid leukemia. Cancer Cell 2:117–125

Shah NP, Tran C, Lee FY, Chen P, Norris D, Sawyers CL (2004) Overriding imatinib resistance with a novel ABL kinase inhibitor. Science 305:399–401

Sick C, Schultheis B, Pasternak G, Kottke I, Horner S, Heissig B, Hehlmann R (2001) Predominantly BCR-ABL negative myeloid precursors in interferon-alpha treated chronic myelogenous leukemia: a follow-up study of peripheral blood colony-forming cells with fluorescence in situ hybridization. Ann Hematol 80:9–16

Sinclair PB, Green a R, Grace C, Nacheva EP (1997) Improved sensitivity of BCR-ABL detection: a triple-probe three-color fluorescence in situ hybridization system. Blood 90:1395–1402

Sorel N, Bonnet M L, Guillier M, Guilhot F, Brizard A, Turhan AG (2004) Evidence of ABL-kinase domain mutations in highly purified primitive stem cell populations of patients with chronic myelogenous leukemia. Biochem Biophys Res Commun 323:728–730

Soverini S, Martinelli G, Amabile M, Poerio A, Bianchini M, Rosti G, Pane F, Saglio G, Baccarani M (2004) Denaturing-HPLC-based assay for detection of ABL mutations in chronic myeloid leukemia patients resistant to Imatinib. Clin Chem 50:1205–1213

Soverini S, Martinelli G, Rosti G, Bassi S, Amabile M, Poerio A, Giannini B, Trabacchi E, Castagnetti F, Testoni N, Luatti S, De Vivo A, Cilloni D, Izzo B, Fava M, Abruzzese E, Alberti D, Pane F, Saglio G, Baccarani M (2005) ABL mutations in late chronic phase chronic myeloid leukemia patients with up-front cytogenetic resistance to imatinib are associated with a greater likelihood of progression to blast crisis and shorter survival: a study by the GIMEMA Working Party on Chronic Myeloid Leukemia. J Clin Oncol 23:4100–4109

Stahlberg A, Hakansson J, Xian X, Semb H, Kubista M (2004) Properties of the reverse transcription reaction in mRNA quantification. Clin Chem 50:509–515

Talpaz M, Silver RT, Druker BJ, Goldman JM, Gambacorti-Passerini C, Guilhot F, Schiffer CA, Fischer T, Deininger MW, Lennard AL, Hochhaus A, Ottmann OG, Gratwohl A, Baccarani M, Stone R, Tura S, Mahon FX, Fernandes-Reese S, Gathmann I, Capdeville R, Kantarjian HM, Sawyers CL (2002) Imatinib induces durable hematologic and cytogenetic responses in patients with accelerated phase chronic myeloid leukemia: results of a phase 2 study. Blood 99:1928–1937

Van Der Velden VH, Hochhaus A, Cazzaniga G, Szczepanski T, Gabert J, Van Dongen JJ (2003) Detection of minimal residual disease in hematologic malignancies by real-time quantitative PCR: principles, approaches, and laboratory aspects. Leukemia 17:1013–1034

Von Bubnoff N, Schneller F, Peschel C, Duyster J (2002) BCR-ABL gene mutations in relation to clinical resistance of Philadelphia-chromosome-positive leukaemia to STI571: a prospective study. Lancet 359:487–491

Wang L, Pearson K, Pillitteri L, Ferguson JE, Clark RE (2002) Serial monitoring of BCR-ABL by peripheral blood real-time polymerase chain reaction predicts the marrow cytogenetic response to imatinib mesylate in chronic myeloid leukaemia. Br J Haematol 118:771–777

Westgard JO, Barry PL, Hunt MR, Groth T (1981) A multi-rule Shewhart chart for quality control in clinical chemistry. Clin Chem 27:493–501

Yamamoto M, Kurosu T, Kakihana K, Mizuchi D, Miura O (2004) The two major imatinib resistance mutations E255K and T315I enhance the activity of BCR/ABL fusion kinase. Biochem Biophys Res Commun 319:1272–1275.

New Therapies for Chronic Myeloid Leukemia

Alfonso Quintás-Cardama, Hagop Kantarjian and Jorge Cortes

Contents

Abstract. Despite the excellent clinical results with imatinib in chronic myeloid leukemia, most patients have minimal residual disease and others will develop resistance and may eventually progress. Thus there is a need for developing approaches to overcome and prevent resistance to imatinib. The "second generation" of more potent tyrosine kinase inhibitors have shown significant activity in the laboratory and in the clinic. However, there is considerable interest in developing agents that may act on different pathways that could either be combined with these inhibitors to better overcome and eventually prevent the development of resistance, to deal with mechanisms of resistance common to all inhibitors, or to deal with the problem of residual disease, that could be mediated by a stem cell insensitive to tyrosine kinase inhibitors. To this effect, many agents have been developed and have already entered the clinical arena, such as hypomethylating agents, farnesyl transferase inhibitors, and homoharringtonine, with promising preclinical and clinical results. Others may have been tested only at a preclinical level but have shown important activity. In addition, the use of immune modulation, for example, in the form of "vaccines," is evolving as a major strategy to achieve eradication of minimal residual disease. This chapter will discuss some of the different agents currently under development, with particular attention to those already in clinical trials. The challenge for the future is to incorporate them into effective strategies that can eliminate the disease and cure all patients with chronic myeloid leukemia.

10.1 Introduction

The hybrid gene BCR-ABL resulting from the t(9;22) is crucial in the pathogenesis of CML (Daley et al. 1990; Faderl et al. 1999; Sawyers 1999). BCR-ABL encodes an 8.5-kb chimeric mRNA that translates into a 210-kDa protein with constitutively activated tyrosine kinase. Importantly, the $p210^{BCR-ABL}$ protein is distinctly restricted to CML cells, thus making it an optimal target for targeted therapeutic approaches. Imatinib mesylate (Gleevec) has ushered in the era of molecular therapeutics in CML and has become the standard in CML treatment due to its potent and selective Bcr-Abl tyrosine kinase inhibitory activity (Kantarjian et al. 2002; O'Brien et al. 2003b; Sawyers et al. 2002; Talpaz et al. 2002). Eighty to 90% of patients with CML in early chronic phase achieve a complete cytogenetic response with imatinib (Kantarjian et al. 2002; O'Brien et al. 2003b). These unprecedented results notwithstanding, imatinib may not eliminate all detectable BCR-ABL-positive cells in a substantial proportion of patients (Hughes et al. 2003); this may eventually lead to the development of resistance to imatinib and transformation to the advanced stages of the disease (Cortes et al. 2005). Mutations in the BCR-ABL tyrosine kinase domain, BCR-ABL overexpression or amplification, and overexpression of Src-related kinases are some of the mechanisms invoked in imatinib resistance (Branford et al. 2004; Corbin et al. 2003; Donato et al. 2004; Griswold et al. 2004). BCR-ABL kinase domain mutations can be demonstrated in 30 to 90% of patients who become resistant to imatinib. More than 30 different point mutations have been reported with different potential for preventing inhibition by imatinib (Corbin et al. 2003). In addition, patients in major molecular responses in whom therapy with imatinib is interrupted experience recurrence of their disease, providing further evidence that residual disease is still present. This may be due to persistence of a subset of quiescent and primitive BCR-ABL-positive cells. The persistence of this innate imatinib-insensitive cell population could eventually lead to development of clinical relapse and resistance to imatinib. Thus, current efforts in CML therapy are directed towards development of new strategies to overcome the mechanisms of imatinib failure, aiming at complete elimination of leukemic progenitor cells. Herein, we provide a review of the therapy for CML, with emphasis on innovative strategies. A family of new, more potent tyrosine kinase inhibitors, some of them with the dual ability to inhibit Src, have shown significant activity in preclinical and clinical studies. These agents are described elsewhere in this book. Here we focus on agents directed at other targets that have shown promise in preclinical studies and some of them also in clinical trials.

10.2 Farnesyl Transferase Inhibitors

Ras gene mutations are commonly encountered in leukemia. Once activated, Ras can stimulate signal pathways that ultimately promote cellular proliferation (Vojtek and Der 1998). In CML, downstream activation of Ras is one of the main events resulting from the Bcr-Abl tyrosine kinase activity. Ras is initially synthesized in the cytoplasm as an inactive protein and later attaches to the membrane. This latter step is critical in Ras function and is accomplished through a posttranslational reaction termed prenylation. During prenylation a 15-carbon isoprenyl (farnesyl) group is attached to the Ras C-terminal cysteine by an enzyme called farnesyltransferase (Ftase) and to a lesser extent by geranylgeranyl-protein transferases (GGPTases) (Beaupre and Kurzrock 1999). Inhibition of the enzymes responsible for prenylation has been sought as a means of inhibiting Ras. In CML, inhibition of Ras may suppress cellular growth in Bcr-Abl-positive hematopoietic cells. Although the development of Ftase inhibitors (FTIs) was initially designed to block Ras signaling, it has become evident that the biologic and clinical effects of FTIs have little to do with inhibition of Ras. Instead, other regulatory proteins equally dependent on prenylation may be more relevant for this effect. Examples of the latter include RhoB, Rab, and the centromeric proteins CENP-E and CENP-F.

The potential for activity of FTIs in CML was first demonstrated in Bcr-Abl-positive cell lines. Lonafarnib (SCH66336), a nonpeptidomimetic FTI, abrogated in a dose-dependent fashion colony formation and proliferation of Bcr-Abl–transformed BaF3 cells as well as cells from patients with CML (Peters et al. 2001). In Bcr-Abl leukemic mouse models harboring either the $p190^{BCR-ABL}$ or $p210^{BCR-ABL}$ products, treatment with lonafarnib resulted in prolonged survival (Peters et al. 2001; Reichert et al. 2001). Importantly, lonafarnib also inhibits proliferation of imatinib-resistant Bcr-Abl–positive cell lines and colony formation of imatinib-resistant CML cells, and sensitizes imatinib-resistant cells to apoptosis with imatinib, suggesting synergy of these two agents (Hoover et al. 2002; Nakajima et al. 2003). Drug combination studies of lonafarnib and imatinib also produced a decrease in early quiescent CML progenitors insensitive to imatinib (Jorgensen et al. 2005).

10.2.1 Single-Agent Studies

The studies of nonpeptidomimetic FTIs as single agents in patients with CML are summarized in Table 10.1. Cortes et al. reported on 22 patients with CML in all phases treated with tipifarnib (R115777) at a dose of 600 mg orally twice daily for 4 weeks every 6 weeks (Cortes et al. 2003 a). All patients had disease progression after interferon (IFN)-α and 77% had disease progression on imatinib. Six patients in chronic phase and 1 in accelerated phase achieved a hematologic response, being complete in 5 of them. Four patients had also minor albeit transient cytogenetic responses (Cortes et al. 2003 a). In a phase I trial of oral tipifarnib (R115777) at doses ranging from 100 mg to 1200 mg twice daily for up to 21 days in adults with poor-risk acute leukemias, the 2 patients with Philadelphia-chromosome (Ph)-positive blastic phase CML included achieved a partial hematologic response (Karp et al. 2001).

Lonafarnib has also been administered as a single agent in a phase II study to patients with CML who had failed prior therapy with imatinib (Borthakur et al. 2005 a). Eight patients were in chronic phase and 4 in accelerated phase. One patient in chronic phase and 1 in accelerated phase had transient hematologic responses (Borthakur et al. 2006). No cytogenetic responses were achieved. These studies demonstrated that FTIs have activity in CML. However, the responses are modest at best and single-agent FTI therapy is unlikely to benefit a significant number of patients.

10.2.2 Combination Studies

Synergy between imatinib and FTIs has been demonstrated both in imatinib-sensitive and imatinib-insensitive cell lines in vitro (Nakajima et al. 2003). Three ongoing studies are investigating the efficacy of these

Table 10.1. Results with farnesyl transferase inhibitors on CML after failure to imatinib

Agent(s)	CML stage	No.	No. response (%)	
			Hematologic*	Cytogenetic
Tipifarnib (Cortes et al. 2003 a)**	CP	10	6 (60)	3 (30)
	AP	6	1 (17)	1 (17)
	BP	6	0	0
Tipifarnib (Karp et al. 2001)	BP	2	2 (100)	NA
Lonafarnib (Borthakur et al. 2006)	CP	6	1 (17)	0
	AP	7	1 (14)	0
Tipifarnib+Imatinib (Cortes et al. 2004 a)	CP	23	7/11 (64)	6/17 (35)
Tipifarnib+Imatinib (Gotlib et al. 2003)	AP, BP	13	3/9 (33)	1/11 (9)
Lonafarnib+Imatinib (Cortes et al. 2004 b)	CP	9	2/6 (33)	1 (11)
	AP	10	3 (30)	1 (10)
	BP	3	1 (33)	0

CP, chronic phase; AP, accelerated phase; BP, blast phase

* Evaluable patient only (not in CHR at start of therapy)

** 23% had not received prior imatinib

combinations in vivo. In a phase I study, imatinib combined with tipifarnib was administered to patients with CML in chronic phase who had failed prior therapy with single-agent imatinib. Eleven patients were evaluable for hematologic response, and 7 (64%) had a complete or partial hematologic response. In addition, 6 of 17 (35%) evaluable patients achieved a cytogenetic response (one complete, one partial, and four minor). Of note, one patient harboring the T315I BCR-ABL kinase domain mutation, which is highly insensitive to imatinib, had a partial cytogenetic response (Cortes et al. 2004a). The same combination in accelerated or blastic phases of CML after imatinib failure rendered hematologic responses in 3 of 9 assessable patients; one patient achieved a minor cytogenetic response (Gotlib et al. 2003b). Lonafarnib has also been combined with imatinib in a phase I study in which CML patients in all phases received both agents after having failed single-agent imatinib. Two of 6 evaluable patients in chronic phase achieved a complete hematologic remission and one had a complete cytogenetic response. Among 13 patients with advanced phase CML, 4 responded, including 1 patient who had a partial cytogenetic response (Cortes et al. 2004b). Pharmacokinetic data from this study suggested no apparent increase in exposure to either lonafarnib or imatinib when administered concomitantly. Despite the small sample size of the 3 previous studies, the results obtained suggest that the combination of imatinib and FTIs has activity in CML, including patients with advanced phase and patients harboring imatinib-resistant Bcr-Abl mutations.

10.3 Hypomethylating Agents

Cytosine methylation is an epigenetic phenomenon that occurs after DNA replication whereby cytosine gains a methyl group at the 5′ position of the pyrimidine ring in areas where cytosine is followed by guanosine. These so-called CpG islands, in which the frequency of CpG is higher than predicted, are present in at least half of all human genes. In differentiated cells, the pattern of DNA methylation is relatively constant and preserved due to the high affinity of DNA methyltransferase for hemimethylated DNA. DNA methylation leads to changes in the organization of chromatin that result in gene silencing (Santini et al. 2001). Aberrant CpG island hypermethylation in regulatory areas of selected genes has been described as a common event in several neoplasia (Baylin et al. 1998), and is associated with inactivation of tumor suppressor genes in cancer (Baylin et al. 1998; Jones and Laird 1999). Conversely, inhibition of methylation in animal models results in abrogation of tumor growth (Laird et al. 1995). These data have triggered interest in the use of hypomethylating agents in human cancer. Methylation of certain genes has been associated with progression and/or adverse prognosis in CML. The Pa promoter of Abl and the p15 promoter are hypermethylated in 81% and 24% of patients, respectively (Nguyen et al. 2000). Interestingly, hypermethylation of p15, but not of the Pa promoter, is associated with disease progression. In addition, both events occur de novo and are acquired separately (Nguyen et al. 2000). An association between hypermethylation and CML progression has been suggested by other studies (Asimakopoulos et al. 1999; Issa et al. 1999; Zion et al. 1994). Differential patterns of p15 methylation have been reported for myeloid and lymphoid blastic phases (Nguyen et al. 2000). In addition, methylation of the cadherin-13 gene occurs at an early stage in CML and is associated with high-risk features and lower probability of response to IFN-α (Roman-Gomez et al. 2003).

Several cytosine analogs have been studied in hematologic malignancies due to their DNA methylation inhibition properties. 5-azacytidine (5-AZA) and 5-aza-2′-deoxycitidine (decitabine) are clinically available and have been tested in CML. Decitabine can demethylate 55% of DNA at concentrations tenfold lower than those of 5-AZA and incorporates into DNA, whereas 5-AZA incorporates primarily into RNA and to a lesser extent into DNA. In addition to their demethylating properties, both drugs also have cytotoxic activity (Santini et al. 2001). 5-AZA has showed significant activity in acute myeloid leukemia and myelodysplastic syndromes (Silverman et al. 2002; Wijermans et al. 2000). In CML, it has been used mostly in combination with other chemotherapeutic agents (etoposide or mitoxantrone) in patients with advanced disease, with reported response rates (i.e., return to chronic phase) of 25–60%. A pilot study of single-agent 5-AZA in 14 patients with CML produced responses in 2 patients (Kantarjian, personal communication, 2004). Decitabine has been used in CML more extensively than 5-AZA (Table 10.2). In one study, decitabine was administered at a dose of 100 mg/m^2 every 12 h for 5 days to 13 patients, at 75 mg/m^2 in the subsequent 33 patients, and at 50 mg/m^2 in 84 patients (Kantarjian et al. 2003a). Of 64 patients in blastic phase, 18 (28%) achieved objective re-

Table 10.2. Response to decitabine in CML according to dose schedule

Decitabine total dose (mg/m^2)	CML Phase	No.	No. response (%)	
			Hematologic	Cytogenetic
500–1000* (Kantarjian et al. 2003a)	CP	8	5 (63)	
	AP	51	28 (55)	7 (14)
	BP	64	18 (28)	5 (8)
150** (Issa et al. 2005)	CP	12	10 (83)	7 (58)
	AP	17	10 (59)	7 (41)
	BP	6	3 (6)	2 (33)

* After interferon failure, no prior imatinib

** After imatinib failure

sponses: 6 complete hematologic responses, 2 partial hematologic responses, 7 hematologic improvements, and 3 returned to a second chronic phase. Among 51 patients with CML in accelerated phase, 28 (55%) had objective responses (12 complete hematologic responses, 10 partial hematologic responses, 3 hematologic improvement, and 3 second chronic phase). Cytogenetic responses were obtained in 5 of 64 (8%) patients in blastic phase (2 partial and 3 minor) and in 7 of 51 (14%) patients in accelerated phase (3 complete, 3 partial, and 1 minor), respectively. Five of 8 patients (63%) treated in chronic phase had objective responses: 1 complete hematologic and minor cytogenetic response, and 4 partial hematologic responses. The most significant toxicity with this regimen was severe delayed myelosuppression, which was prolonged and dose related. Febrile episodes, documented infections and treatment-related deaths occurred in 37%, 34%, and 3% of patients, respectively. Notably, no dose-response correlation could be established. One explanation for this is that decitabine at high doses leads to arrest of DNA synthesis, which results in cytotoxicity, whereas lower doses can provide optimal levels of demethylation without severe cytotoxic effects (Kantarjian et al. 2003a). To establish the minimal effective dose of decitabine, a recent phase I study used doses of 5–20 mg/m^2. A dose of 15 mg/m^2 daily administered for 10 days was well tolerated and provided the best response in patients with a variety of relapsed or refractory myeloid malignancies (Issa et al. 2004). This low-dose, prolonged schedule of decitabine has been investigated in a phase II study which included 35 patients with CML (12 in chronic phase, 17 in accelerated phase, and 6 in blastic phase) after failure or intolerance to imatinib therapy (Table 10.2) (Issa et al. 2005). Decitabine was administered at 15 mg/m^2, 5 days a week for 2 consecutive weeks. Complete hematologic responses were reported in 12 patients (34%) and partial hematologic responses in 7 patients (20%). Sixteen patients (46%) had a cytogenetic response (major in 6 and minor in 10 patients). Again, neutropenic fever was the major adverse effect, occurring in 23% of decitabine courses. Interestingly, reduction in methylation at day 12 but not at 2 weeks of treatment discriminated between responders and non-responders (Issa et al. 2005). Overall, these results suggest a role for decitabine in the treatment of CML. Preclinical studies have shown a synergistic effect between imatinib and decitabine (La Rosee et al. 2004), leading to an ongoing study of this combination therapy in CML.

10.4 Histone Deacetylase Inhibitors

In addition to methylation, other epigenetic phenomena may be relevant in cancer and leukemogenesis. Histone acetylation is involved in regulation of gene transcription (Thiagalingam et al. 2003). Aberrant patterns of acetylation have been demonstrated in several cancers (Timmermann et al. 2001). Silencing of gene expression is associated with deacetylated histones, and this is often associated with regions of DNA methylation (Thiagalingam et al. 2003). Activation of gene expression has been linked to histone acetylation and reactivation of silenced tumor suppressor genes could be used in leukemia therapy. The enzymes histone deacetylases (HDACs) play a major role in keeping the balance between acetylated and deacetylated states of chromatin and are therefore potential therapeutic targets. Several agents that inhibit histone acetylation are currently in clinical trials, including several in CML. Suberoylanilide hydroxamic acid (SAHA) has been linked to downregulation of Bcr-Abl protein levels, resulting in apoptosis of BCR-ABL-positive cell lines and of leukemic cells from imatinib-resistant cell models (Nimmanapalli et al. 2003b; Yu, et al. 2003). Therapy with SAHA in combination with the heat shock protein 90 antagonist 17-AAG exerted growth inhibition and apoptosis in imatinib-resistant and imatinib-sensitive CML cell lines and in cells from patients with CML (Rahmani et al. 2005). Therapy with LAQ824, a cinnamyl hydroxamic acid analogue histone deacetylase inhibitor, depleted the mRNA and protein expression of Bcr-Abl in cells from patients with CML in blastic phase. LAQ824 downregulated the levels of Bcr-Abl-positive cells carrying the highly imatinib-insensitive mutation T315I and induced apoptosis of imatinib-refractory CML blastic phase cells (Nimmanapalli et al. 2003a). Studies with combinations of histone deacetylase inhibitors and imatinib are being undertaken.

10.5 Homoharringtonine

Albeit not a novel agent in CML therapy, homoharringtonine (HHT) might experience a "renaissance" due to its potential in imatinib-resistant CML. HHT is a cephalotaxus alkaloid obtained by alcoholic extraction from an evergreen tree from China. HHT has shown activity against myeloid malignancies by inhibiting protein synthesis, promoting cell differentiation, and inducing apoptosis via a caspase-3-dependent mechanism (Fresno et al. 1977; Kuliczkowski 1989; Yinjun et al. 2004). Before the advent of imatinib, HHT appeared to be the most effective salvage strategy for patients with CML post IFN-α failure, outside the setting of stem cell transplantation. HHT therapy in patients with late phase CML after IFN-α failure was associated with a complete hematologic response rate of 67% and a cytogenetic response rate of 33% (O'Brien et al. 1995). Preclinical studies have demonstrated synergy between HHT, IFN-α, and Ara-C (Visani et al. 1997). In clinical studies, combinations of HHT with low-dose Ara-C or IFN-α were associated with a significant survival advantage relative to single-agent HHT therapy (Kantarjian et al. 2000; O'Brien et al. 2002). Triple therapy combining HHT, IFN-α, and Ara-C used as frontline therapy for patients with early chronic phase CML induced complete hematologic response rates of 94% and cytogenetic response rates of 74%, of which 22% were complete (O'Brien et al. 2003a). The estimated 5-year survival in that study was 88%. Subcutaneous (SC) administration of HHT has been investigated, aiming particularly at more convenient schedules. In a phase I study including 10 patients in accelerated or blastic phase, HHT was administered at a maximum dose of 1.25 mg/m^2 twice daily for 14 days every month (i.e., the same dose used intravenously). Five patients experienced hematologic improvement (Cortes et al. 2003c). Preclinical studies suggest that HHT has synergistic or additive effects with imatinib in vitro against imatinib-resistant cell lines (Chen et al. 2003; Kano et al. 2001; Scappini et al. 2002; Tipping et al. 2002) and against cells from patients with CML in blastic phase (Tipping et al. 2002). A recent phase I/II trial studied 10 CML patients who had received imatinib for at least 2 years and achieved at least a minor cytogenetic response but had reached a plateau in BCR-ABL transcripts. In addition to continuing imatinib therapy, HHT was also administered at 1.25 mg/m^2 SC twice daily for 1–3 days every 28 days (Marin et al. 2005). BCR-ABL transcript level reductions greater than 0.5 log occurred in 7 patients; 5 had a decline greater than 1 log, and 2 patients who had failed to achieve a complete cytogenetic response on imatinib, became 100% Ph negative. In a study designed to treat patients with CML in late chronic phase who had failed single-agent imatinib, therapy with single-agent HHT was initiated with an initial intravenous loading dose of 2.5 mg/m^2 over 24 h, followed by 1.25 mg/m^2 SC twice daily for 14 days every 28 days. All five assessable patients achieved a complete hematologic remission and three had also cytogenetic response, 1 complete and 2 minor (Quintas-Cardama et al. 2005). Interestingly, two patients with imatinib-resistant ABL kinase domain mutations (Y253H and F359I, respectively) responded to HHT, achieving a minor and a complete cytogenetic response, respectively.

Overall, HHT is clinically active in CML and remains an attractive option, particularly in the setting of imatinib failure and for patients harboring imatinib-insensitive mutations (i.e., T315I). Ongoing trials will determine the role of HHT in this particular subset of CML patients, as well as in combination with imatinib.

Table 10.3. Response to vaccinations in CML

Vaccine	No.	Concomitant therapy	No. with response		
			Immune*	Clinical	
				Cytogenetic	Molecular
Junction peptide					
Pinilla-Ibarz et al. 2000	12	IFN and/or Hy	3	1	1
Cathcart et al. 2004	14	IFN (5), DLI (3), none (3), imatinib (2)	14	4 (3 IFN, 1 imatinib)	3 (2 DLI)
Bocchia et al. 2005	16	Imatinib (10), IFN (6)	16	14/15 (9/9 imatinib, 5/6 IFN)	9 (4 complete) (6 imatinib, 3 IFN)
PR1					
Qazilbash et al. 2004	10	Imatinib	6	4	4 (1 complete)
HSP70PC					
Li et al. 2005	20	Imatinib	9/16	9/16	4/4

* Immune response determined by different methods

10.6 Immune Approaches to CML Therapy

Immune-mediated events play an important role in the suppression of CML. Several studies of patients with CML in early chronic phase showed that IFN-α induced a complete cytogenetic response in 10–35%. Of these, approximately 5–10% remain durable despite discontinuation of therapy (Kantarjian et al. 2003b). Immune modulation has been assumed to account at least in part for these durable responses frequently even in the presence of minimal residual disease measured by PCR (Guilhot and Lacotte-Thierry 1998). Moreover, graft-versus-leukemia effect is important in the eradication of CML after allogeneic stem cell transplantation (SCT) (Barrett 2003). Therefore, developing immunologic approaches in CML is an appealing strategy. One approach to stimulate leukemia-specific immune modulation is the use of vaccines directed towards CML-restricted tumor antigens. At least 3 main types of vaccines have been tested in clinical studies (Table 10.3). Some other immune approaches for the treatment of CML, e.g., cell-based therapies, are also in development.

10.6.1 Bcr-Abl Breakpoint Fusion Peptide Vaccines

The fusion-region of the p210$^{BCR-ABL}$ chimeric protein contains unique sequences of amino acids that are expressed exclusively in CML cells. This novel sequence may be a possible antigenic target. Administration to mice of a synthetic peptide composed of 6 BCR, 1 fusion, and 5 ABL amino acids derived from the fusion region, elicited a peptide-specific CD4+, class II major histocompatibility complex (MHC)-restricted, T-cell response (Chen et al. 1992). These specific T cells recognized only the combined sequence of BCR and ABL amino acids but not BCR or ABL amino acid sequences alone (Chen et al. 1992). Several of these BCR-ABL junction-spanning sequences have been tested in vitro for their ability to bind to class I and II MHC molecules in human cell lines (Cullis et al. 1994) and some of them induce MCH class II-restricted T-cell-mediated cytotoxicity from lymphocytes of normal individuals and patients with CML (Pawelec et al. 1996; Yotnda et al. 1998). It has been recently shown that peptides derived from the Bcr-Abl protein can be processed in the cytoplasm and transported to the surface of the CML cell for T-cell presentation and recognition in conjunction with HLA molecules (Clark et al. 2001). A vaccine with a mixture of 5 junction peptides with binding motifs to various HLA molecules has been tested in a phase I dose-escalating trial (Pinilla-Ibarz et al. 2000). Four peptides (9 and 10 amino acids long) could bind class I HLA, whereas one (25 amino acids long) could bind to class II HLA. Twelve patients with CML in partial or complete remission after therapy with IFN-α and/or hydroxyurea received the vaccine at different dose levels (50, 150, 500, and 1500 μg). No major toxicities were recorded. Two of the 6 patients treated at the highest dose level developed significant delayed-type hypersensitivity (DTH) and 3 developed peptide-specific T-cell proliferation, but no cytotoxic T-lymphocytes were identified. One patient had a transient molecular response and another had a transient partial cytogenetic response (Pinilla-Ibarz et al. 2000). A subsequent phase II trial employed a mixture of 6 fusion peptides (5 CML class I and 1 CML class II peptides) (Cathcart et al. 2004). All 14 patients vaccinated developed immune responses represented by DTH and CD4+ proliferative response, whereas 11 had IFN-gamma release as evidenced by CD4 ELISPOT (Enzyme-linked ImmunoSPOT). All patients continued their previous therapy while receiving the vaccine, and 4 patients experienced a decrease in the percentage of Ph-positive metaphases after vaccination while on IFN-α (n=3) or imatinib (n=1). Among 3 patients with molecular evidence of disease after allogeneic stem-cell transplantation and not receiving concomitant therapy while receiving the vaccine, one experienced intermittent negativity in the BCR-ABL transcript level in the bone marrow (3 out of 6 tests), but not in the peripheral blood. Recently, Bocchia et al. have reported on 16 patients with stable residual disease after more than 12 months on imatinib therapy (n=10) or 24 months of IFN-α therapy (n=6) who were vaccinated with similar peptides. Patients received 6 vaccinations with a peptide vaccine derived from the sequence p210-b3a2 (Bocchia et al. 2005). Five of 9 patients on imatinib with persistent Ph-positive metaphases obtained a complete cytogenetic response after the addition of the vaccine, and 3 had undetectable levels of b3a2 transcripts by real-time quantitative reverse-transcriptase polymerase chain reaction (RT-PCR). Among the patients treated with IFN-α, 2 achieved a complete cytogenetic response and 3 had improvement in the percentage of Ph-positive metaphases. Peptide-specific DTH was detected in 11 of 16 patients and CD4+ T cell proliferation in 13 of 14 patients assessed (Bocchia et al. 2005). These studies suggest that this peptide vaccine may have value in managing CML minimal residual disease.

10.6.2 Heat Shock Protein-Based Vaccines

Heat shock proteins (HSPs) encompass a group of chaperone proteins that function as intercellular signaling molecules with a wide range of immunoregulatory activities when released to the extracellular environment (Pockley 2003). Normally, exogenously generated antigens are presented through MHC class II molecules whereas endogenous antigens are presented on MHC class I molecules. However, exogenous peptides chaperoned by HSP can be presented via MHC class I molecules and recognized by CD8(+) cytotoxic T lymphocytes (Suto and Srivastava 1995). When purified from cells, HSPs GP96, HSP90, and HSP70 are associated with a broad range of peptides, thus potentially chaperoning an antigenic repertoire specific for that particular cell. Immunization with cell lysates containing heat-shock protein-peptide complexes demonstrated that protein fragments chaperoned by HSP and nonintact proteins are a sufficient source of antigen transferred to antigen-presenting cells for priming CD8(+) T-cell responses (Binder and Srivastava 2005). Hence, immunization with HSP-peptide complexes derived from neoplastic cells elicits T-cell responses against the chaperoned peptides and against the tumor cells. This approach has been tested in different murine models with favorable results (Udono and Srivastava 1993; Udono et al. 1994). Recently, an autologous vaccine of leukocyte-derived HSP70-peptide complexes (HSP70PC) in conjunction with imatinib was administered to 20 patients with CML in chronic phase who had received imatinib for a median time of 15 months (Li et al. 2005). Four patients had achieved a complete, 4 a major, and 9 none or a minor cytogenetic response prior to vaccination and all had evidence of BCR-ABL transcripts by RT-PCR (Li et al. 2005). Autologous HSP70-peptide complexes were purified from CML cells, collected by leukapheresis and administered intradermally weekly for 8 weeks. Thirteen of 20 patients experienced some degree of response. Nine patients had cytogenetic improvements, including 7 who achieved a complete cytogenetic response. Of 4 patients who only had residual molecular disease prevaccination, 1 obtained a complete molecular response and 3 had reductions of Bcr-Abl transcript levels. These studies are currently being expanded.

10.6.3 PR1 Vaccine

Proteinase 3 (PRO3) is a 26-kDa-neutral serine protease that is stored in primary azurophil granules and is maximally expressed at the promyelocyte stage of myeloid differentiation (Chen et al. 1994). PR1 is a nonapeptide derived from proteinase 3 that is overexpressed in several myeloid malignancies with variable frequency, and almost universally in CML cells (Molldrem et al. 2000). PR1 is presented through HLA-A2.1 molecules (Dengler et al. 1995). PR1 can elicit cytotoxic T lymphocytes (CTL) from HLA-A2.1+ normal donors in vitro and nearly all patients with CML in IFN-α-induced remission (Molldrem et al. 2003). PR1-specific CTL show preferential cytotoxicity toward allogeneic HLA-A2.1+ myeloid leukemia cells over HLA-identical normal donor marrow (Molldrem et al. 2000, 2003) and inhibition of colony-forming unit granulocyte-macrophage (CFU-GM) from the marrow of CML patients, but not CFU-GM from normal HLA-matched donors (Molldrem et al. 1997). PR1-specific CTLs may be responsible, at least in part, for the suppression of CML. Indeed, these CTLs have been identified in most patients with CML who have responded to IFN-α or allogeneic SCT, but not in nonresponding patients, or in those treated with chemotherapy (Molldrem et al. 2000). A phase I trial of vaccination with PR1 peptide included 35 patients with myeloid malignancies who had failed prior therapies (Qazilbash et al. 2004). Patients were assigned at random to receive 0.25 mg, 0.50 mg, or 1.0 mg PR1 peptide SC every 3 weeks for a total of 3 injections. The study included 10 patients with CML of whom 1 achieved a complete cytogenetic response and 3 had improvement in the percentage of Ph-positive metaphases. Responses were also observed among patients with AML and MDS. Clinical responses correlated with immune responses (Qazilbash et al. 2004). It has been suggested that imatinib can downregulate the expression of PRO3, therefore posing a potential risk of a diminished CTL-mediated clearance of CML cells (Burchert et al. 2003). However, the expression of PRO3 is upregulated by IFN-α and current studies are investigating whether the PR1 vaccine alone or in combination with IFN-α may be of benefit for patients with CML with minimal residual disease.

10.6.4 Other Vaccines

All the aforementioned vaccines hold promise and are currently being investigated in larger clinical trials in the setting of imatinib failure or stable persistent minimal residual disease after imatinib therapy. Other peptide-based vaccines are being developed. For instance, there is animal and in vitro evidence suggesting that Wilms' tumor 1 (WT-1), an antigen present in leukemia cells including CML, can generate CML-specific CTLs (Bellantuono et al. 2002), capable of depleting CML cells without affecting normal CD34+ progenitors (Gao et al. 2000, 2003). A WT-1 vaccine is now being introduced in clinical trials in CML. Another approach to vaccination is the GVAX vaccine that has also entered into clinical trials. This vaccine comprises the use of irradiated autologous leukemia cells harvested at diagnosis mixed with GM-CSF-gene-modified K562 cells (CG9962). A phase II trial in patients with AML involved the administration of this vaccine followed by collection of vaccine-primed lymphocytes that were reinfused with the autologous stem cell graft and posttransplant vaccination every 3 weeks starting at week 6 for a total of 8 vaccinations (Borrello et al. 2005). Twenty-seven patients reached the posttransplant vaccination stage of the study. Minimal residual disease monitoring was performed by quantitative RT-PCR of the WT-1 protein. Post transplant, 75% of patients demonstrated clearance of WT-1 from peripheral blood and this was associated with an improved relapse-free survival (90 vs. 20%, $p=0.002$). In a similar approach, a vaccine using K562 cells genetically engineered to produce GM-CSF was used to treat patients with CML who had stable minimal residual disease after at least one year on imatinib. Six of the 17 evaluable patients had improvement of their disease, including 4 who became PCR negative (Smith et al. 2005).

One concern with vaccination approaches directed towards a unique epitope is that they might encounter a phenomenon of immune escape by which the malignant clone downregulates or mutates the target epitope secondary to the "immune pressure" imposed by specific CTLs. Development of vaccines with a wider antigenic scope or through other less specific immunomodulatory strategies, might help to circumvent this potential risk.

10.6.5 Cell-Based Immune Approaches

Dendritic cells (DCs) are at the center of induction of immune responses against cancer cells. In CML, the generation of fully functional DCs is problematic. DCs can be efficiently obtained ex vivo from Ph+ monocyte precursors cultured with GM-CSF and IL-4, IL-13, or IFN-α. Although able to induce CML-specific CTLs with therapeutic potential, these DCs may be functionally compromised (Choudhury et al. 1997). The use of imatinib to obtain Ph-negative DCs may impair their immune function via downregulation of nuclear factor-kappaB (NFκB) (Appel et al. 2004). Autologous Bcr-Abl-positive DCs have been administered in phase I trials with good tolerance but little if any evidence of benefit (Ossenkoppele et al. 2003). An alternative approach is to "prime" or "pulse" DCs with autologous tumor cells lysates or purified peptides (i.e., b3a2), combine them with HSPs, or transfect them with tumor antigen mRNA. Once these primed DCs acquire a mature phenotype, they can secrete IL-2 and IL-12 and express costimulatory molecules (CD80/CD86) and chemokine receptors (CCR7) that enable them to transform nave T cells into CTLs. In a clinical trial, DCs primed with the junction peptide b3a2 were given to 6 patients with CML. No patient experienced clinical improvement although immune responses were elicited in 4 of 6 patients (Takahashi et al. 2003). Osman et al. used donor DCs primed with b3a2 peptide to generate donor CTLs ex vivo to increase the graft-versus-leukemia effect of allogeneic SCT (Osman et al. 1999 a, b). The use of DCs in CML has promise although the techniques to generate ex vivo primed Ph-negative donor DCs need to be streamlined.

10.7 Targeting Bcr-Abl Downstream Signaling Pathways

Intensive research zeroing in on Bcr-Abl biology has provided solid evidence that activation of downstream signaling pathways are an integral part of the transforming activity of the Bcr-Abl fusion oncoprotein. Interference with elements of these pathways could improve on CML therapy, perhaps in combination with Bcr-Abl tyrosine kinase inhibition.

10.7.1 PI3K/Akt Pathway

Several phosphorylated tyrosine residues within the Bcr-Abl fusion protein serve as docking sites for adaptor molecules or signaling mediators to become phosphorylated and hence, activated. Autophosphorylation of BCR-ABL generates phosphorylation of site Tyr177 in the Bcr-Abl protein. This site binds to the SH2 domain of Grb2, which is responsible for the efficient induction of CML-like myeloproliferative disease by BCR/ABL in mice (He et al. 2002; Million and Van Etten 2000). In turn, the scaffolding adaptor protein Gab2 binds to the SH3 domain of Grb2. This leads to tyrosine phosphorylation of Gab2, which is critical for binding to phosphatidylinositol 3-kinase (PI3K) and subsequent activation of the PI3K/Akt pathway (Sattler et al. 2002). Akt promotes antiapoptotic signals required for transformation and ultimately, development of leukemia. The PI3K inhibitor LY294002 markedly increased apoptosis of BCR-ABL-transformed Gab2 (+/+) B lymphoblasts (Klejman et al. 2002). Combinations of imatinib with LY294002 or with the PI3K inhibitor wortmannin were effective in inhibiting clonogenic growth of leukemic CML cells in chronic or blast phase, and more so than any of those drugs alone (Klejman et al. 2002). PI3K signaling is essential for the growth of Ph chromosome-positive CML cells, but not for normal hematopoietic precursors (103–105). For these reasons, PI3K and Akt inhibitors represent rational therapeutic approaches in CML. These compounds are currently being developed.

10.7.2 mTOR Pathway

Rapamycin is a potent immunosuppressive drug whose principal intracellular receptor is termed FKBP. In mammalian cells, the complex of rapamycin and FKBP12 binds with high affinity to the mammalian target of rapamycin (mTOR). mTOR is a serine/threonine kinase which belongs to the family of tyrosine kinases PIKKs (Skorski et al. 1995). Compelling evidence places mTOR downstream of both PI3K and the PI3K-regulated protein kinase, AKT, regulating cell growth and proliferation (Sekulic et al. 2000). This might explain, at least in part, the antitumor effect of the mTOR inhibitor rapamycin. Rapamycin potentiated the inhibitory effect of imatinib on Bcr-Abl-transformed cells, including some imatinib-resistant mutants, but not those carrying the

T315I mutation (Mayerhofer et al. 2005; Mohi et al. 2004). Notably, rapamycin exerted these effects through cell cycle arrest in the G1 phase and by inhibiting the production of vascular endothelial growth factor (VGEF) (Mayerhofer et al. 2005). Anecdotal evidence suggests a favorable clinical effect of rapamycin in vivo: a patient with imatinib-resistant CML in blastic phase was treated with rapamycin at 2 mg daily for 17 consecutive days. This patient had reduction in peripheral blood leukocytes, blasts, and LDH levels, maintained for 4 weeks after discontinuation of rapamycin (Mayerhofer, et al. 2005). Other mTOR inhibitors like RAD001 and CCI779 are currently being evaluated in the clinic.

10.7.3 Raf Kinase Pathway

Raf is a tyrosine kinase protein involved in the Bcr-Abl downstream Ras signaling pathway. BAY 43-9006 (Sorafenib), a Raf-1 inhibitor, abrogates the proliferation of Ba/F3 mouse hematopoietic cells expressing wild-type Bcr-Abl. Sorafenib (BAY 43-9006) also inhibits in vitro growth of cell lines harboring the kinase domain mutants E255K and T315I, with IC_{50} values ranging from 4 to 8 mM (Choi et al. 2002). Studies with sorafenib in hematologic malignancies including CML are ongoing.

10.7.4 MEK/MAPK Pathway

The mitogen-activated protein/extracellular signal-regulated kinase (MEK)/mitogen-activated protein kinase (MAPK) pathway plays an important role in the regulation of apoptosis and survival. The MAPK cascade involves 3 different signal pathways that converge on the serine/threonine kinases JNK, p42/44 MAPK (ERK), and p38 MAPK. These molecules regulate critical cellular events. Whereas activation of JNK and p38 MAPK generally leads to induction of apoptosis, p42/44 MAPK has a cytoprotective effect (Xia et al. 1995). Disruption of MEK/MAPK activation may induce apoptosis in Bcr-Abl-positive leukemia cells (Kang et al. 2000). Several inhibitors of the enzymes that activate MAPK kinases MEK1/2 have been developed, including PD184352, PD98059, and U0126. Concomitant administration of imatinib with these inhibitors induces a marked caspase activation and induction of apoptosis in Bcr-Abl-bearing cells, including imatinib-resistant cell lines (Yu et al. 2002b). These findings confirm that inhibitors of the MEK/MAPK pathway are highly synergistic in vitro with imatinib and may represent a potential therapeutic approach to CML.

10.8 Other Potential Targets in CML

10.8.1 TRAIL

A different approach to induce apoptosis in CML cells is through the tumor necrosis factor (TNF)-related apoptosis-inducing ligand (TRAIL), also known as APO2 ligand (Bhojani et al. 2003; Wiley et al. 1995). Five receptors that bind TRAIL have been identified thus far, of which, two (DR4 and DR5) contain a cytoplasmic 80 amino acid-long death domain capable of transmitting a p53-independent cytotoxic signal (Ashkenazi 2002). The other receptors lack this death domain and act as decoys (decoy receptor-1 [DcR1], DcR2 and osteoprotegerin) competing with DR4 and DR5 for ligands (Ashkenazi 2002; Bhojani et al. 2003). TRAIL suppresses the growth of primary leukemic cells from patients with acute leukemia, CML, and myelodysplastic syndrome (Plasilova et al. 2002) and many imatinib-resistant cell lines (Uno et al. 2003). Imatinib also represses most of the TRAIL-resistant cell lines (Uno et al. 2003), suggesting a potential clinical synergism of a combination of imatinib and recombinant human soluble TRAIL (rhsTRAIL).

10.8.2 Inhibition of Cyclin-Dependent Kinases

Interference with cell cycle regulatory elements is another means to induce apoptosis of malignant cells. Flavopiridol (L86-8275, HMR 1275) is a semisynthetic flavone that exerts a potent inhibitory effect on multiple cyclin-dependent kinases (CDKs) thus causing cell cycle arrest in G1-S and G2-M (Yu et al. 2002a). Flavopiridol is the first of this class of drugs that has entered clinical trials (Senderowicz et al. 1998). In vitro, it potentiated, through mitochondrial injury and caspase activation, imatinib-induced apoptosis in imatinib-resistant K562 cell lines displaying amplification of Bcr-Abl oncoprotein (Yu et al. 2002a). Flavopiridol synergizes with bortezomib to induce apoptosis in CML cells resistant to imatinib through both Bcr-Abl-dependent and -independent mechanisms (Dai et al. 2004).

10.8.3 HSP90 Chaperone Complex

HSP90 is one of the most abundant heat shock proteins and functions as a chaperone protein complex binding a vast array of transcription factors and protein kinases involved in signal transduction, including $p210^{BCR\text{-}ABL}$, MEK, Akt, and others (Goetz et al. 2003). Therefore, HSP90 is an attractive therapeutic target, since disabling the function of this chaperone protein may potentially exert simultaneous inhibitory effects upon several oncogenic signaling pathways. The benzoquinone ansamycin antibiotics herbimycin, geldanamycin, and 17-allylamino-17-demethoxygeldanamycin (17-AAG) represent a class of drugs that specifically bind and disrupt the function of HSP90, inducing the depletion of multiple "client" oncogenic proteins by facilitating their proteasome-mediated degradation (Goetz et al. 2003; Smith et al. 1998; Stancato et al. 1997). 17-AAG is a geldanamycin analog with similar antitumoral efficacy but with an improved toxicity profile that is already in clinical trials (Goetz et al. 2003). In CML, treatment with geldanamycin or 17-AAG of HL-60/Bcr-Abl and K562 cells shifts the binding of Bcr-Abl from HSP90 to HSP70, inducing its proteasomal degradation, and downregulating intracellular levels of c-Raf and Akt kinase activity (Nimmanapalli et al. 2001). 17-AAG also induces degradation of both the wild-type and the highly imatinib-resistant T315I and E255K mutant forms of Bcr-Abl (Gorre et al. 2002). An ongoing clinical trial is exploring the combinations of imatinib and 17-AAG in CML.

10.8.4 RNA Interference

An alternative strategy to prevent $p210^{BCR\text{-}ABL}$ downstream signaling activation is to interfere with the expression of Bcr-Abl itself. This can be accomplished using techniques based on a highly conserved regulatory ontogenetic mechanism that mediates sequence-specific posttranscriptional gene silencing (Hannon 2002; Zamore 2002). This phenomenon is mediated by small interfering RNA (siRNA). siRNAs are small RNA fragments derived from the enzymatic action of the RNase III enzyme Dicer upon double-stranded RNA (Zamore 2002). Recently, the 21-nucleotide siRNAs b3a2_1 and b3a2_3 were found to induce reductions of Bcr-Abl mRNA levels by up to 87% in peripheral blood mononuclear primary cells from patients with CML and Bcr-Abl-positive cell lines. This reduction in mRNA was specific and led to transient inhibition of BCR-ABL-mediated cell proliferation (Scherr et al. 2003). More striking, siRNA homologous to b3a2-fusion site increased the sensitivity to imatinib in Bcr-Abl-overexpressing cells and in cell lines expressing the imatinib-resistant Bcr-Abl kinase domain mutation His396Pro (Wohlbold et al. 2003). Together, these data suggest the potential suitability of RNA interference strategies in combination with imatinib, particularly in the setting of imatinib-resistant CML.

10.8.5 Aurora Kinase Inhibitors

Mutant forms of BCR-ABL confer resistance to tyrosine kinase inhibitors. A highly preserved "gatekeeper" threonine residue near the kinase active site is frequently the target of these mutations, causing deleterious effects on small molecule binding. In CML, this is best exemplified by the mutation T315I that renders CML cells insensitive to imatinib and other kinase inhibitors. Aurora kinases are key elements for chromosome segregation and cytokinesis during the mitotic process (Keen and Taylor 2004). Aurora-A and -B are frequently overexpressed in human cancer leading to aneuploidy and cancer development. The Aurora-kinase inhibitor VX-680 (recently renamed MK-0457) inhibits Aurora-A, -B, -C, and FLT3 with inhibitory constants of 0.6, 18, 4.6, and 30 nM, respectively, inhibiting cells from patients with AML refractory to standard therapies (Doggrell 2004). VX-680 has also led to leukemia regression in an in vivo xenograft model (Harrington et al. 2004). It also has been shown to inhibit a Bcr-Abl T315I mutant that confers resistance to imatinib and the second-generation ATP-competitive Bcr-Abl inhibitors with an IC_{50} value of 30 nM (Carter et al. 2005). VX-680 binds tightly ($Kd \leq 20$ nM) to wild-type Abl and most of its variants, like T315I ($Kd = 5$ nM) (Carter et al. 2005). No effective kinase-targeted therapy is currently available against cells carrying the T315I mutation, suggesting an important therapeutic role of VX-680 in CML. Clinical trials of aurora kinase inhibitors, such as VX-680 and others, in hematologic malignancies including CML are ongoing.

10.8.6 Proteasome Inhibition

IκB, the inhibitor of NF-κB, is likely responsible for the antineoplastic effect of proteasome inhibition. Activated NF-κB translocates to the nucleus and promotes gene transcription (Rothwarf and Karin 1999). Proteasome inhibition may block NF-κB through decreased inactivation of IκB (Adams et al. 1999). In CML, Bcr-Abl activates NF-κB-dependent transcription and NF-κB may be required for BCR-ABL-mediated transformation (Hamdane et al. 1997; Reuther et al. 1998), possibly mediated by the RhoGEF domain of BCR (Korus et al. 2002). Bortezomib (PS341, Velcade), a potent and selective proteasome inhibitor, downregulates in vitro NF-κB DNA binding activity and expression of Bcr-Abl and Bcl-xL in Bcr-Abl-positive cell lines, resulting in apoptosis (Gatto et al. 2003). In a phase II study of bortezomib in imatinib-resistant CML patients in chronic or accelerated phase, 3 of 7 patients had a transient but significant improvement in basophilia (Cortes et al. 2003b).

10.9 Alternative Strategies to Bcr-Abl Inhibition

10.9.1 Bcr-Abl Nuclear Entrapment

Most of the current research endeavors in CML revolve around the direct suppression of the activity of Bcr-Abl. There are alternative ways to counteract the activity of this tyrosine kinase. Bcr-Abl is localized in the cytoplasm of CML cells where it activates antiapoptotic pathways (McWhirter and Wang 1993). However, Bcr-Abl contains nuclear localization sequences (NLS) and a nuclear export sequence (NES) (Vigneri and Wang 2001). Leptomycin B is a drug that blocks the nuclear export of Bcr-Abl through inactivation of the NES-receptor CRM1/exportin-1 (Vigneri and Wang 2001). The Bcr-Abl tyrosine kinase activity in the cell nucleus promotes apoptosis and this cannot be reversed by the cytoplasmic Bcr-Abl. The combined treatment with leptomycin B and imatinib caused the accumulation of 20–25% of the Bcr-Abl inside the nucleus of K562 cells, leading to irreversible cell death via caspase activation (Vigneri and Wang 2001). The proapoptotic effect of both imatinib and leptomycin B, when administered separately, was fully reversible. Nuclear entrapment of just a fraction of the total Bcr-Abl is sufficient to cause cell death. However, leptomycin B caused important neuronal toxicity. Development of new inhibitors of Bcr-Abl nuclear export must be pursued.

10.9.2 Non-ATP-Competitive Bcr-Abl Inhibitors

The currently available tyrosine kinase inhibitors are ATP-competitive inhibitors. All are affected in their ability to inhibit the kinase activity by the T315I mutation, which is considered the "gatekeeper" of the kinase domain. To overcome this problem, new compounds targeting binding-sites outside the ATP-binding domain of Bcr-Abl are being developed. ON012380 is a molecule that targets the substrate-binding site of Bcr-Abl, competing with its natural substrates like Crkl but not with ATP (Gumireddy et al. 2005a). This drug induces cell death of Ph-positive CML cells at a concentration of 10 nM (> tenfold more potent than imatinib), and causes regression of leukemias induced by intravenous injection of 32DcI3 cells expressing the Bcr-Abl mutant T315I (Gumireddy et al. 2005a). This drug also inhibits Lyn kinase activity in the nanomolar range (85 nM), making it suitable to overcome resistance conferred by this pathway. In addition, ON012380 works synergistically with imatinib and has a favorable toxicity profile in animal models. ON01910 is a substrate-competitive inhibitor of Plk1, a protein kinase with an important role in cell cycle progression, which induces mitotic arrest in a wide variety of human tumor cells. Interestingly, ON01910 presents cross reactivity with several tyrosine kinases, and inhibits Bcr-Abl and Src with IC_{50} values of 32 and 155 nM, respectively (Gumireddy et al. 2005b). BIRB796 is an inhibitor of the p38 MAP kinase, currently being tested in inflammatory diseases. Interestingly, BIRB796 binds with excellent affinity to the Bcr-Abl mutant T315I (Kd = 40nM) although high concentrations of this compound are necessary to inhibit autophosphorylation of this mutant in Ba/F3 cells (IC_{50} 1–2 µM) (Carter et al. 2005). In this regard, VX680 (MK-0457) seems to have a more favorable profile against T315I (Carter et al. 2005). Of note, this compound has significantly less affinity for wild-type and other Bcr-Abl mutants (Kd > 1 M) and an IC_{50} > 10 µM, suggesting its possible selectivity in patients who develop the imatinib-insensitive T315I mutation.

10.10 Other Targets and Strategies

VEGF plasma levels and bone marrow vascularity are significantly increased in CML (Aguayo et al. 2000). High VEGF plasma levels have been associated with shorter survival in chronic phase CML (Verstovsek et al. 2002). VEGF suppresses dendritic cell function, which in turn may downmodulate autologous anti-CML T-cell response (Gabrilovich et al. 1996). Therefore, suppression of VGEF might enhance specific immune responses to CML. Anti-VGEF monoclonal antibodies and VEGF receptor inhibitors are available and may be investigated in CML, including the monoclonal antibody bevacizumab and receptor tyrosine kinase inhibitors directed at the VEGF receptor family (e.g., SU5416, PTK787).

Preclinical data support the use of arsenic trioxide (As_2O_3) in CML. Incubation of Bcr-Abl-positive cell lines with As_2O_3 induces a decline in Bcr-Abl protein levels (Perkins et al. 2000) and apoptosis (Puccetti et al. 2000). As_2O_3 is synergistic with imatinib. Of 3 patients with imatinib-resistant, accelerated phase CML treated in a pilot study with As_2O_3 and imatinib, one patient had a major and another a minor cytogenetic response (Ravandi-Kashani et al. 2003). In a phase I trial, imatinib was given in combination with tetra-arsenic tetra-sulfide (As_4S_4) to 9 patients in accelerated or blastic phases (Li et al. 2004). Seven patients (77.8%) achieved a complete hematological response and 3 a cytogenetic response (2 major and 1 minor).

ZRCM5 is a novel triazene compound with a dual mechanism of action. The 2-phenylaminopyrimido-pyridine moiety enables this molecule to directly target Bcr-Abl, whereas a triazene tail exerts alkylating effects inducing DNA breaks and impairing DNA repairing activity. ZRCM5 was found to block Bcr-Abl autophosphorylation in a dose-dependent manner in K562 cell lines; it is fivefold less potent than imatinib (Katsoulas et al. 2005). Studies aiming at increasing the affinity of this drug for Bcr-Abl-positive cells are underway.

Gu et al. reported on the synergistic effect of mycophenolic acid (MA) with imatinib in inducing apoptosis in Bcr-Abl-expressing cell lines (Gu et al. 2005). MA is a specific inosine monophosphate dehydrogenase inhibitor that results in intracellular depletion of guanine nucleotides. The addition of this compound to imatinib reduces the phosphorylation of Stat5 and Lyn, suggesting that this combination in vivo might have additive results.

Zoledronate has showed antileukemic effects (Chuah et al. 2005) and synergism with imatinib via inhibition of Ras-related proteins in cell lines (Kimura et al. 2004; Kuroda et al. 2003). In NOD-SCID mice transplanted with Ph-positive ALL and blastic phase CML cells, intravenous zoledronate reduced significantly the prenylation of Rap1A (a Ras-related protein) and prolonged the survival of mice (Segawa et al. 2005). Overall survival was dramatically improved when imatinib and zoledronate were administered together. Zoledronate was not synergic with imatinib against the Ph-positive mutants T315I and E255K (Segawa et al. 2005).

Heme oxygenase-1 (HO-1) has been identified as a novel BCR/ABL-dependent survival-molecule in primary CML cells (Mayerhofer et al. 2004). Silencing of the expression of HO-1 by siRNAs resulted in apoptosis of K562 cells. Pegylated zinc protoporphyrin (PEG-ZnPP), a competitive inhibitor of HO-1, induces apoptosis in CML-derived cell lines K562 and KU812 with IC_{50} values ranging between 1 and 10 μM and in imatinib-resistant K562 and Ba/F3 cells expressing several Abl kinase domain mutations such as T315I, E255K, M351T, Y253F, Q252H, and H396P. Imatinib and PEG-ZnPP had synergistic growth inhibitory effects in imatinib-resistant leukemic cells.

10.11 Conclusion

Imatinib represents a historical landmark in cancer therapy. Accumulating clinical evidence suggests that most patients with CML in advanced stages and some in chronic phase may develop some form of imatinib resistance. As research on the pathophysiology of CML unfolds, new potential targets are being identified, leading to the development of novel agents with potential to overcome or prevent the development of resistance. The specificity and efficacy of imatinib in CML is uncovering additional heterogeneity of this disease. As the molecular mechanisms responsible for this heterogeneity are discovered, new therapeutic targets are identified. Complete eradication of the disease in most patients may require combinations of agents, and different cocktails may be required in different patients based on their CML molecular fingerprints. Besides the development of new therapies, a major future challenge is to design the adequate models to design the optimal treatment strategy for each patient based on their own CML biology rather than on population averages.

References

Adams J, Palombella VJ, Sausville EA, Johnson J, Destree A, Lazarus DD, Maas J, Pien CS, Prakash S, Elliott PJ (1999) Proteasome inhibitors: a novel class of potent and effective antitumor agents. Cancer Res 59:2615–2622

Aguayo A, Kantarjian H, Manshouri T, Gidel C, Estey E, Thomas D, Koller C, Estrov Z, O'Brien S, Keating M, Freireich E, Albitar M (2000) Angiogenesis in acute and chronic leukemias and myelodysplastic syndromes. Blood 96:2240–2245

Appel S, Boehmler AM, Grunebach F, Muller MR, Rupf A, Weck MM, Hartmann U, Reichardt VL, Kanz L, Brummendorf TH, Brossart P (2004) Imatinib mesylate affects the development and function of dendritic cells generated from CD34+ peripheral blood progenitor cells. Blood 103:538–544

Ashkenazi A (2002) Targeting death and decoy receptors of the tumour-necrosis factor superfamily. Nat Rev Cancer 2:420–430

Asimakopoulos FA, Shteper PJ, Krichevsky S, Fibach E, Polliack A, Rachmilewitz E, Ben-Neriah Y, Ben-Yehuda D (1999) ABL1 methylation is a distinct molecular event associated with clonal evolution of chronic myeloid leukemia. Blood 94:2452–2460

Barrett J (2003) Allogeneic stem cell transplantation for chronic myeloid leukemia. Semin Hematol 40:59–71

Baylin SB, Herman JG, Graff JR, Vertino PM, Issa JP (1998) Alterations in DNA methylation: a fundamental aspect of neoplasia. Adv Cancer Res 72:141–196

Beaupre DM, Kurzrock R (1999) RAS and leukemia: from basic mechanisms to gene-directed therapy. J Clin Oncol 17:1071–1079

Bellantuono I, Gao L, Parry S, Marley S, Dazzi F, Apperley J, Goldman JM, Stauss HJ (2002) Two distinct HLA-A0201-presented epitopes of the Wilms tumor antigen 1 can function as targets for leukemia-reactive CTL. Blood 100:3835–3837

Bellen DW, Graeven U, Elmaagacli AH, Niederle N, Kloke O, Opalka B, Schaefer UW (1995) Prolonged administration of interferon-alpha in patients with chronic-phase Philadelphia chromosome-positive chronic myelogenous leukemia before allogeneic bone marrow transplantation may adversely affect transplant outcome. Blood 85:2981–2990

Bhojani MS, Rossu BD, Rehemtulla A (2003) TRAIL and anti-tumor responses. Cancer Biol Ther 2:S71–78

Binder RJ, Srivastava PK (2005) Peptides chaperoned by heat-shock proteins are a necessary and sufficient source of antigen in the cross-priming of CD8+ T cells. Nat Immunol 6:593–599

Bocchia M, Gentili S, Abruzzese E, Fanelli A, Iuliano F, Tabilio A, Amabile M, Forconi F, Gozzetti A, Raspadori D (2005) Effect of a p210 multipeptide vaccine associated with imatinib or interferon in patients with chronic myeloid leukaemia and persistent residual disease: a multicentre observational trial. Lancet 365:657–662

Borrello H, Levitsky H, Damon L, Linker C, DeAngelo D, Elyea E, Stock W, Sher D, Donnelly A, Hege K (2005) Vaccine-associated immune and WT-1 responses are associated with better relapse-free survival in patients with AML in remission treated with a GM-CSF secreting leukemia vaccine and autologous stem cell transplant. J Clin Oncol, 23:569 s (abstract no 6539)

Borthakur G, Kantarjian H, Daley GQ, Talpaz M, O'Brien M, Garcia-Manero G, Giles F, Faderl S, Sugrue M, Cortes J (2006) Pilot study of lonafarnib (SCH66336, Sarasar), a farnesyl transferase inhibitor, in patients with chronic myeloid leukemia in chronic or accelerated phase resistant or refractory to imatinib. Cancer 106:346–352

Branford S, Rudzki Z, Parkinson I, Grigg A, Taylor K, Seymour JF, Durrant S, Browett P, Schwarer AP, Arthur C, Catalano J, Leahy MF, Filshie R, Bradstock K, Herrmann R, Joske D, Lynch K, Hughes T (2004) Real-time quantitative PCR analysis can be used as a primary screen to identify patients with CML treated with imatinib who have BCR-ABL kinase domain mutations. Blood 104:2926–2932

Burchert A, Wolfl S, Schmidt M, Brendel C, Denecke B, Cai D, Odyvanova L, Lahaye T, Muller MC, Berg T, Gschaidmeier H, Wittig B, Hehlmann R, Hochhaus A, Neubauer A (2003) Interferon-alpha, but not the ABL-kinase inhibitor imatinib (STI571), induces expression of myeloblastin and a specific T-cell response in chronic myeloid leukemia. Blood 101:259–264

Carter TA, Wodicka LM, Shah NP, Velasco AM, Fabian MA, Treiber DK, Milanov ZV, Atteridge CE, Biggs WH, 3rd, Edeen PT, Floyd M, Ford JM, Grotzfeld RM, Herrgard S, Insko DE, Mehta SA, Patel HK, Pao W, Sawyers CL, Varmus H, Zarrinkar PP, Lockhart DJ (2005) Inhibition of drug-resistant mutants of ABL, KIT, and EGF receptor kinases. Proc Natl Acad Sci USA, 102:11011–11016

Cathcart K, Pinilla-Ibarz J, Korontsvit T, Schwartz J, Zakhaleva V, Papadopoulos EB, Scheinberg DA (2004) A multivalent bcr-abl fusion peptide vaccination trial in patients with chronic myeloid leukemia. Blood 103:1037–1042

Chen R, Benaissa S, Plunkett W (2003) A sequential blockade strategy to target the Bcr/Abl oncoprotein in chronic myelogenous leukemia with STI571 and the protein synthesis inhibitor homoharringtonine. Proc Am Assoc Cancer Res 44:34 (abstract no 3788)

Chen T, Meier R, Ziemiecki A, Fey MF, Tobler A (1994) Myeloblastin/proteinase 3 belongs to the set of negatively regulated primary response genes expressed during in vitro myeloid differentiation. Biochem Biophys Res Commun, 200:1130–1135

Chen W, Peace DJ, Rovira DK, You SG, Cheever MA (1992) T-cell immunity to the joining region of p210BCR-ABL protein. Proc Natl Acad Sci USA 89:1468–1472

Choi Y.-J, Wang Q, White S, Gorre ME, Sawyers CL, Bollag G (2002) Imatinib-resistant cell lines are sensitive to the Raf inhibitor BAY 43-9006. Blood 100:369a (abstract no 1427)

Choudhury A, Gajewski JL, Liang JC, Popat U, Claxton DF, Kliche KO, Andreeff M, Champlin RE (1997) Use of leukemic dendritic cells for the generation of antileukemic cellular cytotoxicity against Philadelphia chromosome-positive chronic myelogenous leukemia. Blood 89:1133–1142

Chuah C, Barnes DJ, Kwok M, Corbin A, Deininger MW, Druker BJ, Melo JV (2005) Zoledronate inhibits proliferation and induces apoptosis of imatinib-resistant chronic myeloid leukaemia cells. Leukemia 19:1896–1904

Clark RE, Dodi IA, Hill SC, Lill JR, Aubert G, Macintyre AR, Rojas J, Bourdon A, Bonner PL, Wang L, Christmas SE, Travers PJ, Creaser CS, Rees RC, Madrigal JA (2001) Direct evidence that leukemic cells present HLA-associated immunogenic peptides derived from the BCR-ABL b3a2 fusion protein. Blood 98:2887–2893

Corbin AS, Rosee PL, Stoffregen EP, Druker BJ, Deininger MW (2003) Several Bcr-Abl kinase domain mutants associated with imatinib mesylate resistance remain sensitive to imatinib. Blood 101:4611–4614

Cortes J, Albitar M, Thomas D, Giles F, Kurzrock R, Thibault A, Rackoff W, Koller C, O'Brien S, Garcia-Manero G, Talpaz M, Kantarjian H (2003 a) Efficacy of the farnesyl transferase inhibitor R115777 in chronic myeloid leukemia and other hematologic malignancies. Blood 101:1692–1697

Cortes J, Giles F, O'Brien S, Beran M, McConkey D, Wright J, Scheinkein D, Patel G, Verstovsek S, Pate O, Talpaz M, Kantarjian H (2003 b) Phase II study of bortezomib (VELCADE, formerly PS341) for patients with imatinib-refractory chronic myeloid leukemia in chronic or accelerated phase. Blood 102:312b (abstract no 4971)

Cortes J, O'Brien M, Verstovsek S, Thomas D, Giles F, Garcia-Manero G, Murgo A, Newman R, Rios MB, Talpaz M, Kantarjian H (2003c) Phase I study of subcutaneous homoharringtonine for patients with chronic myelogenous leukemia. Blood 102:322b (abstract no 5010)

Cortes J, Garcia-Manero G, O'Brien S, Hernandez I, Rackoff W, Faderl S, Thomas D, Ferrajoli A, Talpaz M, Kantarjian H (2004a) A phase i study of tipifarnib in combination with imatinib mesylate (IM) for patients (Pts) with chronic myeloid leukemia (CML) in chronic phase (CP) who failed IM therapy. Blood 104:(abstract no 1011)

Cortes J, O'Brien S, Verstovsek S, Daley GQ, Koller C, Ferrajoli A, Pate O, Faderl S, Ravandi F, Talpaz M, Zhu Y, Statkevich P, Sugrue M, Kantarjian H (2004b) Phase I study of lonafarnib (SCH66336) in combination with imatinib for patients (Pts) with chronic myeloid leukemia (CML) after failure to imatinib. Blood 104:(abstract no 1009)

Cortes J, Talpaz M, O'Brien S, Jones D, Luthra R, Shan J, Giles F, Faderl S, Verstovsek S, Garcia-Manero G, Rios MB, Kantarjian H (2005) Molecular responses in patients with chronic myelogenous leukemia in chronic phase treated with imatinib mesylate. Clin Cancer Res 11:3425–3432

Cullis JO, Barrett AJ, Goldman JM, Lechler RI (1994) Binding of BCR/ABL junctional peptides to major histocompatibility complex (MHC) class I molecules: studies in antigen-processing defective cell lines. Leukemia 8:165–170

Dai Y, Rahmani M, Pei XY, Dent P, Grant S (2004) Bortezomib and flavopiridol interact synergistically to induce apoptosis in chronic myeloid leukemia cells resistant to imatinib mesylate through both Bcr/Abl-dependent and -independent mechanisms. Blood 104:509–518

Daley GQ, Van Etten RA, Baltimore D (1990) Induction of chronic myelogenous leukemia in mice by the P210bcr/abl gene of the Philadelphia chromosome. Science 247:824–830

Dengler R, Munstermann U, Al-Batran S, Hausner I, Faderl S, Nerl C, Emmerich B (1995) Immunocytochemical and flow cytometric detection of proteinase 3 (myeloblastin) in normal and leukaemic myeloid cells. Br J Haematol 89:250–257

Doggrell SA (2004) Dawn of Aurora kinase inhibitors as anticancer drugs. Expert Opin Investig Drugs 13:1199–1201

Donato NJ, Wu JY, Stapley J, Lin H, Arlinghaus R, Aggarwal BB, Shishodin S, Albitar M, Hayes K, Kantarjian H, Talpaz M (2004) Imatinib mesylate resistance through BCR-ABL independence in chronic myelogenous leukemia. Cancer Res 64:672–677

Faderl S, Talpaz M, Estrov Z, O'Brien S, Kurzrock R, Kantarjian HM (1999) The biology of chronic myeloid leukemia. N Engl J Med 341:164–172

Fresno M, Jimenez A, Vazquez D (1977) Inhibition of translation in eukaryotic systems by harringtonine. Eur J Biochem 72:323–330

Gabrilovich DI, Chen HL, Girgis KR, Cunningham HT, Meny GM, Nadaf S, Kavanaugh D, Carbone DP (1996) Production of vascular endothelial growth factor by human tumors inhibits the functional maturation of dendritic cells. Nat Med 2:1096–1103

Gao L, Bellantuono I, Elsasser A, Marley SB, Gordon MY, Goldman JM, Stauss HJ (2000) Selective elimination of leukemic CD34(+) progenitor cells by cytotoxic T lymphocytes specific for WT1. Blood 95:2198–2203

Gao L, Xue SA, Hasserjian R, Cotter F, Kaeda J, Goldman JM, Dazzi F, Stauss HJ (2003) Human cytotoxic T lymphocytes specific for Wilms' tumor antigen-1 inhibit engraftment of leukemia-initiating stem cells in non-obese diabetic-severe combined immunodeficient recipients. Transplantation 75:1429–1436

Gatto S, Scappini B, Pham L, Onida F, Milella M, Ball G, Ricci C, Divoky V, Verstovsek S, Kantarjian HM, Keating MJ, Cortes-Franco JE, Beran M (2003) The proteasome inhibitor PS-341 inhibits growth and induces apoptosis in Bcr/Abl-positive cell lines sensitive and resistant to imatinib mesylate. Haematologica 88:853–863

Goetz MP, Toft DO, Ames MM, Erlichman C (2003) The Hsp90 chaperone complex as a novel target for cancer therapy. Ann Oncol 14:1169–1176

Gorre ME, Ellwood-Yen K, Chiosis G, Rosen N, Sawyers CL (2002) BCR-ABL point mutants isolated from patients with imatinib mesylate-resistant chronic myeloid leukemia remain sensitive to inhibitors of the BCR-ABL chaperone heat shock protein 90. Blood 100:3041–3044

Gotlib J, Mauro MJ, O'Dwyer M, Fechter L, Dugan K, Kuyl J, Yekrang A, Mori M, Rackoff W, Coutre S, Druker BJ, Greenberg PL (2003) Tpipifarnib (Zarnestra) and imatinib (Gleevec) combination therapy in patients with advanced chronic myelogenous leukemia (CML): preliminary results of a phase I study. Blood 102:909a (abstract no 3384)

Griswold IJ, Bumm T, O'Hare T, Moseson EM, Druker B, Deininger MW (2004) Investigation of the biological differences between Bcr-Abl kinase mutations resistant to imatinib. Blood 104:161a (abstract no 555)

Gu JJ, Santiago L, Mitchell BS (2005) Synergy between imatinib and mycophenolic acid in inducing apoptosis in cell lines expressing Bcr-Abl. Blood 105:3270–3277

Guilhot F, Lacotte-Thierry L (1998) Interferon-alpha: mechanisms of action in chronic myelogenous leukemia in chronic phase. Hematol Cell Ther 40:237–239

Gumireddy K, Baker SJ, Cosenza SC, John P, Kang AD, Robell KA, Reddy MV, Reddy EP (2005a) A non-ATP-competitive inhibitor of BCR-ABL overrides imatinib resistance. Proc Natl Acad Sci USA 102:1992–1997

Gumireddy K, Reddy MVR, Cosenza SC, Nathan RB, Baker SJ, Papathi N, Jiang J, Holland J, Reddy EP (2005b) ON01910, a non-ATP-competitive small molecule inhibitor of Plk1, is a potent anticancer agent. Cancer Cell 7:275–286

Hamdane M, David-Cordonnier MH, D'Halluin JC (1997) Activation of p65 NF-kappaB protein by p210BCR-ABL in a myeloid cell line (P210BCR-ABL activates p65 NF-kappaB). Oncogene 15:2267–2275

Hannon GJ (2002) RNA interference. Nature 418:244–251

Harrington EA, Bebbington D, Moore J, Rasmussen RK, Ajose-Adeogun AO, Nakayama T, Graham JA, Demur C, Hercend T, Diu-Hercend A, Su M, Golec JM, Miller KM (2004) VX-680, a potent and selective small-molecule inhibitor of the Aurora kinases, suppresses tumor growth in vivo. Nat Med 10:262–267

He Y, Wertheim JA, Xu L, Miller JP, Karnell FG, Choi JK, Ren R, Pear WS (2002) The coiled-coil domain and Tyr177 of bcr are required to induce a murine chronic myelogenous leukemia-like disease by bcr/abl. Blood 99:2957–2968

Hoover RR, Mahon F.-X, Melo JV, Daley GQ (2002) Overcoming STI571 resistance with the farnesyl transferase inhibitor SCH66336. Blood 100:1068–1071

Hughes TP, Kaeda J, Branford S, Rudzki Z, Hochhaus A, Hensley ML, Gathmann I, Bolton AE, van Hoomissen IC, Goldman JM, Radich JP (2003) Frequency of major molecular responses to imatinib or interferon alfa plus cytarabine in newly diagnosed chronic myeloid leukemia. N Engl J Med 349:1423–1432

Issa JP, Kantarjian H, Mohan A, O'Brien S, Cortes J, Pierce S, Talpaz M (1999) Methylation of the ABL1 promoter in chronic myelogenous leukemia: lack of prognostic significance. Blood 93:2075–2080

Issa J-PJ, Garcia-Manero G, Giles FJ, Mannari R, Thomas D, Faderl S, Bayar E, Lyons J, Rosenfeld CS, Cortes J, Kantarjian HM (2004) Phase 1 study of low-dose prolonged exposure schedules of the hypomethylating agent 5-aza-2′-deoxycytidine (decitabine) in hematopoietic malignancies. Blood 103:1635–1640

Issa JP, Gharibyan V, Cortes J, Jelinek J, Morris G, Verstovsek S, Talpaz M, Garcia-Manero G, Kantarjian HM (2005) Phase II study of low-dose decitabine in patients with chronic myelogenous leukemia resistant to imatinib mesylate. J Clin Oncol, 23:3948–3956

Jones PA, Laird PW (1999) Cancer epigenetics comes of age. Nat Genet, 21:163–167

Jorgensen HG, Allan EK, Graham SM, Godden JL, Richmond L, Elliott MA, Mountford JC, Eaves CJ, Holyoake TL (2005) Lonafarnib reduces the resistance of primitive quiescent CML cells to imatinib mesylate in vitro. Leukemia 19:1184–1191

Kang CD, Yoo SD, Hwang BW, Kim KW, Kim DW, Kim CM, Kim SH, Chung BS (2000) The inhibition of ERK/MAPK not the activation of JNK/SAPK is primarily required to induce apoptosis in chronic myelogenous leukemic K562 cells. Leuk Res, 24:527–534

Kano Y, Akutsu M, Tsunoda S, Mano H, Sato Y, Honma Y, Furukawa Y (2001) In vitro cytotoxic effects of a tyrosine kinase inhibitor STI571 in combination with commonly used antileukemic agents. Blood 97:1999–2007

Kantarjian H, Sawyers C, Hochhaus A, Guilhot F, Schiffer C, Gambacorti-Passerini C, Niederwieser D, Resta D, Capdeville R, Zoellner U, Talpaz M, Druker B (2002) Hematologic and cytogenetic responses to imatinib mesylate in chronic myelogenous leukemia. N Engl J Med 346:645–652

Kantarjian HM, Talpaz M, Smith TL, Cortes J, Giles FJ, Rios MB, Mallard S, Gajewski J, Murgo A, Cheson B, O'Brien S (2000) Homoharringtonine and low-dose cytarabine in the management of late chronic-phase chronic myelogenous leukemia. J Clin Oncol 18:3513–3521

Kantarjian HM, O'Brien S, Cortes J, Giles FJ, Faderl S, Issa JP, Garcia-Manero G, Rios MB, Shan J, Andreeff M, Keating M, Talpaz M (2003 a) Results of decitabine (5-aza-2′deoxycytidine) therapy in 130 patients with chronic myelogenous leukemia. Cancer 98:522–528

Kantarjian HM, O'Brien S, Cortes JE, Shan J, Giles FJ, Rios MB, Faderl SH, Wierda WG, Ferrajoli A, Verstovsek S, Keating MJ, Freireich EJ, Talpaz M (2003 b) Complete cytogenetic and molecular responses to interferon-alpha-based therapy for chronic myelogenous leukemia are associated with excellent long-term prognosis. Cancer 97:1033–1041

Karp JE, Lancet JE, Kaufmann SH, End DW, Wright JJ, Bol K, Horak I, Tidwell ML, Liesveld J, Kottke TJ, Ange D, Buddharaju L, Gojo I, Highsmith WE, Belly RT, Hohl RJ, Rybak ME, Thibault A, Rosenblatt J (2001) Clinical and biologic activity of the farnesyltransferase inhibitor R115777 in adults with refractory and relapsed acute leukemias: a phase 1 clinical-laboratory correlative trial. Blood 97:3361–3369

Katsoulas A, Rachid Z, Brahimi F, McNamee J, Jean-Claude BJ (2005) Engineering 3-alkyltriazenes to block bcr-abl kinase: a novel strategy for the therapy of advanced bcr-abl expressing leukemias. Leuk Res 29:693–700

Keen N, Taylor S (2004) Aurora-kinase inhibitors as anticancer agents. Nat Rev Cancer 4:927–936

Kimura S, Kuroda J, Segawa H, Sato K, Nogawa M, Yuasa T, Ottmann OG, Maekawa T (2004) Antiproliferative efficacy of the third-generation bisphosphonate, zoledronic acid, combined with other anticancer drugs in leukemic cell lines. Int J Hematol 79:37–43

Klejman A, Rushen L, Morrione A, Slupianek A, Skorski T (2002) Phosphatidylinositol-3 kinase inhibitors enhance the anti-leukemia effect of STI571. Oncogene 21:5868–5876

Korus M, Mahon GM, Cheng L, Whitehead IP (2002) p38 MAPK-mediated activation of NF-kappaB by the RhoGEF domain of Bcr. Oncogene 21:4601–4612

Kuliczkowski K (1989) Influence of harringtonine on human leukemia cell differentiation. Arch Immunol Ther Exp (Warsz), 37:69–76

Kuroda J, Kimura S, Segawa H, Kobayashi Y, Yoshikawa T, Urasaki Y, Ueda T, Enjo F, Tokuda H, Ottmann OG, Maekawa T (2003) The third-generation bisphosphonate zoledronate synergistically augments the anti-Ph+ leukemia activity of imatinib mesylate. Blood 102:2229–2235

La Rosee P, Johnson K, Corbin AS, Stoffregen EP, Moseson EM, Willis S, Mauro MM, Melo JV, Deininger MW, Druker BJ (2004) In vitro efficacy of combined treatment depends on the underlying mechanism of resistance in imatinib-resistant Bcr-Abl-positive cell lines. Blood 103:208–215

Laird PW, Jackson-Grusby L, Fazeli A, Dickinson SL, Jung WE, Li E, Weinberg RA, Jaenisch R (1995) Suppression of intestinal neoplasia by DNA hypomethylation. Cell 81:197–205

Li JM, Wang AH, Sun HP, Shen Y, Zhao RH, Gu BW, Chen B, Xing W, Shen ZX, Wang ZY, Chen SJ, Chen Z (2004) Phase I clinical trial of Glivec in combination with tetra-arsenic tetra-sulfide in the treatment of CML patients in advanced phase. Blood 104:247 b (abstract no 4653)

Li Z, Qiao Y, Liu B, Laska EJ, Chakravarthi P, Kulko JM, Bona RD, Fang M, Hegde U, Moyo V, Tannenbaum SH, Menoret A, Gaffney J, Glynn L, Runowicz CD, Srivastava PK (2005) Combination of imatinib mesylate with autologous leukocyte-derived heat shock protein and chronic myelogenous leukemia. Clin Cancer Res, 11:4460–4468

Marin D, Kaeda JS, Andreasson C, Saunders SM, Bua M, Olavarria E, Goldman JM, Apperley JF (2005) Phase I/II trial of adding semisynthetic homoharringtonine in chronic myeloid leukemia patients who have achieved partial or complete cytogenetic response on imatinib. Cancer 103:1850–1855

Mayerhofer M, Aichberger KJ, Florian S, Krauth MT, Derdak S, Esterbauer H, Wagner O, Pickl WF, Selzer E, Deininger M, Druker BJ, Greish K, Maeda H, Sillaber C, Valent P (2004) The heme oxygenase-1-targeting compound PEG-ZnPP inhibits growth of imatinib-resistant BCR/ABL-transformed cells. Blood 104:548 a (abstract no 1986)

Mayerhofer M, Aichberger KJ, Florian S, Krauth MT, Hauswirth AW, Derdak S, Sperr WR, Esterbauer H, Wagner O, Marosi C, Pickl WF, Deininger M, Weisberg E, Druker BJ, Griffin JD, Sillaber C, Valent P (2005) Identification of mTOR as a novel bifunctional target in chronic myeloid leukemia: dissection of growth-inhibitory and VEGF-suppressive effects of rapamycin in leukemic cells. FASEB J, 19:960–962

McWhirter JR, Wang JY (1993) An actin-binding function contributes to transformation by the Bcr-Abl oncoprotein of Philadelphia chromosome-positive human leukemias. EMBO J 12:1533–1546

Million RP, Van Etten RA (2000) The Grb2 binding site is required for the induction of chronic myeloid leukemia-like disease in mice by the Bcr/Abl tyrosine kinase. Blood 96:664–670

Mohi MG, Boulton C, Gu T.-L, Sternberg DW, Neuberg D, Griffin JD, Gilliland DG, Neel BG (2004) Combination of rapamycin and protein tyrosine kinase (PTK) inhibitors for the treatment of leukemias caused by oncogenic PTKs. PNAS 101:3130–3135

Molldrem JJ, Clave E, Jiang YZ, Mavroudis D, Raptis A, Hensel N, Agarwala V, Barrett AJ (1997) Cytotoxic T lymphocytes specific for a nonpolymorphic proteinase 3 peptide preferentially inhibit chronic myeloid leukemia colony-forming units. Blood 90:2529–2534

Molldrem JJ, Lee PP, Wang C, Felio K, Kantarjian HM, Champlin RE, Davis MM (2000) Evidence that specific T lymphocytes may participate in the elimination of chronic myelogenous leukemia. Nat Med 6:1018–1023

Molldrem JJ, Lee PP, Kant S, Wieder E, Jiang W, Lu S, Wang C, Davis MM (2003) Chronic myelogenous leukemia shapes host immunity by selective deletion of high-avidity leukemia-specific T cells. J Clin Invest 111:639–647

Nakajima A, Tauchi T, Sumi M, Bishop WR, Ohyashiki K (2003) Efficacy of SCH66336, a farnesyl transferase inhibitor, in conjunction with imatinib against BCR-ABL-positive cells. Mol Cancer Ther 2:219–224

Nguyen TT, Mohrbacher AF, Tsai YC, Groffen J, Heisterkamp N, Nichols PW, Yu MC, Lubbert M, Jones PA (2000) Quantitative measure of c-abl and p15 methylation in chronic myelogenous leukemia: biological implications. Blood 95:2990–2992

Nimmanapalli R, O'Bryan E, Bhalla K (2001) Geldanamycin and its analogue 17-allylamino-17-demethoxygeldanamycin lowers Bcr-Abl levels and induces apoptosis and differentiation of Bcr-Abl-positive human leukemic blasts. Cancer Res 61:1799–1804

Nimmanapalli R, Fuino L, Bali P, Gasparetto M, Glozak M, Tao J, Moscinski L, Smith C, Wu J, Jove R, Atadja P, Bhalla K (2003a) Histone deacetylase inhibitor LAQ824 both lowers expression and promotes proteasomal degradation of Bcr-Abl and induces apoptosis of imatinib mesylate-sensitive or -refractory chronic myelogenous leukemia-blast crisis cells. Cancer Res 63:5126–5135

Nimmanapalli R, Fuino L, Stobaugh C, Richon V, Bhalla K (2003b) Cotreatment with the histone deacetylase inhibitor suberoylanilide hydroxamic acid (SAHA) enhances imatinib-induced apoptosis of Bcr-Abl-positive human acute leukemia cells. Blood 101:3236–3239

O'Brien S, Kantarjian H, Keating M, Beran M, Koller C, Robertson LE, Hester J, Rios MB, Andreeff M, Talpaz M (1995) Homoharringtonine therapy induces responses in patients with chronic myelogenous leukemia in late chronic phase. Blood 86:3322–3326

O'Brien S, Talpaz M, Cortes J, Shan J, Giles FJ, Faderl S, Thomas D, Garcia-Manero G, Mallard S, Beth M, Koller C, Kornblau S, Andreeff M, Murgo A, Keating M, Kantarjian HM (2002) Simultaneous homoharringtonine and interferon-alpha in the treatment of patients with chronic-phase chronic myelogenous leukemia. Cancer, 94:2024–2032

O'Brien S, Giles F, Talpaz M, Cortes J, Rios MB, Shan J, Thomas D, Andreeff M, Kornblau S, Faderl S, Garcia-Manero G, White K, Mallard S, Freireich E, Kantarjian HM (2003a) Results of triple therapy with interferon-alpha, cytarabine, and homoharringtonine, and the impact of adding imatinib to the treatment sequence in patients with Philadelphia chromosome-positive chronic myelogenous leukemia in early chronic phase. Cancer, 98:888–893

O'Brien SG, Guilhot F, Larson RA, Gathmann I, Baccarani M, Cervantes F, Cornelissen JJ, Fischer T, Hochhaus A, Hughes T, Lechner K, Nielsen JL, Rousselot P, Reiffers J, Saglio G, Shepherd J, Simonsson B, Gratwohl A, Goldman JM, Kantarjian H, Taylor K, Verhoef G, Bolton AE, Capdeville R, Druker BJ (2003b) Imatinib compared with interferon and low-dose cytarabine for newly diagnosed chronic-phase chronic myeloid leukemia. N Engl J Med, 348:994–1004

Osman Y, Takahashi M, Zheng Z, Koike T, Toba K, Liu A, Furukawa T, Aoki S, Aizawa Y (1999a) Generation of bcr-abl specific cytotoxic T-lymphocytes by using dendritic cells pulsed with bcr-abl (b3a2) peptide: its applicability for donor leukocyte transfusions in marrow grafted CML patients. Leukemia, 13:166–174

Osman Y, Takahashi M, Zheng Z, Toba K, Liu A, Furukawa T, Aizawa Y, Shibata A, Koike T (1999b) Activation of autologous or HLA-identical sibling cytotoxic T lymphocytes by blood derived dendritic cells pulsed with tumor cell extracts. Oncol Rep 6:1057–1063

Ossenkoppele GJ, Stam AG, Westers TM, de Gruijl TD, Janssen JJ, van de Loosdrecht AA, Scheper RJ (2003) Vaccination of chronic myeloid leukemia patients with autologous in vitro cultured leukemic dendritic cells. Leukemia, 17:1424–1426

Pawelec G, Max H, Halder T, Bruserud O, Merl A, da Silva P, Kalbacher H (1996) BCR/ABL leukemia oncogene fusion peptides selectively bind to certain HLA-DR alleles and can be recognized by T cells found at low frequency in the repertoire of normal donors. Blood 88:2118–2124

Perkins C, Kim CN, Fang G, Bhalla KN (2000) Arsenic induces apoptosis of multidrug-resistant human myeloid leukemia cells that express Bcr-Abl or overexpress MDR, MRP, Bcl-2, or Bcl-x(L). Blood 95:1014–1022

Peters DG, Hoover RR, Gerlach MJ, Koh EY, Zhang H, Choe K, Kirschmeier P, Bishop WR, Daley GQ (2001) Activity of the farnesyl protein transferase inhibitor SCH66336 against BCR/ABL-induced murine leukemia and primary cells from patients with chronic myeloid leukemia. Blood 97:1404–1412

Pinilla-Ibarz J, Cathcart K, Korontsvit T, Soignet S, Bocchia M, Caggiano J, Lai L, Jimenez J, Kolitz J, Scheinberg DA (2000) Vaccination of patients with chronic myelogenous leukemia with bcr-abl oncogene breakpoint fusion peptides generates specific immune responses. Blood 95:1781–1787

Plasilova M, Zivny J, Jelinek J, Neuwirtova R, Cermak J, Necas E, Andera L, Stopka T (2002) TRAIL (Apo2L) suppresses growth of primary human leukemia and myelodysplasia progenitors. Leukemia, 16:67–73

Pockley AG (2003) Heat shock proteins as regulators of the immune response. Lancet, 362:469–476

Puccetti E, Guller S, Orleth A, Bruggenolte N, Hoelzer D, Ottmann OG, Ruthardt M (2000) BCR-ABL mediates arsenic trioxide-induced apoptosis independently of its aberrant kinase activity. Cancer Res, 60:3409–3413

Qazilbash MH, Wieder E, Rios R, Lu S, Kant S, Giralt S, Estey E, Thall PF, de Lima M, Couriel D, Champlin R, Komanduri K, Molldrem J (2004)

Vaccination with the PR1 leukemia-associated antigen can induce complete remission in patients with myeloid leukemia. Blood 104:77a (abstract no 259)

Quintas-Cardama A, Cortes J, Verstovsek S, Laddie N, Estrov Z, Kantarjian H (2005) Subcutaneous (SC) Homoharringtonine (HHT) for patients (Pts) with chronic myelogenous leukemia (CML) in chronic phase (CP) after imatinib mesylate failure. Blood 106:290b (abstract no 4839)

Rahmani M, Reese E, Dai Y, Bauer C, Kramer LB, Huang M, Jove R, Dent P, Grant S, George P, Bali P, Annavarapu S, Scuto A, Fiskus W, Guo F, Sigua C, Sondarva G, Moscinski L, Atadja P, Bhalla K (2005) Cotreatment with suberanoylanilide hydroxamic acid and 17-allylamino 17-demethoxygeldanamycin synergistically induces apoptosis in Bcr-Abl+ Cells sensitive and resistant to STI571 (imatinib mesylate) in association with down-regulation of Bcr-Abl, abrogation of signal transducer and activator of transcription 5 activity, and Bax conformational change combination of the histone deacetylase inhibitor LBH589 and the hsp90 inhibitor 17-AAG is highly active against human CML-BC cells and AML cells with activating mutation of FLT-3. Mol Pharmacol, 67:1166–1176

Ravandi-Kashani F, Ridgeway J, Nishimura S, Agarwal M, Feldman L, Salvado A, Kovak MR, Hoffman R (2003) Pilot study of combination of iamtinib mesylate and Trisenox (As2O3) in patients with accelerated and blast phase CML. Blood 102:314b (abstract no 4977)

Reichert A, Heisterkamp N, Daley GQ, Groffen J (2001) Treatment of Bcr/Abl-positive acute lymphoblastic leukemia in P190 transgenic mice with the farnesyl transferase inhibitor SCH66336. Blood 97:1399–1403

Reuther JY, Reuther GW, Cortez D, Pendergast AM, Baldwin AS Jr (1998) A requirement for NF-kappaB activation in Bcr-Abl-mediated transformation. Genes Dev, 12:968–981

Roman-Gomez J, Castillejo JA, Jimenez A, Cervantes F, Boque C, Hermosin L, Leon A, Granena A, Colomer D, Heiniger A, Torres A (2003) Cadherin-13, a mediator of calcium-dependent cell-cell adhesion, is silenced by methylation in chronic myeloid leukemia and correlates with pretreatment risk profile and cytogenetic response to interferon alfa. J Clin Oncol, 21:1472–1479

Rothwarf DM, Karin M (1999) The NF-kappa B activation pathway: a paradigm in information transfer from membrane to nucleus. Sci STKE, 1999, RE1

Santini V, Kantarjian HM, Issa JP (2001) Changes in DNA methylation in neoplasia: pathophysiology and therapeutic implications. Ann Intern Med, 134:573–586

Sattler M, Mohi MG, Pride YB, Quinnan LR, Malouf NA, Podar K, Gesbert F, Iwasaki H, Li S, Van Etten RA (2002) Critical role for Gab2 in transformation by BCR/ABL. Cancer Cell, 1:479–492

Sawyers CL (1999) Chronic myeloid leukemia. N Engl J Med, 340:1330–1340

Sawyers CL, Hochhaus A, Feldman E, Goldman JM, Miller CB, Ottmann OG, Schiffer CA, Talpaz M, Guilhot F, Deininger MWN, Fischer T, O'Brien SG, Stone RM, Gambacorti-Passerini CB, Russell NH, Reiffers JJ, Shea TC, Chapuis B, Coutre S, Tura S, Morra E, Larson RA, Saven A, Peschel C, Gratwohl A, Mandelli F, Ben-Am M, Gathmann I, Capdeville R, Paquette RL, Druker BJ (2002) Imatinib induces hematologic and cytogenetic responses in patients with chronic myelogenous leukemia in myeloid blast crisis: results of a phase II study. Blood 99:3530–3539

Scappini B, Onida F, Kantarjian HM, Dong L, Verstovsek S, Keating MJ, Beran M (2002) In vitro effects of STI 571-containing drug combinations on the growth of Philadelphia-positive chronic myelogenous leukemia cells. Cancer 94:2653–2662

Scherr M, Battmer K, Winkler T, Heidenreich O, Ganser A, Eder M (2003) Specific inhibition of bcr-abl gene expression by small interfering RNA. Blood 101:1566–1569

Segawa H, Kimura S, Kuroda J, Sato K, Yokota A, Kawata E, Kamitsuji Y, Ashihara E, Yuasa T, Fujiyama Y, Ottmann OG, Maekawa T (2005) Zoledronate synergises with imatinib mesylate to inhibit Ph primary leukaemic cell growth. Br J Haematol 130:558–560

Sekulic A, Hudson CC, Homme JL, Yin P, Otterness DM, Karnitz LM, Abraham RT (2000) A direct linkage between the phosphoinositide 3-kinase-AKT signaling pathway and the mammalian target of rapamycin in mitogen-stimulated and transformed cells. Cancer Res 60:3504–3513

Senderowicz AM, Headlee D, Stinson SF, Lush RM, Kalil N, Villalba L, Hill K, Steinberg SM, Figg WD, Tompkins A, Arbuck SG, Sausville EA (1998) Phase I trial of continuous infusion flavopiridol, a novel cyclin-dependent kinase inhibitor, in patients with refractory neoplasms. J Clin Oncol 16:2986–2999

Silverman LR, Demakos EP, Peterson BL, Kornblith AB, Holland JC, Odchimar-Reissig R, Stone RM, Nelson D, Powell BL, DeCastro CM, Ellerton J, Larson RA, Schiffer CA, Holland JF (2002) Randomized controlled trial of azacitidine in patients with the myelodysplastic syndrome: a study of the cancer and leukemia group B. J Clin Oncol 20:2429–2440

Skorski T, Kanakaraj P, Nieborowska-Skorska M, Ratajczak MZ, Wen SC, Zon G, Gewirtz AM, Perussia B, Calabretta B (1995) Phosphatidylinositol-3 kinase activity is regulated by BCR/ABL and is required for the growth of Philadelphia chromosome-positive cells. Blood 86:726–736

Smith BD, Kasamon YL, Miller CB, Chia C, Murphy K, Kowalski J, Tartakovsky I, Biedrzycki B, Jones RJ, Hege K, Levitsky HI (2005) K562/GM-CSF Vaccination reduces tumor burden, including achieving molecular remissions, in chronic myeloid leukemia (CML) patients with residual disease on imatinib mesylate (IM). Blood 106:801a (abstract no 2858)

Smith DF, Whitesell L, Katsanis E (1998) Molecular chaperones: biology and prospects for pharmacological intervention. Pharmacol Rev 50:493–514

Stancato LF, Silverstein AM, Owens-Grillo JK, Chow YH, Jove R, Pratt WB (1997) The hsp90-binding antibiotic geldanamycin decreases Raf levels and epidermal growth factor signaling without disrupting formation of signaling complexes or reducing the specific enzymatic activity of Raf kinase. J Biol Chem 272:4013–4020

Suto R, Srivastava PK (1995) A mechanism for the specific immunogenicity of heat shock protein-chaperoned peptides. Science 269:1585–1588

Takahashi T, Tanaka Y, Nieda M, Azuma T, Chiba S, Juji T, Shibata Y, Hirai H (2003) Dendritic cell vaccination for patients with chronic myelogenous leukemia. Leuk Res 27:795–802

Talpaz M, Silver RT, Druker BJ, Goldman JM, Gambacorti-Passerini C, Guilhot F, Schiffer CA, Fischer T, Deininger MWN, Lennard AL, Hochhaus A, Ottmann OG, Gratwohl A, Baccarani M, Stone R, Tura S, Mahon F-X, Fernandes-Reese S, Gathmann I, Capdeville R, Kantarjian HM, Sawyers CL (2002) Imatinib induces durable hematologic and cytogenetic responses in patients with accelerated phase chronic myeloid leukemia: results of a phase 2 study. Blood 99:1928–1937

Thiagalingam S, Cheng KH, Lee HJ, Mineva N, Thiagalingam A, Ponte JF (2003) Histone deacetylases: unique players in shaping the epigenetic histone code. Ann NY Acad Sci 983:84–100

Timmermann S, Lehrmann H, Polesskaya A, Harel-Bellan A (2001) Histone acetylation and disease. Cell Mol Life Sci 58:728–736

Tipping AJ, Mahon FX, Zafirides G, Lagarde V, Goldman JM, Melo JV (2002) Drug responses of imatinib mesylate-resistant cells: synergism of imatinib with other chemotherapeutic drugs. Leukemia 16:2349–2357

Udono H, Srivastava PK (1993) Heat shock protein 70-associated peptides elicit specific cancer immunity. J Exp Med 178:1391–1396

Udono H, Levey DL, Srivastava PK (1994) Cellular requirements for tumor-specific immunity elicited by heat shock proteins: tumor rejection antigen gp96 primes CD8+ T cells in vivo. Proc Natl Acad Sci USA 91:3077–3081

Uno K, Inukai T, Kayagaki N, Goi K, Sato H, Nemoto A, Takahashi K, Kagami K, Yamaguchi N, Yagita H, Okumura K, Koyama-Okazaki T, Suzuki T, Sugita K, Nakazawa S (2003) TNF-related apoptosis-inducing ligand (TRAIL) frequently induces apoptosis in Philadelphia chromosome-positive leukemia cells. Blood 101:3658–3667

Verstovsek S, Kantarjian H, Manshouri T, Cortes J, Giles FJ, Rogers A, Albitar M (2002) Prognostic significance of cellular vascular endothelial growth factor expression in chronic phase chronic myeloid leukemia. Blood 99:2265–2267

Vigneri P, Wang JY (2001) Induction of apoptosis in chronic myelogenous leukemia cells through nuclear entrapment of BCR-ABL tyrosine kinase. Nat Med 7:228–234

Visani G, Russo D, Ottaviani E, Tosi P, Damiani D, Michelutti A, Manfroi S, Baccarani M, Tura S (1997) Effects of homoharringtonine alone and in combination with alpha interferon and cytosine arabinoside on "in vitro" growth and induction of apoptosis in chronic myeloid leukemia and normal hematopoietic progenitors. Leukemia 11:624–628

Vojtek AB, Der CJ (1998) Increasing complexity of the Ras signaling pathway. J Biol Chem 273:19925–19928

Wijermans P, Lubbert M, Verhoef G, Bosly A, Ravoet C, Andre M, Ferrant A (2000) Low-dose 5-aza-2′-deoxycytidine, a DNA hypomethylating agent, for the treatment of high-risk myelodysplastic syndrome: a multicenter phase II study in elderly patients. J Clin Oncol 18:956–962

Wiley SR, Schooley K, Smolak PJ, Din WS, Huang CP, Nicholl JK, Sutherland GR, Smith TD, Rauch C, Smith CA et al (1995) Identification and characterization of a new member of the TNF family that induces apoptosis. Immunity 3:673–682

Wohlbold L, van der Kuip H, Miething C, Vornlocher HP, Knabbe C, Duyster J, Aulitzky WE (2003) Inhibition of bcr-abl gene expression by small interfering RNA sensitizes for imatinib mesylate (STI571). Blood 102:2236–2239

Xia Z, Dickens M, Raingeaud J, Davis RJ, Greenberg ME (1995) Opposing effects of ERK and JNK-p38 MAP kinases on apoptosis. Science 270:1326–1331

Yinjun L, Jie J, Weilai X, Xiangming T (2004) Homoharringtonine mediates myeloid cell apoptosis via upregulation of pro-apoptotic bax and inducing caspase-3-mediated cleavage of poly(ADP-ribose) polymerase (PARP). Am J Hematol 76:199–204

Yotnda P, Firat H, Garcia-Pons F, Garcia Z, Gourru G, Vernant JP, Lemonnier FA, Leblond V, Langlade-Demoyen P (1998) Cytotoxic T cell response against the chimeric p210 BCR-ABL protein in patients with chronic myelogenous leukemia. J Clin Invest 101:2290–2296

Yu C, Krystal G, Dent P, Grant S (2002 a) Flavopiridol potentiates STI571-induced mitochondrial damage and apoptosis in BCR-ABL-positive human leukemia cells. Clin Cancer Res 8:2976–2984

Yu C, Krystal G, Varticovksi L, McKinstry R, Rahmani M, Dent P, Grant S (2002 b) Pharmacologic mitogen-activated protein/extracellular signal-regulated kinase kinase/mitogen-activated protein kinase inhibitors interact synergistically with STI571 to induce apoptosis in Bcr/Abl-expressing human leukemia cells. Cancer Res 62:188–199

Yu C, Rahmani M, Almenara J, Subler M, Krystal G, Conrad D, Varticovski L, Dent P, Grant S (2003) Histone deacetylase inhibitors promote STI571-mediated apoptosis in STI571-sensitive and -resistant Bcr/Abl+ human myeloid leukemia cells. Cancer Res 63:2118–2126

Zamore PD (2002) Ancient pathways programmed by small RNAs. Science 296:1265–1269

Zion M, Ben-Yehuda D, Avraham A, Cohen O, Wetzler M, Melloul D, Ben-Neriah Y (1994) Progressive de novo DNA methylation at the bcr-abl locus in the course of chronic myelogenous leukemia. Proc Natl Acad Sci USA 91:10722–10726.

Immune Therapy of Chronic Myelogenous Leukemia

Axel Hoos and Robert Peter Gale

Contents

Abstract. Chronic myelogenous leukemia (CML) is a prototype for immune therapy of cancer in humans. CML cells express one or more cancer-specific antigens: peptide sequences spanning the BCR-ABL-related gene product. Substantial data in humans receiving blood cell and bone marrow transplants indicate a strong immune-mediated anti-leukemia effect. Because this effect occurs in an allogeneic setting it is uncertain whether this anti-leukemia effect will operate in other clinical settings. Additional data supporting a role for immune therapy of CML come from clinical trials of interferon and donor lymphocyte infusions. Here, we critically review data in two major areas of vaccine development: (1) peptides like BCR-ABL, Pr-3, and WT-1; and (2) autologous vaccines like dendritic cells and heat shock protein-peptide complexes. We also consider other related approaches. The data we review indicate encouraging results from preliminary uncontrolled clinical trials with some of these approaches. However, a definitive conclusion awaits results of randomized studies.

11.1 Introduction

The immune system is a powerful defense mechanism against disease. Harnessing the immune system to fight disease can be very effective. Best results are seen in the context of prevention of infections: vaccination with attenuated, killed, or altered viruses; recombinant proteins, or viral toxins has dramatically eliminated or improved diseases like smallpox, measles, polio, and hepatitis. The therapeutic use of the immune system is less successful. This is particularly true in cancer, where several decades of intense study have, so far, yielded little benefit from immune therapy.

Some, but not all of the reasons for this disparity are known. Infections are characterized by "foreign" antigens easily recognized by the immune system. In contrast, cancer-related antigens typically arise from "self" and are therefore more likely to be difficult for the immune system to target. Although most cancer cells are likely detected and destroyed by immune cells, others escape immune surveillance and present a difficult therapy challenge. The considerable heterogeneity of most cancers, and our incomplete understanding of immunity combine to hamper development of effective anti-cancer immune therapies.

Despite these caveats there are some examples in humans that immune therapy can be effective against established cancers including: (1) cytokines, like interferon-α in chronic myelogenous leukemia (CML) and melanoma and interleukin-2 in kidney cancer and melanoma; and (2) allogeneic blood cell or bone marrow transplantation in diverse leukemias. Here, transplanting the donor's immune system can eliminate or control the recipient's cancer being "foreign" to this new immune system. Unfortunately, these therapies have substantial toxicities and do not exploit the potential advantage of targeted immune therapy.

There is continuously expanding knowledge about molecular mechanisms of carcinogenesis and the complexity of the immune system. Because of this several new immune therapies have recently emerged. These approaches promise efficacy without substantial toxicity. Examples are summarized elsewhere (Ribas et al. 2003).

CML is the premier model of immune therapy of cancer in humans. Several forms of immune therapy work in this disease and we understand substantially more about the molecular biology and pathophysiology of CML than most other cancers. Here, we review the mechanisms by which modern immune therapies might benefit persons with CML, summarize data about current immune therapies, and suggest future directions.

11.2 Chronic Myelogenous Leukemia – A Model Disease for Immune Therapy

CML is one of the best-understood cancers in humans. It is caused by the BCR-ABL fusion gene product ($P210^{BCR\text{-}ABL}$), a tyrosine kinase present in all affected patients with CML but not in normal persons or most patients with other blood or bone marrow cancers (Goldman and Melo 2003). The BCR-ABL fusion gene is represented on a chromosomal level by a t(9; 22)(q34; q11) translocation which gives origin to the Philadelphia chromosome (Ph-chromosome) and the BCR-ABL fusion gene. This canonical genetic marker permits sensitive molecular monitoring of minimal residual disease (MRD) using polymerase chain reaction (PCR)-techniques (Gabert et al. 2003; Hughes et al. 2003). The unique BCR-ABL gene product is also a potential target for immune therapy (Butturini and Gale 1995).

Persons with newly diagnosed CML typically receive imatinib mesylate (Gleevec), an inhibitor of the tyrosine kinase activity of $P210^{BCR\text{-}ABL}$. Imatinib effectively reduces numbers of leukemia cells in most persons with CML, creating a favorable clinical setting for specific immune therapy (Goldman and Melo 2003; Hughes et al. 2003; Kantarjian et al. 2004). This approach may be clinically important since recent data suggest imatinib does not completely eradicate CML cells and that resistance develops in a substantial proportion of people over time. Immune therapies of CML, like interferon-α, allogeneic blood and bone marrow transplants, and donor leukocyte infusions (DLI), described below, are useful therapies for CML.

Allogeneic bone marrow transplants are the only proved cure for CML. Despite the 70% success rate of typical allotransplants, there remains substantial morbidity and mortality. Also, after allotransplants, there is a continuous 1–2% annual risk of CML-recurrence for intervals exceeding 10–15 years. Furthermore, persons in hematological remission after allotransplants may have Ph-chromosome-positive cells in their bone marrow for years without clinical relapse, suggesting immune control of disease (Butturini and Gale 1992). Despite this success many people with CML cannot receive an allotransplant because of older age, donor unavailability, and other considerations.

Taken together, this offers the possibility that the potential effects of a systemic immune response against imatinib-induced MRD, as exhibited by novel immune therapies, may offer additional benefits beyond imatinib leading to the cure of CML.

One can envision three types of "cure" of CML as characterized by Baccarani: (1) *Biological cure:* eradication of all CML cells; (2) *Clinical cure*: clinical control of CML without need for therapy despite remaining CML cells; (3) *Therapeutic cure*: clinical control of CML using maintenance therapy (Gale et al. 2005). Following therapy with imatinib, small numbers of residual CML cells may be required to achieve such biological or clinical cure through immune therapy.

Current investigations of immune therapies in CML focus on vaccines. Several types of vaccines are being studied and preliminary results suggest some effects on MRD but require further study. Specific results and their prospects for future investigations are discussed below.

11.3 Immune Mechanisms in CML

11.3.1 T-Cells

Most data from experimental models suggest immunity via cytotoxic T-cells is the most effective component of the immune system against cancer. This has led to many studies using T-cells in persons with cancer (Berinstein 2003; Ribas et al. 2003).

Data from studies of allogeneic bone marrow transplants in CML show that T-cell depletion of the graft decreases graft-versus-host disease (GvHD) but increases risk of leukemia relapse after transplantation. Donor lymphocyte infusions (DLI), given to persons with CML with relapse of leukemia post transplant induce remissions (Kolb et al. 2004). These data support the importance of T-cells as mediators of immune-mediated anti-leukemia effects in persons with CML.

T-cells recognize peptide antigens presented through the major histocompatibility complex (MHC) pathway. Antigen-presenting cells (APC) usually process peptides for presentation, load them onto MHC molecules in the endoplasmic reticulum, and present the MHC-peptide complex on the cell surface for T-cells to be recognized. There are two characterized types of MHC-peptide antigen connections: (1) Class I MHC molecules combine with 8–11 amino acid peptides derived from intracellular proteins. These complexes are recognized by $CD8^+$ cytotoxic T-cells. (2) Class II MHC molecules combine with 12–18 amino acid peptides derived from internalized extracellular proteins. These complexes are recognized by $CD4^+$ T-cells (Ribas et al. 2003). The MHC complex in humans is represented by the human leukocyte antigen (HLA) gene cluster encoded on chromosome 6. HLA-antigens can present peptides only to immune cells of the same HLA type, a phenomenon referred to as HLA- or MHC-restriction (Zinkernagel and Doherty 1997). This HLA-restriction is responsible for the effects of GvHD and, at least in part, graft-versus leukemia (GvL; see below) after HLA-haplotype mismatched allogeneic transplants (Butturini and Gale 1995).

T-cells recognize MHC-peptide complexes through T-cell receptors (TCR), which allow for specific recognition of a broad spectrum of antigens due to genetic rearrangement of their building blocks. TCR building blocks are α-, β-, γ-, or δ-chains, which themselves compose, depending on the chain, of V, D, or J segments. One α- and one β-chain or one γ- and one δ-chain form the heterodimer structure of a TCR. $\alpha{:}\beta$ heterodimers represent the vast majority of all TCRs, while only a small subset represents $\gamma{:}\delta$ heterodimers. Rearrangement of the segments of the α- or β-chains result in about 10^{18} unique receptor formations able to recognize distinct antigens (Janeway 2005). In order to avoid reactivity of TCRs against self-antigens of the host, selection of TCRs during the T-cell maturation process eliminates clones with high affinity to such self-antigens. The resulting repertoire of T-cell receptors allows for recruitment of an overall T-cell population equipped with high specificity to recognize a wide spectrum of foreign antigens and a minimized risk to target self-antigens (Janeway 2005).

The effectiveness of specific T-cells against a target disease depends largely on the presence of relevant antigens, their processing and presentation but also on regulatory mechanisms of the immune system occurring after T-cell activation (Caligiuri et al. 2004). Cancer antigens fall into two key groups: (1) cancer-specific antigens, and (2) cancer-associated antigens. The former are unique antigens present only in cancer cells and can either represent a cancer-specific molecular abnormality or a foreign molecule, such as a viral protein. Examples are chromosomal translocations directly involved in carcinogenesis (Goldman and Melo 2003) or human papillomavirus (HPV) proteins involved in cell transformation in cervical cancer cells (zur Hausen 2002). The latter are antigens associated with the cancer through, for example, overexpression compared to normal tissues. Examples are differentiation antigens like gp100 or trp-2 in melanoma or proteasome-related antigens such as Pr-3 in myeloid leukemias (Molldrem et al. 2000; Ribas et al. 2003).

It has been difficult to identify target antigens for most cancers in humans. The best-studied cancer is malignant melanoma where several antigens were identified and used for immune therapy, mostly with peptide vaccines. Lessons learned from these studies may apply to other cancers. Unfortunately, for most cancers, our knowledge about such antigens is very limited.

For CML, several relevant antigens were identified and characterized. Examples are $P210^{BCR\text{-}ABL}$ and Wilms tumor protein 1 (WT-1). While $P210^{BCR\text{-}ABL}$ is a unique, tumor-specific antigen, WT-1 is a transcription factor overexpressed in myelogenous leukemias and is characterized as a cancer-associated rather than cancer-specific antigen. Several studies show humans can develop a T-cell response to these antigens (Pinilla-Ibarz et al. 2000; Rosenfeld et al. 2003). Details are discussed in the following sections, where immune therapy approaches using the respective antigens as targets for immune therapy are reviewed.

Frequently used tools to detect T-cell recognition of cancer-specific antigens in vitro are ELISPOT and tetramer assays. The γ-IFN release ELISPOT assay is used to quantify the specific anticancer response induced by $CD8^+$ T-cells on the single cell level. It is based on the secretion of γ-IFN by antigen-specific cytotoxic T-cells after contact with the cancer-specific antigen or cancer cell. $CD8^+$ T-cells, typically from blood samples, are immobilized on a membrane impregnated with γ-IFN-specific antibodies. Recognition of target antigen through T-cells leads to γ-IFN secretion, binding to γ-IFN-specific antibodies, and subsequent visualization through a fluorochrome reaction. Because T-cells are distributed on the membrane such that each can create a single color spot after antigen-recognition, the read-out is the ratio of spot-inducing cells to total immobilized cells before and after immune therapy (Hobeika et al. 2005; Keilholz et al. 2002).

The tetramer assay is based on the observation that antigen-specific TCRs reversibly bind tetramer molecules composed of MHC-peptide complexes. Specifically, peptide-antigen, MHC heavy chain, and β_2-microglobulin are folded together in vitro and bound to streptavidin. Linking a fluorochrome to streptavidin results in flow-cytometry detection of T-cells bound to tetramers after antigen recognition (Hobeika et al. 2005; Keilholz et al. 2002).

Both assays are frequently used to characterize T-cell reactivity to cancer-specific targets. However, because of their relative complexity there is substantial interassay variance and comparing results between laboratories is often challenging due to lack of assay standardization. Immune responses in clinical trials determined with these assays provide some insight into potential therapy-induced immune reactivity but exclude other aspects of anticancer immunity. Most important, none of these assays is validated in large clinical trials.

11.3.2 Natural Killer-Cells

Natural killer (NK) cells are part of the innate immune system and, compared to T-cells, do not rearrange their receptors to adapt to the constantly changing antigenic challenge. Instead, NK-receptors recognize conserved molecular structures usually specific to pathogens, which they identify as "foreign." A second group of receptors expressed on NK-cells are inhibitory KIR (Killer cell Ig-like Receptor) receptors which recognize determinants of HLA-haplotypes and suppress NK-cell reactivity to "self" (Colonna et al. 1997; Dohring et al. 1996; Wagtmann et al. 1995). Reduced cell surface expression of HLA-molecules results in increased susceptibility to NK-cell-induced cytotoxicity, suggesting a missing "self" recognition (Karre et al. 1986).

Consequently, in the allogeneic transplant setting an HLA-mismatch can also trigger NK-cell alloreactivity (Aversa et al. 1998). More specifically, MHC mismatch between NK-cell KIR receptors and HLA molecules on recipient cells can trigger this reaction (Ruggeri et al. 2002). NK-cells are implicated to be at least part of the effective immune response to blood and bone marrow cancers. Their potential role in immune therapy is reasonably well understood and summarized elsewhere (Caligiuri et al. 2004).

11.3.3 Antibodies

It is generally believed that an effective immune therapy strategy against CML largely must depend on T-cells. However, most responses triggered by immune therapy are complex and activate other elements of the immune system. Some data show anti-CML antibodies after allotransplants and after DLI. Some data suggest that these represent antibody responses against CML-associated antigens and are not found in normal persons or in allotransplant recipients with GvHD and correlate with clinical responses (Wu et al. 2000). Efforts directed towards serological identification of cancer antigens via recombinant cDNA library expression cloning (SEREX) have identified several antigens including CML66, a cancer-associated antigen expressed on CML cells, which is immunogenic and leads to specific antibody responses (Wu et al. 2000; Yang et al. 2001).

Although the role of antibody responses against CML-associated or -specific antigens is not understood, preliminary data suggest careful study of antibody responses in CML may further the identification of novel CML-related antigens that, subsequently, might be used for immune therapy.

11.4 Established Immune Therapies

11.4.1 Interferon-*α*

The cytokine interferon-*α* (IFN-*α*) is active in CML, and usually associated with substantial toxicity. When used as initial therapy, about 5–10% of persons with chronic phase CML achieve a cytogenetic remission, However, most of these persons still have MRD detectable by molecular techniques. This situation is interpreted as *cancer dormancy* supported by the observation, that – despite cytogenetic or molecular detection of leukemia cells – there are long-term survivors free of clinical CML. Based on these data it is postulated IFN-*α* controls CML by activating the immune system (Talpaz 2001). Recent advances in the understanding of the effects of IFN-*α* suggest a contribution in eliciting T-cell responses against self-antigens in CML (Burchert and Neubauer 2005).

Although some data suggest IFN-*α* may induce CML-associated antigen expression supporting immune responses against CML cells (Burchert et al. 2003), it is unclear whether IFN-*α* might also induce expression of minor HLA-antigens adding at least a partial allogeneic effect. At present, it is not certain whether the effect of IFN-*α* results from an immune effect, an antiproliferative effect, or something else.

Because of the substantial cytogenetic response rates to imatinib but the persistence of MRD, a combination of imatinib followed by IFN-*α* was proposed to consolidate imatinib-induced remissions (Talpaz 2001). Data from an exploratory trial shows feasibility but it is not yet possible to evaluate efficacy (Baccarani et al. 2004).

Based on current knowledge, the benefit of IFN-*α* in CML does not appear to involve alloantigens. This furthers the notion that an immune effect from IFN-*α*, if it exists, may be achieved or enhanced by other immune therapies, like cancer vaccines.

11.4.2 Bone Marrow and Blood Cell Transplants

Bone marrow and blood cell transplants (BMT) are the only known cure for CML (Butturini and Gale 1992). The initial focus of allogeneic transplants was to use high-dose chemotherapy and/or radiation to eradicate leukemia followed by rescue from otherwise irreversible bone marrow failure by the graft. Recently, less intensive conditioning regimens have been used based on the notion that immune-mediated anti-leukemia effects rather than high-dose therapy can eradicate CML cells (see below) (Kolb et al. 2004).

The notion that transplants cure CML by immune-mediated mechanisms is based on substantial clinical data. For example, recipients of transplants from genetically-identical twins, allotransplant recipients without graft-versus-host-disease (GvHD), and recipients of T-cell-depleted allotransplants all have increased leukemia-relapse risks higher than appropriate controls (Butturini and Gale 1992, 1995). Also, stopping posttransplant immune suppression and/or infusion of donor lymphocytes produces remission in persons with leukemia-relapse post transplant. Some studies provide data supporting two distinct immune-mediated anti-leukemia effects: (1) GvHD; and (2) an antileukemic effect distinct from clinical GvHD termed graft-versus-leukemia-effect (GvL). Whether GvL is really distinct from GvHD or an anti-leukemia effect of clinically undetectable GvHD is uncertain. The correct answer to this question is of fundamental importance in trying to determine whether the immune-mediated anti-leukemia effects associated with transplants can operate anywhere but in an allogeneic setting. Data relevant for defining the role of the immune system and suggesting a GvL effect are comparisons of relapse rates with occurrence and severity of GvHD in persons with different genetic backgrounds, and the effects of T-cell depletion and immune suppressive drugs such as cyclosporine. Persons with CML, who develop chronic GvHD after allogeneic BMT have about a fourfold reduced relative relapse risk compared with those without GvHD. Additionally, persons receiving syngeneic BMT from a genetically-identical twin have 12-fold higher relative relapse risk than allogeneic BMT recipients with chronic GvHD (Table 11.1) (Butturini and Gale 1991, 1992).

A direct effect of T-cells on relapse rates is apparent when relapse risks after T-cell-depleted and replete allogeneic BMT are compared. The relative risk for relapse in T-cell-depleted transplants is about sevenfold higher than in T-cell-replete transplants. This effect persists after adjusting for GvHD (Table 11.1). Similarly, immune suppression with cyclosporine in GvHD does not reduce the risk of relapse.

The biologic mechanism for this T-cell effect is not understood, but it is hypothesized that the anti-leukemia effect of GvHD is based on reactivity of donor lymphocytes to minor HLA-antigens (Butturini and Gale 1991; Goulmy et al. 1983), whereas the leukemia-specific effect of GvL is attributed to leukemia-specific antigens and differences in their immunogenicity. Cells mediating the GvL effect are proposed to be cytotoxic T-cells and/or NK cells (Butturini and Gale 1991; Kolb et al. 2004).

11.4.3 Donor Lymphocyte Infusion

As suggested above, T-cells are most likely responsible for the anti-leukemia effects associated with GvHD and GvL seen in BMT recipients. For example, T-cell depletion increases leukemia relapse risk even when adjusted for GvHD (Table 11.1) (Horowitz and Gale 1991; Horowitz et al. 1990). Conversely, infusion of T-cells, termed donor lymphocyte infusion (DLI) can reverse posttransplant relapse. DLI is typically given when graft-versus-host tolerance is established as judged by the absence of GvHD (Kolb et al. 2004). However, giving DLI early post transplant before graft-versus-host-tolerance has developed or can be assessed can increase incidence and/or severity of acute GvHD (Sullivan et al. 1989). Persons with chronic phase CML relapsing after allogeneic BMT, have about a 70% response rate to DLI (Kolb et al. 1995). Persons with few leukemia cells (cytogenetic and/or molecular evidence of leukemia) and those with less advanced disease have higher response rates. Response to DLI typically occurs over 4–6 months consistent with expansion of the infused T-cells (Kolb et al. 2004). The contribution of T-cell subsets and/or dendritic cells to this anti-leukemia effect is undefined. Response to DLI is greater in myeloid-versus lymphoid leukemias; it is suggested this difference results from the direct presentation of myeloid-specific antigens to donor T-cells by dendritic cells which are part of the leukemia clone (Kolb et al. 1995). This notion is the basis for dendritic cell (DC) vaccines in CML (Sect. 11.5.2.1).

The anti-leukemia effect associated with DLI is seen after allogeneic BMT but not after transplants from genetically-identical twins (Kolb et al. 1995). This is consistent with data from allogeneic BMT (Table 11.1) and suggests an allogeneic component for the anti-leukemia effect of DLI.

Although it is widely believed T-cells provide the effector mechanism responsible for GvHD that is associated with an anti-leukemia effect, it is less certain which cells mediate the graft-versus-leukemia (GvL) effect. It might be an immune-specific response of T-cells

Table 11.1. Relative risk for relapse after transplants for chronic phase CML (adapted from Bocchia et al. 2005 with permission)

Study group	N	Relative Risk	p-value
Allogeneic, non-T-cell-depleted transplants			
No GvHD*	115	1.00	–
Acute GvHD only	267	1.15	0.75
Chronic GvHD	45	0.28	0.16
Acute and chronic GvHD	164	0.24	0.03
Syngeneic	24	2.95	0.08
Allogeneic, T-cell-depleted transplants			
All patients	154	5.14	0.0001
No GvHD	74	6.91	0.0001
Acute and/or chronic GvHD	80	4.45	0.003

GvHD, graft versus host disease; relative risk is in comparison to reference group;
* reference group

to leukemia-specific or -related antigens or subclinical GvHD. Current data do not distinguish between these possibilities. Resolving this question will have far-reaching impact for future strategies for immune therapy of CML. If the "GvL effect" is not leukemia-specific there would be no scientific basis to expect a leukemia-specific vaccine to work. However, it would also not exclude such a possibility. Well-conducted vaccine trials using leukemia-specific antigens may provide an answer to this question.

11.5 Investigational Immune Therapies

Novel approaches to immune therapy of CML focus on developing vaccines. Cancer vaccines have a history going back more than 100 years when cancer-regression was observed in persons with severe infection (Hoos 2004). Since then knowledge about cancer and about the immune system have increased substantially. Several novel vaccines are now being studied in solid and hematologic cancers. The hypothesized presence of a characterized cancer-associated or -specific antigen in most persons with the target cancer is the basis for most vaccine strategies. Some cancers, like malignant melanoma, have several well-characterized and frequently expressed cancer-associated antigens. However, identifying similar antigens in most other cancers has proven difficult (Berinstein 2003; Ribas et al. 2003).

In CML, several peptide vaccines target single antigens, which are shared by most persons with the disease such as BCR-ABL ($P210^{BCR\text{-}ABL}$), Pr-3, and WT-1. Other vaccine approaches include a broader repertoire of target antigens to minimize the impact of escape variants on vaccine efficacy and eliminate dependence on certain HLA-antigens or -haplotypes thereby increasing applicability of the vaccine to most persons with CML. Such approaches are illustrated by using autologous leukemia cells from persons with CML as the source of target antigens for vaccination.

Features of cancer vaccines that should be considered in evaluating their likelihood of success include: (1) specificity; (2) immunogenicity of target antigen(s); (3) frequency of antigen expression on cancer cells within and between patients; (4) polyclonality of antigens; and (5) toxicity (Hoos 2004).

Modern cancer vaccines have two important features: good specificity and little toxicity. However, many questions remain to be answered before the relevant factors for success of cancer vaccines are known. Several vaccine strategies used in CML are discussed below and summarized in Table 11.2.

11.5.1 Peptide Vaccines

11.5.1.1 BCR-ABL

The BCR-ABL fusion protein $P210^{BCR\text{-}ABL}$ is a CML-specific molecular abnormality, which, because of its canonical character and specificity for CML, represents a model antigen for cancer immune therapy. Several studies of in vitro immunity after in vivo vaccination in humans report immunogenicity of $P210^{BCR\text{-}ABL}$-derived peptides (Bocchia et al. 1996; Pinilla-Ibarz et al. 2000). Scheinberg and coworkers showed that $P210^{BCR\text{-}ABL}$-derived peptides of 9–11 amino acids spanning the b3a2 BCR-ABL breakpoint can elicit specific HLA class I restricted cytotoxic T-cells in vitro in HLA-matched healthy donors and induce T-cells cytotoxic to allogeneic HLA-A3-matched peptide-pulsed leukemia cell lines or induce killing of autologous and allogeneic HLA-matched peptide-pulsed blood mononuclear cells (Bocchia et al. 1996). Vaccination of 12 persons with chronic phase CML with these peptides combined with an immune-adjuvant (saponin adjuvant; QS-21) was safe and immunogenic (Pinilla-Ibarz et al. 2000). Similar findings are reported using a multivalent peptide vaccine study composed of six BCR-ABL b3a2 breakpoint peptides and QS-21 in 14 persons with chronic phase CML. Most had DTH and $CD4^+$ T-cell proliferative and/or γ-IFN release ELISPOT responses, whereas a few showed similar responses for $CD8^+$ T-cells. Although there were clinical responses in this study, concomitant therapy was given precluding a critical analysis of the clinical outcome (Cathcart et al. 2004). Recently, Bocchia and coworkers reported on 16 persons with chronic phase CML in a phase 2 trial. Most had persisting stable cytogenetic evidence of CML after 1 year of imatinib or 2 years of IFN-α therapy and no detectable change in leukemia level for at least 6 months. Persons received six vaccinations with a 5-valent b3a2 peptide vaccine plus molgramostim and QS-21, and were followed by ELISPOT assay for immunity and cytogenetics and BCR-ABL RT-PCR for persisting leukemia. Fifteen had fewer CML cells detected by cytogenetics after vaccination; three achieved a complete molecular response. Immunogenicity of the vaccine was shown in most persons (Bocchia et al. 2005). These data

Table 11.2. Summary of investigational vaccine approaches for CML in humans

Vaccine	Vaccine characteristics; immune mechanism	Institution	Phase of development and clinical setting	Toxicity	Results suggesting clinical activity	Ref.
$P210^{BCR\text{-}ABL}$ peptide + QS-21 + GM-CSF	5-valent b3a2 peptide vaccine; cytotoxic T-Cell activation	University of Siena	Phase 2; CP CML after 12 months of Imatinib or 24 months of IFN-α (concomitant therapy allowed)	No significant toxicity	N = 16; 15 patients with reduced cytogenetic disease burden after vaccination	Bocchia et al. 2005
PR-1 peptide	Single peptide vaccine; cytotoxic T-cell activation	MD Anderson, Houston	Phase I; CP CML (concomitant therapy allowed)	No significant toxicity	N = 38; correlation between; PR-1-specific T-cells and clinical responses	Molldrem et al. 2000
WT-1 peptide	Single peptide vaccine; cytotoxic T-cell activation	University of Berlin	Phase I/II; recurrent AML	No significant toxicity	N = 1; remission of recurrent AML	Mailander et al. 2004
Autologous heat shock protein-peptide complex 70 (HSPPC-70; AG-858)	Personalized, polyvalent vaccine; cytotoxic T-cell activation; innate immunity	University of Connecticut	Phase I; CP CML with cytogenetic or molecular disease (concomitant therapy allowed)	No significant toxicity	N = 20; 13 patients with reduced disease burden; post vaccination	Li et al. 2005
		Antigenics, Boston	Phase II; CP CML; resistant to imatinib; imatinib + AG-858	No significant toxicity	N = 40; trial ongoing	Marin et al. 2005
Autologous; Ph^+ DC	Whole-cell vaccine; cytotoxic T-cell activation	University of Berlin	Phase I; CP CML without major cytogenetic response after imatinib or IFN-α (concomitant therapy allowed)	No significant toxicity	N = 9; 5 patients with reduced disease burden; post vaccination	Westermann et al. 2004

Autologous; Ph^+ DC+KLH+BCG (in some preparations)	Whole-cell vaccine; cytotoxic T-cell activation	University of Amsterdam	Phase II; CP CML resistant to IFN-α; (concomitant therapy allowed)	2 cases of injection site ulceration	N=3; clinical activity cannot be assessed	Ossenkoppele et al. 2003
Autologous; Ph^+ DC	Whole-cell vaccine; cytotoxic T-cell activation	Mayo Clinic, Rochester	Phase I; Late chronic or accelerated phase CML; (concomitant therapy allowed)	No significant toxicity	N=6; clinical activity cannot be assessed	Litzow et al. 2004

CP CML, chronic phase CML; BCG, Bacillus Calmette-Guerin (mycobacterium tuberculosis); GM-CSF, Granulocyte-Macrophage Colony-Stimulating Factor; KLH, Keyhole Limpet Hemocyanin adjuvant; QS-21, saponin adjuvant suggest some effect of vaccination on residual leukemia in chronic phase CML and highlight the need for further study to determine clinical benefit from vaccination.

11.5.1.2 Pr-3 and Pr-1 Vaccination

The primary granule enzyme Protienase-3 (Pr-3) found in granulocytes, is a cancer-associated antigen overexpressed in myeloid leukemias including CML. Pr-3 is normally maximally expressed in promyelocytes. However, Pr-3 is three- to sixfold overexpressed in about three quarters of persons with CML. Pr-1, a 9 amino acid HLA-A*0201-restricted peptide derived from Pr-3, which is a target epitope of CTLs that preferentially kill myeloid leukemia cells in vitro (Molldrem et al. 1997, 1999). Peptides derived from Pr-3, like Pr-1, are presented on MHC class I molecules from CD34+ CML blasts. These data suggest Pr-3-related peptides could be leukemia-associated antigens. Molldrem et al. used PR1/HLA-A2 tetramers to identify PR-1-specific CTLs in 38 subjects with CML who received allogeneic BMT, interferon-α or chemotherapy and reported a correlation between immune and therapy response (Molldrem et al. 2000). Recent data suggest a low frequency of CD8-positive T-cells reactive to Pr-1 in the blood of normals and people with myeloid leukemias including CML (Rezvani et al. 2003). Molldrem et al. reported that people with CML lack high-avidity leukemia-specific T-cells in contrast to normals. Also, high-avidity PR1-specific T-cells were found in IFN-α-sensitive persons with cytogenetic remission but not others (Molldrem et al. 2003). Taken together, these data suggest Pr-3-related peptides as a potential target for immune therapy of CML. However, they also indicate the need for further study of the underlying immune mechanisms in CML to optimize therapy strategies and avoid immune escape mechanisms.

11.5.1.3 WT-1

The Wilms tumor protein WT-1 is a transcription factor expressed in normal tissues during embryonic development. Overexpression was first described in Wilm tumors of the kidney in children and later in some solid cancers and in most cases of myelodysplastic syndrome (MDS), acute myelogenous leukemia (AML), acute lymphocytic leukemia (ALL), and CML (Rosenfeld et al. 2003). A recent study investigated the expression patterns of WT-1 and BCR-ABL via quantitative RT-PCR during follow-up of persons with Ph-chromosome-positive CML or ALL and showed WT-1 expression changed in parallel with BCR-ABL expression and disease state.

Because of its limited normal tissue expression in adults, WT-1 was identified as a target for immune therapy in these cancers. Indirect data suggest little expression of WT-1 on human hematopoietic progenitor cells (Oka et al. 2002).

WT1-specific, HLA-restricted CTLs have been generated against HLA-A0201 and HLA-A2402-restricted epitopes selectively kill WT1-expressing leukemia cells (Gao et al. 2000, Ohminami et al 2000). Anti-WT-1 antibodies are present in people with leukemia, indicating WT-1 is antigenic (Wu et al. 2005). WT1-reactive, CD8-positive T-cells are detected at low frequency in normal persons and at higher frequency in persons with CML (Rezvani et al. 2003).

These studies support the notion that immunization against WT-1 may be helpful in immune therapy of CML; more data are needed.

Because WT-1 is highly conserved between mice and humans, data from mouse models may be useful for drawing some conclusions for human studies. Experiments in mice report that immunization with peptide or DNA-based WT-1 vaccines can protect against challenge with WT-1-expressing cancer cells (Oka et al. 2002). Vaccination with WT-1 peptide BCG cell wall skeleton (BCG-CWS) can eliminate WT-1 expressing cancer cells in mice. Immunization with WT-1-derived peptides or WT-1 DNA elicits WT-1-specific CTLs, that appear not to attack normal tissues, which typically express low levels of WT-1. Based on these data, clinical trials that target WT-1 are beginning (Mailander et al. 2004). Favorable results are reported in several studies but none yet in CML. It is worth noting parenthetically that transfusion of human T-cells transduced with genes coding for a WT-1 specific T-cell receptor can eliminate human CML cells in a murine model system, an observation that adds further support to the notion that WT-1 may be a promising target for immunotherapy (Xue et al. 2005).

In summary, the use of WT1 as a target for vaccination against WT1-positive CML appears promising but requires substantial further study to elucidate the biology of WT1 expression in health and malignancy and vaccination effects on CML in defined populations.

11.5.2 Autologous Vaccines

Random mutations accumulating in cancer cells create large numbers of molecular abnormalities that are potential targets for immune therapy. The randomness of this process makes each cancer unique. Consequently, it is logical to envision an individualized approach to cancer vaccines built on targeting the repertoire of unique antigens.

CML is an exception to this mechanism in that the canonical BCR-ABL translocation is the transforming event in every case. However, progression of CML from chronic to acute phase is typically accompanied by additional genetic abnormalities (Butturini and Gale 1995). These unidentified and presumably individually specific abnormalities, along with those previously discussed (BCR-ABL, Pr-3, and WT-1) are implicated to contribute to a specific GvL effect (Sect. 11.4.3) and suggest that autologous immune therapy of CML may work.

Several autologous vaccine strategies attempt to exploit the foregoing, for example, autologous dendritic cell vaccines with or without the transduction of a GM-CSF gene (Ossenkoppele et al. 2003; Stam et al. 2003; Westermann et al. 2004) or autologous heat shock protein vaccines targeting the specific potential antigen repertoire of each patient's cancer (Hoos and Levey 2003). Others include vaccines of CML-cell lysates (Zeng et al. 2005). These approaches are discussed below.

11.5.2.1 Dendritic Cell Vaccines

Several autologous dendritic cell (DC)-based vaccines were tested in early clinical trials of persons with CML. The rationale is that DCs are progeny of the CML-clone resulting in constitutive expression of presumed cancer-specific or cancer-associated antigens (like BCR-ABL, Pr-3, and WT-1). These antigens may be processed and presented by autologous DC to T-cells. If adequately formulated as a vaccine, DC may induce anti-CML immune responses, which overcome T-cell anergy or other mechanisms that suppress immunity to CML (Ossenkoppele et al. 2003; Westermann et al. 2004).

A phase 1 study conducted by Westermann and colleagues used autologous DC as adjuvant vaccination in persons with chronic phase CML, who did not achieve a major cytogenetic response after receiving imatinib or IFN-α. The study demonstrated feasibility and safety of vaccination with DC collected by leukapheresis and matured in vitro in nine persons. One-third of cultured DCs had the BCR-ABL transcript. Four subcutaneous injections of $1–50\times10^6$ cells/dose were given. T-cell responses to BCR-ABL were detected in low frequency by ELISPOT and tetramer assays in two cases. In five cases, levels of BCR-ABL-positive cells in the blood decreased. Because concomitant anti-leukemia therapies were given it cannot be determined whether this effect resulted from the DC vaccination (Westermann et al. 2004).

Another phase-1 study in three persons with IFN-α-resistant CML was reported (Ossenkoppele et al. 2003). Here, DCs were generated in culture from blood mononuclear cells and given as four intradermal injections. DCs were pulsed with KLH and radiated. In some injections, BCG particles were added. Antikeyhole limpet hemocyanin (KLH) IgG antibody responses and delayed-type hypersensitivity (DTH) responses against KLH, autologous CML cells, or autologous DC were observed. One person had a measurable durable DTH reaction against leukemia cells lasting up to 20 months. Accrual for this study was stopped when imatinib became available (Ossenkoppele et al. 2003).

A third phase-I trial in six persons with late chronic or accelerated phase CML studied DC obtained by leukapheresis and matured monocytes cultured in vitro. $3–15\times10^6$ DC were injected into cervical lymph nodes four times. DCs from three persons were transfected with a recombinant replication-defective adenovirus carrying the IL-2 gene. Results suggested feasibility and safety of this approach. Some clinical improvement was observed but could not be attributed to vaccination due to use of concomitant therapy. Improvements were accompanied by increased DC-specific T-cell reactivity. Also, IL-2 secreted by transfected DC enhanced in vitro T-cell proliferation and IFN-α release (Litzow et al. 2004).

Some data suggest that adenoviral GM-CSF gene transfer into DC induces maturation of DC and may ensure protracted stimulation of CML-specific T-cells in vivo post vaccination (Stam et al. 2003).

In summary, autologous DC vaccination is feasible and can, sometimes, induce in vitro changes that appear specific for CML. However, there are no convincing data showing clinical benefit and DC vaccination is cumbersome for the routine clinical setting.

11.5.2.2 Heat Shock Protein-Peptide Complex Vaccines

Autologous heat shock protein-peptide complex vaccines (HSPPCs) target the distinct antigenic repertoire of each person's cancer (Hoos and Levey 2003; Srivastava 2000). This is achieved through the physiologic role of heat shock proteins (HSPs) to help newly synthesized polypeptides fold into their functional conformation and chaperone proteins and peptides throughout cellular compartments. HSPs isolated from cancer cells bind diverse low molecular weight antigenic peptides including epitopes, recognizable by cytotoxic T-cells. HSPPCs injected intradermally internalize into DC via the CD91 receptor (Binder and Srivastava 2004). Subsequently, peptides and HSPs dissociate and peptides are processed and presented to T-cells through MHC class I and II pathways. T-cell responses activated by HSPPCs reflect the immunogenicity of the unique repertoire of antigenic peptides isolated from the individual cancer including random mutations and other molecular abnormalities. The antigenic peptides used for vaccination through this approach do not need to be identified and the approach is not HLA-dependent. The immune effects of HSPPCs are versatile and include activation of $CD8^+$ and $CD4^+$ lymphocytes, induction of innate immune responses via NK-cell activation and cytokine secretion, and induction and maturation of DC.

Experimental mice with advanced cancers vaccinated with autologous HSPPCs often show slowing of cancer growth or stabilization of disease, whereas animals with minimal residual disease often show long-lasting protection from clinical recurrence and can be cured. These animals are also resistant to subsequent challenge with the same cancer.

HSPPCs have been tested extensively in clinical trials, mostly in solid cancers (Hoos and Levey 2003). Recently, a phase I study in 20 persons with chronic phase CML was reported (Li et al. 2005). Persons received imatinib or other therapies but had persisting CML measured by cytogenetics, fluorescence in situ hybridization (FISH) or RT-PCR. They received an autologous HSPPC vaccine via intradermal injection of eight doses of 50 μg each over 8 weeks while their prior therapy was continued. This study found it was feasible to produce autologous HSPPCs from cells obtained by leukapheresis and supported the assumption that the vaccine was safe. Nine of 16 persons studied had immune responses post vaccination as characterized by an increase of CML-specific IFN-γ-producing cells and IFN-γ-secreting NK cells in the blood. It was also observed that 13 of 20 persons had fewer leukemia cells post vaccination as measured by cytogenetics, FISH, or RT-PCR. Interpretation of these results is confounded by concomitant therapies. A correlation between immune responses and reduction of leukemia levels was also reported (Li et al. 2005). Although these data are encouraging, definitive studies are needed to establish vaccine efficacy in adequate patient populations. A phase II trial in patients with imatinib-resistant CML is ongoing (Marin et al. 2005; see Table 11.2).

11.5.2.3 Other Approaches

Another form of autologous vaccine is the use of CML cell lysates. Some data in mice suggest that chaperone-rich cell lysates (CRCL) from CML cells activate DCs and stimulate leukemia-specific immune responses (Zeng et al. 2003). The rationale for this approach is based on the presence of a variety of heat shock or chaperone proteins in CRCL, which may channel leukemia-specific peptides into the antigen-presentation pathway as described in Sect. 11.5.2.2. BCR-ABL-related peptides were demonstrated in the peptide repertoire of murine leukemia-derived CRCL and immunization with DCs cultured with leukemia-derived CRCL induced BCR-ABL-specific cytotoxic T-cell responses in vivo and better survival compared to immunization with DCs pulsed with BCR-ABL peptide only. This approach is untested in humans (Zeng et al. 2005).

Considerable data show cancer cells transduced with the GM-CSF gene can prime systemic anticancer immune responses (e.g., Sect. 11.5.2.1). However, challenges associated with culturing cancer cells or DC, individualized GM-CSF gene transfer, and large-scale development of vaccines make this approach tedious. As an alternative, an HLA-negative human cell line producing human GM-CSF was created as a universal "bystander" cell to supplement autologous tumor cell vaccines (Borrello et al. 1999). This approach is also untested in humans.

11.6 Immune Competence in CML

Success of immune therapy in CML requires intact immunity. Several recent studies of disease- or therapy-related effects on immunity in persons with CML were reported. Relevant variables, besides the well-known chemotherapy- or DLI-induced bone marrow suppression, include a potentially limited functionality of Ph-chromosome-positive DC and imatinib-related effects on immunity.

In persons with CML, the ability of DC to produce intracellular cytokines and to process and effectively present antigens is impaired (Dong et al. 2003; Eisendle et al. 2003; Wang et al. 1999; Yasukawa et al. 2001). Chemokine-induced migration of these cells is also reduced (Dong et al. 2003). However, some of these effects are reversible in vitro by culturing DC with IFN-α or TNF-α (Eisendle et al. 2003; Wang et al. 1999). Relevance of these data to immune therapy of CML is uncertain and data from clinical trials are needed to provide answers.

Other data showed diverse effects of imatinib on immune function. Sato and colleagues suggested intensified antigen-presentation of DC in persons with CML receiving imatinib; (Sato et al. 2003) others reported restoration of plasmacytoid DC function (Mohty et al. 2004). In contrast, exposing CD-34$^+$ progenitor cells to imatinib in vitro inhibits differentiation into DC (Appel et al. 2004). Since almost everyone with CML today receives imatinib it is important that vaccine therapies have the ability to operate in persons receiving this drug. Several vaccine studies reported immune responses in patients receiving imatinib (Bocchia et al. 2005; Li et al. 2005). However, the relevant impact of chronic imatinib use on the immune system and the ability to translate immune responses induced in this environment into clinical activity need further study.

11.7 Future Directions

The question of the potential efficacy of immune therapy in CML has, in our opinion, far-reaching importance. This is because results of therapies of CML, like allogeneic BMT and DLI, provide the most convincing evidence that immune therapy may benefit persons with cancer.

Unquestionably, an allogeneic anti-leukemia effect operates in persons with CML receiving the above therapies. Often this is associated with clinical GvHD. There also seems to be an allogeneic anti-leukemia effect distinguishable from clinical GvHD. However, there are two important interrelated issues we cannot resolve: (1) Can these anti-leukemia effects operate in settings without allogeneic disparity, for example, in an autologous setting? and (2) Is there an anti-leukemia effect distinct from GvHD?

Answers to these questions are important. For example, if an allogeneic milieu is required for a clinical anti-leukemia effect, autologous vaccines using cancer-specific but nonallogeneic target antigens are unlikely to be effective. This implies, if there is no clinically effective immune response to cancer-related or -specific antigens, but only to alloantigens, vaccines against targets like BCR-ABL, Pr-3, and WT-1 will not be effective.

There are many reports of increased immune responses, in vitro and in vivo, following treatment with cancer vaccines (Berinstein 2003; Ribas et al. 2003). Those in CML vaccine trials are discussed above. However, results of these tests are not convincingly correlated with clinical response and these tests are not validated surrogates. This is due to the lack of sufficiently powered randomized trials that employ these tests and investigate vaccines with sufficient clinical activity to correlate immune response and clinical events.

Although we found convincing data of immune-related anticancer effects of allogeneic BMT and DLI in CML, results of other immune therapies are less convincing. We identified few persons with CML who received cancer vaccines in whom we think a clinical benefit from vaccination is convincing. Because of the early nature of the clinical trials conducted in CML to date and the confounding issues cited, we think the only critical test of a possible benefit of immune therapy of CML other than allogeneic transplants and DLI must come from large, controlled, randomized trials, especially in populations with minimal residual disease.

CML is an excellent candidate disease in which to test immune therapy of cancer in humans. However, it should be recalled that chronic phase CML, where almost all immune therapy trials are done, is more a preleukemia than leukemia. Chronic phase CML cells have regulated growth and respond appropriately to normal physiological stimuli, like G- or GM-CSF and infection. Persons with cyclical neutropenia and CML have typical oscillations in their WBC. Furthermore, many persons with CML would likely survive normally if they did not progress to acute phase. Consequently, even if immune therapy were successful in chronic phase CML, one should be carefully applying this lesson to bona fide cancers, especially advanced cancers.

Because of the clear anti-leukemia effect of alloimmunity in CML, others have tried to apply this approach to other cancers. Data in blood and bone marrow cancers, like lymphoma and multiple myeloma, are similar to CML but less striking in their magnitude. Data supporting this approach in solid cancers are less studied and far less convincing. Renal cancer is the best-studied example. Here, data supporting a benefit of an allogeneic effect are reasonably convincing (Childs et al. 2000; Rini et al. 2002). Again, it has been difficult or impossible to separate an anticancer effect from GvHD, which limits the utility of this approach. Data in other cancers, we think, either are negative or unconvincing (Blaise et al. 2004; Bregni et al. 2002; Ueno et al. 2003). More data are needed. Again, we urge use of large controlled randomized trials. Because of the difficulty in separating an anticancer benefit from GvHD we think this approach is unlikely to be of broad utility in cancer therapy, even if effective.

It is impossible to know presently if immune therapy other than allogeneic BMT and DLI will work in CML. We do not consider the available data in CML critically evaluable and urge conduct of appropriately designed randomized trials. This notion is supported by recent reports of randomized trials with cancer vaccines in prostate or lung cancer, which suggest clinical benefit from vaccines using autologous antigens providing a basis for further vaccine development (Murray et al. 2005; Small et al. 2005).

References

Appel S, Boehmler AM, Grunebach F, Muller MR, Rupf A, Weck MM, Hartmann U, Reichardt VL, Kanz L, Brummendorf TH, Brossart P (2004) Imatinib mesylate affects the development and function of dendritic cells generated from CD34+ peripheral blood progenitor cells. Blood 103:538–544

Aversa F, Tabilio A, Velardi A, Cunningham I, Terenzi A, Falzetti F, Ruggeri L, Barbabietola G, Aristei C, Latini P, Reisner Y, Martelli MF (1998) Treatment of high-risk acute leukemia with T-cell-depleted stem cells from related donors with one fully mismatched HLA haplotype. N Engl J Med 339:1186–1193

Baccarani M, Martinelli G, Rosti G, Trabacchi E, Testoni N, Bassi S, Amabile M, Soverini S, Castagnetti F, Cilloni D, Izzo B, de Vivo A, Messa E, Bonifazi F, Poerio A, Luatti S, Giugliano E, Alberti D, Fincato G, Russo D, Pane F, Saglio G (2004) Imatinib and pegylated human recombinant interferon-alpha2b in early chronic-phase chronic myeloid leukemia. Blood 104:4245–4251

Berinstein N (2003) Overview of therapeutic vaccination approaches for cancer. Semin Oncol 30:1–8

Binder RJ & Srivastava PK (2004) Essential role of CD91 in re-presentation of gp96-chaperoned peptides. Proc Natl Acad Sci USA 101: 6128–6133

Blaise D, Bay JO, Faucher C, Michallet M, Boiron JM, Choufi B, Cahn JY, Gratecos N, Sotto JJ, Francois S, Fleury J, Mohty M, Chabannon C, Bilger K, Gravis G, Viret F, Braud AC, Bardou VJ, Maraninchi D, Viens P (2004) Reduced-intensity preparative regimen and allogeneic stem cell transplantation for advanced solid tumors. Blood 103:435–441

Bocchia M, Korontsvit T, Xu Q, Mackinnon S, Yang SY, Sette A, Scheinberg DA (1996) Specific human cellular immunity to bcr-abl oncogene-derived peptides. Blood 87:3587–3592

Bocchia M, Gentili S, Abruzzese E, Fanelli A, Iuliano F, Tabilio A, Amabile M, Forconi F, Gozzetti A, Raspadori D, Amadori S, Lauria F (2005) Effect of a p210 multipeptide vaccine associated with imatinib or interferon in patients with chronic myeloid leukaemia and persistent residual disease: a multicentre observational trial. Lancet 365:657–662

Borrello I, Sotomayor EM, Cooke S, Levitsky HI (1999) A universal granulocyte-macrophage colony-stimulating factor-producing bystander cell line for use in the formulation of autologous tumor cell-based vaccines. Hum Gene Ther 10:1983–1991

Bregni M, Dodero A, Peccatori J, Pescarollo A, Bernardi M, Sassi I, Voena C, Zaniboni A, Bordignon C, Corradini P (2002) Nonmyeloablative conditioning followed by hematopoietic cell allografting and donor lymphocyte infusions for patients with metastatic renal and breast cancer. Blood 99:4234–4236

Burchert A, Neubauer A (2005) Interferon alpha and T-cell responses in chronic myeloid leukemia. Leuk Lymphoma 46:167–175

Burchert A, Wolfl S, Schmidt M, Brendel C, Denecke B, Cai D, Odyvanova L, Lahaye T, Muller MC, Berg T, Gschaidmeier H, Wittig B, Hehlmann R, Hochhaus A, Neubauer A (2003) Interferon-alpha, but not the ABL-kinase inhibitor imatinib (STI571), induces expression of myeloblastin and a specific T-cell response in chronic myeloid leukemia. Blood 101:259–264

Butturini A, Gale RP (1991) Graft-vs-leukemia in chronic myelogenous leukemia. In: Deisseroth AB, Arlinghaus RB (eds) Chronic myelogenous leukemia: molecular approaches to research and therapy, vol 13. Marcel Dekker, New York, pp 377–386

Butturini A, Gale RP (1992) Graft versus leukemia. Immunol Res 11:24–33

Butturini A, Gale RP (1995) Chronic myelogenous leukemia as a model of cancer development. Semin Oncol 22:374–379

Caligiuri MA, Velardi A, Scheinberg DA, Borrello IM (2004) Immunotherapeutic approaches for hematologic malignancies. Hematology (Am Soc Hematol Educ Program) 337–353

Cathcart K, Pinilla-Ibarz J, Korontsvit T, Schwartz J, Zakhaleva V, Papadopoulos EB, Scheinberg DA (2004) A multivalent bcr-abl fusion peptide vaccination trial in patients with chronic myeloid leukemia. Blood 103:1037–1042

Childs R, Chernoff A, Contentin N, Bahceci E, Schrump D, Leitman S, Read EJ, Tisdale J, Dunbar C, Linehan WM, Young NS, Barrett AJ (2000) Regression of metastatic renal-cell carcinoma after nonmyeloablative allogeneic peripheral-blood stem-cell transplantation. N Engl J Med 343:750–758

Colonna M, Navarro F, Bellon T, Llano M, Garcia P, Samaridis J, Angman L, Cella M, Lopez-Botet M (1997) A common inhibitory receptor for major histocompatibility complex class I molecules on human lymphoid and myelomonocytic cells. J Exp Med 186:1809–1818

Dohring C, Scheidegger D, Samaridis J, Cella M, Colonna M (1996) A human killer inhibitory receptor specific for HLA-A1,2. J Immunol 156:3098–3101

Dong R, Cwynarski K, Entwistle A, Marelli-Berg F, Dazzi F, Simpson E, Goldman JM, Melo JV, Lechler RI, Bellantuono I, Ridley A, Lombardi G (2003) Dendritic cells from CML patients have altered actin organization, reduced antigen processing, and impaired migration. Blood 101:3560–3567

Eisendle K, Lang A, Eibl B, Nachbaur D, Glassl H, Fiegl M, Thaler J, Gastl G (2003) Phenotypic and functional deficiencies of leukaemic dendritic cells from patients with chronic myeloid leukaemia. Br J Haematol 120:63–73

Gabert J, Beillard E, van der Velden VH, Bi W, Grimwade D, Pallisgaard N, Barbany G, Cazzaniga G, Cayuela JM, Cave H, Pane F, Aerts JL, De Micheli D, Thirion X, Pradel V, Gonzalez M, Viehmann S, Malec M, Saglio G, van Dongen JJ (2003) Standardization and quality control studies of "real-time" quantitative reverse transcriptase polymerase chain reaction of fusion gene transcripts for residual disease detection in leukemia – a Europe Against Cancer program. Leukemia 17:2318–2357

Gale RP, Horowitz MM, Talpaz M, Scheinberg DA, Molldrem J, Li Z, Baccarani M, Goldman JM, Tura S (2005) Immune therapy of chronic myelogenous leukemia. Leuk Res 29:583–586

Goldman JM, Melo JV (2003) Chronic myeloid leukemia–advances in biology and new approaches to treatment. N Engl J Med 349: 1451–1464

Goulmy E, Gratama JW, Blokland E, Zwaan FE, van Rood JJ (1983) A minor transplantation antigen detected by MHC-restricted cytotoxic T lymphocytes during graft-versus-host disease. Nature 302:159–161

Hobeika AC, Morse MA, Osada T, Ghanayem M, Niedzwiecki D, Barrier R, Lyerly HK, Clay TM (2005) Enumerating antigen-specific T-cell responses in peripheral blood: a comparison of peptide MHC Tetramer, ELISpot, and intracellular cytokine analysis. J Immunother 28:63–72

Hoos A (2004) The promise of cancer vaccines. Drug Discovery Devel 13

Hoos A, Levey DL (2003) Vaccination with heat shock protein-peptide complexes: from basic science to clinical applications. Expert Rev Vaccines 2:369–379

Horowitz MM, Gale RP (1991) Graft-versus-leukemia. In: Champlin RE, Gale RP (eds) New strategies in bone marrow transplantation: Proceedings of a Sandoz-UCLA Symposium held in Keystone, Colorado, January 20–27, 1990, Wiley-Liss, New York, pp 275–280

Horowitz MM, Gale RP, Sondel PM, Goldman JM, Kersey J, Kolb HJ, Rimm AA, Ringden O, Rozman C, Speck B et al (1990) Graft-versus-leukemia reactions after bone marrow transplantation. Blood 75:555–562

Hughes TP, Kaeda J, Branford S, Rudzki Z, Hochhaus A, Hensley ML, Gathmann I, Bolton AE, van Hoomissen IC, Goldman JM, Radich JP (2003) Frequency of major molecular responses to imatinib or interferon alfa plus cytarabine in newly diagnosed chronic myeloid leukemia. N Engl J Med 349:1423–1432

Janeway C (2005) The generation of lymphocyte antigen receptors. In: Immunobiology: The Immune System in Health and Disease, Garland Science, New York, pp 135–168

Kantarjian H, Talpaz M, O'Brien S, Garcia-Manero G, Verstovsek S, Giles F, Rios MB, Shan J, Letvak L, Thomas D, Faderl S, Ferrajoli A, Cortes J (2004) High-dose imatinib mesylate therapy in newly diagnosed Philadelphia chromosome-positive chronic phase chronic myeloid leukemia. Blood 103:2873–2878

Karre K, Ljunggren HG, Piontek G, Kiessling R (1986) Selective rejection of H-2-deficient lymphoma variants suggests alternative immune defence strategy. Nature 319:675–678

Keilholz U, Weber J, Finke JH, Gabrilovich DI, Kast WM, Disis ML, Kirkwood JM, Scheibenbogen C, Schlom J, Maino VC, Lyerly HK, Lee PP, Storkus W, Marincola F, Worobec A, Atkins MB (2002) Immunologic monitoring of cancer vaccine therapy: results of a workshop sponsored by the Society for Biological Therapy. J Immunother 25:97–138

Kolb HJ, Schattenberg A, Goldman JM, Hertenstein B, Jacobsen N, Arcese W, Ljungman P, Ferrant A, Verdonck L, Niederwieser D, van Rhee F, Mittermueller J, De Witte T, Holler E, Ansari H (1995) Graft-versus-leukemia effect of donor lymphocyte transfusions in marrow grafted patients. Blood 86:2041–2050

Kolb HJ, Simoes B, Schmid C (2004) Cellular immunotherapy after allogeneic stem cell transplantation in hematologic malignancies. Curr Opin Oncol 16:167–173

Li Z, Qiao Y, Liu B, Laska EJ, Chakravarthi P, Kulko JM, Bona RD, Fang M, Hegde U, Moyo V, Tannenbaum SH, Menoret A, Gaffney J, Glynn L, Runowicz C, Srivastava PK (2005) Combination of imatinib mesylate with autologous leukocyte-derived heat shock protein and chronic myelogenous leukemia. Clin Cancer Res 11:4460–4468

Litzow MR, Dietz AB, Bulur PA, Butler GW, Fink SR, Letendre L, Paternoster SF, Tefferi A, Hoering A, Vuk-Pavlovic S (2004) A phase I trial of autologous dendritic cell therapy for chronic myelogenous leukemia [meeting abstract]. Blood, 104:801a (abstract 2931)

Marin D, Mauro M, Goldman J, Druker B, Devine S, Clark RE, Paquette R, Bashey A, Tallman MS, Dovholuk A, Hoos A, Srivastava PK (2005) Preliminary results from a phase 2 trial of AG-858, an autologous heat shock protein-peptide vaccine, in combination with imatinib in patients with chronic phase chronic myeloid leukemia (CML) resistant to prior imatinib monotherapy [meeting abstract]. Blood 106:(abstract 1094)

Mohty M, Jourdan E, Mami NB, Vey N, Damaj G, Blaise D, Isnardon D, Olive D, Gaugler B (2004) Imatinib and plasmacytoid dendritic cell function in patients with chronic myeloid leukemia. Blood 103: 4666–4668

Molldrem JJ, Lee PP, Wang C, Felio K, Kantarjian HM, Champlin RE, Davis MM (2000) Evidence that specific T lymphocytes may participate in the elimination of chronic myelogenous leukemia. Nat Med 6:1018–1023

Molldrem JJ, Lee PP, Kant S, Wieder E, Jiang W, Lu S, Wang C, Davis MM (2003) Chronic myelogenous leukemia shapes host immunity by selective deletion of high-avidity leukemia-specific T cells. J Clin Invest 111:639–647

Murray N, Butts C, Maksymiuk A, Marshall E, Goss G, Soulieres D (2005) A liposomal MUC1 vaccine for treatment of non-small cell lung cancer (NSCLC); updated survival results from patients with stage IIIB disease [meeting abstract]. Proc Am Soc Clin Oncol (abstract 7037)

Oka Y, Tsuboi A, Elisseeva OA, Udaka K, Sugiyama H (2002) WT1 as a novel target antigen for cancer immunotherapy. Curr Cancer Drug Targets 2:45–54

Ossenkoppele GJ, Stam AG, Westers TM, de Gruijl TD, Janssen JJ, van de Loosdrecht AA, Scheper RJ (2003) Vaccination of chronic myeloid leukemia patients with autologous in vitro cultured leukemic dendritic cells. Leukemia 17:1424–1426

Pinilla-Ibarz J, Cathcart K, Korontsvit T, Soignet S, Bocchia M, Caggiano J, Lai L, Jimenez J, Kolitz J, Scheinberg DA (2000) Vaccination of patients with chronic myelogenous leukemia with bcr-abl oncogene breakpoint fusion peptides generates specific immune responses. Blood 95:1781–1787

Rezvani K, Grube M, Brenchley JM, Sconocchia G, Fujiwara H, Price DA, Gostick E, Yamada K, Melenhorst J, Childs R, Hensel N, Douek DC, Barrett AJ (2003) Functional leukemia-associated antigen-specific memory CD8+ T cells exist in healthy individuals and in patients with chronic myelogenous leukemia before and after stem cell transplantation. Blood 102:2892–2900

Ribas A, Butterfield LH, Glaspy JA, Economou JS (2003) Current developments in cancer vaccines and cellular immunotherapy. J Clin Oncol 21:2415–2432

Rini BI, Zimmerman T, Stadler WM, Gajewski TF, Vogelzang NJ (2002) Allogeneic stem-cell transplantation of renal cell cancer after nonmyeloablative chemotherapy: feasibility, engraftment, and clinical results. J Clin Oncol 20:2017–2024

Rosenfeld C, Cheever MA, Gaiger A (2003) WT1 in acute leukemia, chronic myelogenous leukemia and myelodysplastic syndrome: therapeutic potential of WT1 targeted therapies. Leukemia 17:1301–1312

Ruggeri L, Capanni M, Urbani E, Perruccio K, Shlomchik WD, Tosti A, Posati S, Rogaia D, Frassoni F, Aversa F, Martelli MF, Velardi A (2002) Effectiveness of donor natural killer cell alloreactivity in mismatched hematopoietic transplants. Science 295:2097–2100

Sato N, Narita M, Takahashi M, Yagisawa K, Liu A, Abe T, Nikkuni K, Furukawa T, Toba K, Aizawa Y (2003) The effects of STI571 on antigen presentation of dendritic cells generated from patients with chronic myelogenous leukemia. Hematol Oncol 21:67–75

Small EJ, Schellhammer PF, Higano C, Neumanaitis J, Valone F, Herschberg RM (2005) Immunotherapy (APC8015) for Androgen Independent Prostate Cancer (AIPC): Final Survival data from a Phase 3 randomized placebo-controlled trial. [meeting abstract]. Proc Am Soc Clin Oncol (abstract 264)

Srivastava PK (2000) Immunotherapy of human cancer: lessons from mice. Nat Immunol 1:363–366

Stam AG, Santegoets SJ, Westers TM, Sombroek CC, Janssen JJ, Tillman BW, van de Loosdrecht AA, Pinedo HM, Curiel DT, Ossenkoppele GJ, Scheper RJ, de Gruijl TD (2003) CD40-targeted adenoviral GM-CSF gene transfer enhances and prolongs the maturation of human CML-derived dendritic cells upon cytokine deprivation. Br J Cancer 89:1162–1165

Sullivan KM, Storb R, Buckner CD, Fefer A, Fisher L, Weiden PL, Witherspoon RP, Appelbaum FR, Banaji M, Hansen J et al (1989) Graft-versus-host disease as adoptive immunotherapy in patients with advanced hematologic neoplasms. N Engl J Med 320:828–834

Talpaz M (2001) Interferon-alfa-based treatment of chronic myeloid leukemia and implications of signal transduction inhibition. Semin Hematol 38:22–27

Ueno NT, Cheng YC, Rondon G, Tannir NM, Gajewski JL, Couriel DR, Hosing C, de Lima MJ, Anderlini P, Khouri IF, Booser DJ, Hortobagyi GN, Pagliaro LC, Jonasch E, Giralt SA, Champlin RE (2003) Rapid induction of complete donor chimerism by the use of a reduced-intensity conditioning regimen composed of fludarabine and melphalan in allogeneic stem cell transplantation for metastatic solid tumors. Blood 102:3829–3836

Wagtmann N, Rajagopalan S, Winter CC, Peruzzi M, Long EO (1995) Killer cell inhibitory receptors specific for HLA-C and HLA-B identified by direct binding and by functional transfer. Immunity 3:801–809

Wang C, Al-Omar HM, Radvanyi L, Banerjee A, Bouman D, Squire J, Messner HA (1999) Clonal heterogeneity of dendritic cells derived from patients with chronic myeloid leukemia and enhancement of their T-cells stimulatory activity by IFN-alpha. Exp Hematol 27:1176–1184

Westermann J, Kopp J, van Lessen A, Hecker A, Baskaynak G, Le Coutre P, Döhner C, Döhner H, Dörken B, Pezzutto A (2004) Dendritic cells vaccination in BCR/ABL-positive chronic myeloid leukemia – final results of a phase i/ii study [meeting abstract]. Blood 104:802a (abstract 2934)

Wu CJ, Yang XF, McLaughlin S, Neuberg D, Canning C, Stein B, Alyea EP, Soiffer RJ, Dranoff G, Ritz J (2000) Detection of a potent humoral response associated with immune-induced remission of chronic myelogenous leukemia. J Clin Invest 106:705–714

Wu F, Oka Y, Tsuboi A, Elisseeva OA, Ogata K, Nakajima H, Fujiki F, Masuda T, Murakami M, Yoshihara S, Ikegame K, Hosen N, Kawakami M, Nakagawa M, Kubota T, Soma T, Yamagami T, Tsukaguchi M, Ogawa H, Oji Y, Hamaoka T, Kawase I, Sugiyama H (2005) Th1-biased humoral immune responses against Wilms tumor gene WT1 product in the patients with hematopoietic malignancies. Leukemia 19:268–274

Xue A-A, Gao L, Hart D, Gillmore R, Qasim W, Thrasher A, Apperley J, Engels B, Uckert W, Morris E, Stauss H (2005) Elimination of human leukemia cells in NOD/SCID mice by WT1-TCR gene transdused human T-cells. Blood 106:3062–3067

Yang XF, Wu CJ, McLaughlin S, Chillemi A, Wang KS, Canning C, Alyea EP, Kantoff P, Soiffer RJ, Dranoff G, Ritz J (2001) CML66, a broadly immunogenic tumor antigen, elicits a humoral immune response associated with remission of chronic myelogenous leukemia. Proc Natl Acad Sci USA 98:7492–7497

Yasukawa M, Ohminami H, Kojima K, Hato T, Hasegawa A, Takahashi T, Hirai H, Fujita S (2001) HLA class II-restricted antigen presentation of endogenous bcr-abl fusion protein by chronic myelogenous leukemia-derived dendritic cells to CD4(+) T lymphocytes. Blood 98:1498–1505

Zeng Y, Feng H, Graner MW, Katsanis E (2003) Tumor-derived, chaperone-rich cell lysate activates dendritic cells and elicits potent antitumor immunity. Blood 101:4485–4491

Zeng Y, Graner MW, Thompson S, Marron M, Katsanis E (2005) Induction of BCR-ABL-specific immunity following vaccination with chaperone-rich cell lysates derived from BCR-ABL+ tumor cells. Blood 105:2016–2022

Zinkernagel RM, Doherty PC (1997) The discovery of MHC restriction. Immunol Today 18:14–17

zur Hausen H (2002) Papillomaviruses and cancer: from basic studies to clinical application. Nat Rev Cancer 2:342–350

Therapeutic Strategies and Concepts of Cure in CML

Tariq I Mughal and John M Goldman

Contents

Abstract. The molecular basis of chronic myeloid leukemia (CML) has been reasonably well defined in the last 20 years. The acquisition in a hematopoietic stem cell of a *BCR-ABL* fusion gene is generally considered to be the initiating event for the chronic phase of CML. It leads to expansion of a hematopoietic clone that expresses the Bcr-Abl oncoprotein with enhanced tyrosine kinase activity. Oral administration of the tyrosine kinase inhibitor imatinib mesylate (IM) reduces the leukemia cell mass by at least 2 logs and induces complete cytogenetic remissions in most patients with early phase CML. It probably prolongs survival in comparison with previous treatments, but fails to eradicate leukemia stem cells, some of which may be in a "quiescent" or "dormant" phase. IM is now considered to be the best initial therapy for the majority of patients with newly diagnosed CML, though the issues of optimal dose and duration of treatment are not yet resolved. Some patients who respond initially to IM later become resistant as a result of diverse mechanisms, which include the acquisition of mutations in the *BCR-ABL* kinase domain. Efforts to improve on the use of IM as a single agent include combining it with other agents and the introduction of second-generation tyrosine kinase inhibitors, such as dasatinib and nilotinib. The therapy of patients in the advanced phases of CML remains a significant challenge.

12.1 Introduction

In the last 5 years imatinib mesylate (IM, Gleevec; Glivec, Novartis Pharmaceuticals, Basel, Switzerland) has become well established as the optimal initial therapy for the majority of patients with newly diagnosed chronic myeloid leukemia (CML) (Druker et al. 2001; Mughal and Goldman 2006 a). The advent of this "molecularly targeted therapy" marks the beginning of a new era in which relatively nonspecific and often toxic drugs for treating malignant disease are being replaced by safer and better-tolerated agents whose precise mechanism of action is much better defined than that of their predecessors (Druker and Lydon 2000).

IM induces complete hematologic remissions (CHR) in almost all previously untreated patients with CML in chronic phase (CP) and complete cytogenetic responses (CCyR) in over 80% of patients (O'Brien et al. 2003 a; Simonsson 2005). Data showing the effect of IM on survival beyond 5 years are not yet available, but interim analyses of ongoing clinical studies suggest that about 2% of all chronic phase patients progress to advanced phase disease each year, which contrasts with estimated annual progression rates of >15% for patients treated with hydroxyurea and about 8–10% for patients receiving interferon-alfa (IFN-α, be it as a single agent or in combination with cytarabine [Ara-C]). If this annual rate of disease progression does not increase with longer follow-up, imatinib will be confirmed as a truly remarkable advance in the management of this disease.

It now seems clear that the degree of reduction by IM in the total leukemia cell mass as extrapolated from results of studying numbers of Ph-positive metaphases in the bone marrow and *BCR-ABL* transcripts in the blood correlates with progression-free survival (Hughes et al. 2003; Press et al. 2005). However, most of the patients who achieve a CCyR still have measurable numbers of *BCR-ABL* transcripts in their blood and/or bone marrow, which must reflect the persistence of at least small quantities of leukemia cells. Thus it seems probable that IM will not eradicate residual CML in the vast majority of patients. A central issue is therefore whether total eradication of all residual leukemia stem cells is necessary for cure, or whether the survival of small numbers of residual leukemia stem cells is compatible with long-term survival, and is thus tantamount to cure on an operational level, as may well be the case after allogeneic stem cell transplantation (Kaeda et al. 2006).

Another important issue is the precise role of allogeneic stem cell transplantation (SCT) in the IM era. At the time of writing, some "transplant aficionados" favor SCT as initial therapy for selected patients because they believe transplant to be the only currently available "curative" therapy, and the results are best if the procedure is carried out as early in the CP as possible (Gratwohl 2005), while others feel that the case for "upfront" SCT is very weak in almost all cases. This continuing controversy makes it difficult to construct a "consensus" therapeutic algorithm for patients with CML in CP (Mughal and Goldman 2003).

In this chapter we discuss some of what is known of the biology of the CML stem cell and its impact on the concept of cure. We review some current therapeutic strategies, including clinical trials, designed for the newly diagnosed patients, for IM-refractory or -resistant patients in CP, and for IM-naive patients who present in advanced phase disease.

12.2 CML Stem Cell and Concepts of Cure

A stem cell is usually defined as one of a population of cells which individually has the capacity to self-renew or to differentiate along a defined pathway or pathways. Stem cells can be recognized with variable degrees of precision by their molecular, cell surface antigen, and functional characteristics (e.g., capacity to engraft suitable experimental animals or man, vulnerability to damage by cytotoxic agents, etc.). The surface antigenic characteristics of normal hematopoietic stem cells are defined to a certain extent and CML stem cells share the same characteristics to a considerable degree. Normal stem cells capable of engrafting NOD-SCID mice are contained in the CD34+CD38− mononuclear cell fraction, which comprises 1–10% of the total CD34+

population (Bhatia et al. 1997). Some more primitive stem cells may be CD34-negative (Goodell et al. 1997; Guo et al. 2003; Kuci et al. 2003; Marley et al. 2005). A hierarchy of transplantable leukemia stem cells has been shown in CML analogous to that seen in normal stem cells, with CD34+CD38– populations giving rising to durable hemopoiesis in NOD-SCID mice (Eisterer et al. 2005).

It is generally believed that the bulk of cells that comprise the normal hematopoietic stem cell "reservoir" are dormant or quiescent (defined as in deep G_0) but the proportion of stem cells in cycle may be higher than normal in CML (Eaves et al. 1998; Reya et al. 2001). However, the presence in CML of a still significant population of quiescent stem cells may be inferred from the clinical observation that patients cannot be cured by cycle-dependent cytotoxic drugs and from the fact that some primitive leukemia cells do not label with ^{3}H-thymidine. Moreover, laboratory studies have demonstrated the presence in CML patients of a small population of Ph-positive cells that excludes the Hoechst 33342 and pyronin dyes, a finding consistent with their G_0 status (Holyoake et al. 1999). The efflux of dyes is a property associated with expression of the ATP-binding cassette (ABC) transporter proteins on the surface of stem cells, and this is the defining characteristic of the so-called side populations (Zhou et al. 2001). Although the majority of side population cells in various species do not express the CD34 antigen (Goodell et al. 1997), in humans side population cells with the capacity to regenerate hematopoiesis have only been found in the CD34+CD38– compartment of putative hematopoietic stem cells (Preffer et al. 2002; Uchida et al. 2001). The quiescent state is not, however, irreversible, since cell populations containing a majority of cells judged to be quiescent can engraft NOD-SCID mice (Holyoake et al. 1999), and indeed it is likely that individual CML stem cells, like their normal counterparts, exchange between a quiescent and a cycling status (Wang et al. 1998).

One might have assumed also that the absolute number of CML stem cells was increased in comparison with stem cell numbers in a comparable normal person but this assumption has not been confirmed (Udomsakdi et al. 1992). In fact, the increase, if any, in CML stem cell numbers may be quite small (Jamieson et al. 2004). In contrast, numbers of committed progenitors (CFU-GM) are greatly increased and are capable of a considerable amount of self-renewal in CP and in advanced disease (Gordon et al. 1998; Marley et al. 2000, 2001). Interestingly, the acquisition of the ability to self-renew in granulocyte-macrophage progenitor population in advanced phases of CML has been attributed to reactivation of the beta-catenin pathway in these cells (Jamieson et al. 2004).

In contrast to infectious diseases, the concept of cure for malignant disease is somewhat nebulous. Many infectious diseases have a reasonably well-defined incubation period followed by specific clinical manifestations, after which in most cases the patient returns to normality. The relevant microbe usually disappears, never to recur. Occasionally, the pathogenic microorganism remains in the body long-term in an innocuous state, as for example after infection with herpes group viruses. On other occasions, the pathogen may reactivate after months or years of latency and cause significant clinical illness. The analogy is not perfect but the notion that cure of infection and cure of malignancy may both on occasion be difficult or impossible to define is probably valid. In CML the notion that cure necessarily depends on eradication of all leukemia cells, a status that would in practice be impossible to confirm, is undoubtedly simplistic. One may perhaps accept as cure the absence of recognizable leukemia over a long period of time, but this of course will depend in part on the sensitivity of the assay. Experience gained over 25 years suggests that the great majority of patients alive and apparently free of leukemia 10 or even 5 years after allogeneic SCT for CML in CP will probably never relapse, and may therefore be regarded as "cured" for operational purposes. However, some of these patients have measurable levels of *BCR-ABL* transcripts in their blood, albeit usually intermittently, and the annual risk of relapse may still be about 1% (Fig. 12.1) (Kaeda et al. 2006; Mughal et al. 2001). It seems even more certain that treatment with IM as a single agent does not eradicate all residual leukemia cells in any patient (Michor et al. 2005). Thus some patients do not achieve even CCyR on standard dose IM, and of those who do, some never achieve more than a 3-log reduction in blood transcript numbers. Of those with better responses, only a small minority achieves undetectable transcript status, and this is not durable in most cases (Lange et al. 2005). Even those who do achieve undetectable *BCR-ABL* transcript status usually relapse if imatinib is stopped (Cortes et al. 2004; Rousselot et al. 2005). One explanation may be that certain quiescent and nondividing leukemia stem cells escape the effects of imatinib (Graham et al. 2002). The

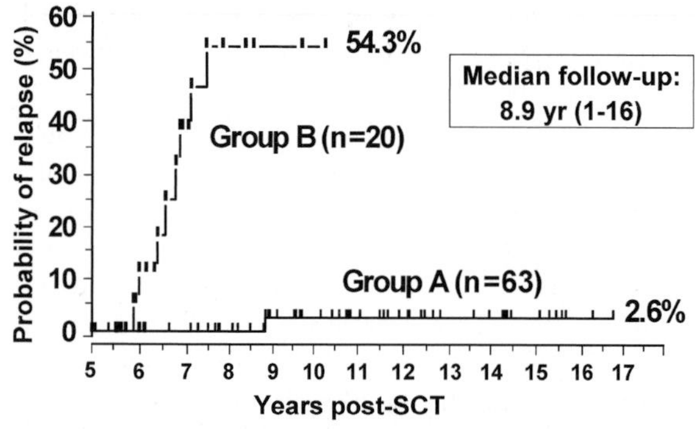

Fig. 12.1. Probability of relapse for 83 patients in remission 5 years after allogeneic SCT for CML in chronic phase. **Group A:** Patients who were continuously negative for BCR-ABL transcripts between 6 months and 5 years post-SCT (n=63). **Group B:** Patients who had one or more low level positive RQ-PCR result during the same time period (n=20) (Adapted from Mughal et al. 2001)

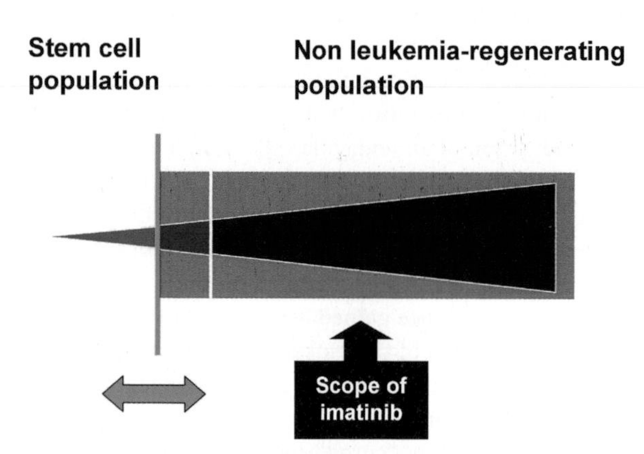

Fig. 12.2. Possible targets for imatinib. Leukemic hematopoiesis is assumed to start from a single stem cell at the *left* of this diagram. The *white vertical line* divides cells with leukemia-regenerating potential (*blue area, at left*) from end-cells with no leukemia regenerating potential (*dark blue area, at right*). It is suggested in some patients imatinib inhibits all the cells with no regenerating potential and some of the cells with leukemia regenerating potential (*red block*). The extent to which cells with leukemia regenerating potential are eliminated is represented by the area between the *green* and *white vertical lines*, but it may vary in different patients (as reflected by the *horizontal green arrow*)

unavoidable conclusion is that small numbers of leukemia cells, possibly only leukemia "stem" cells, survive even in the best IM responders (Fig. 12.2) (Goldman and Gordon 2006; Huntly and Gilliland 2005; Pardal et al. 2003). The challenge is therefore to develop ways of improving the level of response for suboptimal responders and to ensure that those stem cells that do survive have neither the capacity to regenerate CP disease nor any demonstrable vulnerability to acquire the type of mutations, be they in *BCR-ABL* or in other critical genes, that underlie disease progression.

12.3 Cell of Origin for CP

Originally the obvious excess of granulocytes in untreated CML patients led to the conclusion that CML was a disease of the granulocytic series, hence the original designation "chronic granulocytic leukemia." As evidence accumulated in the 1970s that the Ph chromosome could be found also in cells of the erythroid, monocytic, and megakaryocytic series, the concept that the cell of origin was committed to the granulocytic series became untenable. Moreover, the fact that some cases of blastic transformation unequivocally involved cells of the B-lymphocyte lineage and even occasionally of the T-lineage led to the assumption that the acquisition of the Ph-chromosome occurred in a pluripotential stem cell which was entirely equivalent to the most primitive hematopoietic stem cell in man. This remains the most widely accepted view today. However, there are at least some data supporting the notion that acquisition of a Ph chromosome may not be the initial event in the evolution towards CP CML. For example, Fialkow and colleagues in the 1980s adduced evidence of significant chromosomal instability in a Ph-negative cell population in a female with Ph-positive CML who was heterozygous for G6PD, and suggested that the Ph chromosome developed in a clonal population already destined for malignancy (Fialkow et al. 1981). More recently, Vickers calculated that three separate mutational events may contribute towards development of CP CML (Vickers 1996). Of great interest is the recent observation that cytogenetic studies of Ph-negative cells in patients responding to IM show clonal changes in some patients (Bumm et al. 2003; Loriaux and Deininger 2004; O'Dwyer et al. 2002). This too adds weight to the notion, still highly controversial, that some Ph-negative cells in patients with Ph-positive CML are not strictly normal.

It is important to realize that the CML stem cell must have two important properties that distinguish it from its normal counterpart. First, it must have the capacity to produce or reproduce the differentiated myeloid cells that characterize the CP of CML. There must be a mechanism whereby this developing population of Ph-positive cells expresses a proliferative or survival advantage over the residual normal stem cells and induces them to remain quiescent. The results of successful treatment with IM clearly demonstrate that normal stem cells do survive, albeit invisibly, in the newly diagnosed patient. Second, the CML stem cell population must be intrinsically "programmed" to acquire new genetic lesions, some of which underlie progression to advanced phase disease. In other words, it is likely that the leukemia stem cell is genetically unstable and constantly acquiring new genetic lesions, most of which are innocuous, but some of which will eventually harm the patient. Thus the acquisition of mutations in the Bcr-Abl kinase domain is probably just one manifestation of this genetic instability, and the observation that patients in late CP have more such mutations than those newly diagnosed is consistent with the idea that these mutations accumulate with time from disease inception. Finally, it should be stressed that the CML stem cell population defined by their capacity to generate CP disease and the stem cell population vulnerable to acquisition of further genetic changes must overlap but are not necessarily "superimposable;" indeed the recent observation that at least in some cases myeloid blastic transformation appears to originate in a granulocyte-macrophage progenitor population is evidence that they are probably not the same (Jamieson et al. 2004).

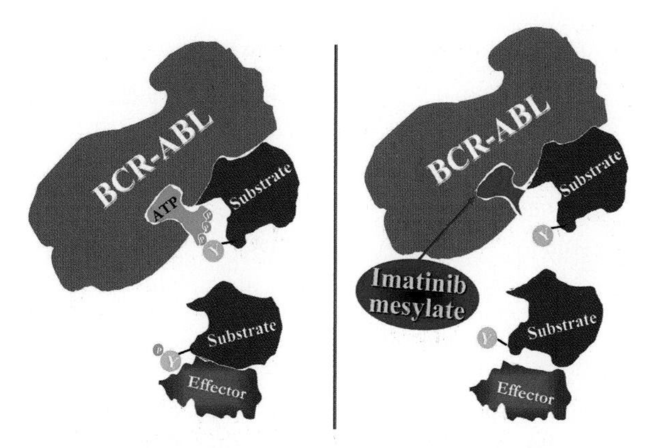

Fig. 12.3. Mode of action of IM: the *left panel* shows the Bcr-Abl oncoprotein with a molecule of ATP in the kinase binding pocket. The relevant substrate is phosphorylated on a tyrosine residue, and this induces changes in its conformation which allow it to interact with other downstream effector molecules. When IM occupies the kinase pocket (*right panel*), the substrate cannot be phosphorylated or change conformation, resulting in prevention of its binding to the next effector and interruption of the oncogenic signal transduction (Diagram prepared by Junia V. Melo and used with permission)

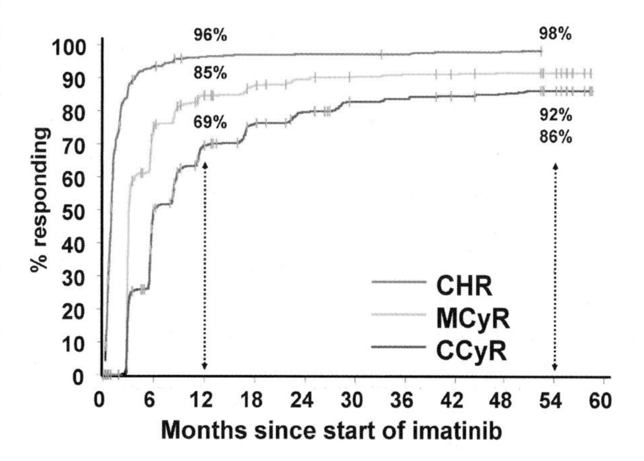

Fig. 12.4. The probability of achieving complete hematological response (CHR), major cytogenetic response (MCyR) and complete cytogenetic response (CCyR) at 12 months and 54 months for 553 patients who started treated with imatinib 400 mg/daily in the IRIS study (Adapted with permission from Simonsson 2005)

12.4 Tyrosine Kinase Inhibitors

12.4.1 Imatinib Mesylate As a Single Agent

IM is a 2-phenylaminopyrimidine compound which inhibits the enzymatic action of the activated Bcr-Abl tyrosine kinase (see Chap. 6 entitled Treatment with Tyrosine Kinase Inhibitors). It acts by occupying the ATP-binding pocket (P-loop) of the Abl kinase component of the Bcr-Abl oncoprotein and thereby blocking the capacity of the enzyme to phosphorylate downstream effector molecules (Fig. 12.3). It also binds to residues outside the P-loop and may act predominantly by holding the Abl component of the Bcr-Abl oncoprotein in an inactive configuration. It entered clinical trials in 1998 (Druker et al. 2001).

The drug rapidly reverses the clinical and hematologic abnormalities of CML and induces CHR responses in over 98% of previously untreated CP patients (Fig. 12.4). It is usually administered orally at a dose of 400 mg/day, though pilot studies suggest that initial treatment with 600 mg or even 800 mg daily may give better results (Kantarjian et al. 2003a, 2004a). Side-effects include nausea, headache, rashes, bone pains, and fluid retention. Significant cytopenias and hepatotoxicity occur less commonly. Very rare cases of severe or fatal cerebral edema have been reported (Ebonether et al. 2002). An interesting non-sinister effect, repigmentation of greying hair, has been reported in a small

Table 12.1. Cytogenetic response to IM by relative risk as defined by Sokal risk score

Sokal risk score	IRIS at 12 months* (Hughes et al. 2003)	IRIS at 42 months* (Guilhot et al. 2004)	IRIS at 54 months* (Simonsson et al. 2005)
Low	76%	91%	94%
Intermediate	67%	84%	88%
High	49%	69%	81%

* p<0.001

group of responders (Burton et al. 2002). The toxicity in general seems to be appreciably less than that associated with IFN-*α*.

A prospective randomized phase III trial designed to compare IM as a single agent with the combination of interferon alpha (IFN-*α*) with cytosine arabinoside (Ara-C) in previously untreated CP patients started in June 2000 and the interim results reported in 2004 showed that 74% of the patients treated with IM had achieved a CCyR compared with 14% of those in the control arm (O'Brien et al. 2003a). Survival without progression to advanced phase disease was significantly better in the IM-treated cohort compared to those who received IFN-*α*/Ara-C (97.2% vs. 90.3%; $p<0.001$). It is still too early to conclude with certainty that patients treated with IM have superior overall survival, though preliminary results based on a 4-year follow-up suggest that only about 2% of patients entered the advanced phases of the disease in each year on treatment. Furthermore, comparing survival in patients treated with imatinib with historical controls treated with IFN-*α* or IFN-*α* plus Ara-C provides strong support for the notion that the survival benefit with IM is likely to be appreciable (Kantarjian et al. 2004b). Several investigators have confirmed that cytogenetic and possibly the molecular response to IM is related to Sokal's risk stratification (Table 12.1) (O'Brien et al. 2003a; Simonsson et al. 2005).

12.4.2 Monitoring Patients on IM Therapy

As detailed in Chap. 9 (Monitoring Disease Response), patients responding to treatment with IM are best monitored by regular, perhaps every 3–6 months, RQ-PCR for *BCR-ABL* transcripts, which may show a steady decline to very low levels, although only a minority achieve a status where transcripts are undetectable (Hughes et al. 2003; Simonsson et al. 2005). In responding patients repeated cytogenetic studies of bone marrow are probably unnecessary, and even fluorescence in situ hybridization studies for the *BCR-ABL* gene are not sufficiently sensitive to quantitate the low levels of residual disease in patients who have achieved CCyR. Instead, RQ-PCR can adequately define the level of response and is unquestionably the best method for identifying incipient relapse, which may indicate the need for a revised therapeutic strategy (Hughes et al. 2006).

12.4.3 For How Long Should IM Therapy Be Continued?

For patients who have achieved a CCyR or near-CCyR state, a seminal question at present is whether IM can be discontinued. Currently there is a paucity of relevant data. Several case reports and a small series of 23 patients suggest that >50% relapse cytogenetically within a short time of discontinuing IM, but very occasional patients who have achieved a "transcript nondetectable" status do not immediately relapse if the drug is stopped (Cortes et al. 2004a; Rousselot et al. 2005). Rarely, patients treated with IM who achieve CCyR proceed directly to blast crisis (Avery et al. 2004; Jabbour et al. 2006). These data add to the notion that CML stem cells with proliferative potential do survive in most or all IM responders. A recent report cited the potential role of cytotoxic T-cells directed against peptides derived from proteinase 3 (myeloblastin) in patients who achieve CCyR with IFN-*α*, but not IM, which could have a significant role in the maintenance of a patient who has discontinued IM (Kurbegov et al. 2004).

12.4.4 High-Dose IM

For CP patients, most clinicians start treatment with IM at a "standard" dose of 400 mg per day. However, in one study patients treated in CP with 800 mg daily achieved more rapid cytogenetic and molecular response than historical controls treated with 400 mg daily. Toxicity was greater in those who received 800 mg daily but this problem was largely overcome by reducing the dose, when necessary, to 600 mg daily (Kantarjian et al. 2004). Along similar lines for patients who have a suboptimal response on 400 mg daily, it is reasonable to increase the dose to 600–800 mg per day; typically this strategy is effective in about a third of the patients, but the toxicity is greater, and > 60% of patients experience severe neutropenia, with > 40% experiencing a serious nonhematologic toxic effect (Cortes et al. 2003a; Kantarjian et al. 2003a). A number of global clinical trials are now comparing results of starting treatment for newly diagnosed CP patients with 400 mg daily with results using 600 or 800 mg daily.

12.4.5 Definition of IM Failure

Failure to respond to IM is in practice difficult to define because it depends on drug dosage, duration of treatment, phase of disease and, most importantly, the response criteria that one chooses to regard as most important, i.e., hematological, cytogenetic, or molecular (Goldman and Marin 2003). Failure may theoretically be primary or secondary. Primary failure describes a situation where a patient has never achieved an adequate response to IM at standard dosage. Thus, Baccarani in conjunction with colleagues on behalf of the European Leukemia-Net has proposed criteria at various time-points after starting treatment with IM that would enable a clinician to classify a given patient as a primary treatment failure (Baccarani et al. 2006). These criteria do not take account of the fact that a patient may achieve a level of response if the IM dose is increased to 600 or 800 mg (Table 12.2). The recognition of IM failure presumably means that treatment strategy should be reassessed, and it may indeed be reasonable to abandon the use of IM completely. Baccarani has also proposed a category "suboptimal response" which implies that the response is "incomplete," and though the patient may still derive substantial benefit from continuing the drug in the short term, the longer-term outlook is not likely to be "optimal." In these cases, other treatment will eventually need to be considered, possibly by an addition to rather than as replacement for imatinib.

Table 12.2. Suggested criteria for IM failure

Time	Criteria for IM failure
3 months	No evidence of an hematologic response (HR)
6 months	Less than complete hematologic response
	No evidence of a cytogenetic response (CyR)
	(Ph-positive metaphases still more than 95%)
12 months	Less than a partial cytogenetic response (PCyR)
	(Ph-positive metaphases still more than 35%)
18 months	Less than a complete cytogenetic response (CCyR)
	Less than a major molecular response (MMolR)

Table based on criteria recommended by Baccarani et al. (2006) on behalf of the European Leukemia-Net (2006).

Secondary failure describes a situation where a patient who has initially responded then loses that response. A patient who has achieved a cytogenetic remission but then relapses to Ph-positivity should be classified as a secondary failure. Likewise, a patient in cytogenetic remission whose transcript numbers rise by 1 log may also be regarded as having lost his/her response to IM (see Chap. 9). About 15% of patients with CML who start IM treatment in early CP become resistant within the first 5 years of treatment (Deininger 2005a; Kantarjian et al. 2003a). Resistance is more common in patients who start IM in "late CP" after prior treatment with other agents. It has been seen in up to 70% of those treated in myeloid blast crisis, and all of those in lymphoid blast crisis relapse within 6 months of their initial response.

12.4.6 Mechanisms of Resistance to IM

Resistance appears to result from a variety of diverse mechanisms, including amplification of the *BCR-ABL* fusion gene, relative overexpression of Bcr-Abl protein, overexpression of P-glycoprotein that enhances the cellular removal of IM, and expansion of a preexisting subclone of Ph-positive cells with point mutations in the Bcr-Abl kinase domain (Deininger et al. 2005b; Gorre et al. 2001; Griffin 2002; Mahon et al. 2000) (See also Chaps. 6 and 9). It is important to note that some CP patients with acquired resistance to IM may still respond well to other agents, such as hydroxyurea or IFN-α, while in other cases the recognition of IM resistance may coincide with or be preceded by only a short interval of clear-cut evidence of disease progression.

Patients who are either refractory or resistant to an increased dose of IM may at present be considered for an allogeneic SCT if their age and the availability of a suitable donor permit. For patients ineligible or reluctant to proceed to SCT, the best current option is to be enrolled in a clinical trial assessing the role of high-dose IM, alternative Bcr-Abl kinase inhibitors, or other investigational agents.

12.4.7 IM-Containing Combinations

Many observations have confirmed the potential synergism between IM and a number of conventional as well as investigational agents (see also Chap. 10 entitled New Therapies for Chronic Myelogenous Leukemia).

12.4.7.1 IM Plus IFN-α

In the pre-IM era, IFN-α, either alone or in combination with Ara-C was generally considered to be the best treatment for all newly diagnosed patients not eligible for allogeneic SCT (Mughal and Goldman 2001). IFN-α treatment induced a CHR in about 70–80% and a CCyR in 15–20% of patients; in those in whom the cytogenetic response was durable, there was a significant overall survival benefit. Most, if not all patients, however, continued to harbor BCR-ABL transcripts. Preliminary results from trials assessing combinations of IM and IFN-α are reasonably encouraging, but only relatively small doses of IFN-α can be tolerated in combination with full-dose IM. More recent efforts are being directed towards use of the long-acting form of IFN-α, pegylated IFN-α, which was introduced a decade ago in the hope of reducing many of the IFN-α-related toxic effects. An Italian study confirmed CCyR in 63% of the cohort, but 58% of the patients experienced toxicity, both hematologic (50%) and nonhematologic (50%) (Baccarani et al. 2004).

12.4.7.2 IM Plus Cytarabine

A small series of patients subjected to combinations of IM and low-dose cytarabine (Ara-C) suggest a CCyR in 57% but an excessive amount of side effects, both hematologic and nonhematologic were noted (Martine et al. 2002). Over 50% of all patients discontinued therapy at 9 months due to toxicity. Clinical trials are comparing the effects of combining IM with IFN-α and IM with Ara-C.

12.4.7.3 IM Plus Hypomethylating Agents

Recently there has been considerable interest in combining IM with hypomethylating agents, such as 5-azacytidine (vidaza) and 5-aza-2′-deoxycytidine (decitabine), both of which disrupt the chromatin by inhibiting DNA methylation and thus lead to gene silencing (Kornblith et al. 2000). Both agents were active when used independently in small pilot studies, and preclinical studies showed synergy when IM was added, particularly with decitabine (Issa et al. 2005; Kantarjian et al. 2003b).

12.4.7.4 IM Plus Farnesyl Transferase Inhibitors

Farnesyl transferase is an enzyme involved in the activation of Ras, an important downstream pathway activated through Bcr-Abl kinase activity. Preclinical studies showed activity of a farnesyl transferase inhibitor (FTI), lonafarnib (SCH66336) (Hoover et al. 2002) and the drug is now being tested in combination with IM in a phase I study (Cortes et al. 2004b). Another FTI, tipifarnib (R115777) has already been tested in a small phase I trial in combination with IM. The study reported cytogenetic responses in 35% of patients, including one CCyR (Cortes et al. 2003b; Gotlib et al. 2003).

12.4.7.5 IM Plus Homoharringtonine

Homoharringtonine (HHT), a semisynthetic plant alkaloid, enhances apoptosis of CML cells (Tipping et al. 2002). As a single agent, the drug has demonstrated activity in IFN-α-resistant/-refractory patients with CML (O'Brien et al. 1995). The drug was also noted to have synergism with IFN-α, and to a lesser degree, with Ara-C. In a small series the combination of HHT with IFN-α produced CCyR in about 25–30% of patients in CP (O'Brien et al. 2003b). Preliminary experience of

HHT in combination with IM in IM-resistant/-refractory patients suggests synergism (Marin et al. 2005, Tipping et al. 2002). In a very small study from the M.D. Anderson Institute, Houston, TX, involving 9 patients who had had a CCyR with IM, the addition of HHT resulted in 2 of 9 patients achieving a 1-log reduction in *BCR-ABL* transcripts (Cortes et al. 2005a). There is a case for considering use of HHT in patients with the highly resistant T315I mutation.

12.4.7.6 IM Plus Arsenic Trioxide

Arsenic trioxide (trisenox) promotes apoptosis and inhibits proliferation of blasts in CML cell lines (Du et al. 2006). Arsenicals, of course, were first introduced as "palliative" therapy of CML in the mid 19th century (see Chap. 1 entitled Chronic Myeloid Leukemia – A Brief History) and were "rediscovered" in the late 1980s for use in a number of hematologic malignancies. Preclinical and two clinical pilot studies using arsenic trioxide in combination with IM, one in IM-refractory patients in CP and the other involving patients in advanced phases, reported cytogenetic responses (Du et al. 2006; Mauro et al. 2002; Ravandi-Kashani et al. 2003). Further studies are on going.

12.4.7.7 IM Plus Bortezomib

Bortezomib (Velcade; PS341), a proteasome inhibitor, has activity in a range of hematologic malignancies (Adams et al. 1999; Cortes et al. 2003c). Preclinical studies established the drug's ability to reduce proliferation and increase apoptosis in CML (Adams et al. 1999). The preliminary results from a phase II study of IM-resistant patients, either in CP or in advanced phase, appear modestly encouraging (Cortes et al. 2003c).

12.4.7.8 IM Plus Anti-VEGF Treatments

In common with patients with other hematologic malignancies, angiogenesis appears to play a role in CML. Patients with CML have increased levels of plasma vascular endothelial growth factor (VEGF) and bone marrow vascularity (Aguayo et al. 2000; Verstovsek et al. 2003). VEGF activity might play a pivotal role in the function of dendritic cells and therefore play an immunomodulatory role. It would be reasonable to assess the combination of anti-VEGF monoclonal antibodies, such as bevacizumab (avastin) and multikinase inhibitors such as AMG706 and SU5416 (Cortes et al. 2004c).

12.4.7.9 IM Plus Leptomycin B

Preclinical studies have shown that the combination of IM and the nuclear export inhibitor leptomycin B traps Bcr-Abl inside the nucleus and leads to death of the leukemic cells (Aloisi et al. 2006). Early ex vivo studies are indicative that the sequential addition of IM and leptomycin B might generate the best response and clinical studies are anticipated in the near future. Clearly the potential neurotoxicity of leptomycin B will have to be borne in mind.

12.4.8 Second Generation Tyrosine Kinase Inhibitors

12.4.8.1 Dasatinib

Dasatinib (Sprycel, BMS-354825) is thiazole-carboxamide structurally unrelated to IM (Shah et al. 2004). It binds to the Abl kinase domain in the active (open) conformation and also inhibits some of the Src family kinases (see Chap. 6). Preclinical studies confirmed that dasatinib was 300-fold more potent than IM and is active against most known IM-resistant mutants, with the notable exception of the T315I mutant (Talpaz et al. 2005). Current results of dasatinib in patients with IM-resistant or IM-intolerant CML in CP from a phase II study of 387 evaluable patients demonstrate a CHR of 90%; major CyRs were noted in 51% with 40% achieving CCyR (Table 12.3 NEW) (Talpaz, et a.l, 2006; Hochhaus et al. 2006). With a median follow-up of 7.8 months, a 10 months progression-free survival was confirmed for 88% of patients.

Myelosuppression was the most common dasatinib-related toxicity. Non-hematological toxicity included fluid retention, in particular superficial edema and pleural and pericardial effusions in 12% of the reported cohort. Other side-effects included diarrhea, headaches, rashes, arthralgias, peripheral neuropathy and cardiac arrhythmias. About 4% of patients, including those with pleural and pericardial effusions, had grade 3-4 side-effects.

Results of dasatinib treatment in patients with the advanced phases of CML were also encouraging, though less robust. In 174 evaluable patients with IM-resistant or IM-intolerant CML in accelerated phase, major HR

Table 12.3. Dasatinib response rates for patients in various phases of CML as reported in Phase II studies. Data collated from various abstracts and published sources in 2006

	Response rate %
Chronic phase CML	
Complete hematologic response	90
Major cytogenetic response	45
Complete cytogenetic response	33
Accelerated phase CM	
Major hematologic response (CHR + NEL)	59
Major cytogenetic response	31
Complete cytogenetic response	21
Myeloid blast phase CML	
Major hematologic response (CHR + NEL)	32
Major cytogenetic response	30
Complete cytogenetic response	27
Lymphoid blast phase CML/Ph + ALL	
Major hematologic response (CHR + NEL)	35
Major cytogenetic response	54
Complete cytogenetic response	50

were observed in 59% with CHR in 33%; major CyRs were noted in 34%, with CCyR in 25% (Talpaz et al. 2006b). In 109 evaluable patients with myeloid BC, major HR were noted in 31%; in 42 evaluable patients with lymphoid BC, 26% achieved a CHR (Cortes et al. 2006; Coutre et al. 2006). The toxicity profile was similar to that seen in patients in CP. Though the follow-up was still relatively short, based on these results, the drug was granted an accelerated approval for its use in IM-resistant or IM-intolerant CML in all phases by the US regulatory agency.

12.4.8.2 Nilotinib

Nilotinib (AMN 107, Tasigna, Novartis Pharmaceuticals, Basel Switzerland) is an aminopyrimidine that is a structural derivative of IM. Compared to IM, it has a 25-fold increased potency to bind the Abl kinase domain in the inactive conformation (Weisberg et al. 2005). Preclinical studies confirmed its efficacy against all known IM-resistant mutants, other than the T315I mutant (Mestan et al. 2005). Preliminary results from 67 patients with CML in CP who were IM-resistant or IM-intolerant were reported recently. MHR were observed in 83% of the cohort, with 19% achieving a major CCyR. The drug was also found in a small series of 22 patients with the more advanced phases of CML (Kantarjian et al. 2006a, b). Major HR were noted in 64% of patients, with 45% achieving CHR. The toxicity profile revealed myelosuppression, in particular thrombocytopenia, diarrhea, rash, myalgia, arthralgia and peripheral edema.

12.5 Immunotherapy

Following the realization that a molecular remission and "cure" might not be possible with IM alone, many efforts were directed to exploring the potential of developing an active specific immunotherapy strategy for patients with CML by inducing an immune response to a tumor-specific antigen (Cathcart et al. 2004; Copland et al. 2004) (see also Chap. 11 entitled Immune Therapy of Chronic Myelogenous Leukemia). The principle involves generating an immune response to the unique amino-acid sequence of p210 at the fusion point. Clinical responses to the Bcr-Abl peptide vaccination, including CCyRs, have been reported in a small series (Bocchia et al. 2005). It is of interest that, in contrast to previous similar unsuccessful attempts, the current series included administration of GM-CSF as an immune adjuvant, and patients were only enrolled if they had measurable residual disease and HLA alleles to which the selected fusion peptides were predicted to bind avidly. If these results can be confirmed, vaccine development against Bcr-Abl and other CML-specific antigens could become an attractive treatment for patients who have achieved a minimal residual disease status with IM. Other targets for vaccine therapy now being studied include peptides derived from the Wilms tumor-1 protein, proteinase-3 and elastase, all of which are overexpressed in CML cells (Molldrem et al. 1996; Oka et al. 2004).

Another vaccine strategy which may prove useful for patients who do not achieve a CCyR to IM is a heat shock protein 70 (Hsp70) peptide complex (Srivastava, 2000; Suto et al. 1995). Heat shock proteins are antiapoptotic proteins which appear to play a major role in the immune response to CML and a number of other malignancies. They do this by inducing maturation of dendritic cells, and by induction of innate immune response including natural killer cell activation and cytokine secretion and activation of CD8+ and CD4+ lymphocytes (Pockley 2003; Srivastava 2002). In CML cells, Bcr-Abl expression is accompanied by an upregulation of Hsp70, leading to induction and activation of STAT 5 and Bcl-x_L. This in turn leads to the activation of several apoptosis signaling pathways, including caspase-9 and caspase-3. Hsp70 inhibits apoptosis and recent observations suggest that attenuated levels of Hsp70 might be a useful target for reversing Bcr-Abl-mediated resistance. A current study is exploring the use of autologous Hsp70-peptide complexes to immunize patients who appear to be either resistant to IM or fail to achieve a CCyR. Preliminary results following the recruitment of 11 patients were encouraging, with 2 of 5 patients who had completed the study achieving a complete molecular remission (Li et al. 2003).

12.6 Other Investigational Approaches

Numerous studies have also tested other specific inhibitors of signal transduction pathways downstream of Bcr-Abl alone and in combination with IM (Cortes et al. 2004c). Many of these agents have not entered formal clinical trials. Histone deacetylase inhibitors, such as LAQ824, reduce Bcr-Abl expression and apoptosis in CML cell lines from patients with advanced phase disease (Nimmanapalli et al. 2003; Yu et al. 2003). Another agent, 17-allylaminogeldanamycin (17-AAG), which degrades the Bcr-Abl oncoprotein by inhibiting the heat shock protein 90 (Hsp90), a molecular chaperone required for stabilization of Bcr-Abl, has just entered phase I studies (Nimmanapalli et al. 2001). 17-AAG appears to have activity in patients with the E255K and T315I mutations. It also downregulates *BCR-ABL* mRNA, though the precise mechanisms remain unclear. Another novel tyrosine kinase inhibitor, PD166326, also appears to have significant activity in patients with the H396P and M351T mutants (Wolff et al. 2005). This agent also appears to be superior to IM in murine models. Other potential agents include rapamycin, an mTOR inhibitor, and wortmannin and LY292004, which are PI3K inhibitors but not currently available in a formulation suitable for clinical use (Mayerhofer et al. 2005; Mohi et al. 2004; Sattler et al. 2002). Rapamycin is synergistic with IM in inhibiting Bcr-Abl-transformed cells, including those that are IM-resistant (Ly et al. 2003). Efforts are also being directed to induce apoptosis in IM-refractory cells through Apo2 ligand (also known as tumor necrosis factor-related apoptosis-inducing ligand or TRAIL) (Uno et al. 2003). Flavopiridol, a potent inhibitor of multiple cyclin-dependent kinases has also been found to potentiate IM-induced apoptosis in *Bcr-Abl*-positive cell lines (Yu et al. 2002).

Very recently a small molecule, ON012380 (Onconova Therapeutics), has been reported as active in suppressing proliferation of murine Ba/F3 cells transfected with BCR-ABL genes bearing all clinically significant mutations, including the highly resistant T315I (Gumireddy et al. 2005). Similarly to adaphostin, this compound acts very differently from the "conventional" tyrosine kinase inhibitors (Mow et al. 2002). Instead of competing with ATP to inhibit the function of the Bcr-Abl oncoprotein, it blocks the substrate binding site and so acts synergistically with IM to inhibit wild-type and mutant forms of Bcr-Abl (Fig. 12.5). In murine models, it appears to have very little toxicity at doses which appear to be maximally effective; importantly, no myelosuppression has been noted so far. The drug is now in a phase I trial. Another small molecule, VX-680 (Aurora kinase inhibitor, Vertex Pharmaceuticals, Cambridge, MA), has significant activity against the T315I BCR-ABL mutant in patient-derived samples. The molecule binds to Abl in a mode that accommodates substitution of isoleucine for threonine at the 315 position, possibly because it avoids contact with the innermost cavity of the Abl kinase domain (Young et al. 2006). A third new agent of interest is SGX-70430 (SGX Pharma, San Diego, CA), designed specifically to inhibit the T315I mutant, but with activity also against the wild-type and most of the other known Bcr-Abl mutants (Burley 2005).

12.7 Stem Cell Transplantation

12.7.1 Allogeneic SCT

For patients with CML in CP treated by allogeneic SCT with marrow from HLA-identical siblings or a matched unrelated donor, the overall leukemia-free survival at 5 years is now 80% and 60%, respectively (Weisdorf et al. 2002) (see also Chap. 7 entitled Allogeneic Transplantation for CML). The transplant-related mortality is about 20% and the chance of relapse is about 15% (Fig. 12.6). Many efforts continue to improve on this, and recently a number of factors, such as increasing

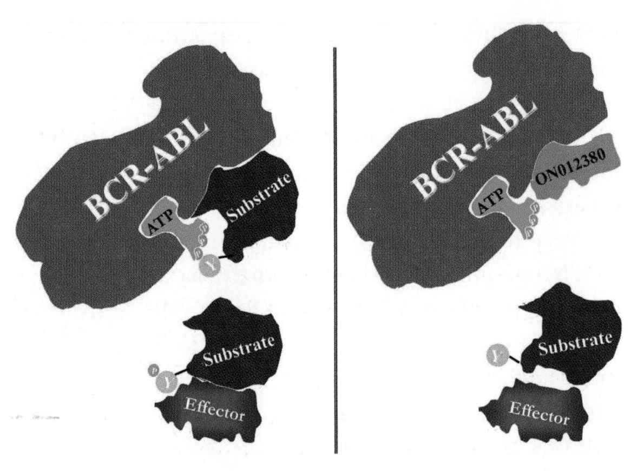

Fig. 12.5. Mode of action of ON102380 (Onconova) which blocks access to the substrate binding site of the Bcr-Abl oncoprotein (Diagram prepared by Junia V. Melo based on data reported by Gumireddy et al. 2005, and used with permission.)

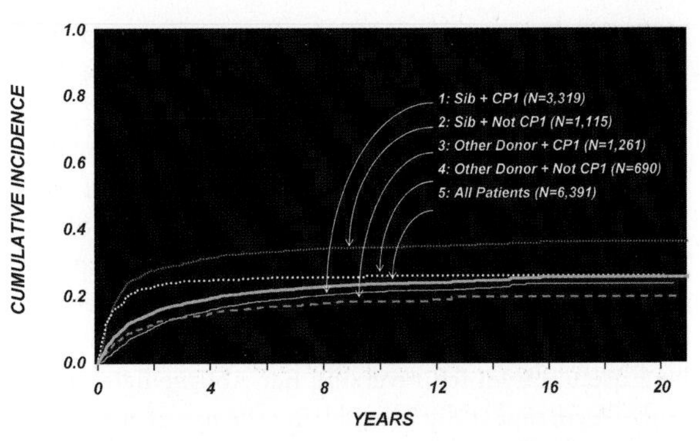

Fig. 12.6. Cumulative incidence of relapse after allogeneic SCT fron CML. Note that very occasional patients relapse more than 10 years after SCT. (Data collated by the International Bone Marrow Transplant Registry, Milwaukee, WI, 2003)

the early recovery of natural killer (NK) cells by transplanting CD34 cell doses greater than 5×10^6/kg, have been shown to be associated with better results (Savani et al. 2006). Most, but not all, patients who are negative for *BCRr-ABL* transcripts at 5 years following the SCT, remain negative for long periods and will probably never relapse (Fig. 12.1) (Mughal et al. 2001).

Currently it appears reasonable to offer a trial of IM therapy to all newly diagnosed patients, though there is conflicting data on a possible adverse effect of prior IM and there is very little information on children (Bornhäuser et al. 2006). Some clinicians feel that adult patients who are classified as "high-risk" by the Sokal criteria and "good-risk" by the European Group for Blood and Marrow Transplantation (EBMT) risk stratification score and all children should still be considered for an allogeneic SCT as a first-line therapy, provided that they have a suitable donor and indeed wish to be transplanted following an informed discussion (Gratwohl et al. 2005).

About 10–30% of patients subjected to allogeneic SCT relapse within the first 3 years post transplant (Barrett 2003). Rare patients in cytogenetic remission relapse directly into advanced phase disease without any identified intervening period of CP. There are various options for the management of relapse to CP, including use of IM, IFN-α, a second transplant using the same or another donor, or lymphocyte transfusions from the original donor. Such donor lymphocyte infusions (DLI) have gained greatly in popularity in recent years and are believed to reflect the capacity of lymphoid cells collected from the original transplant donor to mediate a "graft-versus-leukemia" (GvL) effect even though they may have failed to eradicate the leukemia at the time of the original transplant (Dazzi et al. 2000).

12.7.2 Autologous SCT

Because only a minority of patients are eligible for allogeneic SCT, much interest has focused on the possibility that life may be prolonged and some "cures" effected by autografting CML patients still in CP (Mughal et al. 1994) (see also Chap. 8 entitled Autografting in Chronic Myeloid Leukemia). It is possible that the pool of leukemic stem cells can be substantially reduced by an autograft procedure, and autografting may confer a short-term proliferative advantage on Ph-negative (presumably normal) stem cells (Carella et al. 1999). In practice, some patients have achieved temporary Ph-negative hematopoiesis after autografting. Preliminary studies have been reported in which patients have been autografted with Ph-negative stem cells collected from the peripheral blood in the recovery phase following high-dose combination chemotherapy; some such patients achieved durable Ph-negativity (Apperley et al. 2004). Currently, Ph-negative CD34+ cells have been harvested from a number of patients induced to Ph-negativity with IM, but few patients if any have been autografted with these cells (Kreuzer et al. 2004; Perseghin et al. 2005).

12.8 Treatment Options

12.8.1 Treatment of Chronic Phase Disease

There is still controversy about the best primary management of a patient who presents with CML in CP (as mentioned above). The main issues relate to the starting dose of IM and the timing of allogeneic SCT for a patient who would have been a candidate for the procedure before the advent of IM. There is no doubt that the rare patient fortunate enough to have a syngeneic twin should be considered for "up-front" transplant because the transplant-related mortality (TRM) is negligible and long-term results are excellent. The case for initial treatment with SCT for a child presenting with CML who has an HLA-identical sibling is similarly cogent because such patients have a low risk of TRM.

The optimal starting dose of IM for a new patient is not known at present. Conventionally most patients receive 400 mg daily, but 600 mg daily may give a quicker response on the basis of surrogate markers, and may possibly be associated with better overall survival. For the patient who starts treatment with IM but is subsequently judged to have failed, the choice lies between use of a second-generation tyrosine kinase inhibitor, presently either dasatinib or nilotinib, use of other experimental therapies (as mentioned above), or SCT if the patient is eligible.

12.8.2 Treatment of Advanced Phase Disease

12.8.2.1 Accelerated Phase Disease

It is difficult to make general statements about the optimal management of patients in accelerated phase disease, partly because there is no universal agreement about the definition of this phase. Patients who have not previously been treated with IM may obtain benefit from the introduction of this agent. For patients progressing to accelerated phase on IM, it is best to discontinue this drug and consider alternative strategies. Patients whose disease seems to be moving towards overt blastic transformation may benefit from appropriate cytotoxic drug combinations for acute myelogenous leukemia (AML) or acute lymphoblastic leukemia (ALL) (Mughal and Goldman 2006b). Allogeneic SCT should certainly be considered for younger patients if suitable donors can be identified. Reduced intensity conditioning allografts are probably not indicated since the efficacy of the GvL effecting advanced phase CML is not clearly established. Clinical trials exploring the use of either dasatinib or nilotinib are available for those who wish to enroll in a clinical study and the preliminary results, discussed above, are encouraging (Hochhaus et al. 2005).

12.8.2.2 Blastic Phase Disease

Patients in blastic transformation may be treated with cytotoxic drug combinations analogous to those used for AML or ALL, in the hope of prolonging life, but cure can no longer be a realistic objective. Patients in lymphoid transformation tend to fare slightly better in the short term than those in myeloid transformation (Kantarjian et al. 2002). If intensive therapy is not deemed appropriate, it is not unreasonable to use a relatively innocuous drug such a hydroxyurea at higher than usual dosage; the blast cell numbers will be reduced substantially in most cases but their numbers usually increase again within 3–6 weeks. Combination chemotherapy may restore 20% of patients to a situation resembling CP disease and this benefit may last for 3–6 months. A very small minority, probably less than 10%, may achieve substantial degrees of Ph-negative hemopoiesis. This is most likely in patients who entered blastic transformation very soon after diagnosis (Mughal and Goldman, 2006b).

IM can be remarkably effective in controlling the clinical and hematologic features of CML in advanced phases in the very short term (Sawyers et al. 2003). In some patients in established myeloid blastic transformation who received 600 mg daily massive splenomegaly was entirely reversed and blast cells were eliminated from the blood and marrow, but such responses are almost always short lived. Thus IM should be incorporated into a program of therapy that involves also use of conventional cytotoxic drugs. As in the case of accelerated phase disease, it is useful to consider patients who enter blastic phase while on IM for clinical trials using either dasatinib or nilotinib.

Allogeneic SCT using HLA-matched sibling donors can be performed in accelerated phase; the probability of leukemia-free survival at 5 years is 30–50% (Gratwohl et al. 2001). SCT performed in overt blastic transformation is nearly always unsuccessful. The mortality resulting from graft-versus-host disease is extremely high and the probability of relapse in those who survive the transplant procedure is very considerable. The probability of survival at 5 years is consequently 0–10%.

12.9 Conclusions, Decision Making, and Future Directions

The impressive success of IM in inducing CHR and CCyRs in the majority of newly diagnosed patients with CML in CP has made it the first-line therapy, at least in the developed world. Current molecular data, however, suggest that total eradication of leukemia for these patients is unlikely. Until the longer term results of IM are available, two contrasting therapeutic algorithms for patients based on prognostic factors, both disease-related such as the Sokal risk score, and treatment-related, such as the EBMT transplant risk score, can be considered (Fig. 12.7) (NCCN guidelines version 1.2006). The Sokal risk score, though derived in the pre-IM era, has recently been validated for use in IM-treated patients (Goldman et al. 2005; Simonsson et al. 2005). It is likely that other candidate disease-related prognostic factors, such as genomic profiling, will be found useful in the near future (Radich et al. 2006; Yong et al. 2006). Clearly the most robust prognostic indicators to IM treatment, so far, are the cytogenetic and molecular responses.

One treatment option involves a trial of IM or an IM-containing combination for all newly diagnosed patients. The other involves an early allogeneic SCT to suitable patients, such as those with Sokal high-risk features and EBMT low-risk CP disease, patients with syngeneic donors, and possibly children with CP disease (Baccarani et al. 2006). Patients in advanced phase disease, with the exception of those in accelerated phase based merely on extra cytogenetic changes, might also be considered for a transplant.

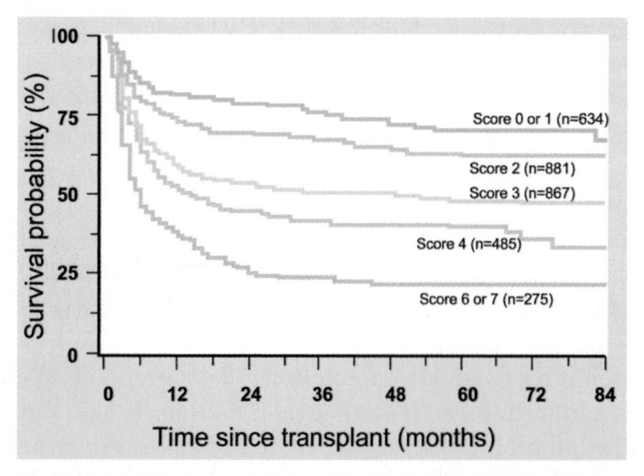

Fig. 12.7. Overall survival probability after allogeneic bone-marrow transplantation for CML according to pretransplant risk score

IM has unequivocally established the principle that molecularly targeted treatment can work and a large number of small, relatively nontoxic agents are now being studied in the laboratory. The second generation of tyrosine kinase inhibitors, such as dasatinib and nilotinib, have already been shown to have significant activity in selected patients, in both CP and the more advanced phases of the disease, who are resistant to IM.

Finally, the notion that the GvL effect is the principal reason for success in patients with CML subjected to an allograft has renewed interest in immunotherapy, and there are plans to test combinations of kinase inhibitors and various immunotherapeutic strategies in the near future.

References

Adams J, Palombella VJ, Sausville EA et al (1999) Proteasome inhibitors: a novel class of potent and effective antitumor agents. Cancer Res 59:2615–2622

Aguayo A, Kantarjian H, Manshouri T et al (2000) Angiogenesis in acute and chronic leukemias and myelodysplastic syndromes. Blood 96:2240–2245

Aloisi A, Gregorio SD, Stagno F et al (2006) BCR-ABL nuclear entrapment kills human CML cells: ex-vivo study on 35 patients with combination of imatinib mesylate and leptomycin B. Blood 107:1591–1598

Apperley JF, Boque C, Carella A et al (2004) Autografting in chronic myeloid leukaemia: a meta-analysis of six randomised trials. Bone Marrow Transplant 33 (Suppl 1):S28

Avery S, Nadal E, Marin D et al (2004) Lymphoid transformation in a CML patient in complete cytogenetic remission following treatment with imatinib. Leukemia Res 28 (Suppl 1):75–77

Baccarani M, Martinelli G, Rosti G et al (2004) Imatinib and pegylated human recombinant interferon-alpha2b in early chronic-phase chronic myeloid leukemia. Blood 104:4245–4251

Baccarani M, Saglio G, Goldman J et al (2006) Evolving concepts in the management of chronic myeloid leukemia. Recommendations from an expert panel on behalf of the European Leukemia-net. Blood 108:1835–1840

Barrett J (2003) Allogeneic stem cell transplantation for chronic myeloid leukemia. Semin Hematol 40:59–71

Bhatia M, Wang JCY, Kapp U et al (1997) Purification of primitive human hematopoietic cells capable of repopulating immune-deficient mice. Proc Nat Acad Sci USA 94:5320–5325

Bocchia M, Gentili S, Abruzzese E et al (2005) Effect of a p210 multipeptide vaccine associated with imatinib or interferon in patients with chronic myeloid leukaemia and persistent residual disease: a multicentre observational trial. Lancet 365:657–659

Bornhäuser M, Kröger N, Schwerdtfeger R et al (2006) Allogeneic haematopoietic cell transplantation for chronic myelogenous leukaemia in the era of imatinib: a retrospective multicentre study. Eur J Haematol 76:9–17

Burton C, Azzi A, Kerridge I (2002) Adverse effects after imatinib mesylate therapy. N Engl J Med 346:713

Bumm T, Muller C, Al Ali HK et al (2003) Emergence of clonal cytogenetic abnormalities in Ph-cells in some CML patients in cytogenetic remission to imatinib but restoration of polyclonal hematopoiesis in the majority. Blood 101:1941–1949

Burley S (2005) Application of FAST Fragment-based lead discovery and structure-guided design to discover small molecule inhibitors of Bcr-Abl tyrosine kinase active against the T315I imatinib-resistant mutant. Blood 106:abstract 698

Carella AM, Lerma E, Corsetti MT et al (1999) Autografting with Philadelphia chromosome negative mobilized hematopoietic progenitor cells in chronic myelogenous leukemia. Blood 83:1534–1539

Cathcart K, Pinilla-Ibarz J, Korontsvit T et al (2004) A multivalent bcr-abl fusion peptide vaccination trial in patients with chronic myeloid leukemia. Blood 103:1037–1042

Clark RE, Dodi IA, Hill SC et al (2001) Direct evidence that leukemic cells present HLA-associated immunogenic peptides from the BCR-ABL b3a2 fusion protein. Blood 98:2887–2893

Copland M, Fraser AR, Harrison SJ, Holyoake TL (2005) Targeting the silent minority: emerging immunotherapeutic strategies for eradication of malignant stem cells in chronic myeloid leukaemia. Cancer Immunol Immunother 54:297–306

Cortes J, Kantarjian H (2005) New targeted approaches in chronic myeloid leukemia. J Clin Oncol 23:6316–6324

Cortes J, Giles F, O'Brien S et al (2003 a) Result of high-dose imatinib mesylate in patients with Philadelphia chromosome-positive chronic myeloid leukemia after failure of interferon-α. Blood 102:83–86

Cortes J, Albitar M, Thomas D et al (2003 b) Efficacy of the farnesyl transferase inhibitor R115777 in chronic myeloid leukemia and other hematologic malignancies. Blood 101:1692–1697

Cortes J, Giles F, O'Brien SM et al (2003 c) Phase II study of bortezomib (Velcade, formerly PS341) for patients with imatinib-refractory chronic myeloid leukemia in chronic or accelerated phase. Blood 102:312 b, abstract 4971

Cortes J, O'Brien S, Kantarjian HM (2004 a) Discontinuation of imatinib therapy after achieving a molecular response. Blood 104:2204–2205

Cortes J, O'Brien S, Verstovsek S et al (2004 b) Phase I study of lonafarnib (SCH66336) in combination with imatinib for patients (pts) with chronic myeloid leukemia (CML) after failure to imatinib. Blood 104:288 a, abstract 1009

Cortes JE, O'Brien SM, Giles F et al (2004 c) Investigational strategies in chronic myelogenous leukemia. Hematol Oncol Clin N Am 18:619–639

Cortes J, Kim DW, Rosti G et al (2006) Dasatinib in patients with chronic myeloid leukemia in myeloid blast crisis who are resistant or intolerant to imatinib: results of the CA1800006 'START-B' Study. J Clin Oncol 24:18S, abstract 6529

Coutre S, Martinelli G, Dombret H et al (2006) Dasatinib in patients with chronic myeloid leukemia in lymphoid blast crisis or Ph-chromosome positive acute lymphoblastic leukemia (Ph+ALL) who are imatinib-resistant or intolerant: Results of the CA180015 'START-L' study. J Clin Oncol 24:18S, abstract 6528

Dazzi F, Szydlo RM, Cross NC et al (2000) Durability of responses following donor lymphocyte infusions for patients who relapse after allogeneic stem cell transplantation for chronic myeloid leukemia. Blood 96:2712–2716

Deininger MWN (2005 a) Can we afford to let sleeping dogs lie? Blood 105:1840–1841

Deininger M, Buchdunger E, Druker BJ (2005 b) The development of imatinib as a therapeutic agent for chronic myeloid leukemia. Blood 105:2640–2653

Druker BJ, Lyndon NB (2000) Lessons learned from the development of an abl tyrosine kinase inhibitor for chronic myeloid leukemia. J Clin Invest 105:3–7

Druker BJ, Tamura S, Buchdunger E et al (1996) Effects of a selective inhibitor of the Abl tyrosine kinase on the growth of BCR-ABL positive cells. Nat Med 2:561–566

Druker BJ, Talpaz M, Resta DJ et al (2001) Efficacy and safety of a specific inhibitor of the BCR-ABL tyrosine kinase in chronic myeloid leukemia. N Engl J Med 344:1031–1037

Druker BJ, Guilhot F, O'Brien S et al (2006) Five-year follow-up of imatinib therapy for newly diagnosed chronic myeloid leukemia in chronic-phase shows sustained responses and high overall survival. New Engl J Med, in press

Du Y, Wang K, Fang H et al (2006) Coordination of intrinsic, extrinsic, and endoplasmic reticulum-mediated apoptosis by imatinib mesylate combined with arsenic trioxide in chronic myeloid leukemia. Blood 107:1582–1590

Eaves AC, Barnett MJ, Ponchio L et al (1998) Differences between normal and CML stem cells: potential targets for clinical exploitation. Stem Cells 16 (Suppl 1):77–83

Ebonether M, Stentoft J, Ford J, Buhl L, Gratwohl A (2002) Cerebral edema as a possible complication of treatment with imatinib. Lancet 359:1751–1752

Eisterer W, Jiang X, Christ O et al (2005) Different subsets of primary chronic myeloid leukemia stem cells engraft immunodeficient mice and produce a model of human disease. Leukemia 19:435–411

El Ouriaghli F, Sloand E, Mainwaring L et al (2003) Clonal dominance in chronic myelogenous leukemia is associated with diminished sensitivity to the antiproliferative effects of neutrophil elastase. Blood 102:3786–3792

Fialkow PJ, Martin PJ, Najfeld, V et al (1981) Multistep origin of chronic myelogenous leukemia. Blood 58:158–163

Goldman JM, Marin D (2003) Management decisions in chronic myeloid leukemia. Semin Hematol 40:97–103

Goldman JM, Gordon MY (2006) Why do stem CML cells survive allogeneic stem cell transplantation or imatinib? Does it really matter? Leuk Lymphoma 47:1–8

Goldman JM, Hughes T, Radich J et al (2005) Continuing reduction in level of residual disease after 4 years in patients with CML in chronic phase responding to first-line imatinib (IM) in the IRIS study. Blood 106:51 a, abstract 163

Goodell MA, Rosenzweig M, Kim H et al (1997) Dye efflux studies suggest that stem cells expressing low or undetectable levels of CD34 antigen exist in multiple species. Nat Med 3:1337–1345

Gordon MY, Marley SB, Lewis JL et al (1998) Treatment with interferon-α preferentially reduces the capacity for amplification of granulocyte-macrophage progenitors (CFU-GM) from patients with chronic myeloid leukemia but spares normal CFU-GM. J Clin Invest 102:710–715

Gorre ME, Mohammed M, Ellwood K, Hsu N, Paquette R, Rao PN, Sawyers CL (2001) Clinical resistance to STI-571 cancer therapy caused by BCR-ABL gene mutation or amplification. Science 293:876–880

Gotlib J, Mauro MJ, O'Dwyer M et al (2003) Tipifarnib (Zarnestra) and imatinib (Gleevec) combination therapy in patients with advanced chronic myelogenous leukemia (CML): Preliminary results of a phase I study. Blood 102:909a, abstract 3384

Gratwohl A, Passweg J, Baldomero H et al (2001) Hematopoietic stem cell transplantation activity in Europe. Bone Marrow Transplant 27:899–916

Gratwohl A et al (2005) Does early stem cell transplant have a role in chronic myeloid leukaemia? Lancet Oncol 6:722–724

Griffin JD (2002) Resistance to targeted therapy in leukaemia. Lancet 359:458–459

Gumireddy K, Baker SJ, Cosenza SC, John P, Kang AD, Robell KA, Reddy MVR, Reddy EP (2005) A non-ATP-competitive inhibitor of BCR-ABL overrides imatinib resistance. Proc Nat Acad Sci USA 102:1992–1997

Guo Y, Lubbert M, Engelhardt M (2003) CD34– hematopoietic stem cells: current concepts. Stem Cells 21:15–20

Hochhaus A, Kantrajian H, Baccarani M et al (2006) Dasatinib in patients with chronic phase chronic myeloid leukemia who are resistant or intolerant to imatinib: Results of the CA180013 'START-C' study. J Clin Oncol 24:18S, abstract 6526

Holyoake T, Jiang X, Eaves C, Eaves A (1999) Isolation of a highly quiescent subpopulation of primitive leukemic cells in chronic myeloid leukemia. Blood 94:2056–2064

Hoover RR, Mahon FX, Melo JV, Daley GQ (2002) Overcoming STI571 resistance with farnesyl transferase inhibitor SCH66336. Blood 100:1068–1071

Hughes TP, Kaeda J, Branford S et al (2003) Frequency of major molecular responses to imatinib or interferon alfa plus cytarabine in newly diagnosed patients with chronic myeloid leukemia. N Engl J Med 349:1423–1432

Hughes TP, Deininger M, Hochhaus A et al (2006) Monitoring CML patients responding to treatment with tyrosine kinase inhibitors: Review and recommendations for harmonizing current methodology for detecting BCR-ABL transcripts and kinase domain mutations and for expressing results. Blood 168:28–37

Huntly BJ, Gilliland DG (2005) Leukemia stem cells and the evolution of cancer-stem cell research. Nat Rev Cancer 5:311–321

Issa J-P, Gharibyan V, Cortes J et al (2005) Phase II study of low-dose decitabine in patients with chronic myelogenous leukemia resistant to imatinib mesylate. J Clin Oncol 23:3948–3956

Jabbour E, Kantarjian H, O'Brien S et al (2006) Sudden blastic transformation in patients with chronic myeloid leukemia treated with imatinib mesylate. Blood 107:480–482

Jamieson CH, Ailles LE, Dylla SJ et al (2004) Granulocyte-macrophage progenitors as candidate leukemic stem cells in blast-crisis CML. N Engl J Med 351:657–667

Kaeda J, O'Shea D, Szydlo RM et al (2006) Serial measurements BCR-ABL transcripts in the peripheral blood after allogeneic stem cell transplant for chronic myeloid leukemia: An attempt to define patients who may not require further therapy. Blood 102:4121–4126

Kantarjian HM, Cortes J, O'Brien S et al (2002) Imatinib mesylate (STI571) therapy for Philadelphia chromosome-positive chronic myelogenous leukaemia in blast phase. Blood 99:3547–3553

Kantarjian HM, Talpaz M, O'Brien S et al (2003 a) Dose escalation of imatinib mesylate can overcome resistance to standard-dose therapy in patients with chronic myelogenous leukemia. Blood 101:473–475

Kantarjian HM, O'Brien S, Cortes J et al (2003 b) Results of decitabine (5-aza-2'deoxycytidine) therapy in 130 patients with chronic myelogenous leukemia. Cancer 98:522–528

Kantarjian H, Talpaz M, O'Brien S et al (2004 a) High-dose imatinib mesylate therapy in newly diagnosed Philadelphia chromosome-positive chronic phase chronic myeloid leukemia. Blood 103:2873–2878

Kantarjian HM, Cortes JE, O'Brien S et al (2004 b) Long-term survival benefit and improved complete cytogenetic and molecular response rates with imatinib mesylate in Philadelphia chromosome-positive chronic myeloid leukemia after failure of interferon-α. Blood 104:1979–1988

Kantarjian HM, Giles F, Wunderle L et al (2006 a) Nilotinib in imatinib-resistant CML and Philadelphia chromosome-positive ALL. N Engl J Med 354:2531–2541

Kantarjian HM, Gatterman N, O'Brien S et al (2006 b) A phase II study of AMN107, a novel inhibitor of bcr-abl, administered to imatinib resistant and intolerant patients with chronic myelogenous leukemia in chronic phase. J Clin Oncol 24:18S, abstract 6534

Kornblith AB, Herndon JE, Silverman LR et al (2000) Impact of azacytidine on the quality of life of patients with myelodysplastic syndrome treated in a randomized phase III trial: A cancer and Leukemia Group B study. J Clin Oncol 18:956–962

Kreuzer KA, Kluhs C, Baskaynak G et al (2004) Filgrastim-induced stem cell mobilization in chronic myeloid leukaemia patients during imatinib therapy: safety, feasibility and evidence for an efficient in vivo purging. Br J Haematol 124:195–199

Kuci S, Wessels JT, Buhring H-J et al (2003) Identification of a novel class of human adherent CD34- stem cells that give rise to SCID-repopulating cells. Blood 101:869–876

Kurbegov D, Molldrem JL (2004) Immunity to chronic myelogenous leukemia. Hematol Oncol Clin North Am 18:733–752

Lange T, Bumm T, Mueller M et al (2005) Durability of molecular remission in chronic myeloid leukemia patients treated with imatinib vs stem cell transplantation. Leukemia 19:1262–1265

Li Z, Qiao Y, Laska E et al (2003) Combination of imatinib mesylate with autologous leukocyte-derived heat shock protein 70 vaccine for chronic myelogenous leukemia. Proc Am Soc Clin Onc 14:664

Loriaux M, Deininger M (2004) Clonal abnormalities in Philadelphia chromosome negative cells in chronic myeloid leukemia patients treated with imatinib. Leuk Lymph 45:2197–2203

Ly C, Arechiga AF, Melo JV, Walsh C, Ong ST (2003) Bcr-Abl kinase modulates the transplantation regulators ribosomal protein S6 and 4E-BP1 in chronic myelogenous leukemia cells via the mammalian target of rapamycin. Cancer Res 63:5716–5722

Mahon FX, Deininger MWN, Schultheis B et al (2000) Selection and characterization of BCR-ABL positive cell lines with differential sensitivity to the tyrosine kinase inhibitor STI571: diverse mechanisms of resistance. Blood 96:1070–1079

Marin D, Kaeda JS, Andreasson C et al (2005) Phase I/II trial of adding semisynthetic homoharringtonine in chronic myeloid leukemia patients who have achieved partial or complete cytogenetic response on imatinib. Cancer 103:1850–1855

Marley SB, Gordon MY (2005) Chronic myeloid leukemia: stem cell derived but progenitor cell driven. Clin Sci (London) 109:13–25

Marley SB, Deininger MW, Davidson RJ et al (2000) The tyrosine kinase inhibitor STI571, like interferon-α, preferentially reduces the capacity for amplification of granulocyte-macrophage progenitors from patients with chronic myeloid leukemia. Exp Hematol 28:551–557

Marley SB, Davidson RJ, Lewis JL et al (2001) Progenitor cells from patients with advanced phase chronic myeloid leukemia respond to ST571 in vitro. Leuk Res 25:997–1002

Martine G, Philippe R, Michel T et al (2002) Imatinib (Gleevec) and cytarabine (Ara-C) is an effective regimen in Philadelphia-positive chronic myelogenous leukemia chronic phase patients. Blood 100:95 a, abstract 351

Mauro MJ, Deininger MWN, O'Dwyer ME et al (2002) Phase I/II study of arsenic trioxide (trisenox) in combination with imatinib mesylate (Gleevec, STI571) in patients with Gleevec-resistant chronic myelogenous leukemia in chronic phase. Blood 100, abstract 3090

Mayerhofer M, Aichberger KJ, Florian S et al (2005) Identification of mTOR as a novel bifunctional target in chronic myeloid leukemia: dissection of growth-inhibitory and VEGF-suppressive effects of rapamycin in leukemic cells. FASEB J 19:960–962

Mestan J, Brueggen J, Fabbro D et al (2005) In vivo activity of AMN107, as selective Bcr-Abl kinase inhibitor, in murine leukemia models. J Clin Oncol 23:565s, abstract 6522

Michor F, Hughes TP, Iwasa Y et al (2005) Dynamics of chronic myeloid leukaemia. Nature 435:1267–1270

Mohi MG, Boulton C, Gu T-L et al (2004) Combination of rapamycin and protein tyrosine kinase (PTK) inhibitors for the treatment of leukemias caused by oncogenic PTKs. Proc Natl Acad Sci USA 101:3130–3135

Molldrem J, Dermime S, Parker K et al (1996) Targeted T-cell therapy for human leukemia: cytotoxic T lymphocytes specific for a peptide derived from proteinase 3 preferentially lyse human myeloid leukemia cells. Blood 88:2450–2457

Molldrem JJ, Lee PP, Wang C et al (2000) Evidence that specific T lymphocytes may participate in the elimination of chronic myelogenous leukemia. Nat Med 6:1018–1023

Mughal TI, Goldman JM (2001) Chronic myeloid leukaemia: STI571 magnifies the therapeutic dilemma. Eur J Cancer 37:561–568

Mughal TI, Goldman JM (2003) Chronic myeloid leukemia: The value of tyrosine kinase inhibition. Am J Cancer 2:305–311

Mughal TI, Goldman JM (2004) Chronic myeloid leukemia: Current status and controversies. Oncology 18:837–847

Mughal TI, Goldman JM (2006 a) Molecularly targeted treatment of chronic myeloid leukemia: Beyond the imatinib era. Front Biosci 1:209–220

Mughal TI, Goldman JM (2006 b) Chronic myeloid leukemia: Why does it evolve from chronic phase to blast transformation? Front Biosci 1:198–208

Mughal TI, Hoyle C, Goldman JM (1994) Autografting for patients with chronic myeloid leukemia – the Hammersmith Experience. Stem Cell 11:20–22

Mughal TI, Yong A, Szydlo RM et al (2001) The probability of long-term leukaemia-free survival for patients in molecular remission 5 years after allogeneic stem cell transplantation for chronic myeloid leukaemia in chronic phase. Br J Haematol 115:569–574

Mow BM, Chandra J, Svingen PA et al (2002) Effects of the Bcr/abl kinase inhibitors STI571 and adaphostin (NSC 680410) on chronic myelogenous leukemia cells in vitro, Blood, 99:664–671

Nimmanapalli R, O'Bryan E, Bhalla K (2001) Geldanamycin and its analogue 17-allylamino-17-demethoxygeldanamycin lowers Bcr-Abl levels and induces apoptosis and differentiation of Bcr-Abl-positive human leukemic blasts. Cancer Res 61:1799–1804

Nimmanapalli R, Fuino L, Bali P et al (2003) Histone deacetylase inhibitor LAQ824 both lowers expression and promotes proteasomal degradation of Bcr-Abl and induces apoptosis of imatinib mesylate-sensitive or -refractory chronic myelogenous leukemia-blast crisis cells. Cancer Res 63:5126–5135

O'Brien S, Kantarjian H, Keating M et al (1995) Homoharringtonine therapy induces responses in patients with chronic myelogenous leukemia in late chronic phase. Blood 86:3322–3326

O'Brien SG, Guilhot F, Larson RA et al (2003 a) Imatinib compared with interferon and low dose cytarabine for newly diagnosed chronic-phase chronic myeloid leukemia. N Engl J Med 348:994–1004

O'Brien S, Giles F, Talpaz M et al (2003 b) Results of triple therapy with interferon-alfa, cytarabine, and homoharringtonine, and the impact of adding imatinib to treatment sequence in patients with Philadelphia chromosome-positive chronic myelogenous leukemia in early chronic phase. Cancer 98:888–893

O'Dwyer ME, Mauro MJ, Kurilik G et al (2002) The impact of clonal evolution on response to imatinib mesylate (STI571) in accelerated phase CML. Blood 100:1628–1633

Ogawa M, Fried J, Sakai A, Clarkson BD (1970) Studies of cellular proliferation in human leukemia. IV. The proliferative activity, generation time and emergence time of neutrophilic granulocytes in chronic granulocytic leukemia. Cancer 25:1031–1049

Oka Y, Tsuboi A, Taguchi T et al (2004) Induction of WTI (Wilms tumor gene)-specific cytotoxic T lymphocytes by WTI peptide vaccine and the resultant cancer regression. PNAS 101:13885–13890

Pardal R, Clark MF, Morrison SJ (2003) Applying the principles of stem-cell biology to cancer. Nat Rev Cancer 3:895–902

Perseghin P, Gambacorti-Passerini C, Tornaghi L et al (2005) Peripheral blood progenitor cell collection in chronic myeloid leukemia patients with complete cytogenetic response after treatment with imatinib mesylate. Transfusion 45:1214–1220

Pockley AG (2003) Heat shock proteins as regulators of the immune response. Lancet 362:469–476

Preffer FI, Dombkowski D, Sykes M et al (2002) Lineage-negative side-population with restricted hematopoietic capacity circulate in normal adult blood: Immunophenoptypic and functional characterization. Stem Cells 20:417–427

Press RD, Love Z, Tronnes AA et al (2006) BCR-ABL mRNA levels at and after the time of complete cytogenetic response (CCR) predict the duration of CCR in imatinib-treated patients with CML. Blood 102:4250–4256

Radich J, Dai HD, Mao M et al (2006) Gene expression changes associated with progression and response in chronic myeloid leukemia. Proc Natl Acad Sci USA 103:2794–2799

Ravandi-Kashani F, Ridgeway J, Nishimura S et al (2003) Pilot study of combination of imatinib mesylate and Trisenox (As2O3) in patients with accelerated and blast phase CML. Blood 102:314 b, abstract 4977

Reya T, Morrison SJ, Clarke MF, Weissman IL (2001) Stem cells, cancer and cancer stem cells. Nature 414:105–111

Rousselot O, Huguet F, Rea D et al (2006) Imatinib mesylate discontinuation in patients with chronic myelogenous leukemia in complete molecular remission for more than 2 years. Blood, DOI 10.1882/blood-2006-03-011239

Sattler M, Mohi MG, Pride YB et al (2002) Critical role for Gab2 in transformation by BCR/ABL. Cancer Cell 1:479–492

Savani BN, Rezvani K, Mielke S et al (2006) Factors associated with early molecular remission after T cell-depleted allogeneic stem cell transplantation for chronic myelogenous leukemia. Blood 107:1688–1695

Sawyers CL, Hochhaus A, Feldman E et al (2002) Imatinib induces hematologic and cytogenetic responses in patients with chronic myelogenous leukemia in myeloid blast crisis: results of a phase II study. Blood 99:3530–3539

Shah NP, Tran C, Lee FY et al (2004) Overriding imatinib resistance with a novel ABL kinase inhibitor. Science 305:399–401

Simonsson B for the IRIS study group (2005) Beneficial effects of cytogenetic and molecular response on long-term outcome in patients with newly diagnosed chronic myeloid leukemia in chronic phase (CML-CP) treated with imatinib (IM): Update from the IRIS study. Blood 106:52a, abstract 166

Srivastava PK (2000) Immunotherapy of human cancer: lessons from mice. Nat Immunol 1:363–366

Srivastava PK (2002) Roles of heat-shock proteins in innate and adaptive immunity. Nat Rev Immunol 2:185–194

Suto R, Srivastava PK (1995) A mechanism for the specific immunogenicity of heat shock protein-chaperoned peptides. Science 269:1585–1588

Talpaz M, Rousselot P, Kim DW et al (2005) A phase II study of dasatinib in patients with chronic myeloid leukemia (CML) in myeloid blast crisis who are resistant or intolerant to imatinib: First results of the CA180006 'START-B' study. Blood 106:16a, abstract 40

Talpaz M, Shah NP, Kantarjian H et al (2006a) Dasatinib in imatinib-resistant Philadelphia chromosome-positive leukemias. N Engl J Med 354:2531–2541

Talpaz M, Apperley JF, Kim DW et al (2006b) Dasatinib in patients with accelerated phase chronic myeloid leukemia who are resistant or intolerant to imatinib: Results of the CA1800006 'START-B' study. J Clin Oncol 24:18S, abstract 6526

Tipping AJ, Mahon FX, Zafiridis G et al (2002) Drug responses of imatinib mesylate-resistant cells: synergism of imatinib with other chemotherapeutic agents. Leukemia 16:2349–2357

Uchida N, Fujisaki T, Eaves AC, Eaves CJ (2001) Transplantable hematopoietic stem cells in human fetal liver have a CD34+ side population (SP) phenotype. J Clin Invest 108:1071–1077

Udomsakdi C, Eaves C, Swolin B et al (1992) Rapid decline of chronic myeloid leukemia cells in long term culture due to a defect at the leukemic stem cell level. Proc Nat Acad Sci USA 89:6192–6196

Uno K, Inukai T, Kayagaki N et al (2003) TNF-related apoptosis-inducing ligand (TRAIL) frequently induces apoptosis in Philadelphia chromosome-positive leukemia cells. Blood 101:3658–3667

Verstovsek S, Lunin S, Kantarjian H et al (2003) Clinical relevance of VEGF receptors 1 and 2 in patients with chronic myeloid leukemia. Leuk Res 27:661–669

Vickers M (1996) Estimation of the number of mutations necessary to cause chronic myeloid leukaemia from epidemiological data. Br J Haematol 94:1–4

Wang JCY, Lapidot T, Cashman JD et al (1998) High level engraftment of NOD/SCID mice by primitive normal and leukemic hematopoietic cells from patients with chronic myeloid leukemia in chronic phase. Blood 91:2406–2414

Weisberg E, Manley PW, Breitenstein W et al (2005) Characterization of AMN 107, a selective inhibitor of native and mutant Bcr-Ab l. Cancer Cell 7:129–141

Weisdorf DJ, Anasetti C, Antin JH et al (2002) Allogeneic bone marrow transplantation for chronic myelogenous leukemia: comparative analysis of unrelated versus matched sibling donor transplantation. Blood 99:1971–1977

Wolff NC, Veach DR, Tong WP et al (2005) PD166326, a novel tyrosine kinase inhibitor, has greater antileukemic activity than imatinib mesylate in a murine model of chronic myelogenous leukemia. Blood 105:3995–4003

Xue S-A, Gao L, Hart D et al (2005) Elimination of human leukemia cells in NOD/SCID mice by WT1-TCR gene transduced human T cells. Blood 106:3062–3067

Yong ASM, Szydlo RM, Goldman JM et al (2005) Molecular profiling of CD34+ cells identifies low expression of CD7 with high expression of proteinase 3 or elastase as predictors for longer survival in CML patients. Blood 107:205–212

Young MA, Shah NP, Chao LH et al (2006) Structure of the kinase domain of an imatinib-resistant Abl mutant in complex with the Aurora kinase inhibitor VX-680. Cancer Res 66:1007–1014

Yu C, Krystal G, Dent P et al (2002) Flavopiridol potentiates STI571-induced mitochondrial damage and apoptosis in BCR-ABL-positive human leukemia cells. Clin Cancer Res 8:2976–2984

Yu C, Rahmani M, Conrad D, Subler M, Dent P, Grant S (2003) The proteasome inhibitor bortezomib interacts synergistically with histone deacetylase inhibitors to induce apoptosis in Bcr/Abl+ cells sensitive and resistant to STI571. Blood 102:3765–3774

Zeng Y, Graner MW, Thompson S et al (2005) Induction of BCR-ABL-specific immunity following vaccination with chaperone rich lysates from BCR-ABL+ tumor cells. Blood 105:2016–2022

Zhou S, Schuetz JD, Bunting KD et al (2001) The ABC transporter Bcrp1/ABCG2 is expressed in a wide variety of stem cells and is a molecular determinant of the side-population phenotype. Nat Med 7:1028–1034

BCR-ABL-Negative Chronic Myeloid Leukemia

Nicholas C. P. Cross and Andreas Reiter

Contents

Abstract. Acquired constitutive activation of protein tyrosine kinases is a central feature of myeloproliferative disorders, including *BCR-ABL*-negative chronic myeloid leukaemia (CML). Genes that are most commonly involved are those encoding the receptor tyrosine kinases *PDGFRA*, *PDGFRB*, *FGFR1*, and the nonreceptor tyrosine kinases *JAK2* and *ABL*, although no abnormality is specific to BCR-ABL-negative CML. Activation occurs as a consequence of specific point mutations or fusion genes generated by chromosomal translocations, insertions or deletions. Mutant kinases are constitutively active in the absence of the natural ligands and are generally believed to be primary abnormalities that deregulate hemopoiesis in a manner analogous to BCR-ABL. With the advent of targeted signal transduction therapy, an accurate molecular diagnosis of BCR-ABL-negative CML and related disorders by morphology, karyotyping, and molecular genetics has become increasingly important. Imatinib induces high response rates in patients associated with activation of ABL, PDGFR and PDGFR. Other inhibitors under development are promising candidates for effective treatment of patients with constitutive activation of other tyrosine kinases.

13.1 Classification and Identification of *BCR-ABL*-Negative CML

The chronic myeloproliferative disorders (CMPD) are clonal diseases characterized by excess proliferation of cells from one or more myeloid lineages. Proliferation is accompanied by relatively normal maturation, resulting in increased numbers of leukocytes in the peripheral blood. The most common CMPDs are chronic myeloid leukaemia (CML), polycythaemia vera (PV), essential thrombocythaemia (ET), and idiopathic myelofibrosis (IMF). The majority of cases can be categorized as one of these entities by standard clinical and morphological investigations plus, in the case of CML, the detection of the Philadelphia (Ph) chromosome and/or the *BCR-ABL* fusion (Vardiman et al. 2002).

Although conventional cytogenetic analysis reveals the classic t(9;22)(q34;q11) in most CML cases, about 10% have a variant translocation (De Braekeleer 1987). These are usually complex variants involving one or more chromosomes in addition to chromosomes 9 and 22, or simple variants that typically involve chromosomes 22 and a chromosome other than 9 (Chase et al. 2001). The overwhelming majority of these cases are positive for *BCR-ABL*, and confirmation of the presence of this fusion is usually made by reverse transcription polymerase chain reaction (RT-PCR) to detect *BCR-ABL* mRNA in cell extracts, or fluorescence in situ hybridization (FISH) to detect the juxtaposition of the *BCR* and *ABL* genes in fixed metaphase or interphase cells. It is important to be aware of the existence of rare variant *BCR-ABL* mRNA fusions in roughly 1% of cases (Barnes and Melo 2002) that may not be detectable by some commonly used PCR primer sets, and also that it is possible for FISH to miss *BCR-ABL* positive cases, although this seems to be very uncommon. In addition, some translocations that look like simple variants of the Ph-chromosome, e.g., the t(4;22)(q12;q11), t(8;22)(p11;q11) or t(9;22)(p24;q11) do not actually involve *ABL*, but instead result in *BCR-PDGFRA*, *BCR-FGFR1*, or *BCR-JAK2* fusions, respectively (Baxter et al. 2002; Demiroglu et al. 2001; Griesinger et al. 2005).

A further 10% of patients with clinical and morphological features of CML are Ph negative without apparent rearrangement of chromosomes 9 or 22. In roughly half of these cases *BCR-ABL* is detected by molecular methods and thus the term "Ph-negative CML" should be avoided (Chase et al. 2001; Hild and Fonatsch 1990). The remaining 5% of cases have historically been referred to as "*BCR-ABL*-negative CML," although this entity is not formally recognized under the current World Health Organization (WHO) classification. The features of these cases are heterogeneous and overlap with other WHO-recognized subtypes of CMPD or myelodysplastic/myeloproliferative disorders (MDS/MPD), particularly atypical CML (aCML), chronic eosinophilic leukemia (CEL), and chronic myelomonocytic leukemia (CMML). *BCR-ABL*-negative CML can thus be viewed as part of a spectrum of clinically related disorders which share a related molecular pathogenesis.

13.2 Mutated Tyrosine Kinases in *BCR-ABL*-Negative CML

13.2.1 Cytogenetic Abnormalities

The great majority of *BCR-ABL*-negative MPDs present with a normal or aneuploid karyotype, i.e., gains or losses of whole chromosomes, and thus there are no clues at this level of analysis to indicate what underlying abnormalities are driving aberrant proliferation of myeloid cells. A small subset of cases, however, present with

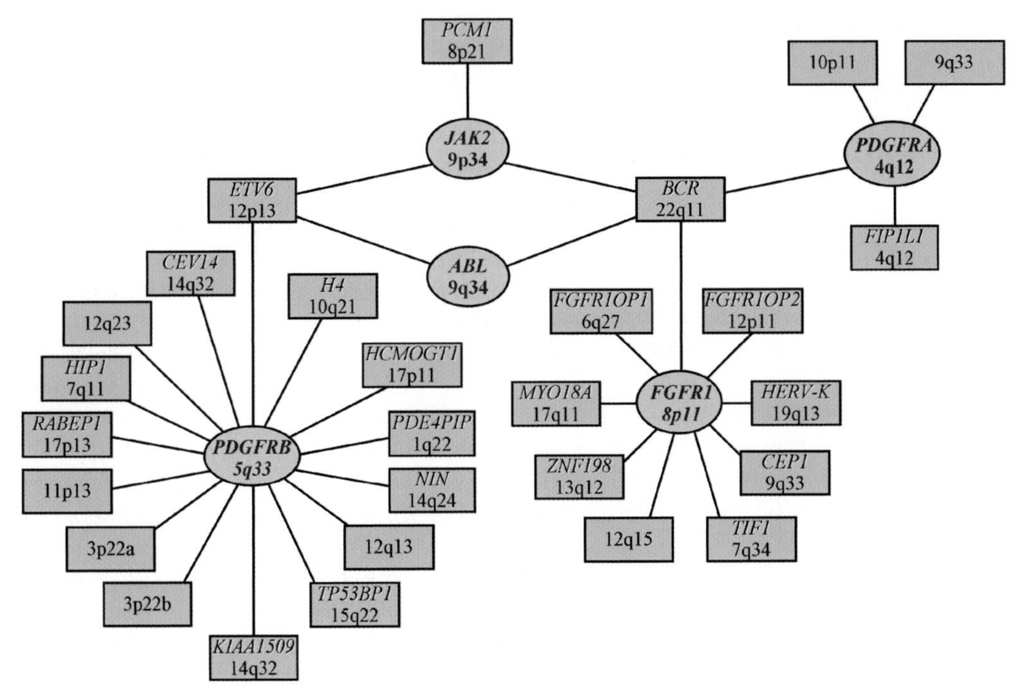

Fig. 13.1. Network of tyrosine kinase fusion genes in *BCR-ABL*-negative CML and related conditions. Tyrosine kinases are shown in *blue* with partner genes in *green* and the cytogenetic location of each gene is indicated. Partner genes that are unpublished as of January 2006 are indicated by cytogenetic location only

reciprocal chromosomal translocations, and although these are uncommon, they have turned out to be highly informative. The first recurrent abnormality to be identified was the t(5;12)(p13;q31-33) and to date more than 50 cases have been described in association with atypical CML, CMML, CEL, MDS, IMF, acute myeloid leukemia (AML), and unclassified CMPD (Greipp et al. 2004; Steer and Cross 2002). Many other translocations have been reported that are apparently unique but accumulating reports indicated the presence of at least four recurrent breakpoint clusters at 4q11-12, 5q31-33, 8p11-12 and 9p24. Molecular analysis has shown that these translocations target the tyrosine kinase genes *PDGFRA*, *PDGFRB*, *FGFR1*, and *JAK2*, respectively (Fig. 13.1). Tyrosine kinases are enzymes that catalyze the transfer of phosphate from ATP to tyrosine residues in their own cytoplasmic domains (autophosphorylation) and tyrosines of other intracellular proteins. Tyrosine kinases are normally tightly regulated signaling proteins that impact on proliferation, differentiation, and apoptosis (Hunter 1998). Overall there are believed to be in the region of 90 receptor tyrosine kinases (RTKs) and nonreceptor tyrosine kinases (NRTKs) in the human genome (Manning et al. 2002). Translocations that target tyrosine kinases produce fusions genes encoding novel chimeric proteins with a common generic structure: an amino terminal "partner" protein that retains one or more dimerization/oligomerization motifs fused to the carboxy terminal part of the protein tyrosine kinase, and including the entire catalytic domain.

13.2.2 *PDGFRA* Fusion Genes

13.2.2.1 *BCR-PDGFRA*

The first reported fusion gene to involve *PDGFRA* was cloned from two patients with atypical *BCR-ABL*-negative CML, both of whom had a t(4;22)(q12;q11) (Baxter et al. 2002). Two further patients have been reported (Safley et al. 2004; Trempat et al. 2003) and we are aware of three additional cases with this fusion. One patient progressed to B-cell acute lymphoblastic leukemia (ALL), another presented with B-ALL and a third had T-lymphoid extramedullary disease, clearly indicating that the disease, like CML, is a stem cell disorder. The breaks within *BCR* were variable and unusually the genomic breakpoints in two of the three characterized cases fell within a *PDGFRA* exon, with *BCR* intron sequence being incorporated into the mature fusion mRNA (Baxter et al. 2002).

13.2.2.2 *FIP1L1-PDGFRA*

To date, the most common known PDGFR fusion is *FIP1L1-PDGFRA*, which is generated by a cytogenetically invisible 800-kb interstitial deletion on chromosome 4q12 (Cools et al. 2003a; Griffin et al. 2003). This abnormality is normally associated with CEL (typically presenting as idiopathic hypereosinophilic syndrome; HES or systemic mastocytosis with eosinophilia), although it also seen in very occasional cases with atypical CML (NCPC, unpublished observations). As above, the breakpoints within *FIP1L1* are variable and a number of different exons are fused to *PDGFRA*. Of note, *PDGFRA* breakpoints in the fusion mRNA for both *FIP1L1-PDGFRA* and *BCR-PDGFRA* are located within *PDGFRA* exon 12, a highly unusual finding that is presumably strongly selected for (see below). In addition to the breakpoint variability, *FIP1L1* is subject to a high level of alternative splicing and, furthermore, a number of different cryptic splice sites may be utilized during splicing of the fusion transcripts (Cools et al. 2003a; Walz et al. 2004). Consequently patients may express several different mRNA fusions of variable length, some of which do not preserve the correct reading frame. This has important implications for strategies for molecular detection and development of quantitative RT-PCR assays to determine response to treatment. Furthermore, variant breakpoints may result in mRNA fusions that are difficult to amplify with standard primer sets, even in untreated patients (NCPC and AR, unpublished data). Comprehensive screening for *FIP1L1-PDGFRA* should therefore include fluorescence in situ hybridization analysis to detect *CHIC* deletion (a surrogate marker for the fusion; Cools et al., 2003) in addition to RT-PCR.

13.2.3 *PDGFRB* Fusion Genes

13.2.3.1 Multiple *PDGFRB* Partner Genes

To date, nine *PDGFRB* gene fusions have been described in MPDs: the t(5;12)(q33;p12), t(5;7)(q33;q11), t(5;10)(q33;q21), t(5;17)(q33;p13), t(1;5)(q23;q33), t(5;17) (q33;p11), t(5;14)(q33;q24), t(5;14)(q33;q32) and t(5;15) (q33;q22) fuse *ETV6* (*TEL*), *HIP1*, *H4/D10S170*, *RABEP1*, *PDE4DIP* (Myomegalin), *HCMOGT*, *NIN*, *KIAA1509*, and *TP53BP1*, respectively, to *PDGFRB* (Golub et al. 1994; Grand et al. 2004b; Kulkarni et al. 2000; Levine et al. 2005b; Magnusson et al. 2001; Morerio et al. 2004; Ross et al. 1998; Schwaller et al. 2001; Vizmanos et al. 2004b; Wilkinson et al. 2003). Of these, *ETV6-PDGFRB* is the best characterized and most frequently observed, although it is very rare (Greipp et al. 2004). All of the other *PDGFRB* fusions are extremely uncommon and most have only been reported in single individuals. A tenth fusion, *TRIP11-PDGFRB* (formerly *CEV14-PDGFRB*) has been described in a patient who acquired a t(5;14)(q33;q32) as a secondary abnormality at relapse of AML (Abe et al. 1997).

13.2.3.2 Clinical Features of Cases with *PDGFRB* Rearrangements

Patients with a rearrangement of the *PDGFRB* gene have a very wide age range (3–84 years), can present with a variable degree of monocytosis and thus have features that are generally suggestive of both CML and CMML (Apperley et al. 2002; Bain 1996; Gotlib 2005; Greipp et al. 2004; Steer and Cross 2002). Both *PDGFRA* and *PDGFRB* fusions are predominantly associated with males (approximately 8:1 male:female ratio). Because of broader clinical and laboratory findings, patients have typically been diagnosed as having aCML, CMML, MDS/MPD, or juvenile myelomonocytic leukemia (JMML). Eosinophilia is usually present but a lack of eosinophilia does not exclude involvement of *PDGFRB*. Other typical features of MPDs such as elevated hematocrit, thrombocytosis, or basophilia are uncommon. Since the number of cases reported with variant translocations is so small, it is not possible to discern if there are any phenotypic differences between patients with different *PDGFRB* fusions.

13.2.3.3 Cytogenetics and *PDGFRB* Rearrangements

The chromosomal 5q breakpoints underlying these fusion genes are variable and have been assigned from 5q31-33. Furthermore, alternative fusion genes with rearrangements of 5q31-35 but without involvement of *PDGFRB* have been described in a variety of related hematological disorders, including MDS and AML (Borkhardt et al. 2000; Jaju et al. 2001; Taki et al. 1999; Yoneda-Kato et al. 1996). This means that the involvement of the *PDGFRB* gene can neither be confirmed nor excluded by cytogenetic analysis. Dual-color FISH can confirm rearrangement of *PDGFRB*; however, the interpretation of results may sometimes be difficult and potentially lead to false-negative results in occasional cases due to complex translocations (Kulkarni et al. 2000). FISH analysis has nevertheless demonstrated disruption of *PDGFRB* in patients with thus far uncharacterized 5q translocations, suggesting that several other partner genes remain to be identified (Baxter et al. 2003).

13.2.3.4 Breakpoints in *PDGFR* Fusion Genes

Despite sharing extensive homology, different breakpoint patterns have emerged for fusions involving *PDGFRA* and *PDGFRB* fusion genes. The genomic breakpoints for *PDGFRA* fall within intron 11 or exon 12 which, after splicing, leads to an mRNA fusion of the partner gene to a truncated *PDGFRA* exon 12. The predicted fusion proteins therefore lack part of the WW domain within the juxtamembrane region, a protein–protein interaction motif that is believed to mediate both positive and negative regulatory roles (Chen et al. 2004c). In contrast, the genomic breakpoints in *PDGFRB* are intronic and consequently fusions involving this gene retain the WW domain. A variant breakpoint has been reported in only a single case in which *NIN* is fused to *PDGFRB* exon 12 and therefore the WW domain is lost (Vizmanos et al. 2004b). This indicates that the WW domain is not required for transformation by *PDGFRB* fusion genes, but why disruption of this motif appears to be selected for in *PDGFRA* but not *PDGFRB* fusions is currently unclear.

13.2.4 *FGFR1* Fusion Genes

13.2.4.1 Clinical Presentation

The terms "8p11 myeloproliferative syndrome (EMS)" or "stem cell leukemia-lymphoma syndrome (SCLL)" have been suggested for the distinctive and again very rare disease associated with 8p11-12 translocations and rearrangement of *FGFR1* (Inhorn et al. 1995; Macdonald et al. 1995, 2002). The majority of EMS patients present with typical features of MDS/MPD like disease including leukocytosis, a hypercellular marrow, and splenomegaly. Marked eosinophilia in the peripheral blood and/or bone marrow is usually but not always present. EMS can resemble CMML and aCML, but the distinguishing feature of this condition is the strikingly high incidence of coexisting non-Hodgkins lymphoma that may be either of B- or, more commonly, T-cell phenotype. In many cases lymphadenopathy is present at diagnosis, whereas in others it appears during the course of the disease. EMS is an aggressive disease and rapidly transforms to acute leukemia, usually of myeloid phenotype, within 1 or 2 years of diagnosis. The median time to transformation is only 6–9 months and thus far the only effective treatment for this condition appears to be allogeneic bone marrow transplantation (Inhorn et al. 1995, 2002).

13.2.4.2 Diversity of *FGFR1* Fusions

To date, eight different *FGFR1* fusions have been described in EMS: the t(6;8)(q27;p11), t(7;8)(q34;q11), t(8;9)(p11;q33), ins(12;8)(p11;p11p21), t(8;13)(p11;q12), t(8;17) (p11;q25), t(8;19)(p12;q13) and t(8;22)(p11;q22) fuse *FGFR1OP* (also known as *FOP*), *TIF1*, *CEP1*, *FGFR1OP2*, *ZNF198*, *MYO18A*, *HERV-K*, and *BCR* to *FGFR1*, respectively (Belloni et al. 2005; Demiroglu et al. 2001; Fioretos et al. 2001; Grand et al. 2003; Guasch et al. 2000; 2003b; Popovici et al. 1998, 1999; Reiter et al. 1998; Smedley et al. 1998b; Walz et al. 2005; Xiao et al., 1998). All mRNA fusions described to date involve *FGFR1* exon 9.

13.2.4.3 Influence of the Partner Gene on Disease Phenotype

Despite the small number of cases reported in the literature there has been increasing evidence that different *FGFR1* partner genes are associated with subtly different disease phenotypes. For example, some patients with a t(6;8) and a *FGFR1OP-FGFR1* fusion were diagnosed initially as having PV (Popovici et al. 1999; Vizmanos et al. 2004a). Thrombocytosis and monocytosis have been described relatively frequently in patients with a t(8;9), and thus the disease with this translocation resembles CMML but without major dysplastic signs in either lineage (Guasch et al. 2000; Macdonald et al. 2002). The incidence of T-cell non-Hodgkin's lymphoma (T-NHL) appears to be considerably higher in cases that present with a t(8;13) compared to patients with variant translocations (Macdonald et al. 2002). Strikingly, patients that have been described with a t(8;22) and a *BCR-FGFR1* fusion had a clinical and morphological picture that was very similar to typical, *BCR-ABL*-positive CML (Demiroglu et al. 2001; Fioretos et al. 2001; Pini et al. 2002), although one case that was studied in detail also showed evidence of lymphoproliferation (Murati et al. 2005a). These patients also had basophilia, a feature that is uncommon in *BCR-ABL*-negative MPDs and is rare in EMS with other *FGFR1* partner genes. It was proposed therefore that the BCR moiety of the fusion might directly contribute to the specific clinical features that are characteristic of CML, a hypothesis that has been borne out by detailed studies using murine models (see below).

13.2.5 *JAK2* Fusions Genes

13.2.5.1 *JAK2* Fusions in CML-Like Diseases

The first evidence that *JAK2* is causally involved in the development of a MPD stems from the discovery of the *ETV6-JAK2* as a consequence of the t(9;12)(p24; p13) in aCML and ALL (Lacronique et al. 1997; Peeters et al. 1997). Recently, we identified a series of patients, including five with aCML or CEL, with a t(8;9)(p21-23;p23-24) and *PCM1-JAK2* fusion (Reiter et al. 2005). Other cases have subsequently been reported and this fusion is also seen in association with ALL or AML (Murati et al. 2005b). A single patient has also been described with a CML-like disease and a *BCR-JAK2* fusion (Griesinger et al. 2005). As described above for *PDGFR* fusion genes, *JAK2* fusions are predominantly seen in males and currently the reasons for these marked sex biases remain obscure. A much smaller but nevertheless significant male excess is also seen in *BCR-ABL*-positive CML (Ries et al. 2003), but no obvious differences have been seen for patients with *FGFR1* fusions (Macdonald et al. 2002). Significant male excesses have also been described in subsets of other hematological malignancies, for example young patients with non-Hodgkin's lymphoma or Hodgkin's disease and middle aged patients with chronic lymphocytic leukemia or lymphocytic lymphoma (Cartwright et al. 2002).

13.2.6 The V617F *JAK2* Mutation

13.2.6.1 V617F Is the Most Common Abnormality in *BCR-ABL*-Negative CML

Very recently, *JAK2* has emerged as the single most important factor in MPDs (see Chaps. 15 Chronic Idiopathic Myelofibrosis, 16 Polycythemia Vera – Clinical Aspects, and 18 Essential Thrombocythemia). A single point mutation in exon 12 (or exon 14 depending on the reference sequence used for numbering) encoding for the pseudokinase (JH2) domain was identified in >80% of patients with PV and roughly 40–50% of patients with ET and IMF, respectively (Baxter et al. 2005; James et al. 2005; Kralovics et al. 2005; Levine et al. 2005a). The mutation occurs at nucleotide 1849 (amino acid residue 617) where a guanine is replaced with a thymine resulting in a valine to phenylalanine substitution at codon 617 (V617F). In addition to classical MPDs, we and others have observed V617F *JAK2* in 17–19% of patients with *BCR-ABL*-negative CML and 3–13% of cases with CMML (Jelinek et al. 2005; Jones et al. 2005; Steensma et al. 2005). V617F was not seen in patients with *BCR-ABL*-positive CML, nor in any case with any other tyrosine kinase fusion (Jones et al. 2005). The mutation is thus the most common abnormality described to date in *BCR-ABL*-negative CML. Peripheral

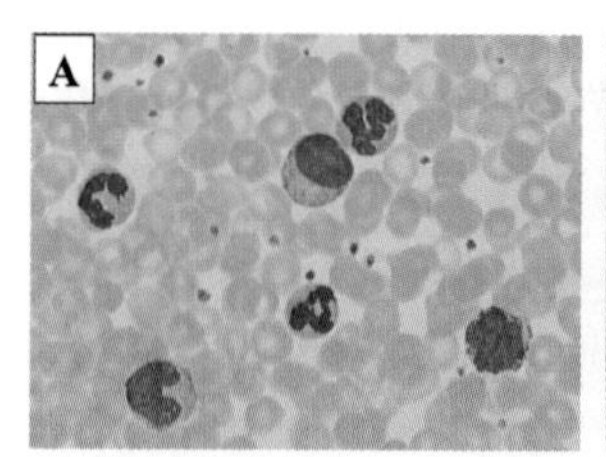

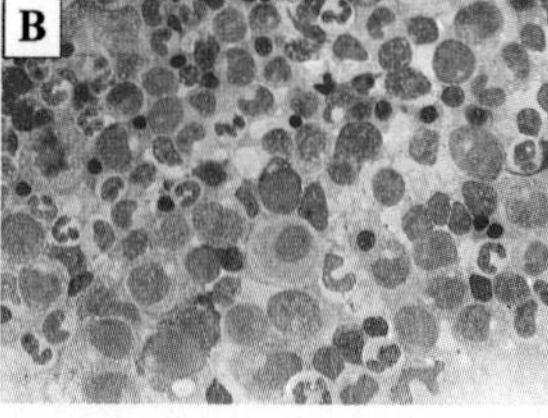

Fig. 13.2. Bone marrow and peripheral blood morphology in a case of V617F *JAK2*-positive atypical CML. **(A)** Peripheral blood smear showing a leukocytosis with pathological left shift of granulopoiesis and an increase of basophils (May-Grünwald-Giemsa, Zeiss Plan-Apochromat ×63). **(B)** Bone marrow smear showing an increased cellularity with prominent neutrophil granulopoiesis and abnormal micromegakaryocytes (May-Grünwald-Giemsa, Zeiss Plan-Apochromat×63)

blood and bone marrow morphology for a V617F-positive, *BCR-ABL*-negative CML case is shown on Fig. 13.2.

13.2.6.2 The Role of V617F *JAK2*

Whether V617F is the primary abnormality initiating diverse MPDs or a secondary change associated with disease evolution remains unclear. Jak2 is a nonreceptor tyrosine kinase that plays a major role in myeloid development by transducing signals from diverse cytokines and growth factor receptors, including those for IL-3, IL-5, erythropoietin, GM-CSF, G-CSF, and thrombopoietin (Parganas et al. 1998; Verma et al. 2003). V617F is located within a highly conserved region of the JH2 domain, a region that is homologous to the true tyrosine kinase domain but lacks key catalytic residues. The JH2 domain is believed to negatively regulate Jak2 signaling by direct interaction with the kinase domain (Saharinen et al. 2000) and V617F is believed to disrupt this interaction. Whether the mutation results in hypersensitivity to growth factor stimulation or true growth factor independent signaling remains a matter of debate. Furthermore it is not at all clear why different individuals with V617F show preferential expansion of erythroid, granulocyte, megakaryocyte, monocyte, or eosinophil lineages. Potentially, this could be due to the identity of the cell in which the mutation arises, the constitutional genetic background of the individual, or to other, acquired changes that may precede or be subsequent to V617F. An alternative viewpoint is that the presence of the *JAK2* V617F itself defines a unique disease entity with variable clinical features.

13.2.7 Transforming Properties of Activated Tyrosine Kinases

13.2.7.1 Structure and Activity of Tyrosine Kinase Fusions

Balanced chromosomal translocations, insertions, or deletions that target genes encoding RTKs generate fusion proteins in which the extracellular ligand-binding domain is replaced by the N-terminal part of a partner protein. For fusion genes involving NRTKs, a variable portion of N-terminal sequence (that may or may not include regions responsible for interaction with normal upstream or regulatory components) is replaced by the partner protein. In all cases the entire catalytic domain of the kinase is retained and, although the chimeric proteins are no longer responsive to their natural ligands, they have constitutive tyrosine kinase activity, i.e., they are continuously sending proliferative and antiapoptotic signals to the cell in which they reside. Structurally and functionally, these fusion proteins are very similar to *BCR-ABL* in CML. Although mRNA encoding the reciprocal fusion is detectable in some cases, there is no evidence to suggest that these products play any important pathogenetic role in the disease process.

13.2.7.2 Assays for Activated Tyrosine Kinases

The activity of tyrosine kinase fusion genes and other mutations have been assayed extensively by their ability to transform growth-factor-dependent cells lines, most commonly Ba/F3 cells, to growth-factor independence. Artificial mutants have been used to show that transformation typically depends on the catalytic activity of the kinase and the presence of dimerization or oligomerization domains of the partner protein (see below). Retroviral transfection of tyrosine kinase fusion genes into mouse bone marrow followed by transplantation into syngeneic recipient mice typically induces a rapidly fatal MPD (Carroll et al. 1997; Guasch et al. 2003a; Liu et al. 2000; Million et al. 2004; Roumiantsev et al. 2004; Schwaller et al. 1998; Tomasson et al. 1999), whereas introduction of V617F *JAK2* resulted in PV-like abnormalities (James et al. 2005). Murine models have proved to be crucial tools for understanding the molecular basis for phenotypic differences between different fusions, for evaluating new treatments, and for investigating the precise molecular mechanisms by which transformation occurs. Signal transduction cascades induced by activated tyrosine kinases have been reviewed in detail elsewhere, but broadly it appears that there are very few qualitative differences in signaling between different fusions. However subtle dependencies on specific pathways may be apparent in murine systems despite the fact that no differences in transforming ability can be discerned in cell lines.

13.2.7.3 Role of Partner Proteins in Transformation Mediated by Tyrosine Kinase Fusions

The partner proteins are generally unrelated in sequence but have some structural and functional properties in common. The vast majority of partner genes contain one or more dimerization domains that are required for the transforming activity of the fusion proteins. Homotypic interaction between specific domains of the partner protein leads to dimerization or oligomerization of the fusion protein mimicking the normal process of ligand-mediated dimerization and resulting in constitutive activation of the tyrosine kinase moiety. Since the elements that control the expression of the partner gene will largely or completely control expression of the tyrosine kinase fusion gene, the partner gene must be normally expressed in hemopoietic progenitor cells. In fact, most partner genes appear to serve a housekeeping role in that they are universally or widely expressed. Of note, some of these genes have been found as recurrent fusion partners for different tyrosine kinases, e.g., *BCR* (*BCR-ABL*, *BCR-PDGFRA*, *BCR-JAK2* or *BCR-FGFR1*) or *ETV6* (*ETV6-PDGFRB*, *ETV6-ABL*, *ETV6-SYK*) (Baxter et al. 2002; Demiroglu et al. 2001; Golub et al. 1994; Griesinger et al. 2005; Kuno et al. 2001; Lacronique et al. 1997; Peeters et al. 1997). Detailed modeling in mice has shown that the partner protein may play additional roles in transformation. For example, *ZNF198-FGFR1* induced an MPD with T-cell lymphoma, whereas *BCR-FGFR1* induced a CML-like disease without lymphoma, i.e., the two fusions induced murine diseases that were strikingly similar to their human counterparts (Roumiantsev et al. 2004). Interestingly, the CML-like disease was dependent on the Bcr Y177 Grb2 binding site, confirming the hypothesis that the partner protein is not always a passive component that serves only to constitutively activate the kinase moiety of the fusion, but may also contribute directly to the disease phenotype. Grb2 is also bound by Etv6, an interaction that is important for transformation by Etv6-Abl (Million et al. 2004).

Although the partner proteins are involved in a wide range of cellular processes, it is notable that several (e.g., Nin, Fgfr1OP/Fop, Cep1, Pcm1) are components of the centrosome. It remains to be established whether centrosomal proteins are recurrent partners for tyrosine kinases in malignancy simply because they are widely expressed and contain dimerization motifs, or whether the fusions also result in a pathological alteration of centrosome function. Recent data have suggested that an unidentified centrosomal mechanism controls the number of neurons generated by neural precursor cells and it is possible that similar mechanisms operate during hemopoiesis (Bond et al. 2005). Interestingly, the Fop-Fgfr1 fusion protein is located almost exclusively at centrosomes and actively signals from this position. Delavel et al. hypothesize that the centrosome, which is linked to the microtubules, is close to the nucleus, and is connected to the Golgi apparatus and the proteasome, could serve to integrate multiple signaling pathways controlling cell division, cell migration, and cell fate. Abnormal kinase activity at the centrosome may be an efficient way to pervert cell division in malignancy (Delaval et al. 2005).

13.2.8 Summary of Molecular Abnormalities

Although more than 20 tyrosine kinase fusion genes have been described in cases of *BCR-ABL*-negative CML, collectively these cases are rare. In addition to the fusions described above, sporadic MPD cases have been reported in association with other tyrosine kinase fusion genes such as *ETV6-ABL* (Andreasson et al. 1997; Keung et al. 2002). Despite their rarity, these fusion genes have highlighted the fundamental role of deregulated tyrosine kinases in MPDs, and paved the way for the finding of the much more common mutation V617F *JAK2*. We have also determined that activating mutations of *FLT3* are seen in a small proportion (approximately 5%) of *BCR-ABL*-negative CML cases (Jones et al. 2005).

Despite these findings, the molecular pathogenesis of the majority of *BCR-ABL*-negative CML cases remains obscure (Fig. 13.3) and several groups, including ours, are performing systematic screens to search for new abnormalities of tyrosine kinase genes. It should be noted, however, that the association between MPD and constitutively activated tyrosine kinases is not absolute and a few cases of CML-like diseases have been reported in conjunction with translocations that are normally associated with AML, for example the t(6;9)(p23;q24) and the t(7;11)(p15;p15), which result in *DEK-CAN* and *NUP98-HOXA9* fusions, respectively (Hild and Fonatsch 1990; Soekarman et al. 1992; Takeda et al. 1986; Wong et al. 1999). In addition, *NRAS* mutations are found in approximately 13% of *BCR-ABL*-negative CML cases (Jones et al. 2005). N-Ras acts downstream of tyrosine kinase and we have found that tyrosine kinase fusions genes, tyrosine kinase mutations (V617F *JAK2* and *FLT3* internal tandem duplications), and *NRAS* mutations are mutually exclusive, i.e., only one of these changes is generally found in any given case, presumably because of functional redundancy

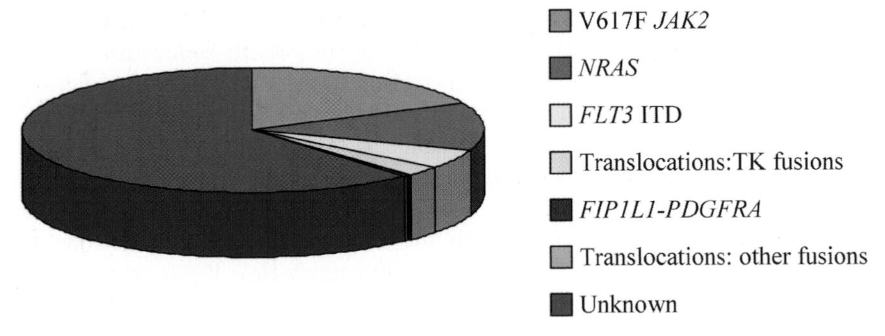

Fig. 13.3. Molecular pathogenesis of *BCR-ABL*-negative CML. The largest category (unknown) corresponds to patients for which no causative mutations can be identified. Causative or likely causative mutations are seen in approximately one third of cases. In order of prevalence these are V617F *JAK2*; activating mutations of *NRAS*; *FLT3* internal tandem duplication (ITD); tyrosine kinase fusion genes seen caused by cytogenetically visible chromosomal translocations (translocations: TK fusions), *FIP1L1-PDGFRA*; visible translocations that generate nontyrosine kinase gene fusions (translocations: other fusions). It should be noted that since *BCR-ABL*-negative CML is rare and no large, truly prospective series are available the prevalence of specific changes are only approximations

(Jones et al. 2005). Activation of tyrosine kinases is not specific to MPDs and tyrosine fusion genes have also been reported in other malignancies, notably ALL and B-cell lymphoma (Pulford et al. 2004), and also in nonhematological diseases such as papillary thyroid carcinoma (Pierotti et al. 1992; Santoro et al. 1994) and secretory breast cancer (Tognon et al. 2002). Within the MPDs, however, most tyrosine kinase fusion genes are associated with relatively aggressive, CML-like diseases rather than more indolent disorders.

13.3 Clinical Implications of Molecular Abnormalities

13.3.1 Responses to Imatinib

Imatinib, a 2-phenylaminopyrimidine molecule, occupies the ATP binding site and inhibits the tyrosine kinase activities of Abl, Arg (Abl2), Kit, Pdgfr*α*, Pdgfr*β*, Fms, and Lck protein tyrosine kinases (Buchdunger et al. 1996, 2000; Dewar et al. 2005; Druker et al. 1996; Fabian et al. 2005). Following the extraordinary success of imatinib in the treatment of patients with *BCR-ABL*-positive CML, there has been considerable interest in extending its clinical use to diseases in which other activated tyrosine kinases are implicated. Dramatic responses to imatinib treatment have been reported in MPDs with constitutive activation of both Pdgfr*α* or Pdgfr*β*. Apperley et al. reported four patients who had an MPD and an associated *PDGFRB* rearrangement and who were treated with 400 mg imatinib. After 4 weeks of treatment all patients responded with a normalization of blood counts and responses were durable with follow-up of 9–12 months or longer (Apperley et al. 2002; David et al., submitted). Response to imatinib has also been documented in individuals with other *PDGFRB* fusion genes (Garcia et al. 2003; Grand et al. 2004b; Gunby et al. 2003; Levine et al. 2005b; Magnusson et al. 2002; Pitini et al. 2003; Vizmanos et al. 2004b; Wilkinson et al. 2003), two patients with a *BCR-PDGFRA* fusion gene (Safley et al. 2004; Trempat et al. 2003), and many patients with *FIP1L1-PDGFRA*-positive disease (Cools et al. 2003a; Gotlib 2005). Overall, these results suggest that imatinib should be the treatment of choice in all MPDs which are associated with *PDGFRA* or *PDGFRB* fusion genes.

Occasional patients have been reported to be responsive to imatinib even though no underlying tyrosine kinase mutation has been identified, suggesting that additional acquired imatinib-sensitive abnormalities remain to be identified. Imatinib is not active against Fgfr1, Jak2, or Flt3 and the few anecdotal CML-like patients with activating fusions or mutations involving these genes that have been treated have not shown any significant clinical response.

13.3.2 Identification of Candidates for Imatinib Treatment

To date, all patients with *PDGFRB* fusion genes have had a visible abnormality of chromosome 5q in bone marrow metaphases and thus standard cytogenetic analysis remains the front-line test for identification of these individuals. Most cases show simple reciprocal translocations, but more complex events are seen in some cases. We have screened more than 100 CML-like MPDs without 5q abnormalities for the *ETV6-PDGFRB* fusion and have not seen a single positive case. Consequently, we feel that it is not worthwhile screening cases by RT-PCR unless there is cytogenetic evidence that a *PDGFRB* fusion might be present. As mentioned above, the presence of a 5q31-33 translocation in a patient with a CML-like disease does not definitely mean that *PDGFRB* is involved. Indeed, roughly half of cases who present with a t(5;12)(q31-33;p13) do not have *ETV6-PDGFRB* and, instead, it appears that elements controlling the expression of *ETV6* are acting to upregulate the *IL-3* gene (Cools et al. 2002). These latter cases would not be expected to be responsive to imatinib.

BCR-PDGFRA and other, as yet unpublished fusions involving *PDGFRA* are also associated with cytogenetic abnormalities, in this case of chromosome 4q. *FIP1L1-PDGFRA*, however, is cytogenetically cryptic and we believe that all cases of *BCR-ABL*-negative CML-like disease with eosinophilia should be screened for this fusion by RT-PCR and/or FISH for *CHIC2* deletion (Cools et al. 2003a; Pardanani et al. 2003).

13.3.3 New Tyrosine Kinase and Other Inhibitors

Several other TK inhibitors have been developed and recently entered phase I/II trials, e.g., dasatinib (BMS354825), a synthetic small-molecule ATP-competitive inhibitor of Src and Abl tyrosine kinases (Shah et al., 2004), and nilotinib (AMN107), a novel aminopyrimidine inhibitor (Weisberg et al. 2005). Preliminary results have shown that these molecules are highly active against a number of different imatinib-resistant Abl kinase domain mutations seen in *BCR-ABL*-positive CML (see Chaps. 5 Signal Transduction Inhibitors in Chronic Myeloid Leukemia and 6 Treatment with Tyrosine Kinase Inhibitors). In addition, activity of these compounds against *PDGFRA* and *PDGFRA* fusions in cell lines and mice has been documented (Chen et al. 2004a; Cools et al. 2003b; Growney et al. 2005; Shah et al. 2004; Weisberg et al. 2005) although treatment of *PDGFR*-rearranged patients has not thus far been described (Lombardo et al. 2004; Shah et al. 2004; Stover et al. 2005; Weisberg et al. 2005).

Currently, there are no specific Fgfr1 or Jak2 inhibitors that are generally available for clinical use, although proof of principle experiments suggesting the possibility of targeted therapy for patients with activating mutations of these kinases have been performed using model systems and a variety of compounds (Demiroglu et al. 2001; Grand et al. 2004a). PKC412, a staurosporine derivative which inhibits protein kinase C, Vegf, and Pdgf receptors, induced a partial response in a single patient with the *ZNF198-FGFR1* fusion (Chen et al. 2004a) but it is not entirely clear if this response was really a consequence of targeting the activated tyrosine kinase or not. A number of Jak inhibitors have been developed with a view to their use as immunosuppressants by blocking the action of Jak3 and it is possible that these or other compounds may be developed to selectively interfere with Jak2 (Borie et al. 2004). There is also considerable interest is developing kinase inhibitors that block interactions with substrates rather than the ATP binding pocket (Gumireddy et al. 2005), inhibitors that interfere with downstream signal transduction pathways (for recent reviews see Chalandon and Schwaller, 2005 or Krause and Van Etten, 2005), and alternative strategies such as siRNA (Chen et al. 2004b; Withey et al. 2005). Overall, the advent of effective, targeted signal transduction therapy is rapidly pushing the classification of MPDs away from traditional hematological groupings and towards a genetic-based structure that directs specific treatment.

References

Abe A, Emi N, Tanimoto M, Terasaki H, Marunouchi T, Saito H (1997) Fusion of the platelet-derived growth factor receptor beta to a novel gene CEV14 in acute myelogenous leukemia after clonal evolution. Blood 90:4271–4277

Andreasson P, Johansson B, Carlsson M, Jarlsfelt I, Fioretos T, Mitelman F, Hoglund M (1997) BCR/ABL-negative chronic myeloid leukemia with ETV6/ABL fusion. Genes Chromosomes Cancer 20:299–304

Apperley JF, Gardembas M, Melo JV, Russell-Jones R, Bain BJ, Baxter J, Chase A, Chessells JM, Colombat M, Dearden CE, Dimitrijevic S, Mahon FX, Marin D, Nikolova Z, Olavarria E, Silberman S, Schultheis B, Cross NCP, Goldman JM (2002) Response to imatinib mesylate in patients with chronic myeloproliferative diseases with rearrangements of the platelet-derived growth factor receptor beta. N Engl J Med 347:481–487

Bain BJ (1996) Eosinophilic leukaemias and the idiopathic hypereosinophilic syndrome. Br J Haematol 95:2–9

Barnes DJ, Melo JV (2002) Cytogenetic and molecular genetic aspects of chronic myeloid leukaemia. Acta Haematol 108:180–202

Baxter EJ, Hochhaus A, Bolufer P, Reiter A, Fernandez JM, Senent L, Cervera J, Moscardo F, Sanz MA, Cross NCP (2002) The t(4;22)(q12;q11) in atypical chronic myeloid leukaemia fuses BCR to PDGFRA. Hum Mol Genet 11:1391–1397

Baxter EJ, Kulkarni S, Vizmanos JL, Jaju R, Martinelli G, Testoni N, Hughes G, Salamanchuk Z, Calasanz MJ, Lahortiga I, Pocock CF, Dang R, Fidler C, Wainscoat JS, Boultwood J, Cross NCP (2003) Novel translocations that disrupt the platelet-derived growth factor receptor beta (PDGFRB) gene in BCR-ABL-negative chronic myeloproliferative disorders. Br J Haematol 120:251–256

Baxter EJ, Scott LM, Campbell PJ, East C, Fourouclas N, Swanton S, Vassiliou GS, Bench AJ, Boyd EM, Curtin N, Scott MA, Erber WN, Green AR (2005) Acquired mutation of the tyrosine kinase JAK2 in human myeloproliferative disorders. Lancet 365:1054–1061

Belloni E, Trubia M, Gasparini P, Micucci C, Tapinassi C, Confalonieri S, Nuciforo P, Martino B, Lo-Coco F, Pelicci PG, Di Fiore PP (2005) 8p11 myeloproliferative syndrome with a novel t(7;8) translocation leading to fusion of the FGFR1 and TIF1 genes. Genes Chromosomes Cancer 42:320–325

Bond J, Roberts E, Springell K, Lizarraga S, Scott S, Higgins J, Hampshire DJ, Morrison EE, Leal GF, Silva EO, Costa SM, Baralle D, Raponi M, Karbani G, Rashid Y, Jafri H, Bennett C, Corry P, Walsh CA, Woods CG (2005) A centrosomal mechanism involving CDK5RAP2 and CENPJ controls brain size. Nat Genet 37:353–355

Borie DC, O'Shea JJ, Changelian PS (2004) JAK3 inhibition, a viable new modality of immunosuppression for solid organ transplants. Trends Mol Med 10:532–541

Borkhardt A, Bojesen S, Haas OA, Fuchs U, Bartelheimer D, Loncarevic IF, Bohle RM, Harbott J, Repp R, Jaeger U, Viehmann S, Henn T, Korth P, Scharr D, Lampert F (2000) The human GRAF gene is fused to MLL in a unique t(5;11)(q31;q23) and both alleles are disrupted in three cases of myelodysplastic syndrome/acute myeloid leukemia with a deletion 5q. Proc Natl Acad Sci USA 97:9168–9173

Buchdunger E, Cioffi CL, Law N, Stover D, Ohno-Jones S, Druker BJ, Lydon NB (2000) Abl protein-tyrosine kinase inhibitor STI571 inhibits in vitro signal transduction mediated by c-kit and platelet-derived growth factor receptors. J Pharmacol Exp Ther 295:139–145

Buchdunger E, Zimmermann J, Mett H, Meyer T, Muller M, Druker BJ, Lydon NB (1996) Inhibition of the Abl protein-tyrosine kinase in vitro and in vivo by a 2-phenylaminopyrimidine derivative. Cancer Res 56:100–104

Carroll M, Ohno-Jones S, Tamura S, Buchdunger E, Zimmermann J, Lydon NB, Gilliland DG, Druker BJ (1997) CGP 57148, a tyrosine kinase inhibitor, inhibits the growth of cells expressing BCR-ABL, TEL-ABL, and TEL-PDGFR fusion proteins. Blood 90:4947–4952

Cartwright RA, Gurney KA, Moorman AV (2002) Sex ratios and the risks of haematological malignancies. Br J Haematol 118:1071–1077

Chalandon Y, Schwaller J (2005) Targeting mutated protein tyrosine kinases and their signaling pathways in hematologic malignancies. Haematologica 90:949–968

Chase A, Huntly BJ, Cross NCP (2001) Cytogenetics of chronic myeloid leukaemia. Best Pract Res Clin Haematol 14:553–571

Chen J, DeAngelo DJ, Kutok JL, Williams IR, Lee BH, Wadleigh M, Duclos N, Cohen S, Adelsperger J, Okabe R, Coburn A, Galinsky I, Huntly B, Cohen PS, Meyer T, Fabbro D, Roesel J, Banerji L, Griffin JD, Xiao S, Fletcher JA, Stone RM, Gilliland DG (2004a) PKC412 inhibits the zinc finger 198-fibroblast growth factor receptor 1 fusion tyrosine kinase and is active in treatment of stem cell myeloproliferative disorder. Proc Natl Acad Sci USA 101:14479–14484

Chen J, Wall NR, Kocher K, Duclos N, Fabbro D, Neuberg D, Griffin JD, Shi Y, Gilliland DG (2004b) Stable expression of small interfering RNA sensitizes TEL-PDGFbetaR to inhibition with imatinib or rapamycin. J Clin Invest 113:1784–1791

Chen J, Williams IR, Kutok JL, Duclos N, Anastasiadou E, Masters SC, Fu H, Gilliland DG (2004c) Positive and negative regulatory roles of the WW-like domain in TEL-PDGFbetaR transformation. Blood 104:535–542

Cools J, Mentens N, Odero MD, Peeters P, Wlodarska I, Delforge M, Hagemeijer A, Marynen P (2002) Evidence for position effects as a variant ETV6-mediated leukemogenic mechanism in myeloid leukemias with a t(4;12)(q11-q12;p13) or t(5;12)(q31;p13). Blood 99: 1776–1784

Cools J, DeAngelo DJ, Gotlib J, Stover EH, Legare RD, Cortes J, Kutok J, Clark J, Galinsky I, Griffin JD, Cross NCP, Tefferi A, Malone J, Alam R, Schrier SL, Schmid J, Rose M, Vandenberghe P, Verhoef G, Boogaerts M, Wlodarska I, Kantarjian H, Marynen P, Coutre SE, Stone R, Gilliland DG (2003a) A tyrosine kinase created by fusion of the PDGFRA and FIP1L1 genes as a therapeutic target of imatinib in idiopathic hypereosinophilic syndrome. N Engl J Med 348:1201–1214

Cools J, Stover EH, Boulton CL, Gotlib J, Legare RD, Amaral SM, Curley DP, Duclos N, Rowan R, Kutok JL, Lee BH, Williams IR, Coutre SE, Stone RM, DeAngelo DJ, Marynen P, Manley PW, Meyer T, Fabbro D, Neuberg D, Weisberg E, Griffin JD, Gilliland DG (2003b) PKC412 overcomes resistance to imatinib in a murine model of FIP1L1-PDGFR alpha-induced myeloproliferative disease. Cancer Cell 3:459–469

De Braekeleer M (1987) Variant Philadelphia translocations in chronic myeloid leukemia. Cytogenet Cell Genet 44:215–222

Delaval B, Létard S, Lelievre H, Chevrier V, Daviet L, Dubreuil P, Birnbaum D (2005) Oncogenic tyrosine kinase of malignant hemopathy targets the centrosome. Cancer Res 65:7231–7240

Demiroglu A, Steer EJ, Heath C, Taylor K, Bentley M, Allen SL, Koduru P, Brody JP, Hawson G, Rodwell R, Doody ML, Carnicero F, Reiter A, Goldman JM, Melo JV, Cross NCP (2001) The t(8;22) in chronic myeloid leukemia fuses BCR to FGFR1: transforming activity and specific inhibition of FGFR1 fusion proteins. Blood 98:3778–3783

Dewar AL, Cambareri AC, Zannettino AC, Miller BL, Doherty KV, Hughes TP, Lyons AB (2005) Macrophage colony-stimulating factor receptor c-fms is a novel target of imatinib. Blood 105:3127–3132

Druker BJ, Tamura S, Buchdunger E, Ohno S, Segal GM, Fanning S, Zimmermann J, Lydon NB (1996) Effects of a selective inhibitor of the Abl tyrosine kinase on the growth of Bcr-Abl positive cells. Nat Med 2:561–566

Fabian MA, Biggs WH, III, Treiber DK, Atteridge CE, Azimioara MD, Benedetti MG, Carter TA, Ciceri P, Edeen PT, Floyd M, Ford JM, Galvin M, Gerlach JL, Grotzfeld RM, Herrgard S, Insko DE, Insko MA, Lai AG, Lelias JM, Mehta SA, Milanov ZV, Velasco AM, Wodicka LM, Patel HK, Zarrinkar PP, Lockhart DJ (2005) A small molecule-kinase interaction map for clinical kinase inhibitors. Nat Biotechnol 23:329–336

Fioretos T, Panagopoulos I, Lassen C, Swedin A, Billstrom R, Isaksson M, Strombeck B, Olofsson T, Mitelman F, Johansson B (2001) Fusion of the BCR and the fibroblast growth factor receptor-1 (FGFR1) genes as a result of t(8;22)(p11;q11) in a myeloproliferative disorder: the first fusion gene involving BCR but not ABL. Genes Chromosomes Cancer 32:302–310

Garcia JL, Font dM, Hernandez JM, Queizan JA, Gutierrez NC, Hernandez JM, San Miguel JF (2003) Imatinib mesylate elicits positive clinical response in atypical chronic myeloid leukemia involving the platelet-derived growth factor receptor beta. Blood 102:2699–2700

Golub TR, Barker GF, Lovett M, Gilliland DG (1994) Fusion of PDGF receptor beta to a novel ets-like gene, tel, in chronic myelomonocytic leukemia with t(5;12) chromosomal translocation. Cell 77:307–316

Gotlib J (2005) Molecular classification and pathogenesis of eosinophilic disorders: 2005 update. Acta Haematol 114:7–25

Grand EK, Grand FH, Chase AJ, Ross FM, Corcoran M, Oscier DG, Cross NCP (2003) Identification of a novel gene, FGFR1OP2, fused to FGFR1 in the 8p11 myeloproliferative syndrome. Genes Chromosomes Cancer 40:78–83

Grand EK, Chase AJ, Heath C, Rahemtulla A, Cross NCP (2004 a) Targeting FGFR3 in multiple myeloma: inhibition of t(4;14)-positive cells by SU5402 and PD173074. Leukemia 18:962–966

Grand FH, Burgstaller S, Kuhr T, Baxter EJ, Webersinke G, Thaler J, Chase AJ, Cross NCP (2004 b) p53-Binding protein 1 is fused to the platelet-derived growth factor receptor beta in a patient with a t(5;15)(q33;q22) and an imatinib-responsive eosinophilic myeloproliferative disorder. Cancer Res 64:7216–7219

Greipp PT, Dewald GW, Tefferi A (2004) Prevalence, breakpoint distribution, and clinical correlates of t(5;12). Cancer Genet Cytogenet 153:170–172

Griesinger F, Hennig H, Hillmer F, Podleschny M, Steffens R, Pies A, Wormann B, Haase D, Bohlander SK (2005) A BCR-JAK2 fusion gene as the result of a t(9;22)(p24;q11.2) translocation in a patient with a clinically typical chronic myeloid leukemia. Genes Chromosomes Cancer 44:329–333

Griffin JH, Leung J, Bruner RJ, Caligiuri MA, Briesewitz R (2003) Discovery of a fusion kinase in EOL-1 cells and idiopathic hypereosinophilic syndrome. Proc Natl Acad Sci USA 100:7830–7835

Growney JD, Clark JJ, Adelsperger J, Stone R, Fabbro D, Griffin JD, Gilliland DG (2005) Activation mutations of human c-KIT resistant to imatinib are sensitive to the tyrosine kinase inhibitor PKC412. Blood 106:721–724

Guasch G, Mack GJ, Popovici C, Dastugue N, Birnbaum D, Rattner JB, Pebusque MJ (2000) FGFR1 is fused to the centrosome-associated protein CEP110 in the 8p12 stem cell myeloproliferative disorder with t(8;9)(p12;q33). Blood 95:1788–1796

Guasch G, Delaval B, Arnoulet C, Xie MJ, Xerri L, Sainty D, Birnbaum D, Pebusque MJ (2003 a) FOP-FGFR1 tyrosine kinase, the product of a t(6;8) translocation, induces a fatal myeloproliferative disease in mice. Blood 103:309–312

Guasch G, Popovici C, Mugneret F, Chaffanet M, Pontarotti P, Birnbaum D, Pebusque MJ (2003 b) Endogenous retroviral sequence is fused to FGFR1 kinase in the 8p12 stem-cell myeloproliferative disorder with t(8;19)(p12;q13.3). Blood 101:286–288

Gumireddy K, Baker SJ, Cosenza SC, John P, Kang AD, Robell KA, Reddy MV, Reddy EP (2005) A non-ATP-competitive inhibitor of BCR-ABL overrides imatinib resistance. Proc Natl Acad Sci USA 102:1992–1997

Gunby RH, Cazzaniga G, Tassi E, le Coutre P, Pogliani E, Specchia G, Biondi A, Gambacorti-Passerini C (2003) Sensitivity to imatinib but low frequency of the TEL/PDGFR beta fusion protein in chronic myelomonocytic leukemia. Haematologica 88:408–415

Hild F, Fonatsch C (1990) Cytogenetic peculiarities in chronic myelogenous leukemia. Cancer Genet Cytogenet 47:197–217

Hunter T (1998) The Croonian Lecture 1997. The phosphorylation of proteins on tyrosine: its role in cell growth and disease. Philos Trans R Soc Lond B Biol Sci 353:583–605

Inhorn RC, Aster JC, Roach SA, Slapak CA, Soiffer R, Tantravahi R, Stone RM (1995) A syndrome of lymphoblastic lymphoma, eosinophilia, and myeloid hyperplasia/malignancy associated with t(8;13)(p11;q11): description of a distinctive clinicopathologic entity. Blood 85:1881–1887

Jaju RJ, Fidler C, Haas OA, Strickson AJ, Watkins F, Clark K, Cross NCP, Cheng JF, Aplan PD, Kearney L, Boultwood J, Wainscoat JS (2001) A novel gene, NSD1, is fused to NUP98 in the t(5;11)(q35;p15.5) in de novo childhood acute myeloid leukemia. Blood 98:1264–1267

James C, Ugo V, Le Couedic JP, Staerk J, Delhommeau F, Lacout C, Garcon L, Raslova H, Berger R, Bennaceur-Griscelli A, Villeval JL, Constantinescu SN, Casadevall N, Vainchenker W (2005) A unique clonal JAK2 mutation leading to constitutive signalling causes polycythaemia vera. Nature 434:1144–1148

Jelinek J, Oki Y, Gharibyan V, Bueso-Ramos C, Prchal JT, Verstovsek S, Beran M, Estey E, Kantarjian HM, Issa JP (2005) JAK2 mutation 1849G>T is rare in acute leukemias but can be found in CMML, Philadelphia-chromosome negative CML and megakaryocytic leukemia. Blood 106:3370–3373

Jones AV, Cross NCP (2004) Oncogenic derivatives of platelet-derived growth factor receptors. Cell Mol Life Sci 61:2912–2923

Jones AV, Kreil S, Zoi K, Waghorn K, Curtis C, Zhang L, Score J, Seear R, Chase AJ, Grand FH, White H, Zoi C, Loukopoulos D, Terpos E, Vervessou EC, Schultheis B, Emig M, Ernst T, Lengfelder E, Hehlmann R, Hochhaus A, Oscier D, Silver RT, Reiter A, Cross NCP (2005) Widespread occurrence of the JAK2 V617F mutation in chronic myeloproliferative disorders. Blood 106:2162–2168

Keung YK, Beaty M, Steward W, Jackle B, Pettnati M (2002) Chronic myelocytic leukemia with eosinophilia, t(9;12)(q34;p13), and ETV6-ABL gene rearrangement: case report and review of the literature. Cancer Genet Cytogenet 138:139–142

Kralovics R, Passamonti F, Buser AS, Teo SS, Tiedt R, Passweg JR, Tichelli A, Cazzola M, Skoda RC (2005) A gain-of-function mutation of JAK2 in myeloproliferative disorders. N Engl J Med 352:1779–1790

Krause DS, Van Etten RA (2005) Tyrosine kinases as targets for cancer therapy. N Engl J Med 353:172–187

Kulkarni S, Heath C, Parker S, Chase A, Iqbal S, Pocock CF, Kaeda J, Cwynarski K, Goldman JM, Cross NCP (2000) Fusion of H4/D10S170 to the platelet-derived growth factor receptor beta in BCR-ABL-negative myeloproliferative disorders with a t(5;10)(q33;q21). Cancer Res 60:3592–3598

Kuno Y, Abe A, Emi N, Iida M, Yokozawa T, Towatari M, Tanimoto M, Saito H (2001) Constitutive kinase activation of the TEL-Syk fusion gene in myelodysplastic syndrome with t(9;12)(q22;p12). Blood 97:1050–1055

Lacronique V, Boureux A, Valle VD, Poirel H, Quang CT, Mauchauffe M, Berthou C, Lessard M, Berger R, Ghysdael J, Bernard OA (1997) A TEL-JAK2 fusion protein with constitutive kinase activity in human leukemia. Science 278:1309–1312

Levine RL, Wadleigh M, Cools J, Ebert BL, Wernig G, Huntly BJ, Boggon TJ, Wlodarska I, Clark JJ, Moore S, Adelsperger J, Koo S, Lee JC, Gabriel S, Mercher T, D'Andrea A, Frohling S, Dohner K, Marynen P, Vandenberghe P, Mesa RA, Tefferi A, Griffin JD, Eck MJ, Sellers

WR, Meyerson M, Golub TR, Lee SJ, Gilliland DG (2005a) Activating mutation in the tyrosine kinase JAK2 in polycythemia vera, essential thrombocythemia, and myeloid metaplasia with myelofibrosis. Cancer Cell 7:387–397

Levine RL, Wadleigh M, Sternberg DW, Wlodarska I, Galinsky I, Stone RM, DeAngelo DJ, Gilliland DG, Cools J (2005b) KIAA1509 is a novel PDGFRB fusion partner in imatinib-responsive myeloproliferative disease associated with a t(5;14)(q33;q32). Leukemia 19:27–30

Liu Q, Schwaller J, Kutok J, Cain D, Aster JC, Williams IR, Gilliland DG (2000) Signal transduction and transforming properties of the TEL-TRKC fusions associated with t(12;15)(p13;q25) in congenital fibrosarcoma and acute myelogenous leukemia. EMBO J 19:1827–1838

Lombardo LJ, Lee FY, Chen P, Norris D, Barrish JC, Behnia K, Castaneda S, Cornelius LA, Das J, Doweyko AM, Fairchild C, Hunt JT, Inigo I, Johnston K, Kamath A, Kan D, Klei H, Marathe P, Pang S, Peterson R, Pitt S, Schieven GL, Schmidt RJ, Tokarski J, Wen ML, Wityak J, Borzilleri RM (2004) Discovery of N-(2-chloro-6-methyl- phenyl)-2-(6-(4-(2-hydroxyethyl)-piperazin-1-yl)-2-methylpyrimidin-4 ylamino)thiazole-5-carboxamide (BMS-354825), a dual Src/Abl kinase inhibitor with potent antitumor activity in preclinical assays. J Med Chem 47:6658–6661

Macdonald D, Aguiar RC, Mason PJ, Goldman JM, Cross NCP (1995) A new myeloproliferative disorder associated with chromosomal translocations involving 8p11: a review. Leukemia 9:1628–1630

Macdonald D, Reiter A, Cross NCP (2002) The 8p11 myeloproliferative syndrome: a distinct clinical entity caused by constitutive activation of FGFR1. Acta Haematol 107:101–107

Magnusson MK, Meade KE, Brown KE, Arthur DC, Krueger LA, Barrett AJ, Dunbar CE (2001) Rabaptin-5 is a novel fusion partner to platelet-derived growth factor beta receptor in chronic myelomonocytic leukemia. Blood 98:2518–2525

Magnusson MK, Meade KE, Nakamura R, Barrett J, Dunbar CE (2002) Activity of STI571 in chronic myelomonocytic leukemia with a platelet-derived growth factor beta receptor fusion oncogene. Blood 100:1088–1091

Manning G, Whyte DB, Martinez R, Hunter T, Sudarsanam S (2002) The protein kinase complement of the human genome. Science 298:1912–1934

Million RP, Harakawa N, Roumiantsev S, Varticovski L, Van Etten RA (2004) A direct binding site for Grb2 contributes to transformation and leukemogenesis by the Tel-Abl (ETV6-Abl) tyrosine kinase. Mol Cell Biol 24:4685–4695

Morerio C, Acquila M, Rosanda C, Rapella A, Dufour C, Locatelli F, Maserati E, Pasquali F, Panarello C (2004) HCMOGT-1 is a novel fusion partner to PDGFRB in juvenile myelomonocytic leukemia with t(5;17)(q33;p11.2). Cancer Res 64:2649–2651

Murati A, Arnoulet C, Lafage-Pochitaloff M, Adelaide J, Derre M, Slama B, Delaval B, Popovici C, Vey N, Xerri L, Mozziconacci MJ, Boulat O, Sainty D, Birnbaum D, Chaffanet M (2005a) Dual lympho-myeloproliferative disorder in a patient with t(8;22) with BCR-FGFR1 gene fusion. Int J Oncol 26:1485–1492

Murati A, Gelsi-Boyer V, Adelaide J, Perot C, Talmant P, Giraudier S, Lode L, Letessier A, Delaval B, Brunel V, Imbert M, Garand R, Xerri L, Birnbaum D, Mozziconacci MJ, Chaffanet M (2005b) PCM1-JAK2 fusion in myeloproliferative disorders and acute erythroid leukemia with t(8;9) translocation. Leukemia 19:1692–1696

Pardanani A, Ketterling RP, Brockman SR, Flynn HC, Paternoster SF, Shearer BM, Reeder TL, Li CY, Cross NCP, Cools J, Gilliland DG, Dewald GW, Tefferi A (2003) CHIC2 deletion, a surrogate for FIP1L1-PDGFRA fusion, occurs in systemic mastocytosis associated with eosinophilia and predicts response to Imatinib therapy. Blood 102:3093–3096

Parganas E, Wang D, Stravopodis D, Topham DJ, Marine JC, Teglund S, Vanin EF, Bodner S, Colamonici OR, van Deursen JM, Grosveld G, Ihle JN (1998) Jak2 is essential for signaling through a variety of cytokine receptors. Cell 93:385–395

Peeters P, Raynaud SD, Cools J, Wlodarska I, Grosgeorge J, Philip P, Monpoux F, Van Rompaey L, Baens M, Van den BH, Marynen P (1997) Fusion of TEL, the ETS-variant gene 6 (ETV6), to the receptor-associated kinase JAK2 as a result of t(9;12) in a lymphoid and t(9;15;12) in a myeloid leukemia. Blood 90:2535–2540

Pierotti MA, Santoro M, Jenkins RB, Sozzi G, Bongarzone I, Grieco M, Monzini N, Miozzo M, Herrmann MA, Fusco A, Hay I, Della Porta G, Vecchio G (1992) Characterization of an inversion on the long arm of chromosome 10 juxtaposing D10S170 and RET and creating the oncogenic sequence RET/PTC. Proc Natl Acad Sci USA 89:1616–1620

Pini M, Gottardi E, Scaravaglio P, Giugliano E, Libener R, Baraldi A, Muzio A, Cornaglia E, Saglio G, Levis A (2002) A fourth case of BCR-FGFR1 positive CML-like disease with t(8;22) translocation showing an extensive deletion on the derivative chromosome 8p. Hematol J 3:315–316

Pitini V, Arrigo C, Teti D, Barresi G, Righi M, Alo G (2003) Response to STI571 in chronic myelomonocytic leukemia with platelet derived growth factor beta receptor involvement: a new case report. Haematologica 88:ECR18

Popovici C, Adelaide J, Ollendorff V, Chaffanet M, Guasch G, Jacrot M, Leroux D, Birnbaum D, Pebusque MJ (1998) Fibroblast growth factor receptor 1 is fused to FIM in stem-cell myeloproliferative disorder with t(8;13). Proc Natl Acad Sci USA 95:5712–5717

Popovici C, Zhang B, Gregoire MJ, Jonveaux P, Lafage-Pochitaloff M, Birnbaum D, Pebusque MJ (1999) The t(6;8)(q27;p11) translocation in a stem cell myeloproliferative disorder fuses a novel gene, FOP, to fibroblast growth factor receptor 1. Blood 93:1381–1389

Pulford K, Lamant L, Espinos E, Jiang Q, Xue L, Turturro F, Delsol G, Morris SW (2004) The emerging normal and disease-related roles of anaplastic lymphoma kinase. Cell Mol Life Sci 61:2939–2953

Reiter A, Sohal J, Kulkarni S, Chase A, Macdonald DH, Aguiar RC, Goncalves C, Hernandez JM, Jennings BA, Goldman JM, Cross NCP (1998) Consistent fusion of ZNF198 to the fibroblast growth factor receptor-1 in the t(8;13)(p11;q12) myeloproliferative syndrome. Blood 92:1735–1742

Reiter A, Walz C, Watmore A, Schoch C, Blau I, Schlegelberger B, Berger U, Telford N, Aruliah S, Yin JA, Vanstraelen D, Barker HF, Taylor PC, O'Driscoll A, Benedetti F, Rudolph C, Kolb HJ, Hochhaus A, Hehlmann R, Chase A, Cross NCP (2005) The t(8;9)(p22;p24) is a recurrent abnormality in chronic and acute leukemia that fuses PCM1 to JAK2. Cancer Res 65:2662–2667

Ries LAG, Eisner MP, Kosary CL (2003) SEER Cancer Statistic Review, 1975–2000 National Cancer Institute. Bethesda, MD. 2003

Ross TS, Bernard OA, Berger R, Gilliland DG (1998) Fusion of Huntingtin interacting protein 1 to platelet-derived growth factor beta receptor (PDGFbetaR) in chronic myelomonocytic leukemia with t(5;7)(q33;q11.2). Blood 91:4419–4426

Roumiantsev S, Krause DS, Neumann CA, Dimitri CA, Asiedu F, Cross NCP, Van Etten RA (2004) Distinct stem cell myeloproliferative/T lymphoma syndromes induced by ZNF198-FGFR1 and BCR-FGFR1 fusion genes from 8p11 translocations. Cancer Cell 5:287–298

Safley AM, Sebastian S, Collins TS, Tirado CA, Stenzel TT, Gong JZ, Goodman BK (2004) Molecular and cytogenetic characterization of a novel translocation t(4;22) involving the breakpoint cluster region and platelet-derived growth factor receptor-alpha genes in a patient with atypical chronic myeloid leukemia. Genes Chromosomes Cancer 40:44–50

Saharinen P, Takaluoma K, Silvennoinen O (2000) Regulation of the Jak2 tyrosine kinase by its pseudokinase domain. Mol Cell Biol 20:3387–3395

Santoro M, Dathan NA, Berlingieri MT, Bongarzone I, Paulin C, Grieco M, Pierotti MA, Vecchio G, Fusco A (1994) Molecular characterization of RET/PTC3; a novel rearranged version of the RETproto-oncogene in a human thyroid papillary carcinoma. Oncogene 9:509–516

Schwaller J, Frantsve J, Aster J, Williams IR, Tomasson MH, Ross TS, Peeters P, Van Rompaey L, Van Etten RA, Ilaria R, Jr., Marynen P, Gilliland DG (1998) Transformation of hematopoietic cell lines to growth-factor independence and induction of a fatal myelo- and lymphoproliferative disease in mice by retrovirally transduced TEL/JAK2 fusion genes. EMBO J 17:5321–5333

Schwaller J, Anastasiadou E, Cain D, Kutok J, Wojiski S, Williams IR, LaStarza R, Crescenzi B, Sternberg DW, Andreasson P, Schiavo R, Siena S, Mecucci C, Gilliland DG (2001) H4(D10S170), a gene frequently rearranged in papillary thyroid carcinoma, is fused to the platelet-derived growth factor receptor beta gene in atypical chronic myeloid leukemia with t(5;10)(q33;q22). Blood 97:3910–3918

Shah NP, Tran C, Lee FY, Chen P, Norris D, Sawyers CL (2004) Overriding imatinib resistance with a novel ABL kinase inhibitor. Science 305:399–401

Smedley D, Hamoudi R, Clark J, Warren W, Abdul-Rauf M, Somers G, Venter D, fagan K, Cooper C, Shipley J (1998a) The t(8;13)(p11;q11–12) rearrangement associated with an atypical myeloproliferative disorder fuses the fibroblast growth factor receptor 1 gene to a novel gene RAMP. Hum Mol Genet 7:637–642

Smedley D, Somers G, Venter D, Chow CW, Cooper C, Shipley J (1998b) Characterization of a t(8;13)(p11;q11–12) in an atypical myeloproliferative disorder. Genes Chromosomes Cancer 21:70–73

Soekarman D, von Lindern M, Daenen S, de Jong B, Fonatsch C, Heinze B, Bartram C, Hagemeijer A, Grosveld G (1992) The translocation (6;9) (p23;q34) shows consistent rearrangement of two genes and defines a myeloproliferative disorder with specific clinical features. Blood 79:2990–2997

Steensma DP, Dewald GW, Lasho TL, Powell HL, McClure RF, Levine RL, Gilliland DG, Tefferi A (2005) The JAK2 V617F activating tyrosine kinase mutation is an infrequent event in both "atypical" myeloproliferative disorders and the myelodysplastic syndrome. Blood 106:1207–1209

Steer EJ, Cross NCP (2002) Myeloproliferative disorders with translocations of chromosome 5q31-35: role of the platelet-derived growth factor receptor Beta. Acta Haematol 107:113–122

Stover EH, Chen J, Lee BH, Cools J, McDowell E, Adelsperger J, Cullen D, Coburn A, Moore SA, Okabe R, Fabbro D, Manley PW, Griffin JD, Gilliland DG (2005) The small molecule tyrosine kinase inhibitor AMN107 inhibits TEL-PDGFRbeta and FIP1L1-PDGFRalpha in vitro and in vivo. Blood 106:3206–3213

Takeda T, Ikebuchi K, Zaike Y, Mori M, Ohyashiki K, Ikeuchi T (1986) Ph-negative chronic myelocytic leukemia with a complex translocation involving chromosomes 7 and 11. Cancer Genet Cytogenet 21:123–127

Taki T, Kano H, Taniwaki M, Sako M, Yanagisawa M, Hayashi Y (1999) AF5q31, a newly identified AF4-related gene, is fused to MLL in infant acute lymphoblastic leukemia with ins(5;11)(q31;q13q23). Proc Natl Acad Sci USA 96:14535–14540

Tognon C, Knezevich SR, Huntsman D, Roskelley CD, Melnyk N, Mathers JA, Becker L, Carneiro F, MacPherson N, Horsman D, Poremba C, Sorensen PH (2002) Expression of the ETV6-NTRK3 gene fusion as a primary event in human secretory breast carcinoma. Cancer Cell 2:367–376

Tomasson MH, Williams IR, Hasserjian R, Udomsakdi C, McGrath SM, Schwaller J, Druker B, Gilliland DG (1999) TEL/PDGFbetaR induces hematologic malignancies in mice that respond to a specific tyrosine kinase inhibitor. Blood 93:1707–1714

Trempat P, Villalva C, Laurent G, Armstrong F, Delsol G, Dastugue N, Brousset P (2003) Chronic myeloproliferative disorders with rearrangement of the platelet-derived growth factor alpha receptor: a new clinical target for STI571/Glivec. Oncogene 22:5702–5706

Vardiman JW, Harris NL, Brunning RD (2002) The World Health Organization (WHO) classification of the myeloid neoplasms. Blood 100:2292–2302

Verma A, Kambhampati S, Parmar S, Platanias LC (2003) Jak family of kinases in cancer. Cancer Metastasis Rev 22:423–434

Vizmanos JL, Hernandez R, Vidal MJ, Larrayoz MJ, Odero MD, Marin J, Ardanaz MT, Calasanz MJ, Cross NCP (2004a) Clinical variability of patients with the t(6;8)(q27;p12) and FGFR1OP-FGFR1 fusion: two further cases. Hematol J 5:534–537

Vizmanos JL, Novo FJ, Roman JP, Baxter EJ, Lahortiga I, Larrayoz MJ, Odero MD, Giraldo P, Calasanz MJ, Cross NCP (2004b) NIN, a gene encoding a CEP110-like centrosomal protein, is fused to PDGFRB in a patient with a t(5;14)(q33;q24) and an imatinib-responsive myeloproliferative disorder. Cancer Res 64:2673–2676

Walz C, Cilloni D, Soverini S, Roche C, Ottovani E, Martinelli G, Saglio G, Preudhomme C, Paschka P, Apperley J, Hochaus A, Hehlmann R, Cross NCP, Grimwade D, Reiter A (2004) Molecular Heterogeneity of the FIP1L1-PDGFRA Fusion Gene in Chronic Eosinophilic Leukemia (CEL) and Systemic Mastocytosis with Eosinophilia (SME): A Study of 43 Cases. Blood 104:667a

Walz C, Chase A, Schoch C, Weisser A, Schlegel F, Hochhaus A, Fuchs R, Schmitt-Graff A, Hehlmann R, Cross NCP, Reiter A (2005) The t(8;17)(p11;q23) in the 8p11 myeloproliferative syndrome fuses MYO18A to FGFR1. Leukemia 19:1005–1009

Weisberg E, Manley PW, Breitenstein W, Bruggen J, Cowan-Jacob SW, Ray A, Huntly B, Fabbro D, Fendrich G, Hall-Meyers E, Kung AL, Mestan J, Daley GQ, Callahan L, Catley L, Cavazza C, Mohammed A, Neuberg D, Wright RD, Gilliland DG, Griffin JD (2005) Characterization of AMN107, a selective inhibitor of native and mutant Bcr-Abl. Cancer Cell 7:129–141

Wilkinson K, Velloso ER, Lopes LF, Lee C, Aster JC, Shipp MA, Aguiar RC (2003) Cloning of the t(1;5)(q23;q33) in a myeloproliferative disorder associated with eosinophilia: involvement of PDGFRB and response to imatinib. Blood 102:4187–4190

Withey JM, Marley SB, Kaeda J, Harvey AJ, Crompton MR, Gordon MY (2005) Targeting primary human leukaemia cells with RNA interference: Bcr-Abl targeting inhibits myeloid progenitor self-renewal in chronic myeloid leukaemia cells. Br J Haematol 129:377–380

Wong KF, So CC, Kwong YL (1999) Chronic myelomonocytic leukemia with t(7;11)(p15;p15) and NUP98/HOXA9 fusion. Cancer Genet Cytogenet 115:70–72

Xiao S, Nalabolu SR, Aster JC, Ma J, Abruzzo L, Jaffe ES, Stone R, Weissman SM, Hudson TJ, Fletcher JA (1998) FGFR1 is fused with a novel zinc-finger gene, ZNF198, in the t(8;13) leukaemia/lymphoma syndrome. Nat Genet 18:84–87

Yoneda-Kato N, Look AT, Kirstein MN, Valentine MB, Raimondi SC, Cohen KJ, Carroll AJ, Morris SW (1996) The t(3;5)(q25.1;q34) of myelodysplastic syndrome and acute myeloid leukemia produces a novel fusion gene, NPM-MLF1. Oncogene 12:265–275

Hypereosinophilic Syndrome

Elizabeth H. Stover, Jason Gotlib, Jan Cools and D. Gary Gilliland

Contents

Abstract. Hypereosinophilic syndrome (HES) is characterized by persistent overproduction of eosinophils, and the exclusion of other known causes of eosinophilia. Clinical manifestations of HES are related to eosinophilic infiltration of end organs that may include the skin, heart, lung, central nervous system, and gastrointestinal tract. Treatment has been largely empirically derived, and may include steroids, cytotoxic agents, and immunomodulatory agents. It was recently observed that a subset of patients diagnosed with HES demonstrated remarkable clinical responses to empiric treatment with the small molecule tyrosine kinase inhibitor imatinib. These responses suggested that an imatinib-sensitive tyrosine kinase contributed to pathogenesis of HES in these cases, and led to the cloning of FIP1L1-PDGFRA. FIP1L1-PPDGFRA is a constitutively activated tyrosine kinase that is imatinib sensitive, and is expressed as a consequence of an interstitial chromosomal deletion on chromosome 4. In addition to imatinib, other targeted therapies have evolved for treatment of HES, including monoclonal antibody therapy directed against IL-5. Thus, significant progress has been made in our understanding of the pathogenesis and therapy of HES in recent years, and has had an impact on approach to classification and clinical management.

14.1 Introduction

The term hypereosinophilic syndrome (HES) was first suggested by Hardy and Anderson in 1968 to describe patients with prolonged eosinophilia of unknown cause (Hardy and Anderson 1968). Subsequently, Chusid and colleagues suggested in 1975 three diagnostic criteria for HES that are still utilized today, and include (1) persistent eosinophilia arbitrarily defined as $>1500/mm^3$; (2) absence of evidence for other causes of eosinophilia that include infection, especially parasitic infection, allergic hypersensitivity disease, or connective tissue disease among others; and (3) signs and symptoms of end-organ involvement due to eosinophilic infiltration (Chusid et al. 1975). Clinically, HES is comprised of a heterogeneous group of disorders, and the etiology is not known in many cases. Indeed, it is often difficult even to delineate between reactive versus neoplastic cases of HES. Recent findings indicate that at least a subset of patients diagnosed with HES will harbor a recurrent FIP1L1-PDGFRA gene rearrangement that accounts for the eosinophilia (Cools et al. 2003 a). The fusion protein has important therapeutic implications as a target for imatinib therapy, and may alter the approach to classification of the eosinophilias. However, the cause of the broad spectrum of cases of HES that are FIP1L1-PDGFRA negative remains elusive, and warrants further investigation. In this chapter, we will review the epidemiology, diagnosis, and classification of the syndrome, and discuss strategies for integration of the disease due to FIP1L1-PDGFRA gene rearrangement into current algorithms. The clinicopathologic findings will be overviewed as well as therapeutic approaches to HES.

14.2 Epidemiology

HES is a rare disorder that has been reported to have a striking male predominance (9:1) and is most often diagnosed in individuals between the ages of 20 and 50 (Fauci et al. 1982). Rare pediatric cases have been reported (Alfaham et al. 1987; Wynn et al. 1987), but the median age at diagnosis in one series of 50 patients characterized at the NIH was 33 years (Fauci et al. 1982).

14.3 Classification

The most recent World Health Organization (WHO) criteria follow the earlier diagnostic criteria iterated above, and require exclusion of reactive causes of eosinophilia for a diagnosis of HES or chronic eosinophilic leukemia (CEL). A list of reactive causes of eosinophilia that comprises a differential diagnosis for HES is shown in Table 14.1. In addition, a diagnosis of HES or CEL requires exclusion of malignancies in which eosinophilia is reactive or part of the neoplastic clone – a feature that is complicated by elucidation of the FIP1L1-PDGFRA fusion as an etiology of HES/CEL. Lastly, it is necessary to exclude T-cell disorders associated with abnormalities of immunophenotype and cytokine production, with or without evidence of lymphocyte clonality (Bain et al. 2001).

CEL is distinguished from HES by WHO criteria that include the presence of increased blasts in the peripheral blood (>2%) or bone marrow (5–19%), or the demonstration of a clonality in the myeloid lineage (Bain et al. 2001). It is likely that these criteria for CEL will underestimate the number of cases, in that assessment of clonal markers of disease is a challenge in the context of hypereosinophilia. Clonal cytogenetic abnormalities in purified eosinophils that are identified by conventional karyotyping (Goldman et al. 1975), or by fluorescent in situ analysis (FISH) (Forrest et al. 1998), are definitive. However, the absence of such aberrations does not preclude clonal derivation of eosinophils. X-inactivation analysis may demonstrate clonal derivation of cells in patients with hypereosinophilia, but can only be informative in the less common female patients (Chang et al. 1999; Luppi et al. 1994).

Apart from the WHO criteria for diagnosis of HES and CEL, it has been suggested that HES may be further subdivided into distinctive clinical entities. These include a myeloproliferative variant, a lymphoproliferative

Table 14.1. Reactive causes of eosinophilia (reproduced from Gotlib et al. 2004)

Allergic/hypersensitivity diseases
Asthma, rhinitis, drug reactions, allergic broncho-pulmonary aspergillosis, allergic gastroenteritis
Infections
Parasitic
Strongyloidiasis, Toxocara canis, Trichinella spiralis, visceral larva migrans, filariasis, schistosomiasis, Ancylostoma duodenale, Fasciola hepatica, echinococcus, other parasitic diseases
Bacterial/Mycobacterial
Fungal (coccidioidomycosis, cryptococcus)
Viral (HIV, HSV, HTLV-II)
Rickettsial
Connective tissue diseases
Churg-Strauss syndrome, Wegener's granulomatosis, rheumatoid arthritis, polyarteritis nodosa, systemic lupus erythematosus, scleroderma, eosinophilic fasciitis
Pulmonary diseases
Bronchiectasis, cystic fibrosis, Loeffler's syndrome, eosinophilic granuloma of the lung
Cardiac diseases
Tropical endocardial fibrosis, eosinophilic endomyocardial fibrosis or myocarditis
Skin diseases
Atopic dermatitis, urticaria, eczema, bullous pemphigoid, dermatitis herpetiformis, Gleich syndrome (episodic angioedema with eosinophilia)
Gastrointestinal diseases
Eosinophilic gastroenteritis, celiac disease
Immune system diseases/abnormalities
Wiskott-Aldrich syndrome, hyper-IgE with infections, hyper-IgM syndrome, IgA deficiency
Metabolic abnormalities
Addison's disease
Other
Il-2 therapy, L-tryptophan ingestion, toxic oil syndrome, renal graft rejection

variant, and other primary hypereosinophilias that include Gleich's syndrome, familial hypereosinophilia, and organ-specific hypereosinophilias.

14.3.1 The Myeloproliferative Variant of HES

A designation of myeloproliferative variant of HES, which has a disease presentation similar to chronic myelogenous leukemia (CML), has been suggested, with clinical features that included hepatomegaly, splenomegaly, anemia, thrombocytopenia, bone marrow dysplasia or fibrosis, and elevated levels of cobalamin (Roufosse et al. 2003). It has been noted that the myeloproliferative variant is often unresponsive to steroid therapy and is associated with a more aggressive form of disease with a poor prognosis, and that these patients often have elevated serum tryptase levels (Klion et al. 2003). As discussed below, it is this subset of patients that is most likely to be imatinib responsive as a consequence of the presence of FIP1L1-PDGFRA. This subgroup is also notable for a striking male predominance of ~9:1.

14.3.2 The Lymphoproliferative Variant of HES

There is an abnormal, clonal expansion of T-lymphocyte populations in a proportion of patients diagnosed with HES, as first reported by Cogan and colleagues (Cogan et al. 1994), and subsequent findings suggest that this is a distinct clinical entity (Roufosse et al. 2004). Disease pathophysiology in these cases has been attributed to expression of cytokines, in particular IL-5, by the aberrant T-cell clone that enhance proliferation and survival of eosinophilic progenitors. Immunophenotypic analysis of these patients may demonstrate a double-negative population of immature T-cells (CD3+CD4–CD8– or CD3–CD4+CD8–) (Brugnoni et al. 1997; Cogan et al. 1994), and elevated levels of IgE, IL-5, and in some cases IL-4 and IL-13, suggesting that these T-cells have a helper type 2 (Th2) profile (Brugnoni et al. 1996; Cogan et al. 1994; Roufosse et al. 1999; 2003). T-cell clonality, as assessed by T-cell receptor gene rearrangement, strongly supports the diagnosis.

Lymphoproliferative HES may have highly variable clinical manifestations, with dermatologic involvement being the most common. Gastrointestinal and pulmonary involvement may also be observed, but fibrotic changes in the endomyocardium and bone marrow are uncommon by comparison with the myeloproliferative variant. The prevalence of the syndrome among cases of HES is difficult to assess, in part because of variability in the diagnostic criteria employed, and portal of entry into the health care system. For example, patients with lymphoproliferative HES may more often be evaluated in dermatology clinics, whereas those with myeloproliferative HES are frequently treated in hematology/oncology clinics. Lymphoproliferative HES may progress to lymphoma, with an increased risk reported in patients with the CD3–CD4+CD8– immunophenotype and with clonal cytogenetic abnormalities (Bank et al. 2001; Brugnoni et al. 1997; Roufosse et al. 2000).

14.3.3 Other Primary Eosinophilia Syndromes

Other syndromes characterized by primary overproduction of eosinophils include Gleich's syndrome, a rare disorder associated with cyclical episodes of eosinophilia and angioedema that is associated with increased levels of IL-5 (Gleich et al. 1984). In addition, there are rare cases of autosomal dominant familial eosinophilia that map to 5q31-33 (Klion et al. 2004a), though affected individuals often have indolent clinical courses. There are also a spectrum of organ-specific eosinophilic disorders that include eosinophilic gastroenteritis, eosinophilic cystitis, and chronic eosinophilic pneumonia.

14.3.4 Hematologic Malignancies Associated with Eosinophilia

A spectrum of hematologic malignancies are associated with eosinophilia that is thought to be due to production of cytokines from the neoplastic clone, including IL-3 and IL-5 (Table 14.2). Examples include T-cell lymphomas (Kawasaki et al. 1991), acute lymphoblastic leukemia (Catovsky et al. 1980; Takai and Sanada 1991), and Hodgkin's disease (Endo et al. 1995). In other hematologic malignancies, eosinophils are part of the malignant clone. Examples include AML with karyotypic abnormalities involving chromosome 16q22, including inv(16)(p13q22) or t(16;16)(p13;q22) associated with the M4Eo phenotype (Le Beau et al. 1983), or less commonly with t(8;21)(q22:q22) (Swirsky et al. 1984). Other karyotypes that have been associated with eosinophilia in AML patients include monosomy 7 (Song and Park 1987), trisomy 1 (Harrington et al. 1988), t(10;11)(p14;q21) (Broustet et al. 1986; Fischkoff et al. 1988), and t(16;21)(p11;q22) (Mecucci et al. 1985).

Table 14.2. Malignancies associated with reactive or clonal eosinophilias

Lymphomas
Hodgkin's disease
Non-Hodgkin's lymphoma
T-cell lymphoma/mycosis fungoides/Sézary syndrome
Angioimmunoblastic lymphadenopathy
Angiolymphoid hyperplasia with eosinophilia
Vascular tumors
Myelodysplastic syndrome
Myeloproliferative disorders
Chronic myelogenous leukemia
Polycythemia vera
Essential thrombocythemia
Systemic mastocytosis
Acute leukemias
Acute lymphoblastic leukemia
Acute myelogenous leukemia
Various solid tumors (breast, lung, GI, renal, metastatic neoplasms)
Langerhans cell histiocytosis

Chronic myeloproliferative disorders may also be associated with pronounced eosinophilia. These include chronic myelomonocytic leukemia associated with expression of the TEL-PDGFRB fusion as a consequence of t(5;12)(q31;p12) (Golub et al. 1994) or the TEL-ABL fusion in patients with t(9;12)(q34;p12). Eosinophilia has also been reported in the spectrum of other CMML patients with involvement of PDGFRB or PDGFRA, suggesting that there are specific signal transduction pathways that are activated by the respective constitutively activated tyrosine kinases that enhance eosinophil proliferation and survival. In addition, patients with a phenotype referred to as stem-cell myeloproliferative disease that have rearrangements involving the *FGFR1* gene almost invariably have associated eosinophilia (Demiroglu et al. 2001; Guasch et al. 2000; Popovici et al. 1998, 1999). It is also worth noting that small molecule tyrosine kinase inhibitors are useful in treating many of these diseases, including imatinib for treatment of

PDGFRB and *ABL* rearranged disease (Apperley et al. 2002), and PKC412 for treatment of patients with rearrangements involving the *FGFR1* gene (Chen et al. 2004).

Eosinophilia has been reported in ~13% of patients with myelodysplastic syndrome (MDS) (Matsushima et al. 2003), in some cases due to clonal involvement of the eosinophil lineage (Forrest et al. 1998; Matsushima et al. 1995), and is associated with lower overall survival and higher likelihood of leukemia progression (Matsushima et al. 2003). In addition to association of eosinophilia with T-cell malignancies, rare cases of B-cell ALL are associated with eosinophilia due to translocations that result in overexpression of IL5 (Meeker et al. 1990).

14.4 Cytogenetic Abnormalities in HES

By WHO criteria, any patient that meets diagnostic criteria for HES, but has a clonal chromosomal abnormality, should be reclassified as chronic eosinophilic leukemia (CEL). With this caveat, there is a spectrum of cytogenetic abnormalities that have been reported in patients with HES or CEL. Careful inspection of these cytogenetic abnormalities suggests that the majority of them target known loci involved in myeloproliferative disease with associated eosinophilia, including the *PDGFRB* locus at 5q31-33 (Granjo et al. 2002; Lepretre et al. 2002; Luciano et al. 1999; Yakushijin et al. 2001; Yamada et al. 1998; Yates and Potter 1991), the *PDGFRA* locus at 4q11-12 (Cools et al. 2003a; Duell et al. 1997; Myint et al. 1995; Schoffski et al. 2000), or the *ABL* locus at 9q34 (Bakhshi et al. 2003; Quiquandon et al. 1995; Yamada et al. 1998). It is important to characterize such karyotypic abnormalities at the molecular level, in that all three of these alleles are targets for therapy with imatinib.

14.5 Molecular Genetics of HES

14.5.1 The *FIP1L1-PDGFRA* Fusion Gene

Several studies, beginning with a case report in 2001, reported remarkable clinical responses in HES patients treated with imatinib (Ault et al. 2002; Cools et al. 2003a; Cortes et al. 2003; Gleich et al. 2002; Pardanani et al. 2003; Schaller and Burkland 2001) (Table 14.3). These observations prompted molecular analysis of genomic loci that encode the five known imatinib-sensitive tyrosine kinases in the human genome, *ABL*, *ARG*, *KIT*, *PDGFRA*, and *PDGFRB*. The molecular basis for response in the majority of patients treated with imatinib was ultimately shown to be due to expression of a

Table 14.3. Published reports on the use of imatinib in HES and CEL (reproduced from Gotlib et al. 2004)

Author	No. patients treated with imatinib	Responses	Comments
Schaller and Burkland 2001*	1	CR	Initial report: rapid hematologic remission on imatinib 100 mg/d
Gleich et al. 2002*	5	4 CR	IL-5 levels normal in responders
Ault et al. 2002*	1	CR	Resolution of 70% eosinophilia in 18 days on imatinib 100 mg/d
Pardanani et al. 2003*	7	3 CR, 1 PR	IL-5 levels elevated in responders
Cortes et al. 2003*	9	4 CR, 1 PR	4 responses at imatinib 100 mg/d; 1 response at 400 mg/d
Cools et al. 2003	11	9 CR	*FIP1L1-PDGFRA* fusion present in 5/9 responders
Klion et al. 2003	6	6 CR	HES patients with elevated serum tryptase levels treated with imatinib

* FIP1L1-PDGFRA fusion not assessed

CR, complete hematologic remission; PR, partial hematologic remission

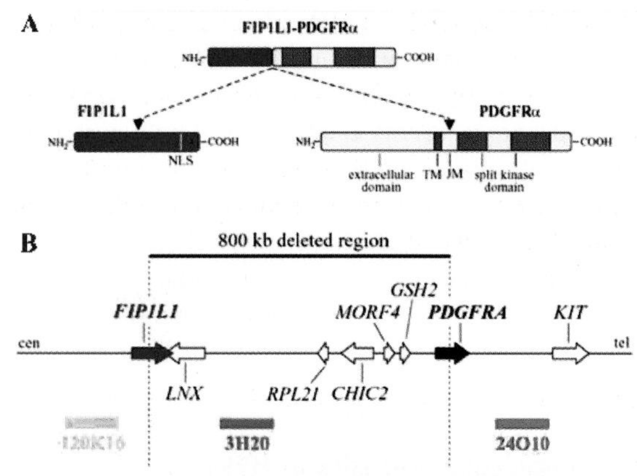

Fig. 14.1. Fusion of *FIP1L1* to *PDGFRA*. (**A**) FIP1L1, PDGFRα and FIP1L1-PDGFRα fusion proteins. NLS, nuclear localization signal; TM, transmembrane region; JM, juxtamembrane region. (**B**) 4q12 chromosomal region around the *FIP1L1* and *PDGFRA* genes. The 800-kb deletion, resulting in the fusion of the 5′ part of *FIP1L1* to the 3′ part of *PDGFRA*, and the location of 3 BAC probes (RPCI11-120K16, RPCI11-3H20 and RPCI11-24O10) is indicated. cen, centromeric side; tel, telomeric side (Reproduced from Gotlib et al. 2004)

novel imatinib-sensitive, constitutively activated tyrosine kinase, FIP1L1-PDGFRA (Cools et al. 2003a).

FIP1L1-PDGFRA is a fusion tyrosine kinase that is similar to other activated tyrosine kinases associated with myeloproliferative disease in humans, such as the *BCR-ABL* and *TEL-PDGFRB* fusion genes. However, it is generated by a novel mechanism of interstitial chromosomal deletion rather than chromosomal translocation (Fig. 14.1). *FIP1L1* coding sequences are fused to *PDGFRA* by virtue of an ~800-Kb deletion on chromosome 4q12 that is not evident by conventional cytogenetic banding techniques.

FIP1L1 (Fip1-like-1) is a 520-amino-acid protein with homology to Fip1, a yeast protein with synthetic lethal function that is involved in polyadenylation (Helmling et al. 2001; Preker et al. 1995). Recent data suggest that the human homolog FIP1L1 has a similar function in polyadenylation. Based on the abundance of FIP1L1 expressed sequence tags in the databases that are derived from different tissues and cell types, FIP1L1 expression appears to be under the control of a ubiquitous promoter. PDGFRA is a member of the Type III transmembrane cytokine receptor family that has extracellular immunoglobulin-like domains, transmembrane and juxtamembrane domains, and a so-called split tyrosine kinase domain. The genomic breakpoints that generate the fusion gene are variable among different HES patients within FIP1L1, but generally occur between exons 7 and 10. In contrast, the breakpoint in PDGFRA always involves exon 12. The resulting FIP1L1-PDGFRA fusion includes coding sequences for the entire PDGFRA tyrosine kinase domain, but invariably disrupts the PDGFRA juxtamembrane domain.

The mechanism of activation of the PDGFRA tyrosine kinase is not fully understood. Most fusion tyrosine kinases are constitutively activated by virtue of a 5′ partner gene with a dimerization or oligomerization motif, such as the coiled-coil motif in BCR. However, such motifs are lacking in the FIP1L1 sequences incorporated into the fusion. Recent data indicate that the mechanism of activation is likely to be disruption of a negative regulatory domain, the juxtamembrane domain, and loss of autoinhibition of kinase activation (Stover et al. 2006).

FIP1L1-PDGFRA transforms hematopoietic cell lines to factor independent growth, and activates the downstream effector molecule STAT5. Expression of the fusion gene in a murine bone marrow transplantation model (Cools et al. 2003b) results in a myeloproliferative phenotype characterized by marked leukocytosis, but without prominent eosinophilia. At this juncture, the basis for the lineage predilection of the fusion is not understood. Sensitive probes for the fusion indicate that it is present in all myeloid lineages. Thus, it is possible that eosinophils are particularly sensitive to the proliferative and survival signals generated by FIP1L1-PDGFRA. In addition, a recent animal model of disease indicates that coexpression of IL-5 with the FIP1L1-PDGFRA fusion recapitulates many of the features of HES including eosinophilia, suggesting that there may be cell nonautonomous contributions and interactions that potentiate the human phenotype (Yamada et al. 2006).

14.5.2 Resistance to Imatinib

Two patients have been reported that developed resistance to imatinib (Cools et al. 2003a; von Bubnoff et al. 2005). In each case the patients had progressed to an acute leukemia, and acquired a T674I substitution in the PDGFRA catalytic domain at the time of developing clinical resistance to imatinib. T674I is homologous to the T315I substitution that confers resistance to imatinib in the context of the BCR-ABL fusion. FIP1L1-PDGFRA T674I is highly resistant to imatinib as well, in both in vitro and in vivo models of disease. These data provide the most compelling evidence that FIP1L1-PDGFRA is the cause of HES, and the basis for responsiveness to imatinib.

These findings also suggest that proactive strategies for identification of compounds that can overcome resistance to imatinib are warranted. One report indicates that the small molecule kinase inhibitor PKC412 can effectively inhibit the FIP1L1-PDGFRA T674I kinase both in vitro and in vivo (Cools et al. 2003b).

14.5.3 Diagnosis of FIP1L1-PDGFRA-Positive HES

Data that support the presence of FIP1L1-PDGFRA include presence of a fusion transcript by RT-PCR and/or deletion of the *CHIC2* locus that is contained within the ~800-Kb deletion on chromosome 4q12 (Fig. 14.1 and Fig. 14.2). In addition, patients with the FIP1L1-PDGFRA fusion have elevated serum tryptase that reflects concomitant involvement of the mast cell lineages. Lastly, patients with the myeloproliferative variant of HES are more likely than those with the lymphoproliferative variant to have the fusion gene.

The invariable elevation of tryptase reflects abnormalities of the mast cell lineage in patients diagnosed with HES, and is usually associated with abnormal collections of mast cells in the bone marrow of affected patients. These observations have suggested that FIP1L1-PDGFRA-positive patients previously diagnosed as having HES might best be considered as having systemic mast cell disease (SMCD) with associated eosinophilia. Regardless of nomenclature, patients with these phenotypic characteristics are likely to be responsive to imatinib therapy.

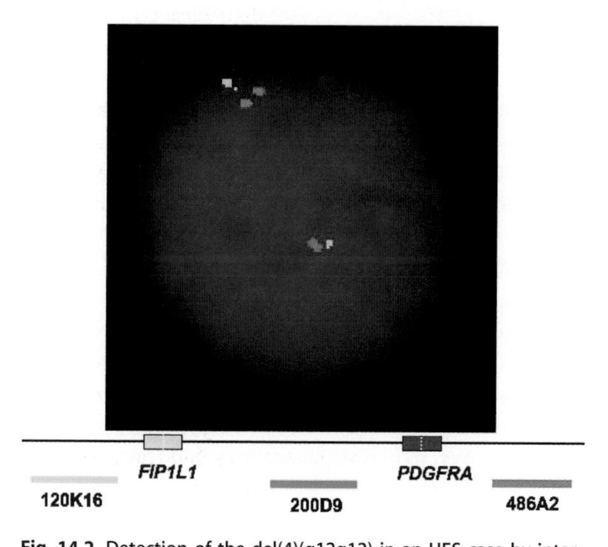

Fig. 14.2. Detection of the del(4)(q12q12) in an HES case by interphase FISH BAC probes used are shown. Absence of probe *200D9* (green) and presence of the 2 flanking probes is indicative for the presence of this specific deletion on one of the chromosomes 4. (FISH picture kindly provided by Dr. Iwona Wlodarska, Center for Human Genetics, Leuven, Belgium) (see also Fig. 14.1)

14.6 Clinicopathologic Manifestations of HES

14.6.1 Hematologic Abnormalities

Although the diagnosis of HES requires pronounced eosinophilia (>1500/mm^3), the range in absolute eosinophil count is highly variable, ranging from <10,000 to >100,000 (Fauci et al. 1982; Lefebvre et al. 1989; Spry et al. 1983; Weller and Bubley 1994). In addition to eosinophilia, neutrophilia, and basophilia, immaturity and/or dysplasia of myeloid and eosinophil progenitors and mast cells may be observed. These features may complicate the delineation of HES from other hematologic malignancies associated with similar findings, such as chronic myelomonocytic leukemia with eosinophilia, or systemic mast cell disease. Other characteristic findings include anemia in as many as 53% of patients, thrombocytopenia (31%), and bone marrow eosinophilia ranging from 7 to 57%. Charcot-Leyden crystals, the condensates of lysophospholipase from eosinophil granules, are observed in most patients.

14.6.2 Other Organ System Involvement in HES

In addition to hematologic manifestations of disease, there is variable end-organ involvement in HES that most frequently involves the skin, heart, lungs, and central nervous system (Fauci et al. 1982; Lefebvre et al. 1989; Spry et al. 1983; Weller and Bubley 1994) (Table 14.4). Cardiac disease is initiated by damage to the endomyocardium due to eosinophilic infiltration. In the thrombotic stage of the disease, local platelet thrombi may lead to development of mural thrombi that have the potential to embolize. Contents of eosinophilic granules may be released locally, including major basic protein and eosinophilic cationic protein that further promote endothelial damage and hypercoagulability, thereby further increasing thromboembolic risk (Tai et al.

Table 14.4. Organ involvement in hypereosinophilic syndrome (modified from Weller et al. 1994 and Brito-Babapulle 1997)

Organ system	Cumulative freq*	Organ-specific manifestations
Hematologic	100	Leukocytosis with eosinophilia, neutrophilia, basophilia, myeloid immaturity, dysplastic and/or immature eosinophils, anemia, thrombocytopenia or thrombocytosis, increased marrow blasts, myelofibrosis.
Cardiovascular	58	Cardiomyopathy, constrictive pericarditis, endomydocarditis, mural thrombi, valvular dysfunction, endomyocardial fibrosis
Dermatologic	56	Angioedema, urticaria, papules, nodules, plaques, erythroedema, mucosal ulcers, vesico-bullous lesions, microthrombi, vasculitis
Neurologic	54	Thromboembolism, peripheral neuropathy, encephalopathy, seizures, dementia, eosinophilic meningitis, cerebellar disease
Pulmonary	49	Pulmonary infiltrates, effusions, fibrosis, emboli, nodules, acute respiratory distress syndrome
Splenic	43	Hypersplenism, infarct
Liver/gall bladder	30	Hepatomegaly, focal or diffuse hepatic lesions on imaging, chronic active hepatitis, hepatic necrosis, Budd-Chiari syndrome, sclerosing cholangitis, cholecystitis, cholestasis
Ocular	23	Microthrombi, choroidal infarcts, retinal arteritis, episcleritis, kerato-conjunctivitis sicca, Adie's syndrome
Gastrointestinal	23	Ascites, diarrhea, gastritis, colitis, pancreatitis
Musculoskeletal	N/A	Arthritis, effusions, bursitis, synovitis, Raynaud's syndrome, digital necrosis, polymyositis/myopathy
Renal		Acute renal failure with Charco-Leyden crystalluria, nephrotic syndrome, crescentic glomerulonephritis

* Cumulative frequency from three studies (%)

1987; Venge et al. 1980). As thrombi organize, fibrosis ensues, with thickening of the endocardial lining that may result in end-stage restrictive cardiomyopathy. Valvular insufficiency may occur due to mural endocardial thrombosis and fibrosis involving either the tricuspid or mitral valves. (Ommen et al. 2000; Radford et al. 2002; Tanino et al. 1983). Dermatologic involvement is observed in more than half of patients, and may be manifest with pleiotropic signs and symptoms that can include angioedema, urticaria, papules or nodules, or plaques due to eosinophilic infiltration (DeYampert and Beck 1997; Kazmierowski et al. 1978). In addition, mucosal ulceration, vesico-bullous lesions, and vasculitis have been observed (Leiferman et al. 1982; Parker 1988; Sanchez and Padilla 1982). Pulmonary involvement in HES may include development of pulmonary infiltrates (Chusid et al. 1975; Slabbynck et al. 1992), pleural effusions (Chusid et al. 1975; Cordier et al. 1990), fibrosis, and emboli due to similar eosinophilic infiltration pathophysiology as observed in the heart. Acute respiratory distress syndrome may ensue in some patients (Winn et al. 1994), and pulmonary involvement may be exacerbated by concomitant cardiac disease. Neurologic manifestations of disease may be due to thromboembolism from cardiovascular involvement, but peripheral neuropathy, encephalopathy, and eosinophilic meningitis have been observed due to eosinophilic infiltration (Kwon et al. 2001; Moore et al. 1985; Weingarten et al. 1985; Wichman et al. 1985). Other organ systems with less frequent clinical manifestations of disease include the liver, pancreas, gastrointestinal tract, and kidneys.

14.7 Prognosis

It is difficult to generate accurate predictors of outcome due in part to the rarity of HES and to variation in approaches to treatment. Furthermore, it is likely that the use of imatinib, or other PDGFRA-selective small molecule inhibitors, will influence the outcome. In one review of 57 HES cases reported between 1919 and 1973 (Chusid et al. 1975), the median survival was 9 months, with a 3-year survival of only 12%. Most patients had advanced disease, and congestive heart failure was the cause of death in 65% of autopsied cases. A correlate of poor prognosis included WBC >100,000/mm^3. In a more recent study conducted on patients who were not treated with imatinib, 40 patients had a 5-year survival of 80%, with a 42% 15-year survival. Poor prognostic factors included the presence of a myeloproliferative phenotype, poor response to corticosteroids, cardiac disease, male sex, and the absolute eosinophil count (Lefebvre et al. 1989). These are also clinical features that currently define the FIP1L1-PDGFRA-positive group of HES patients (Klion et al. 2003) and it is likely that imatinib therapy will have a favorable impact in this poor prognosis group.

14.8 Treatment

14.8.1 Corticosteroids

Steroids will continue to be a mainstay of therapy for many patients with HES, in particular those who are not responsive to imatinib therapy (Fauci et al. 1982; Parrillo et al. 1978; Weller and Bubley 1994). Steroids should also be considered in FIP1L1-PDGFRA-positive patients who are treated with imatinib (see below) if they have evidence of active myocarditis as assessed by EKG, echocardiography, or elevated serum troponin levels (Pitini et al. 2003). It is appropriate to maintain patients at the lowest possible dose that ameliorates clinical symptoms and end-organ involvement, since some patients require long duration of treatments. Most patients will develop relative steroid resistance with time, and require consideration for other therapeutic intervention, such as conventional cytotoxic agents.

14.8.2 Cytotoxic Therapy for HES

Many of the same agents are employed for treatment of HES as for chronic myelogenous leukemia prior to the advent of imatinib. Hydroxyurea is an effective treatment for patients with steroid resistant disease, or as a steroid-sparing agent (Chambers et al. 1990; Fauci et al. 1982; Parrillo et al. 1978), but is not effective for inducing rapid reduction in eosinophil count, since its effects may take 10–14 days to be fully manifest. Second-line agents that have been employed include vincristine (Chusid and Dale 1975; Cofrancesco et al. 1984; Sakamoto et al. 1992), pulse-dosing of chlorambucil, cyclophosphamide, and etoposide (Bourrat et al. 1994; Lee et al. 2002; Smit et al. 1991; Weller and Bubley 1994).

14.8.3 Biological Response Modifiers for Treatment of HES

Interferon-alpha (IFN-α) can engender long-term clinical responses in patients with HES or CEL, even in cases of disease that is resistant to steroids or hydroxyurea (Butterfield and Gleich 1994; Ceretelli et al. 1998; Luciano et al. 1999; Yamada et al. 1998; Yoon et al. 2000), and has been advocated as a front-line therapy (Ceretelli et al. 1998). IFN-α has been reported to induce improvement in virtually all organ systems involved in HES, including hepatosplenomegaly (Ceretelli et al. 1998; Luciano et al. 1999), cardiac and thromboembolism (Schoffski et al. 2000; Yamada et al. 1998), mucosal ulcers (Butterfield and Gleich 1994), and skin (Yoon et al. 2000). The proposed mechanisms of action of IFN-α include inhibition of eosinophil proliferation and differentiation (Broxmeyer et al. 1983), as well as suppression of mediators of inflammation from eosinophils such as cationic protein, neurotoxin, and IL-5 through the IFN-α receptor (Aldebert et al. 1996). Efficacy in the lymphoproliferative variant of HES has been attributed to inhibition of IL-5 production by CD4+ helper T-cells (Schandene et al. 1996). Other immunomodulatory agents that have been reported to have efficacy in HES include cyclosporin A (Nadarajah et al. 1997; Zabel and Schlaak 1991) and 2-chlorodeoxyadenosine (Ueno et al. 1997).

14.8.4 Anticoagulation and Antiplatelet Agents

Anticoagulation is indicated in patients with thromboembolic disease, with agents including warfarin, heparin, and antiplatelet agents. However, even with therapeutic dosing, success in preventing recurrent thromboembolism is variable, and it may be most important to focus on treatment of the underlying etiology (Johnston and Woodcock 1998; Moore et al. 1985; Narayan et al. 2003; Spry et al. 1983).

14.8.5 Cardiac Surgery

Consideration for surgical intervention is warranted in patients with cardiac complications of HES that include defects in valvular function, endomyocardial thrombosis, or fibrosis, and appears to carry modest risk of disease recurrence at operative sites (Fauci et al. 1982; Weller and Bubley 1994). Mitral and tricuspid valve repair or replacement (Cameron et al. 1985; Harley et al. 1982; Hendren et al. 1988; Tanino et al. 1983; Weyman et al. 1977), and endomyocardectomy (Cameron et al. 1985; Chandra et al. 1996) for late-stage fibrotic heart disease may improve cardiac function. Mechanical valves may increase risk of recurrent thrombosis, and thus bioprosthetic devices are recommended.

14.8.6 Stem Cell Transplantation

Allogeneic stem cell transplantation has been used as treatment for patients with aggressive disease using both conventional and nonmyeloablative approaches. Disease-free survivals in case reports range from 8 months to 5 years (Basara et al. 1998; Chockalingam et al. 1999; Esteva-Lorenzo et al. 1996; Sigmund and Flessa 1995; Vazquez et al. 2000). There are few data and shorter follow-up on patients receiving nonmyeloablative conditioning regimens, but remission durations of 3–12 months have been reported (Juvonen et al. 2002; Ueno et al. 2002). The considerable risks of stem cell transplantation may outweigh the potential benefits in most patients with HES, but should be considered in patients with refractory disease. It remains a clinical challenge to identify appropriate candidates for stem cell transplantation prior to progressive end-organ damage that would preclude this approach.

14.8.7 Therapies with Limited Value

Leukapheresis has not proven to be useful except in rare emergencies in which acute reduction of eosinophils is warranted, but eosinophil counts rebound rapidly (Blacklock et al. 1979; Chambers et al. 1990; Davies and Spry 1982). Antihistamines, anabolic steroids, methotrexate, busulfan, azathioprine, and cyclophosphamide are thought to have limited, if any, value in the treatment of HES. Splenectomy may be considered for complications related to hypersplenism, including splenic infarction, refractory cytopenias related to splenic sequestration, or splenic pain, but is not considered a mainstay of therapy (Ault et al. 2002; Spry et al. 1983).

14.8.8 Molecularly Targeted Therapies for HES

14.8.8.1 Small Molecule Tyrosine Kinase Inhibitors

A trial of imatinib is warranted in HES patients who have evidence for the FIP1L1-PDGFRA gene rearrangement (see Sect. 14.5 above). Most patients will respond to low doses of imatinib (100 mg/day), in contrast to imatinib therapy for *BCR-ABL*-positive CML that typically requires 400–600 mg/day. The differential clinical sensitivity has been attributed to a ~100-fold higher sensitivity of Fip1L1-PDGFRA to imatinib compared to BCR-ABL.

Imatinib response rates in FIP1L1-PDGFRA-positive patients approach 100% (Klion et al. 2004b), and most patients have dramatic reductions in eosinophil count within 1 week of initiation of therapy. Signs and symptoms of disease frequently regress within 1 month, and reversal of virtually all organ involvement has been reported, even in severely affected individuals. An exception is patients who have developed fibrotic cardiomyopathy prior to initiation of therapy. Side effects of therapy are modest, and rarely lead to cessation of therapy. However, there has been a case report of a patient with abrupt cardiac decompensation shortly after initiation of imatinib that was attributed to eosinophil lysis in the endomyocardium. The patient was treated effectively with steroids and resumed imatinib treatment without further complications. However, it has been recommended that patients with elevated serum troponin levels be pretreated with steroids prior to initiation of imatinib.

Although imatinib (100 mg/day) is sufficient to induce complete remission, some patients will remain PCR positive. One reported experience suggests that increasing the dose to 400 mg/day is effective in inducing clinical hematologic and molecular remission (Klion et al. 2004b), and it has been suggested that patients be treated at this higher dose to achieve molecular remission, and then carefully dose reduced while monitoring for molecular relapse (Klion et al. 2004b).

A significant proportion of patients have been reported to respond to imatinib in the absence of detectable FIP1L1-PDGFRA fusion. These findings suggest either that there are other complex rearrangements involving PDGFRA (Walz et al. 2006; Score et al. 2006) that have not been detected, or that there may be other imatinib-responsive alleles in patients with HES. Therefore, it is reasonable to consider a trial of imatinib in patients with the myeloproliferative variant that are FIP1L1-PDGFRA negative. If there is no significant response within 1 month of treatment at doses as high as 400 mg/day, it is unlikely that further therapy or dose escalation will be effective. In addition, in the absence of the FIP1L1-PDGFRA fusion, it appears that patients with the lymphoproliferative variant of HES are unlikely to respond to imatinib.

Resistance to imatinib has not yet emerged as a major clinical problem in HES, and to date has only been observed in 2 patients with the FIP1L1-PDGFRA fusion associated with an acute myeloid leukemia phenotype. It is possible that the high potency of imatinib for inhibition of FIP1L1-PDGFRA will effectively suppress emergence of resistance clones. However, it seems likely that with long-term follow-up resistance will eventually ensue. Several novel tyrosine kinase inhibitors are being developed that may be effective for resistance due to the T674I mutation, including PKC412 that inhibits FIP1L1-PDGFRA T674I in vitro and in vivo (Cools et al. 2003b).

14.8.8.2 Monoclonal Antibody Therapy

Because IL-5 is thought to contribute to the pathogenesis of IL-5 in at least a proportion of cases of HES, in particular the lymphoproliferative variant, and may potentiate eosinophilia induced by the FIP1L1-PDGFRA fusion, antibodies directed against IL-5 epitopes are attractive candidates for therapeutic intervention. Preliminary data indicate that two different anti-IL5 monoclonal antibodies, SCH55700 and mepolizumab, can result in dramatic and prolonged reduction in circulating eosinophil levels. There were responders among a broad spectrum of HES patients, even among patients with low basal IL5 levels (Kay and Klion 2004). Such agents may have value alone or in combination, and may be useful as steroid sparing agents, especially in patients that lack the Fip1L1-PDGFRA fusion.

14.9 Therapeutic Approach and Classification Revisited

There have been significant strides in the past several years in our understanding of the pathogenesis and treatment of HES. These include a molecular marker for a subtype of disease that is imatinib responsive, and insights into contributions of the lymphoid lineage to phenotype. The current WHO classification scheme requires that identification of a clonal marker of disease in the eosinophil lineage mandates reclassification of a patient diagnosed with HES as having CEL. Thus, a patient who has HES, but is subsequently found to have the FIP1L1-PDGFRA fusion, would be reclassified as having CEL.

An alternative approach to diagnosis and classification is outlined in Fig. 14.3 (Gotlib et al. 2004). Patients who do not have secondary causes of eosinophilia would be screened for the presence of the FIP1L1-PDGFRA fusion. Patients who are positive, and have less than 20% bone marrow blasts, would be classified as *FIPL1-PDGFRA-positive chronic eosinophilic leukemia* (F-P+ CEL). As for *BCR-ABL-positive* CML these cases would be highly likely to respond to therapy with imatinib.

Patients who are negative for the fusion gene would be stratified into one of three diagnostic groups. Those who are negative for the FIP1L1-PDGFRA fusion but have clonal cytogenetic abnormalities, clonal eosinophils, or increased bone marrow blasts (5–19%) would be categorized as *CEL, unclassified*. These two categories correspond to the myeloproliferative variant phenotype. Those who are FIP1L1-PDGFRA negative without clonal abnormalities would be grouped as *hypereosinophilic syndrome (HES)*. Finally, in patients with eosinophilia associated with an abnormal population of T-cells characterized by either abnormal immunophenotype or clonal T cell gene rearrangement by PCR would be classified as *T-cell-associated HES*. This last category would correspond to the lymphoproliferative phenotypic variant.

A rationale for superimposing these categories on HES and CEL as defined by WHO criteria is that it permits rational application of currently available therapies. For example, *F-P-positive CEL* patients should be considered candidates for treatment with imatinib. Patients categorized as *CEL, unclassified*, or HES, especially those with characteristics of the myeloproliferative variant may respond to imatinib, and a therapeutic

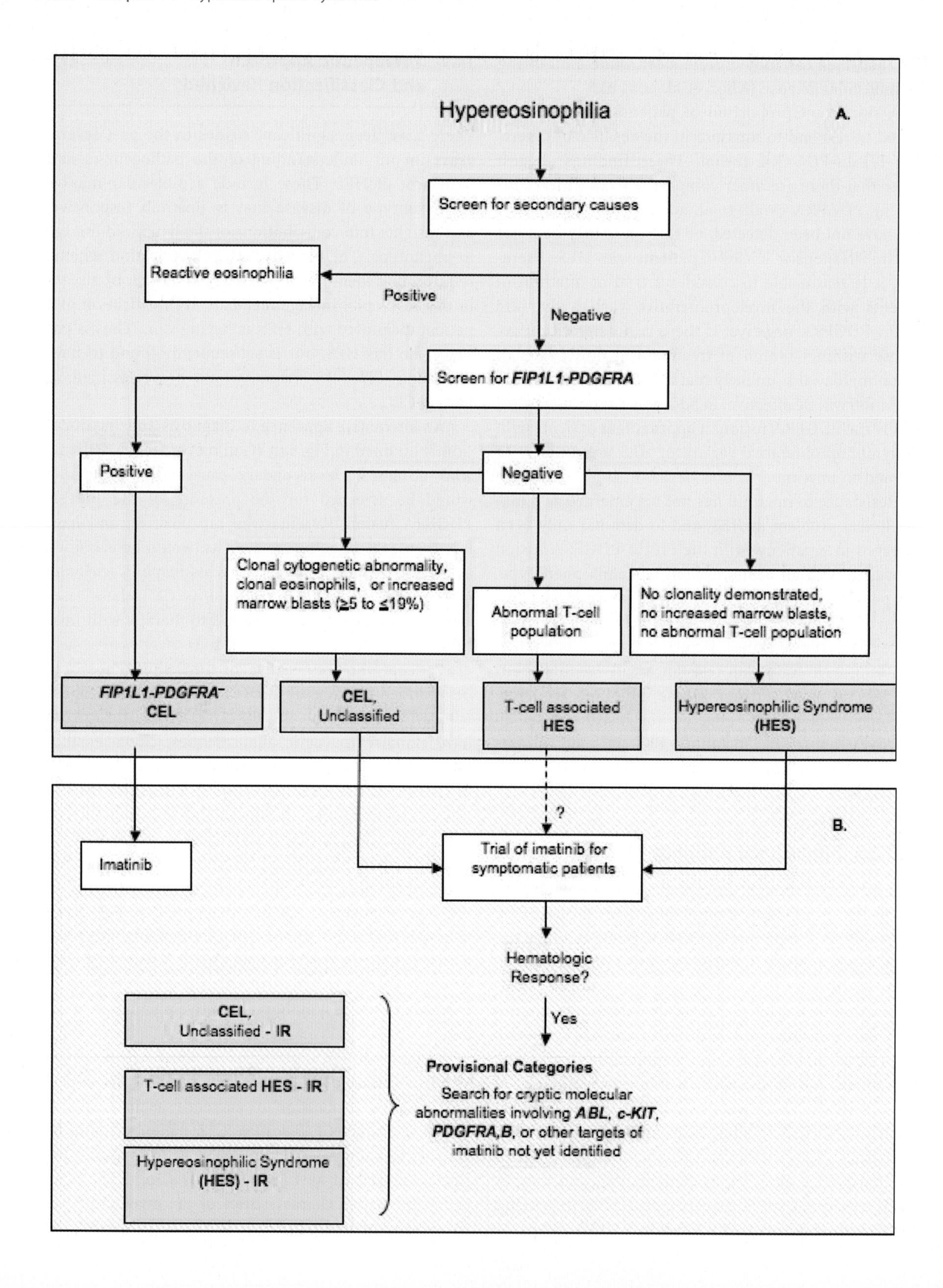
Hypereosinophilia
A.
Screen for secondary causes
Reactive eosinophilia
Positive
Negative
Screen for FIP1L1-PDGFRA
Positive
Negative
Clonal cytogenetic abnormality, clonal eosinophils, or increased marrow blasts (≥5 to ≤19%)
Abnormal T-cell population
No clonality demonstrated, no increased marrow blasts, no abnormal T-cell population
FIP1L1-PDGFRA⁻ CEL
CEL, Unclassified
T-cell associated HES
Hypereosinophilic Syndrome (HES)
?
B.
Imatinib
Trial of imatinib for symptomatic patients
Hematologic Response?
Yes
CEL, Unclassified - IR
T-cell associated HES - IR
Hypereosinophilic Syndrome (HES) - IR
Provisional Categories
Search for cryptic molecular abnormalities involving ABL, c-KIT, PDGFRA,B, or other targets of imatinib not yet identified

trial could be considered. Patients in these categories who respond to imatinib should be carefully studied to attempt to identify the imatinib-responsive allele. Finally, those patients with *T-cell HES* are less likely to respond to therapy with imatinib, but may be candidates for treatment with antibodies directed against IL5.

14.10 Summary and Conclusions

Although major strides have been made in recent years in our understanding of the molecular pathophysiology and treatment of hypereosinophilic syndromes there are a number of important problems and challenges that remain. These include developing standard treatment algorithms for FIP1L1-PDGFRA-positive patients. Further investigation is necessary to understand the optimal dose and duration of therapy with imatinib, and the clinical importance of establishing molecular remission. It will be important to characterize the genetic basis for imatinib responsiveness in patients who are FIP1L1-PDGFRA negative, and to develop strategies to overcome resistance to imatinib when it develops. Finally, it will be of interest to ascertain the basis for the lineage predilection of the FIP1L1-PDGFRA fusion to selectively stimulate eosinophils, although it is expressed in multiple myeloid lineages.

It will be important to determine the genetic basis of other eosinophilia syndromes, and whether these are also imatinib responsive, such as Churg-Strauss syndrome or eosinophilic gastroenteritis, although initial data indicates that these disorders are pathophysiologically distinct from HES. The role of T-cells in HES through both cell-autonomous and nonautonomous effects needs to be further investigated, as well as the potential role for combination therapy with anti-IL5 and imatinib in selected cases.

References

Aldebert D, Lamkhioued B, Desaint C, Gounni AS, Goldman M, Capron A, Prin L, Capron M (1996) Eosinophils express a functional receptor for interferon alpha: inhibitory role of interferon alpha on the release of mediators. Blood 87:2354–2360

Alfaham MA, Ferguson SD, Sihra B, Davies J (1987) The idiopathic hypereosinophilic syndrome. Arch Dis Child 62:601–613

Apperley JF, Gardembas M, Melo JV, Russell-Jones R, Bain J, Baxter EJ, Chase A, Chessells JM, Colombat M, Dearden CE, Dimitrijevic S, Mahon FX, Marin D, Nikolova Z, Olavarria E, Silberman S, Schultheis B, Cross NC, Goldman JM (2002) Response to imatinib mesylate in patients with chronic myeloproliferative diseases with rearrangements of the platelet-derived growth factor receptor beta. N Engl J Med 347:481–487

Ault P, Cortes J, Koller C, Kaled ES, Kantarjian H (2002) Response of idiopathic hypereosinophilic syndrome to treatment with imatinib mesylate. Leuk Res 26:881–884

Bain B, Pierre R, Imbert M, Vardiman JW, Brunning RD, Flandrin G (2001) Chronic eosinophilic leukemia and the hyperesoinpohilic syndrome. In: Jaffe ES, Harris NL, Stein H, Vardiman JW (eds) World Health Organization of tumours: tumours of the haematopoietic and lymphoid tissues. IARC Press, Lyon, France, pp 29–31

Bakhshi S, Hamre M, Mohamed AN, Feldman G, Ravindranath Y (2003) t(5;9)(q11;q34): a novel familial translocation involving Abelson oncogene and association with hypereosinophilia. J Pediatr Hematol Oncol 25:82–84

Bank I, Amariglio N, Reshef A, Hardan I, Confino Y, Trau H, Shtrasburg S, Langevitz P, Monselise Y, Shalit M, Rechavi G (2001) The hypereosinophilic syndrome associated with CD4+CD3-helper type 2 (Th2) lymphocytes. Leuk Lymphoma 42:123–133

Basara N, Markova J, Schmetzer B, Blau IW, Kiehl MG, Bischoff M, Kirsten D, Fauser AA (1998) Chronic eosinophilic leukemia: successful treatment with an unrelated bone marrow transplantation. Leuk Lymphoma 32:189–193

Blacklock HA, Cleland JF, Tan P, Pillai VM (1979) The hypereosinophilic syndrome and leukapheresis. Ann Intern Med 91:650–651

Bourrat E, Lebbe C, Calvo F (1994) Etoposide for treating the hypereosinophilic syndrome. Ann Intern Med 121:899–900

Brito-Babapulle F (1997) Clonal eosinophilic disorders and the hypereosinophilic syndrome. Blood Rev 11:129–145

Broustet A, Bernard P, Dachary D, David B, Marit G, Lacombe F, Issanchou AM, Reiffers J (1986) Acute eosinophilic leukemia with a translocation (10p+;11q–). Cancer Genet Cytogenet 21:327–333

Broxmeyer HE, Lu L, Platzer E, Feit C, Juliano L, Rubin BY (1983) Comparative analysis of the influences of human gamma, alpha and beta interferons on human multipotential (CFU-GEMM), erythroid

Fig. 14.3 A, B. An algorithm for approach to diagnosis and management of hypereosinophilia as it relates to the FIP1L1-PDGFRA allele. After exclusion of secondary causes of eosinophilia, patients should be screened for the presence of the FIP1L1-PDGFRA fusion. Those patients who are positive are classified as FIP1L1-PDGFRA-positive chronic eosinophilic syndrome (CEL) and are candidates for therapy with imatinib as a single agent. Those without the fusion, but with clonal cytogenetic abnormalities are classified as CEL, unclassified; those with clonal T-cell rearrangements as T-cell associated HES; and those lacking any of these features as HES. In any of the latter categories, symptomatic patients may also be candidates for imatinib therapy in that not all responding patients have a detectable FIP1L1-PDGFRA fusion. Patients can then be furthered classified as indicated based on imatinib responsiveness. In any of these circumstances, conventional therapy may be appropriate and may include steroids, cytoreductive therapy, and/or biological response modifiers. Certain patients may be candidates for experimental protocols that could include agents that target IL-5

(BFU-E) and granulocyte-macrophage (CFU-GM) progenitor cells. J Immunol 131:1300–1305

Brugnoni D, Airo P, Rossi G, Bettinardi A, Simon HU, Garza L, Tosoni C, Cattaneo R, Blaser K, Tucci A (1996) A case of hypereosinophilic syndrome is associated with the expansion of a CD3-CD4+ T-cell population able to secrete large amounts of interleukin-5. Blood 87:1416–1422

Brugnoni D, Airo P, Tosoni C, Taglietti M, Lodi-Rizzini F, Calzavara-Pinton P, Leali C, Cattaneo R (1997) CD3-CD4+ cells with a Th2-like pattern of cytokine production in the peripheral blood of a patient with cutaneous T cell lymphoma. Leukemia 11:1983–1985

Butterfield JH, Gleich GJ (1994) Response of six patients with idiopathic hypereosinophilic syndrome to interferon alfa. J Allergy Clin Immunol 94:1318–1326

Cameron J, Radford DJ, Howell J, O'Brien MF (1985) Hypereosinophilic heart disease. Med J Aust 143:408–410

Catovsky D, Bernasconi C, Verdonck PJ, Postma A, Hows J, van der Does-van den Berg A, Rees JK, Castelli G, Morra E, Galton DA (1980) The association of eosinophilia with lymphoblastic leukaemia or lymphoma: a study of seven patients. Br J Haematol 45:523–534

Ceretelli S, Capochiani E, Petrini M (1998) Interferon-alpha in the idiopathic hypereosinophilic syndrome: consideration of five cases. Ann Hematol 77:161–164

Chambers LA, Leonard SS, Whatmough AE, Weller PF, Bubley GJ, Kruskall MS (1990) Management of hypereosinophilic syndrome with chronic plasma- and leukapheresis. Prog Clin Biol Res 337:83–85

Chandra M, Pettigrew RI, Eley JW, Oshinski JN, Guyton RA (1996) Cine-MRI-aided endomyocardectomy in idiopathic hypereosinophilic syndrome. Ann Thorac Surg 62:1856–1858

Chang HW, Leong KH, Koh DR, Lee SH (1999) Clonality of isolated eosinophils in the hypereosinophilic syndrome. Blood 93:1651–1657

Chen J, Deangelo DJ, Kutok JL, Williams IR, Lee BH, Wadleigh M, Duclos N, Cohen S, Adelsperger J, Okabe R, Coburn A, Galinsky I, Huntly B, Cohen PS, Meyer T, Fabbro D, Roesel J, Banerji L, Griffin JD, Xiao S, Fletcher JA, Stone RM, Gilliland DG (2004) PKC412 inhibits the zinc finger 198-fibroblast growth factor receptor 1 fusion tyrosine kinase and is active in treatment of stem cell myeloproliferative disorder Proc Natl Acad Sci USA 101:14479–14484

Chockalingam A, Jalil A, Shadduck RK, Lister J (1999) Allogeneic peripheral blood stem cell transplantation for hypereosinophilic syndrome with severe cardiac dysfunction. Bone Marrow Transplant 23:1093–1094

Chusid MJ, Dale DC (1975) Eosinophilic leukemia. Remission with vincristine and hydroxyurea. Am J Med 59:297–300

Chusid MJ, Dale DC, West BC, Wolff SM (1975) The hypereosinophilic syndrome: analysis of fourteen cases with review of the literature. Medicine (Baltimore) 54:1–27

Cofrancesco E, Cortellaro M, Pogliani E, Boschetti C, Salvatore M, Polli EE (1984) Response to vincristine treatment in a case of idiopathic hypereosinophilic syndrome with multiple clinical manifestations. Acta Haematol 72:21–25

Cogan E, Schandene L, Crusiaux A, Cochaux P, Velu T, Goldman M (1994) Brief report: clonal proliferation of type 2 helper T cells in a man with the hypereosinophilic syndrome. N Engl J Med 330:535–538

Cools J, DeAngelo DJ, Gotlib J, Stover EH, Legare RD, Cortes J, Kutok J, Clark J, Galinsky I, Griffin JD, Cross NC, Tefferi A, Malone J, Alam R, Schrier SL, Schmid J, Rose M, Vandenberghe P, Verhoef G, Boogaerts M, Wlodarska I, Kantarjian H, Marynen P, Coutre SE, Stone R, Gilliland DG (2003 a) A tyrosine kinase created by fusion of the PDGFRA and FIP1L1 genes as a therapeutic target of imatinib in idiopathic hypereosinophilic syndrome. N Engl J Med 348:1201–1214

Cools J, Stover EH, Boulton CL, Gotlib J, Legare RD, Amaral SM, Curley DP, Duclos N, Rowan R, Kutok JL, Lee BH, Williams IR, Coutre SE, Stone RM, DeAngelo DJ, Marynen P, Manley PW, Meyer T, Fabbro D, Neuberg D, Weisberg E, Griffin JD, Gilliland DG (2003 b) PKC412 overcomes resistance to imatinib in a murine model of FIP1L1-PDGFRalpha-induced myeloproliferative disease. Cancer Cell 3:459–469

Cordier JF, Faure M, Hermier C, Brune J (1990) Pleural effusions in an overlap syndrome of idiopathic hypereosinophilic syndrome and erythema elevatum diutinum. Eur Respir J 3:115–118

Cortes J, Ault P, Koller C, Thomas D, Ferrajoli A, Wierda W, Rios MB, Letvak L, Kaled ES, Kantarjian H (2003) Efficacy of imatinib mesylate in the treatment of idiopathic hypereosinophilic syndrome. Blood 101:4714–4716

Davies J, Spry C (1982) Plasma exchange or leukapheresis in the hypereosinophilic syndrome. Ann Intern Med 96:791

Demiroglu A, Steer EJ, Heath C, Taylor K, Bentley M, Allen SL, Koduru P, Brody JP, Hawson G, Rodwell R, Doody ML, Carnicero F, Reiter A, Goldman JM, Melo JV, Cross NC (2001) The t(8;22) in chronic myeloid leukemia fuses BCR to FGFR1: transforming activity and specific inhibition of FGFR1 fusion proteins. Blood 98:3778–3783

DeYampert NM, Beck LA (1997) Eosinophilia and multiple erythematous indurated plaques. Idiopathic hypereosinophilic syndrome (IHS). Arch Dermatol 133:1581–1584

Duell T, Mittermuller J, Schmetzer HM, Kolb HJ, Wilmanns W (1997) Chronic myeloid leukemia associated hypereosinophilic syndrome with a clonal t(4;7)(q11;q32). Cancer Genet Cytogenet 94:91–94

Endo M, Usuki K, Kitazume K, Iwabe K, Okuyama Y, Urabe A (1995) Hypereosinophilic syndrome in Hodgkin's disease with increased granulocyte-macrophage colony-stimulating factor. Ann Hematol 71:313–314

Esteva-Lorenzo FJ, Meehan KR, Spitzer TR, Mazumder A (1996) Allogeneic bone marrow transplantation in a patient with hypereosinophilic syndrome. Am J Hematol 51:164–165

Fauci AS, Harley JB, Roberts WC, Ferrans VJ, Gralnick HR, Bjornson BH (1982) NIH conference. The idiopathic hypereosinophilic syndrome. Clinical, pathophysiologic, and therapeutic considerations. Ann Intern Med 97:78–92

Fischkoff SA, Testa JR, Schiffer CA (1988) Acute eosinophilic leukemia with a (10;11) chromosomal translocation. Leukemia 2:394–397

Forrest DL, Horsman DE, Jensen CL, Berry BR, Dalal BI, Barnett MJ, Nantel SH (1998) Myelodysplastic syndrome with hypereosinophilia and a nonrandom chromosomal abnormality dic(1;7):confirmation of eosinophil clonal involvement by fluorescence in situ hybridization. Cancer Genet Cytogenet 107:65–68

Gleich GJ, Schroeter AL, Marcoux JP, Sachs MI, O'Connell EJ, Kohler PF (1984) Episodic angioedema associated with eosinophilia. N Engl J Med 310:1621–1626

Gleich GJ, Leiferman KM, Pardanani A, Tefferi A, Butterfield JH (2002) Treatment of hypereosinophilic syndrome with imatinib mesylate. Lancet 359:1577–1578

Goldman JM, Najfeld V, Th'ng KH (1975) Agar culture and chromosome analysis of eosinophilic leukaemia. J Clin Pathol 28:956–961

Golub TR, Barker GF, Lovett M, Gilliland DG (1994) Fusion of PDGF receptor beta to a novel ets-like gene, tel, in chronic myelomonocytic leukemia with t(5;12) chromosomal translocation. Cell 77:307–316

Gotlib J, Cools J, Malone JM3, Schrier SL, Gilliland DG, Coutre SE (2004) The FIP1L1-PDGFRalpha fusion tyrosine kinase in hypereosinophilic syndrome and chronic eosinophilic leukemia: implications for diagnosis, classification, and management. Blood 103:2879–2891

Granjo E, Lima M, Lopes JM, Doria S, Orfao A, Ying S, Barata LT, Miranda M, Cross NC, Bain BJ (2002) Chronic eosinophilic leukaemia presenting with erythroderma, mild eosinophilia and hyper-IgE: clinical, immunological and cytogenetic features and therapeutic approach. A case report. Acta Haematol 107:108–112

Guasch G, Mack GJ, Popovici C, Dastugue N, Birnbaum D, Rattner JB, Pebusque MJ (2000) FGFR1 is fused to the centrosome-associated protein CEP110 in the 8p12 stem cell myeloproliferative disorder with t(8;9)(p12;q33). Blood 95:1788–1796

Hardy WR, Anderson RE (1968) The hypereosinophilic syndromes. Ann Intern Med 68:1220–1229

Harley JB, McIntosh CL, Kirklin JJ, Maron BJ, Gottdiener J, Roberts WC, Fauci AS (1982) Atrioventricular valve replacement in the idiopathic hypereosinophilic syndrome. Am J Med 73:77–81

Harrington DS, Peterson C, Ness M, Sanger W, Smith DM, Vaughan W (1988) Acute myelogenous leukemia with eosinophilic differentiation and trisomy-1. Am J Clin Pathol 90:464–469

Helmling S, Zhelkovsky A, Moore CL (2001) Fip1 regulates the activity of Poly(A) polymerase through multiple interactions. Mol Cell Biol 21:2026–2037

Hendren WG, Jones EL, Smith MD (1988) Aortic and mitral valve replacement in idiopathic hypereosinophilic syndrome. Ann Thorac Surg 46:570–571

Johnston AM, Woodcock BE (1998) Acute aortic thrombosis despite anticoagulant therapy in idiopathic hypereosinophilic syndrome. J R Soc Med 91:492–493

Juvonen E, Volin L, Koponen A, Ruutu T (2002) Allogeneic blood stem cell transplantation following non-myeloablative conditioning for hypereosinophilic syndrome. Bone Marrow Transplant 29:457–458

Kawasaki A, Mizushima Y, Matsui S, Hoshino K, Yano S, Kitagawa M (1991) A case of T-cell lymphoma accompanying marked eosinophilia, chronic eosinophilic pneumonia and eosinophilic pleural effusion. A case report. Tumori 77:527–530

Kay AB, Klion AD (2004) Anti-interleukin-5 therapy for asthma and hypereosinophilic syndrome. Immunol Allergy Clin North Am 24:645–666

Kazmierowski JA, Chusid MJ, Parrillo JE, Fauci AS, Wolff SM (1978) Dermatologic manifestations of the hypereosinophilic syndrome. Arch Dermatol 114:531–535

Klion AD, Noel P, Akin C, Law MA, Gilliland DG, Cools J, Metcalfe DD, Nutman TB (2003) Elevated serum tryptase levels identify a subset of patients with a myeloproliferative variant of idiopathic hypereosinophilic syndrome associated with tissue fibrosis, poor prognosis, and imatinib responsiveness. Blood 101:4660–4666

Klion AD, Law MA, Riemenschneider W, McMaster ML, Brown MR, Horne M, Karp B, Robinson M, Sachdev V, Tucker E, Turner M, Nutman TB (2004a) Familial eosinophilia: a benign disorder? Blood 103:4050–4055

Klion AD, Robyn J, Akin C, Noel P, Brown M, Law M, Metcalfe DD, Dunbar C, Nutman TB (2004b) Molecular remission and reversal of myelofibrosis in response to imatinib mesylate treatment in patients with the myeloproliferative variant of hypereosinophilic syndrome. Blood 103:473–478

Kwon SU, Kim JC, Kim JS (2001) Sequential magnetic resonance imaging findings in hypereosinophilia-induced encephalopathy. J Neurol 248:279–284

Le Beau MM, Larson RA, Bitter MA, Vardiman JW, Golomb HM, Rowley JD (1983) Association of an inversion of chromosome 16 with abnormal marrow eosinophils in acute myelomonocytic leukemia. A unique cytogenetic-clinicopathological association. N Engl J Med 309:630–636

Lee JH, Lee JW, Jang CS, Kwon ES, Min HY, Jeong S, Kwon KS, Lee DH, Cho HG, Kim PS, Kim HG, Shin YW, Kim YS (2002) Successful cyclophosphamide therapy in recurrent eosinophilic colitis associated with hypereosinophilic syndrome. Yonsei Med J 43:267–270

Lefebvre C, Bletry O, Degoulet P, Guillevin L, Bentata-Pessayre M, Le Thi Huong D, Godeau P (1989) [Prognostic factors of hypereosinophilic syndrome. Study of 40 cases]. Ann Med Interne (Paris) 140:253–257

Leiferman KM, O'Duffy JD, Perry HO, Greipp PR, Giuliani ER, Gleich GJ (1982) Recurrent incapacitating mucosal ulcerations. A prodrome of the hypereosinophilic syndrome. JAMA 247:1018–1020

Lepretre S, Jardin F, Buchonnet G, Lenain P, Stamatoullas A, Kupfer I, Courville P, Callat MP, Contentin N, Bastard C, Tilly H (2002) Eosinophilic leukemia associated with t(2;5)(p23;q31). Cancer Genet Cytogenet 133:164–167

Luciano L, Catalano L, Sarrantonio C, Guerriero A, Califano C, Rotoli B (1999) AlphaIFN-induced hematologic and cytogenetic remission in chronic eosinophilic leukemia with t(1;5). Haematologica 84:651–653

Luppi M, Marasca R, Morselli M, Barozzi P, Torelli G (1994) Clonal nature of hypereosinophilic syndrome. Blood 84:349–350

Matsushima T, Murakami H, Kim K, Uchiumi H, Murata N, Tamura J, Sawamura M, Karasawa M, Naruse T, Tsuchiya J (1995) Steroid-responsive pulmonary disorders associated with myelodysplastic syndromes with der(1q;7p) chromosomal abnormality. Am J Hematol 50:110–115

Matsushima T, Handa H, Yokohama A, Nagasaki J, Koiso H, Kin Y, Tanaka Y, Sakura T, Tsukamoto N, Karasawa M, Itoh K, Hirabayashi H, Sawamura M, Shinonome S, Shimano S, Miyawaki S, Nojima Y, Murakami H (2003) Prevalence and clinical characteristics of myelodysplastic syndrome with bone marrow eosinophilia or basophilia. Blood 101:3386–3390

Mecucci C, Bosly A, Michaux JL, Broeckaert-Van Orshoven A, Van den Berghe H (1985) Acute nonlymphoblastic leukemia with bone marrow eosinophilia and structural anomaly of chromosome 16. Cancer Genet Cytogenet 17:359–363

Meeker TC, Hardy D, Willman C, Hogan T, Abrams J (1990) Activation of the interleukin-3 gene by chromosome translocation in acute lymphocytic leukemia with eosinophilia. Blood 76:285–289

Moore PM, Harley JB, Fauci AS (1985) Neurologic dysfunction in the idiopathic hypereosinophilic syndrome. Ann Intern Med 102:109–114

Myint H, Chacko J, Mould S, Ross F, Oscier DG (1995) Karyotypic evolution in a granulocytic sarcoma developing in a myeloproliferative disorder with a novel (3;4) translocation. Br J Haematol 90:462–464

Nadarajah S, Krafchik B, Roifman C, Horgan-Bell C (1997) Treatment of hypereosinophilic syndrome in a child using cyclosporine: implication for a primary T-cell abnormality. Pediatrics 99:630–633

Narayan S, Ezughah F, Standen GR, Pawade J, Kennedy CT (2003) Idiopathic hypereosinophilic syndrome associated with cutaneous infarction and deep venous thrombosis. Br J Dermatol 148:817–820

Ommen SR, Seward JB, Tajik AJ (2000) Clinical and echocardiographic features of hypereosinophilic syndromes. Am J Cardiol 86:110–113

Pardanani A, Reeder T, Porrata LF, Li CY, Tazelaar HD, Baxter EJ, Witzig TE, Cross NC, Tefferi A (2003) Imatinib therapy for hypereosinophilic syndrome and other eosinophilic disorders. Blood 101:3391–3397

Parker CJ (1988) Hypereosinophilic syndrome with cutaneous blisters and bowel necrosis. Australas J Dermatol 29:103–106

Parrillo JE, Fauci AS, Wolff SM (1978) Therapy of the hypereosinophilic syndrome. Ann Intern Med 89:167–172

Pitini V, Arrigo C, Azzarello D, La Gattuta G, Amata C, Righi M, Coglitore S (2003) Serum concentration of cardiac Troponin T in patients with hypereosinophilic syndrome treated with imatinib is predictive of adverse outcomes. Blood 102:3456–3457

Popovici C, Adelaide J, Ollendorff V, Chaffanet M, Guasch G, Jacrot M, Leroux D, Birnbaum D, Pebusque MJ (1998) Fibroblast growth factor receptor 1 is fused to FIM in stem-cell myeloproliferative disorder with t(8;13). Proc Natl Acad Sci USA 95:5712–5717

Popovici C, Zhang B, Gregoire MJ, Jonveaux P, Lafage-Pochitaloff M, Birnbaum D, Pebusque MJ (1999) The t(6;8)(q27;p11) translocation in a stem cell myeloproliferative disorder fuses a novel gene, FOP, to fibroblast growth factor receptor 1. Blood 93:1381–1389

Preker PJ, Lingner J, Minvielle-Sebastia L, Keller W (1995) The FIP1 gene encodes a component of a yeast pre-mRNA polyadenylation factor that directly interacts with poly(A) polymerase. Cell 81:379–389

Quiquandon I, Claisse JF, Capiod JC, Delobel J, Prin L (1995) alpha-Interferon and hypereosinophilic syndrome with trisomy 8: karyotypic remission. Blood 85:2284–2285

Radford DJ, Garlick RB, Pohlner PG (2002) Multiple valvar replacements for hypereosinophilic syndrome. Cardiol Young 12:67–70

Roufosse F, Schandene L, Sibille C, Kennes B, Efira A, Cogan E, Goldman M (1999) T-cell receptor-independent activation of clonal Th2 cells associated with chronic hypereosinophilia. Blood 94:994–1002

Roufosse F, Schandene L, Sibille C, Willard-Gallo K, Kennes B, Efira A, Goldman M, Cogan E (2000) Clonal Th2 lymphocytes in patients with the idiopathic hypereosinophilic syndrome. Br J Haematol 109:540–548

Roufosse F, Cogan E, Goldman M (2003) The hypereosinophilic syndrome revisited. Annu Rev Med 54:169–184

Roufosse F, Cogan E, Goldman M (2004) Recent advances in pathogenesis and management of hypereosinophilic syndromes. Allergy 59:673–689

Sakamoto K, Erdreich-Epstein A, deClerck Y, Coates T (1992) Prolonged clinical response to vincristine treatment in two patients with idiopathic hypereosinophilic syndrome. Am J Pediatr Hematol Oncol 14:348–351

Sanchez JL, Padilla MA (1982) Hypereosinophilic syndrome. Cutis 29:490–492

Schaller JL, Burkland GA (2001) Case report: rapid and complete control of idiopathic hypereosinophilia with imatinib mesylate. MedGenMed 3:9

Schandene L, Del Prete GF, Cogan E, Stordeur P, Crusiaux A, Kennes B, Romagnani S, Goldman M (1996) Recombinant interferon-alpha selectively inhibits the production of interleukin-5 by human CD4+ T cells. J Clin Invest 97:309–315

Schoffski P, Ganser A, Pascheberg U, Busche G, Gaede B, Hertenstein B (2000) Complete haematological and cytogenetic response to interferon alpha-2a of a myeloproliferative disorder with eosinophilia associated with a unique t(4;7) aberration. Ann Hematol 79:95–98

Score J, Curtis C, Waghorn K, Stalder M, Jotterand M, Grand FH, Cross NC (2006) Identification of a novel imatinib responsive KIF5B-PDGFRA fusion gene following screening for PDGFRA overexpression in patients with hypereosinophilia. Leukemia 20(5):827–832

Sigmund DA, Flessa HC (1995) Hypereosinophilic syndrome: successful allogeneic bone marrow transplantation. Bone Marrow Transplant 15:647–648

Slabbynck H, Impens N, Naegels S, Dewaele M, Schandevyl W (1992) Idiopathic hypereosinophilic syndrome-related pulmonary involvement diagnosed by bronchoalveolar lavage. Chest 101:1178–1180

Smit AJ, van Essen LH, de Vries EG (1991) Successful long-term control of idiopathic hypereosinophilic syndrome with etoposide. Cancer 67:2826–2827

Song HS, Park SK (1987) A case of monosomy-7 eosinophilic leukemia and neurofibromatosis, terminated with disseminated cryptococcosis. Korean J Intern Med 2:131–134

Spry CJ, Davies J, Tai PC, Olsen EG, Oakley CM, Goodwin JF (1983) Clinical features of fifteen patients with the hypereosinophilic syndrome. Q J Med 52:1–22

Stover EH, Chen J, Folens C, Lee BH, Mentens N, Marynen P, Williams IR, Gilliland DG, Cools J (2006) Activation of FIP1L1-PDGFRα requires disruption of the juxtamembrane domain of PDGFRα and is FIP1L1-independent. Proc Natl Acad Sci USA 103:8078–8083

Swirsky DM, Li YS, Matthews JG, Flemans RJ, Rees JK, Hayhoe FG (1984) 8;21 translocation in acute granulocytic leukaemia: cytological, cytochemical and clinical features. Br J Haematol 56:199–213

Tai PC, Ackerman SJ, Spry CJ, Dunnette S, Olsen EG, Gleich GJ (1987) Deposits of eosinophil granule proteins in cardiac tissues of patients with eosinophilic endomyocardial disease. Lancet 1:643–647

Takai K, Sanada M (1991) Hypereosinophilic syndrome evolving to acute lymphoblastic leukemia. Int J Hematol 54:231–239

Tanino M, Kitamura K, Ohta G, Yamamoto Y, Sugioka G (1983) Hypereosinophilic syndrome with extensive myocardial involvement and mitral valve thrombus instead of mural thrombi. Acta Pathol Jpn 33:1233–1242

Ueno NT, Zhao S, Robertson LE, Consoli U, Andreeff M (1997) 2-Chlorodeoxyadenosine therapy for idiopathic hypereosinophilic syndrome. Leukemia 11:1386–1390

Ueno NT, Anagnostopoulos A, Rondon G, Champlin RE, Mikhailova N, Pankratova OS, Zoubarovskaya LS, Semenova EV, Afanasyev BV, O'Brien S, Andreeff M, Zaritskey AY (2002) Successful non-myeloablative allogeneic transplantation for treatment of idiopathic hypereosinophilic syndrome. Br J Haematol 119:131–134

Vazquez L, Caballero D, Canizo CD, Lopez C, Hernandez R, Gonzalez I, Flores T, San Miguel JF (2000) Allogeneic peripheral blood cell transplantation for hypereosinophilic syndrome with myelofibrosis. Bone Marrow Transplant 25:217–218

Venge P, Dahl R, Hallgren R, Ollson I 1980, Cationic proteins of human eosinophils and their role in the inflammatory reaction. In: Mahmoud A, Austen KF (eds) The eosinophil in health and disease. Grune and Stratton, New York, pp 131–144

von Bubnoff N, Sandherr M, Schlimok G, Andreesen R, Peschel C, Duyster J (2005) Myeloid blast crisis evolving during imatinib treatment of an FIP1L1-PDGFR alpha-positive chronic myeloproliferative disease with prominent eosinophilia. Leukemia 19:286–287

Walz C, Curtis S, Schnittger S, Schultheis B, Metzgeroth G, Schoch C, Lengfelder E, Erben P, Muller MC, Haferlach T, Hochhaus A, Hehlmann R, Cross NC, Reiter A (2006) Transient response to imatinib in a chronic eosinophilic leukemia associated with ins(9;4)(q33;q12q25) and a CDK5RAP2-PDGFRA fusion gene. Genes Chromosomes Cancer 45(10):950–956

Weingarten JS, O'Sheal SF, Margolis WS (1985) Eosinophilic meningitis and the hypereosinophilic syndrome. Case report and review of the literature. Am J Med 78:674–676

Weller PF, Bubley GJ (1994) The idiopathic hypereosinophilic syndrome. Blood 83:2759–2779

Weyman AE, Rankin R, King H (1977) Loeffler's endocarditis presenting as mitral and tricuspid stenosis. Am J Cardiol 40:438–444

Wichman A, Buchthal F, Pezeshkpour GH, Fauci AS (1985) Peripheral neuropathy in hypereosinophilic syndrome. Neurology 35:1140–1145

Winn RE, Kollef MH, Meyer JI (1994) Pulmonary involvement in the hypereosinophilic syndrome. Chest 105:656–660

Wynn SR, Sachs MI, Keating MU, Ostrom NK, Kadota RP, O'Connell EJ, Smithson WA (1987) Idiopathic hypereosinophilic syndrome in a 5 1/2-month-old infant. J Pediatr 111:94–97

Yakushijin K, Murayama T, Mizuno I, Sada A, Koizumi T, Imoto S (2001) Chronic eosinophilic leukemia with unique chromosomal abnormality, t(5;12) (q33;q22). Am J Hematol 68:301–302

Yamada O, Kitahara K, Imamura K, Ozasa H, Okada M, Mizoguchi H (1998) Clinical and cytogenetic remission induced by interferon-alpha in a patient with chronic eosinophilic leukemia associated with a unique t(3;9;5) translocation. Am J Hematol 58:137–141

Yates P, Potter MN (1991) Eosinophilic leukaemia with an abnormality of 5q31, the site of the IL-5 gene. Clin Lab Haematol 13:211–215

Yoon TY, Ahn GB, Chang SH (2000) Complete remission of hypereosinophilic syndrome after interferon-alpha therapy: report of a case and literature review. J Dermatol 27:110–115

Zabel P, Schlaak M (1991) Cyclosporin for hypereosinophilic syndrome. Ann Hematol 62:230–231

Chronic Idiopathic Myelofibrosis

John T. Reilly

Contents

Abstract. Chronic idiopathic myelofibrosis (CIMF) is a clinico-pathological entity characterized by a stem-cell-derived clonal myeloproliferation, extramedullary hematopoiesis, proliferation of bone marrow stromal components, splenomegaly, and ineffective erythropoiesis. It is the least common of the chronic myeloproliferative disorders and carries the worst prognosis with a median survival of only 4 years. Treatment for most cases is supportive, while androgens, recombinant erythropoietin, steroids and immuno-modulatory drugs are effective approaches for the management of anemia. Splenectomy and involved field irradiation may also be beneficial in carefully selected patients. Cure is only possible following bone marrow transplantation and a number of practical prognostic scores are available for identifying patients that would benefit from this approach. Recently, the use of low intensity conditioning has resulted in prolonged survival and lower transplant-related mortality. Finally, the recent reports of the association of CIMF with a gain-of-function JAK2 mutation opens the door to targeted therapies as well as molecular monitoring of treatment response.

15.1 Introduction

Chronic idiopathic myelofibrosis (CIMF), or myelofibrosis with myeloid metaplasia (MMM), is a chronic stem cell disorder characterized by bone marrow fibrosis, extramedullary hematopoiesis, splenomegaly, and a leuko-erythroblastic blood picture. It is an uncommon disorder, with a reported annual incidence ranging from 0.5 to 1.3 per 100,000 (Dougan et al. 1981; Mesa et al. 1997), with the highest rates being found among the Ashkenazi Jews in northern Israel (Chaiter et al. 1992). The etiology of CIMF is unknown, although environmental factors may be relevant as the disorder has been linked in a small number of patients to radiation (Andersen et al. 1964) and benzene exposure (Hu 1987). Although first described by Heuck in 1879, it was not until 1951, following Dameshek's seminal publication (Dameshek 1951), that the disease was regarded as one of the chronic myeloproliferative disorders. Recently, considerable progress has been made in understanding its pathogenesis, although this has yet to result in significant therapeutic advances. Indeed, its prognosis remains poor when compared to other *BCR-ABL*-negative chronic myeloproliferative disorders (Rozman et al. 1991), with death resulting from cardiac failure, infection, hemorrhage, and leukemic transformation.

15.2 Pathogenesis

15.2.1 Clonality

It has been appreciated for many years that CIMF is a clonal disorder and that the disease arises from the proliferation of malignant pluripotential stem cells. Such a conclusion was first suggested by early studies of the X-chromosome inactivation patterns of G-6-PD in patients who were heterozygous for this gene (Jacobson et al. 1978; Kahn et al. 1975). However, the low frequency of G-6-PD heterozygotes in the general population has led several groups to analyze the more informative X-linked genes, hypoxanthine phosphoribosyl transferase (HPRT) and phosphoglycerate kinase (PGK). In these studies, monoclonal hematopoiesis was documented in all patients irrespective of whether they had early cellular phase disease or more advanced myelofibrosis (Kreipe et al. 1991; Tsukamoto et al. 1994). Recently, Reeder and colleagues (2003), using fluorescent in situ hybridization (FISH), have provided evidence that both B and T cells can be involved, while karyotypic analysis has shown that the stromal proliferation is polyclonal, or reactive, and not part of the underlying clonal hematopoiesis (Jacobson et al. 1978; Wang et al. 1992). Involvement of the B and T lymphocytic lineage was also suggested by an earlier study that utilized N-*Ras* gene mutational analysis, again supporting the pluripotent stem cell origin of the disease (Buschle et al. 1988). An increased number of circulating hematopoietic precursors, including pluripotent (CFU-GEMM) and lineage restricted progenitor cells (BFU-E, CFU-GM, and CFU-MK), is a feature of CIMF (Carlo-Stella et al. 1987; Han et al. 1988; Hibbin et al. 1984) and is likely to result from the proteolytic release of stem cells from the marrow (Zu et al. 2005). It is also possible that the spleen and liver contribute to the circulating progenitor pool (Wolf and Neiman 1987) as splenectomy temporarily normalizes levels (Craig et al. 1991). The high level of circulating progenitor cells is reflected in the significantly increased peripheral blood $CD34^+$ cell count (Andreasson et al. 2002; Arora et al. 2004). Indeed, it has been proposed that not only can the absolute number of $CD34^+$ cells be used to differentiate CIMF from other Philadelphia (Ph)-negative CMPDs, but the levels may also predict evolution to blast transformation (Barosi et al. 2001). Increased sensitivity of committed erythroid progenitors to erythropoietin has been reported (Carlo-Stella et al. 1987), while CFU-MK may exhibit autonomous growth (Han et al. 1988; Taksin et al. 1999) and/or hypersensitivity to interleukin-3 (Kobayashi et al. 1993). Such findings, coupled with the fact that autonomous megakaryocyte growth is not related to *MPL* mutations or autocrine stimulation by Mpl-L (Taksin et al. 1999), suggest that events downstream from receptor-ligand binding are likely to be pathogenetically important (Taksin et al. 1999). Finally, indirect evidence for the involvement of the pluripotential stem cell is provided by the rare reports of acquired hemoglobin H disease (Veer et al. 1979), paroxysmal nocturnal hemoglobinuria (Nakahata et al. 1993; Shaheen et al. 2005), acquired Pelger-Huet anomaly and neutrophil dysfunction (Perianin et al. 1984), as well as many abnormalities of platelet function (Cunietti et al. 1981; Schafer 1982).

15.2.2 Cytogenetics

Cytogenetic studies have played a pivotal role in the elucidation of pathogenetically important oncogenes in many hematological malignancies although, until recently, the data for CIMF has been sparse and confusing. However, over the last 15 years the publication of three large studies, involving a total of 256 well-characterized patients, has helped to clarify the situation (Demory et al. 1988; Reilly et al. 1997; Tefferi et al. 2001a). All three studies, as well as a literature review of 157 abnormal cases (Bench et al. 1998), have revealed that deletions of 13q and 20q, trisomy 8 and abnormalities of chromosomes 1, 7, and 9 constitute more than 80% of all chromosomal changes in CIMF. Deletions of 13q are the most common cytogenetic abnormality, occurring in approximately 25% of cases with an abnormal cytogenetic analysis (Demory et al. 1988; Reilly et al. 1997). The genetic loss is large and involves the gene-rich region around RB-1, D13S319, and D13S25 (Sinclair et al. 2001). It is possible that more than one gene is involved on chromosome 13 since Macdonald and colleagues (1999) reported a case of CIMF with a t(4;13)(q25;q12) and provided evidence for the involvement of a novel gene located at 13q12. The second and third most common abnormalities are deletions of 20q and partial duplication of the long arm of chromosome 1, respectively (Demory et al. 1988; Reilly et al. 1997). Amplifications of 1q follow a nonrandom pattern and, although it may involve the whole of 1q, it always appears to include the specific segment, 1q23-1q32 (Donti et al. 1990). The inability to identify common breakpoints, or a preferential translocation site, suggests that an increase in gene(s) copy number located on 1q is more important than the position effect due to the juxtaposition of specific DNA sequences. In support of this view, Zanke and colleagues (1994) have demonstrated amplification and overexpression of a hematopoietic protein tyrosine phosphatase (HePTP) in patients with partial trisomy 1q. The underlying molecular consequences of 13q- and 20q- remain to be determined, although extensive mapping and mutational screening have not identified any candidate genes and suggest that haplo-insufficiency may be a mechanism (reviewed Reilly 2005). These three lesions, however, are not specific for CIMF and have also been reported in polycythemia vera, myelodysplastic syndrome, and other hematological malignancies. In contrast, the abnormality der(6)t(1;6)(q23-25;p21-22) has been recently identified as a possible marker for CIMF, although it is scarce, occurring in less than 3% of cases (Dingli et al. 2005). The incidence of chromosomal abnormalities in CIMF is significantly lower in younger patients (Cervantes et al. 1998), a fact that may explain their better prognosis. Indeed, normal cytogenetic findings are characteristic of pediatric cases, which, coupled with their long-term survival, suggests that they may have a different pathogenesis and require a more conservative management (Altura et al. 2000). Comparative genomic hybridization (CGH) studies have revealed that genomic aberrations are much more common than indicated by standard cytogenetic analysis and occur in the majority of cases. Gains of 9p appear to be the most frequent finding, occurring in 50% of cases, and suggests that genes on 9p may play a crucial role in the pathogenesis of CIMF (Al-Assar et al. 2005). A third of patients with CIMF possess an abnormal karyotype at diagnosis (Okamura et al. 2001; Reilly et al. 1994), although this increases to approximately 90% following acute transformation, a finding that supports the multistep process of leukemogenesis (Mesa et al. 2005; Reilly et al. 1994). The majority of leukemic transformations exhibit "high risk" cytogenetic changes, including -5/5q- and -7/-7q and, as a result, respond dismally to chemotherapy (Mesa et al. 2005).

Chromosomal abnormalities have been associated with a poor prognosis in several studies (Demory et al. 1988; Reilly et al. 1997), although the prognostic impact of specific cytogenetic lesions has been difficult to define. A recent report addressed this issue and indicated that only certain clonal abnormalities, such as trisomy 8 and deletion of 12p, carry an adverse prognosis, in contrast to the majority of changes which have little survival effect (Tefferi et al. 2001a). In addition, a number of rare karyotypic abnormalities, unrelated to therapy, have been associated with a poor outcome. Trisomy 13, a nonrandom aberration in myelofibrosis, confers a poor prognosis due to early blast transformation (Zojer et al. 1999), as appears also to be the case for del(1)t(1;9) (Rege-Cambrin et al. 1991) and t(6;10)(q27;q11) (Cox et al. 2001). Recently, Strasser-Weipel et al. (2004) reported the association of chromosome 7 deletions (-7/7q-) with an unfavorable prognosis, although surprisingly not with leukemic transformation. Finally, cytogenetic abnormalities have also been linked to treatment response, with anemia responding less well in patients with chromosomal abnormalities (Besa et al. 1982).

15.2.3 Molecular Studies

Recently, an acquired somatic point mutation in the *JAK2* gene (Val617Phe) has been reported in 49% of a total of 88 CIMF patients by four independent groups (Baxter et al. 2005; James et al. 2005; Kralovics et al. 2005; Levine et al. 2005). This mutation, which also occurs in approximately 90% of patients with polycythemia vera and 40% of patients with essential thrombocythemia, almost certainly contributes to the myeloproliferative state, as cellular expression has been shown to lead to growth factor independence (James et al. 2005) as well as myelofibrosis in a murine bone marrow transplant model (Wernig et al. 2006). Interestingly, 22% of CIMF cases are homozygous for the *JAK2* mutation, a feature that appears linked to loss of heterozygosity of 9p (Kralovics et al. 2005). Initial clinical studies suggest that CIMF patients possessing the *JAK2* mutation have a higher total white cell and neutrophil count, are less likely to require blood transfusions and have a poorer survival (Campbell et al. 2006). It is to be hoped that this novel finding will lead to the future development of targeted therapy for use in this group of related disorders. The molecular defects in the remaining cases remain essentially unknown. Intriguingly, STAT5 has been reported to be constitutively activated in the majority of CIMF $CD34^+$ cells and megakaryocytes (Komura et al. 2003), and suggests that STAT5 activation may occur by mechanisms other than by acquired *JAK2* mutations. However, mutational screening of candidate receptor tyrosine kinase (RTK) genes that activate JAK2, namely *c-KIT*, *c-FMS*, and *FLT3*, has been unhelpful (Abu-Duhier et al. 2003). A possible clue to alternative STAT5 activation mechanisms in CIMF is the reported overexpression of FK506 binding protein 56 (FKBP51) in megakaryocytes. This immunophilin is known to induce sustained activation of the JAK2/STAT5 pathway as well as being able to induce an antiapoptotic phenotype (Giraudier et al. 2002). Overexpression of FKBP51 may also have a role in the activation of NF-κB, a feature of CIMF megakaryocytes and circulating CD34 cells (Komura et al. 2005). The mechanism by which FKBP51 is upregulated in CIMF, however, remains to be determined. *RAS* mutations, predominantly affecting codon 12 of *N-RAS*, have been described, but appear rare, occurring in approximately 6% of patients in chronic phase (Reilly et al. 1994). Mutations involving *p53* and *p16* are also rare in the chronic phase of the disease, although they may be associated with transformation of a variety of BCR-ABL-negative chronic myeloproliferative disorders, including myelofibrosis (Gaidano et al. 1993; Tsuruni et al. 2002; Wang and Chen 1999). Kimura and colleagues (1997) reported *KIT* mutations (Asp52Asn) in two patients and suggested that this acquired abnormality resulted in enhanced sensitivity to KIT ligand. However, a detailed study did not confirm these findings, suggesting that such mutations are rare (Abu-Duhier et al. 2003). Loss of heterozygosity (LOH) studies have highlighted RARβ2 to be a candidate tumor suppressor gene in CIMF, although for most patients epigenetic changes rather than gene deletion may be the most significant determinant of reduced activity (Jones et al. 2004). Finally, a recent study, using oligonucleotide microarrays on purified $CD34^+$ cells, has highlighted the potential underlying complexity in CIMF by identifying 95 genes that were aberrantly expressed (Jones et al. 2005)

15.2.4 Role of Growth Factors

Myelofibrotic stroma has a complex structure, characterized by an increase in total collagen, that includes both the interstitial and basement membrane collagens, types I, III, IV, V, and VI (Apaja-Sarkkinen et al. 1986; Gay et al. 1984; Reilly, et al. 1985a, 1995b). In addition, there is an excessive deposition of fibronectin (Reilly et al. 1985a), laminin (Reilly et al. 1985b) tenascin (Reilly et al. 1995), and vitronectin (Reilly and Nash 1988) as well as a marked neo-vascularization and an associated endothelial cell proliferation (Mesa et al. 2000; Reilly et al. 1985b). Indeed, the hypervascularity and sinusoidal hyperplasia leads to a marked increase in bone marrow blood flow (Charbord 1986). The increased deposition of interstitial and basement membrane antigens is supported by the findings of raised serum markers for laminin and collagen types I, III, and IV, especially in patients with active disease (Hasselbalch et al. 1986; Reilly et al. 1995). These complex structural features and the wealth of stromal proteins are now believed to result from the abnormal release of growth factors, especially PDGF and TGF-β, from clonally involved megakaryocytes (Fig. 15.1).

15.2.4.1 Platelet-Derived Growth Factor

A number of observations support the concept that the megakaryocytic lineage plays a pivotal role in the pathogenesis of myelofibrotic stroma. Structural and matura-

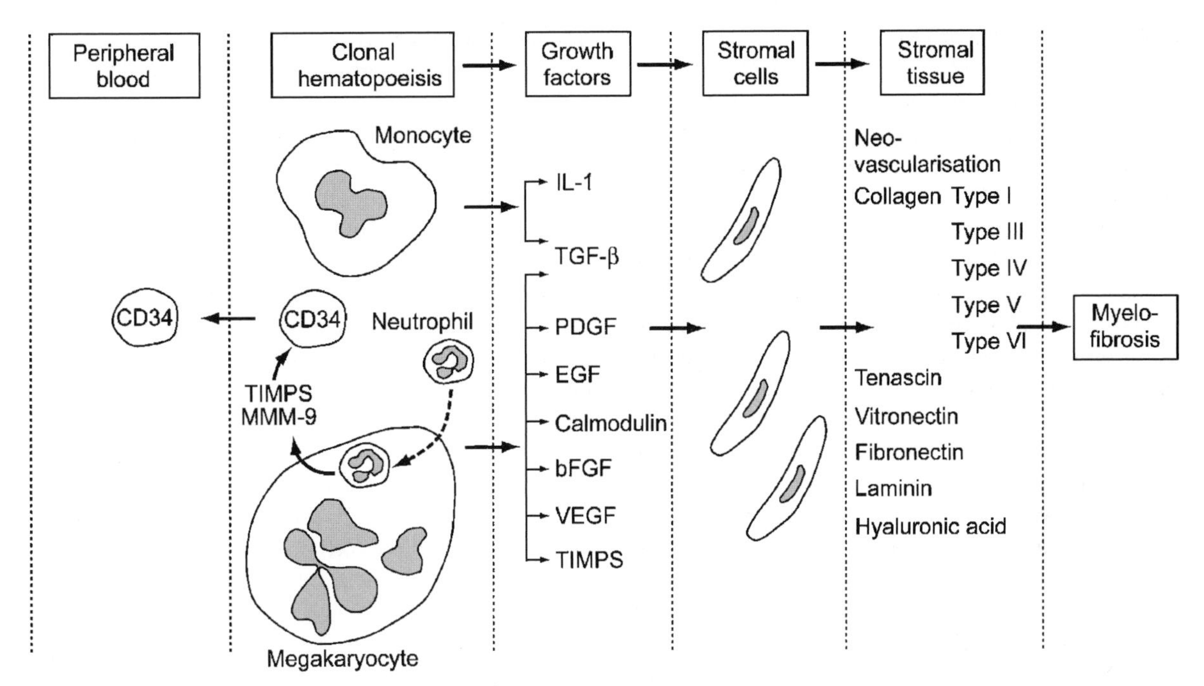

Fig. 15.1. The current pathogenetic model for the development of myelofibrotic stroma. bFGF, basic fibroblast growth factor; EGF, epidermal growth factor; IL-1, interleukin-1; PDGF, Platelet-derived growth factor; TGF-β, transforming growth factor-β; TIMPs, Tissue inhibitors of metalloproteins; VEGF, vascular growth factor. (Modified from Reilly 1997, Blood Reviews 11:233–242)

tional defects of megakaryocytes are well-recognized features, including conspicuous proliferation and clustering, and with accumulation of fibrotic tissue often being associated with necrotic and/or dysplastic megakaryocytes (Thiele et al. 1991). In addition, bone marrow fibrosis is a well-described feature of patients with megakaryocytic leukemia (Den Ottolander et al. 1979) and the rare Gray Platelet Syndrome (Jantunen et al. 1994), disorders that are thought to affect platelet alpha granule packaging. However, the first tangible evidence for the role of megakaryocytic-derived growth factors was provided by Castro-Malaspina and colleagues (1981), who demonstrated that megakaryocytic homogenates stimulated the proliferation of bone marrow fibroblasts and that this effect was the result of PDGF. Subsequently, decreased platelet PDGF levels (Bernabei et al. 1986; Dolan et al. 1991; Katoh et al. 1988) associated with increased plasma and urinary levels (Gersuk et al. 1989) were reported in patients, a finding thought to reflect an abnormal release and/or leakage of PDGF from bone marrow megakaryocytes. In addition, similar findings for platelet β-thromboglobulin and platelet factor 4 favor a platelet and/or megakaryocyte release mechanism (Romano et al. 1990; Sacchi et al. 1986). However, the release of PDGF, while undoubtedly inducing fibroblast growth, cannot account totally for the observed complexity of the stromal tissue. PDGF, for example, does not have angiogenic properties, nor does it increase the transcription of stromal proteins. Additional growth factors must play a role, the most important of which is probably transforming growth factor-β.

15.2.4.2 Transforming Growth Factor-β (TGF-β)

Like PDGF, TGF-β is synthesized by megakaryocytes, stored in platelet alpha granules and released at sites of injury (Fava et al. 1990). The pathological relevance of TGF-β lies in its ability to regulate extracellular matrix synthesis. It increases, for example, transcription of genes that code for fibronectin, collagens I, III and IV, and tenascin. It possesses powerful angiogenetic properties, with neovascularization occurring within 48 h of injection and, in addition, it can decrease the activity of metalloproteinases, enzymes that degrade extracellular stromal tissue (Overall et al. 1989; Roberts et al. 1986). In addition, TGF-β promotes endothelial cell migration, enhances stromal cell synthesis of vascular endothelial growth factor (VEGF), and may also inhibit the production of antiangiogenic molecules (Harmey et al. 1998; O'Mahoney et al. 1998). The combined effect of these activities is the increased synthesis and accumulation of extracellular matrix. Evidence for a pathogenetic role in CIMF include the report of significantly increased intraplatelet TGF-β levels when compared to normal platelets (Martyr et al. 1991), the finding of active TGF-β synthesis by megakaryoblasts (Terui et al. 1990), and the finding of increased plasma concentrations in a case of acute micromegakaryocytic leukemia that correlated with enhanced stromal turnover (Reilly et al. 1993). In addition, TGF-β expression is increased in patients' peripheral blood mononuclear cells at the mRNA level and/or at the secreted protein level (Martyré et al. 1994). Megakaryocytes, however, may not be the only cellular source of TGF-β, since TGF-β deposition appears to correlate with fibrosis even in cases with normal or reduced megakaryocyte numbers (Johnson et al. 1995). Interestingly, macrophages are frequently increased in myelofibrosis (Thiele et al. 1992; Titius et al. 1994) as is serum M-CSF, a growth factor which regulates the survival, proliferation, differentiation, and activation of macrophages (Gilbert et al. 1989). Furthermore, it has been shown that circulating monocytes in CIMF may be preactivated and contain increased levels of cytoplasmic TGF-β and IL-1 (Rameshwar et al. 1994). It has also been hypothesized that extracellular matrix protein-adhesion molecule interactions, involving CD44, may induce overproduction of fibrogenic cytokines in CIMF monocytes and contribute to stromal fibrosis in the bone marrow (Rameshwar et al. 1996). However, TGF-β is known to negatively regulate the cycling status of primitive progenitor cells and yet CIMF is characterized by an increased number of circulating CD34+ cells. This apparent paradox has been addressed by Le Bousse-Kerdiles and colleagues, who suggest that the explanation may, in part, be due to an acquired reduction in TGF-β type II receptor expression on myelofibrotic CD34+ progenitor cells. This fact, coupled with increased expression of basic fibroblast growth factor (bFGF) on the same cells, could explain the impaired inhibition by TGF-β (Le Bousse-Kerdiles et al. 1996).

15.2.4.3 Additional Growth Factors and Cytokines

A number of additional growth factors have been implicated in the pathogenesis of myelofibrotic stroma, including the calcium binding protein calmodulin, basic fibroblast growth factor (bFGF), vascular endothelial growth factor (VEGF), and the tissue inhibitors of metalloproteinases (TIMPS) (Fig. 15.1). Several facts suggest a role for extracellular calmodulin, including the finding of elevated urinary levels in CIMF, the knowledge that platelets are a rich source of calmodulin, and the fact that the protein acts as a fibroblast mitogen in the absence other growth factors (Dalley et al. 1996; Eastham et al. 1994). The finding of elevated plasma levels of VEGF in CIMF (Novetsky et al. 1997), coupled with the fact that megakaryocytes produce and secrete large amounts (Brogi et al. 1994), suggests that this multifunctional cytokine may also contribute to the pathogenesis of the characteristic neoangiogenesis. In addition, bFGF has been reported by Martyré and colleagues (1997) to be elevated in platelets and megakaryocytes from CIMF patients, while urinary excretion is similarly increased (Dalley et al. 1996). Megakaryocytes and platelets are also rich sources of releasable TIMPS, with serum levels being significantly higher than those found in plasma. These proteins may contribute to the induction of marrow fibrosis by inhibiting connective tissue breakdown by members of the matrix metalloproteinase family and by functioning as growth factors for marrow fibroblasts. Indeed, Murate and colleagues (1997) have shown that the combined effects of TIMP-1 and TIMP-2 are almost equal to the fibrogenic effects of TGF-β. Recently, Emadi and colleagues (2005) have provided evidence for the involvement of IL-8 and its receptors (CXCR1 and CXCR2) in the altered megakaryocytic proliferation, differentiation and ploidization characteristic of CIMF, while IL-6 is also likely to be involved (Wang et al. 1997). The study of the pathogenesis of osteosclerosis typical of advanced CIMF has been limited, but it may be related to the overproduction of osteoprotegerin (OPG) (Wang et al. 2004).

Finally, an underlying mechanism for megakaryocyte-derived growth factor release has recently been proposed, in addition to the standard model of dysplasia and defective alpha granule packaging. CIMF, for example, is characterized by enhanced neutrophil and eosinophil emperipolesis by megakaryocytes, with the latter expressing both abnormal amounts and distribution of P-selectin, an important mediator of neutrophil rolling (Schmitt et al. 2002). Activation of the engulfed neutrophils results in release of their proteolytic enzymes leading both to death of cells and the release of megakaryocytic TGF-β and PDGF. This phenomenon could also underlie the increased neutrophil elastase and active MMP-9 present in CIMF which, as a result of their multiple proteolytic activities, may enhance the release of $CD34^+$ progenitor cells from the bone marrow (Schmitt et al. 2002; Xu et al. 2003) (Fig. 15.1).

15.2.5 Animal Models

Several mouse models support the pivotal role of megakaryocytes in the development of the stromal proliferation, or myelofibrosis, that characterizes CIMF. These models were originally developed to investigate the role of thrombopoietin (TPO) and its receptor (Mpl), as well as the transcription factor GATA-1, in the control of megakaryocytopoiesis (Vannuchi et al. 2004; Yan et al. 1996). It was noted, however, that mice that overexpressed TPO, or underexpressed GATA-1, developed a clinical state similar to myelofibrosis, with tear drop poikilocytosis, increased circulating progenitors, and extramedullary hematopoiesis. The linking event appears to be a block in megakaryocyte differentiation, associated with an abnormal localization of P-selectin, which leads to neutrophil emperipolesis and the eventual release of TGF-β1 from megakaryocytic alpha granules (Vannucchi et al. 2005). These animal models support clinical observations and imply that myelofibrosis may not have a single cause, but may be the consequence of any perturbation that leads to increased neutrophil emperipolesis within the megakaryocyte. Although such models do not provide any insight into the pathogenesis of the underlying clonal hematopoiesis, they do support the link between TGF-β and stromal tissue development and may be of value for identifying novel antifibrotic agents for use in reversing clinical myelofibrosis.

15.3 Diagnosis

Classical CIMF is characterized by bone marrow fibrosis, extramedullary hematopoiesis, splenomegaly, and a leuko-erythroblastic blood picture. However, in contrast to CML, there is no specific biological marker and many

Table 15.1. Conditions associated with bone marrow fibrosis

Malignant	Non-malignant
Chronic idiopathic myelofibrosis	Infections (e.g., TB, visceral leischmaniasis
Other chronic myeloproliferative disorders, histoplasmosis, HIV) (e.g., PV, CML, ET)	Renal osteodystrophy
Acute megakaryoblastic leukemia	Vitamin D deficiency
(Acute myelofibrosis)	Hypothyroidism
Myelodysplastic syndromes	Hyperthyroidism
Acute myeloid leukemia	Gray platelet syndrome
Acute lymphoblastic leukemia	Systemic lupus erythematosus
Hairy cell leukemia	Scleroderma
Hodgkin's disease	Radiation exposure
Non-Hodgkin's lymphoma	Benzene exposure
Multiple myeloma	Gaucher's disease
Systemic mastocytosis	Osteopetrosis
Metastatic carcinoma (e.g., breast, prostate, stomach)	

Table 15.2. Italian Consensus Diagnostic criteria

Necessary criteria
Diffuse bone marrow fibrosis
Absence of Ph-chromosome or *BCR-ABL*
Optional criteria
Splenomegaly of any grade
Aniso-poikilocytosis
Presence of immature circulating myeloid cells
Presence of circulating erythroblasts
Clusters of megakaryocytes and abnormal megakaryocytes in the bone marrow
Myeloid metaplasia

Diagnosis of CIMF is acceptable if the following combinations are present: the two necessary criteria plus any other two optional criteria when splenomegaly is present, or the two necessary criteria plus any other four criteria if splenomegaly is absent.

studies have included a heterogeneous population of patients. The inappropriate inclusion of cases with secondary myelofibrosis, postpolycythemic myelofibrosis, and myelodysplasia with myelofibrosis and related disorders (Table 15.1) may explain the discrepancies in the early literature relating to cytogenetic abnormalities, therapeutic response, and prognosis. To address these difficulties, the "Italian Consensus Conference on Diagnostic Criteria for Myelofibrosis with Myeloid Metaplasia" proposed a definition of CIMF that has >80% sensitivity and specificity (Barosi et al. 1999). The definition requires two necessary criteria, namely diffuse bone marrow fibrosis and the absence of the Ph chromosome or *BCR-ABL* rearrangement, as well as a number of optional criteria (see Table 15.2). However, although this definition of CIMF encompasses a wide spectrum of the disease, from the early stages with slight reticulin fibrosis to the late osteomyelosclerotic phase (CIMF-1 to 3), it fails to include the recently recognized initial prefibrotic stage (CIMF-0) (see Figs. 15.2–15.4).

The concept of a prefibrotic stage of classical CIMF, that is distinguishable from essential thrombocythemia, has been stressed by a number of European histopathologists (Buhr et al. 2003; Georgii et al. 1998; Thiele and Kvasnicka 2004; Thiele et al. 1999) with the result that prefibrotic CIMF has been incorporated in the WHO classification of hematopoietic and lymphoid tumors

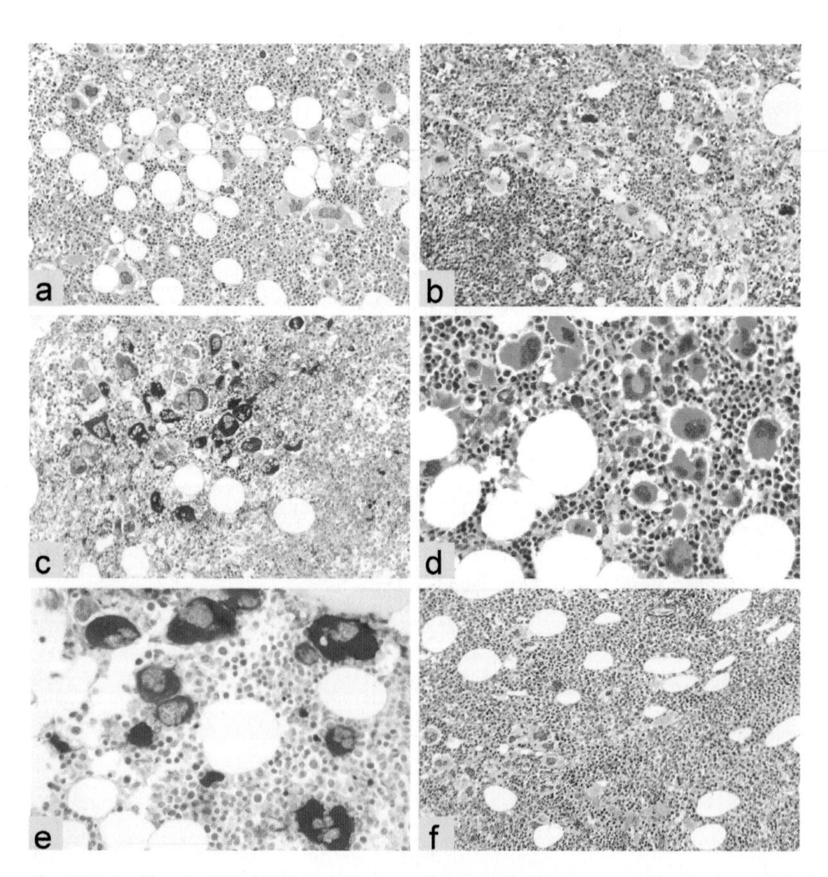

Fig. 15.2. Prefibrotic CIMF (CIMF-0). (**a**) An overall hypercellularity is evident including prominent growth of abnormally differentiated megakaryocytes (i.e., false ET). (**b**) There is a mixed neutrophil granulocytic and megakaryocytic proliferation with loose to dense clustering. (**c**) Atypias of megakaryopoiesis include histotopography (dense clustering) besides maturation defects revealing hypolobulated (bulbous) and hyperchromatic nuclei. (**d**) A prevalence of abnormal megakaryocytes with deviation of nuclear-cytoplasmic maturation is detectable. (**e**) Megakaryocytic abnormalities are highlighted by application of immunohistochemistry. (**f**) No increase in the reticulin fiber content may be observed. (**a**, **b**, **c**, **f**) ×70; (**d**, **e**) ×380; (**a**). hematoxylin-eosin, (**b**). AS-D-chloroacetate esterase, (**c**) and (**e**). CD61 immunostaining, (**d**). PAS (periodic acid Schiff reagent), (**d**). Silver immunostaining after Gomori (courtesy of Dr. Kvasnicka)

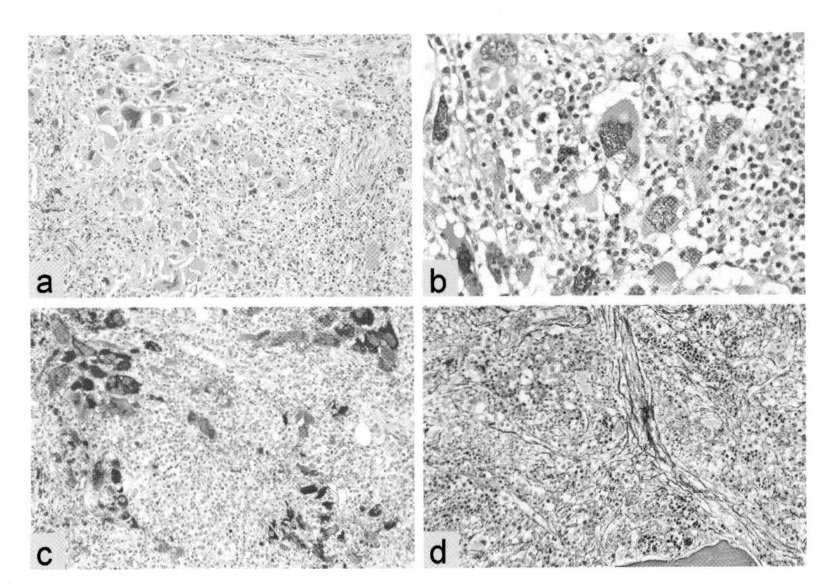

Fig. 15.3. Manifest CIMF. (**a**) In addition to a still slighty hypercellular bone marrow and a prominent granulopoiesis there are clusters of atypical megakaryocytes trapped in a fibrous meshwork. (**b**) Megakaryocytes show abnormal cloud-like (bulbous) nuclei and maturation defects (**c**) Dense clustering of atypical megakaryocytes is a conspicuous feature. (**d**) A dense increase in reticulin and some collagen fibers are characteristic. (**a**, **c**, **d**) ×170; (**b**) ×380; (**a**) Hematoxylin-eosin, (**b**) PAS. (**c**) CD61 immunostaining (**d**) Silver impregnation after Gomori (courtesy of Dr. Kvasnicka

(Thiele et al. 2001b). It has been estimated that approximately 25% of patients with CIMF initially present with a hypercellular bone marrow characterized by granulocytic and megakaryocytic proliferation and with little or no reticulin. The diagnosis requires careful examination of the bone marrow trephine and relies on the identification of morphologically atypical megakaryocytes, including dense clustering with hypolobulated (bulbous) and hyperchromatic nuclei. Other diagnostically important parameters include the frequency and shape of microvasculature (Kvasnicka et al. 2004), the level of $CD34^+$ progenitor cells (Thiele and Kvasnicka 2002), and abnormalities of cell kinetics (Kvasnicka et al. 1999). Prefibrotic CIMF is likely to have been misdiagnosed as essential thrombocythemia in many studies since it is characterized by thrombocythemia, borderline anemia, mild splenomegaly, and an absence of a leuko-erythroblastic blood picture (Thiele and Kvasnicka 2004; Thiele et al. 2001a). The natural history of prefibrotic CIMF remains unclear since prospective studies are lacking. However, preliminary data suggest that the rate of progression to advanced disease may depend on the degree of megakaryocytic dysplasia (Buhr et al. 2003; Thiele et al. 2003).

15.4 Clinical Manifestations

CIMF characteristically occurs after the age of 50, with a median age at diagnosis of approximately 60 years. About 25% of patients are asymptomatic at diagnosis and are identified following routine examination. The most common symptoms in classical CIMF are the consequence of anemia, namely fatigue, weakness, dyspnea, and palpitations. Splenomegaly is characteristic and when massive can lead to a variety of complaints including abdominal discomfort and early satiety (Fig. 15.5). Splenic infarction, due to the inability of the blood supply to match organ growth, usually produces transient discomfort although rarely can result in severe abdominal pain simulating an abdominal emergency (Fig. 15.6). Hepatomegaly occurs in approximately 70% of cases and portal hypertension may result from increased hepatic blood flow or intrahepatic obstruction (Tsao et al. 1989; Wanless et al. 1990). Nonspecific symptoms may dominate the clinical picture in CIMF, including low-grade fever, night sweats, and weight loss, and are associated with a poor prognosis (Cervantes et al. 1998). Patients may also complain of bone pain, especially in the lower extremities. Bleeding may complicate the clinical course and although often mild, manifesting

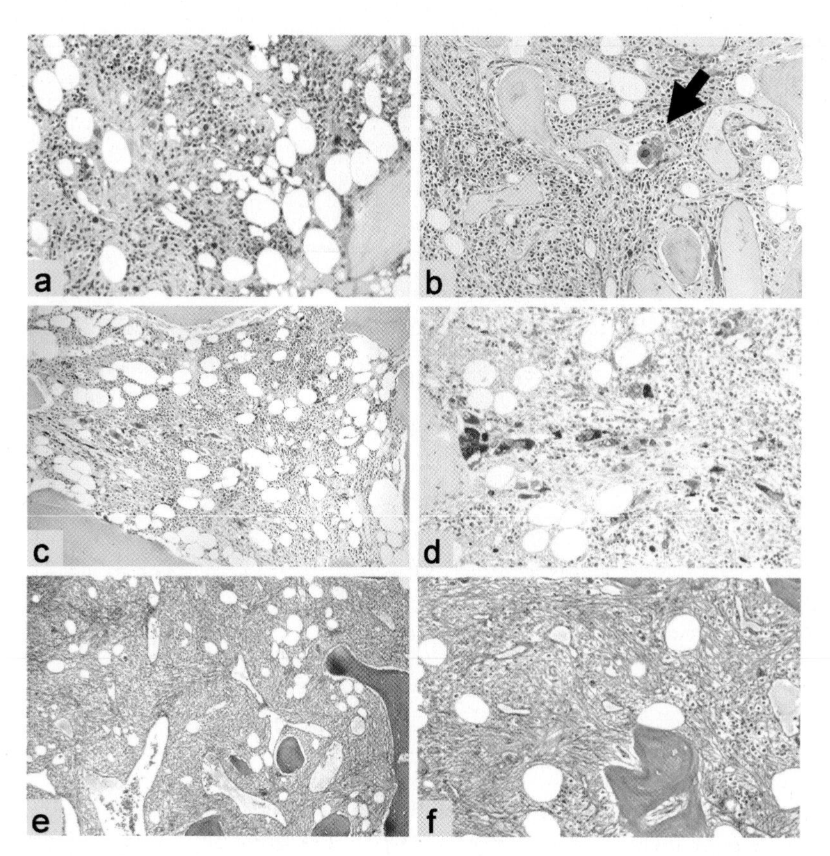

Fig. 15.4. Advanced CIMF. (**a**) Patchy hematopoiesis shows megakaryocyte clusters besides a reduction of granulo- and erythropoiesis and bundles of fibers. (**b**) Prominent dilated sinuses with intraluminally dislocated megakaryopoiesis (*arrow*) may be observed. (**c**) In addition to differences in cellularity there are initial plaque-like osteosclerotic changes and a meshwork of fibers. (**d**) Megakaryocytes reveal abnormalities of histopography (endosteal translocation and clustering) apparently in close association with bud-like endophytic bone formation – osteosclerosis may usually be found. (**a**, **b**, **d**) ×170; (**c**, **e**, **f**) ×80; (**a**) AS-D-chloroacteta esterase, (**b**) PAS, (**c**) Haematoxylin-eosin, (**d**) CD61 immunostaining; (**e**, **f**) Silver impregnation after Gomori (courtesy of Dr. Kvasnicka)

as petechiae and ecchymoses, can be life threatening due to massive gastrointestinal hemorhage. The hemorrhagic diathesis may result from a combination of thrombocytopenia, acquired platelet dysfunction, and low-grade disseminated intravascular coagulation.

Extramedullary hematopoiesis (EMH), or myeloid metaplasia, may result in a bewildering array of symptoms which depend on the specific organ involved. EMH, for example, may affect the central nervous system and result in spinal cord compression (Horwood et al. 2003; Price and Bell 1985), delirium (Cornfield et al. 1983), diabetes insipidus (Badon et al. 1985), serious headaches and exophthalmos due to meningeal infiltration (Ayyildiz et al. 2004; Landolfi et al. 1988), as well as raised intracranial hypertension with papilledema and ultimately coma (Cameron et al. 1981; Ligumski et al. 1979; Lundh et al. 1982). Involvement of lymph nodes can lead to generalized and marked lymphadenopathy (Williams et al. 1985). Pleural infiltration may result in hemothoraces (Kupferschmid et al. 1993) and pleural effusions (Jowitt et al. 1997) (Fig. 15.7), while massive ascites may result from ectopic implants of peritoneal or mesenteric extramedullary hematopoiesis (Yotsumoto et al. 2003). The effusions often contain a variety of hematopoietic elements, including megakaryocytes, immature myeloid cells, and erythroblasts. The gastrointestinal tract may be involved and this results in abdominal pain and intestinal obstruction (Mackinnon et al. 1986; Sharma et al. 1986), while infiltration of the kidneys (Fig. 15.8), prostate, and gallbladder have been reported to result in chronic renal failure, bladder outlet obstruction, and chronic cholecystitis, respectively

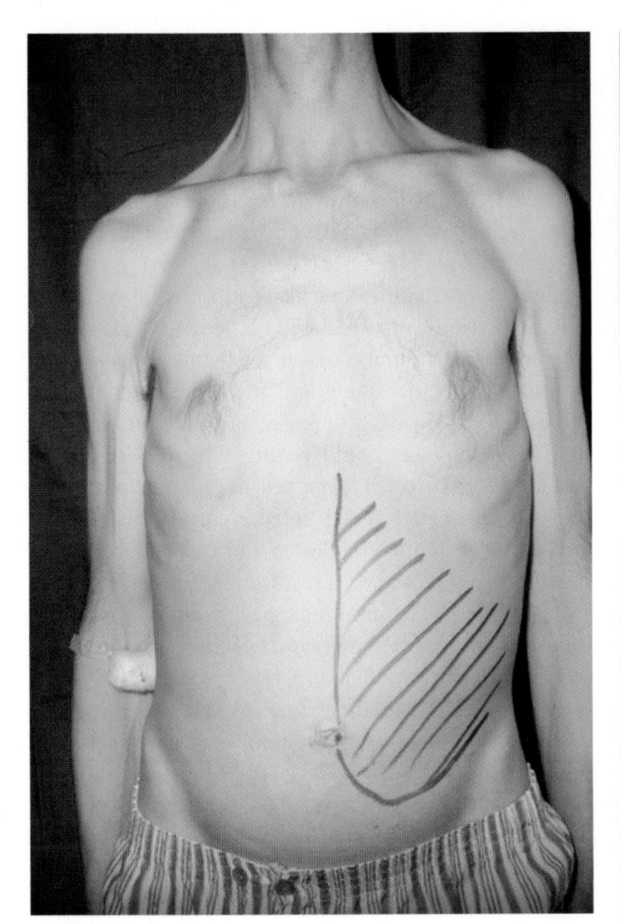

Fig. 15.5. Gross splenomegaly (extending 22 cm below the left costal margin) and associated cachexia

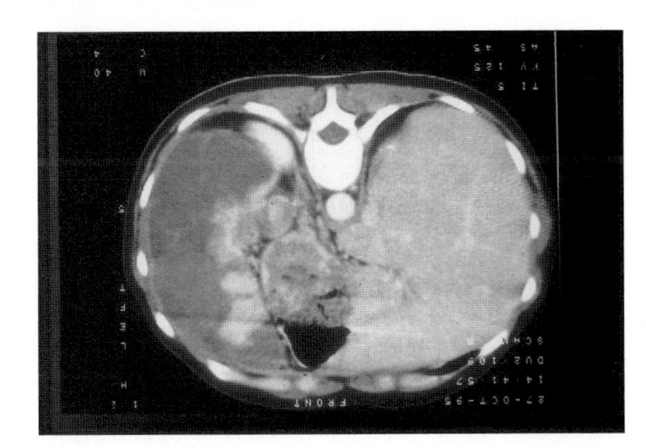

Fig. 15.6. Massive splenic infarction necessitating splenectomy

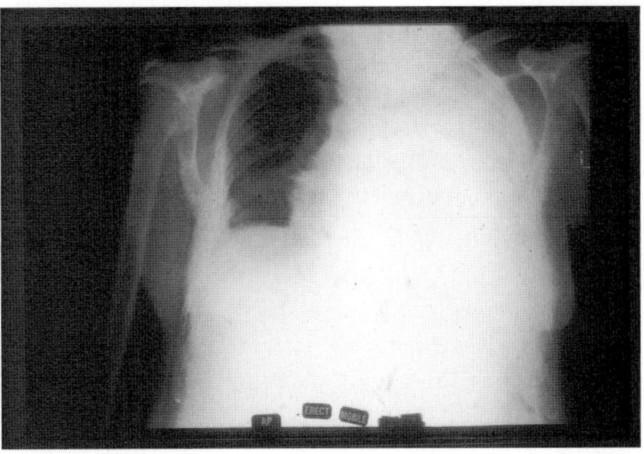

Fig. 15.7. Pleural effusion in a patient with myelofibrosis and extramedullary hematopoiesis involving the pleura

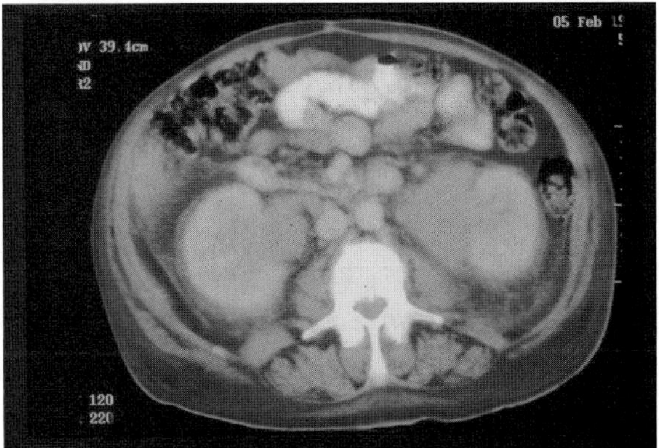

Fig. 15.8. Extramedullary hematopoiesis involving both kidneys

(Humphrey and Vollmer 1991; Schnuelle et al. 1999; Thorns et al. 2002). Involvement of breast tissue may mimic carcinoma (Martinelli et al. 1983), while urethral infiltration has been reported to masquerade as a caruncle (Balogh and O'Hara 1986) and synovial involvement can give rise to arthritis (Heinicke et al. 1983). Skin manifestations are rare and include erythematous plaques (Fig. 15.9), nodules, diffuse or papular erythema, ulcers, and bullae (Loewy et al. 1994). Rarely, the development of CIMF can be preceded by the presence of neutrophilic dermatosis, or "Sweet's syndrome" while pyoderma gangrenosum and leukemic infiltrations have been reported (Gibson et al. 1985).

The major causes of death are infection, hemorrhage, cardiac failure, and acute leukemic transformation. The latter, which occurs in approximately 15% of patients (Silverstein et al. 1973) are commonly myeloblastic or myelomonoblastic, but may involve the megakaryocytic (Reilly et al. 1993), erythroid (Garcia et al. 1989), lymphoid (Polliak et al. 1980), and basophilic

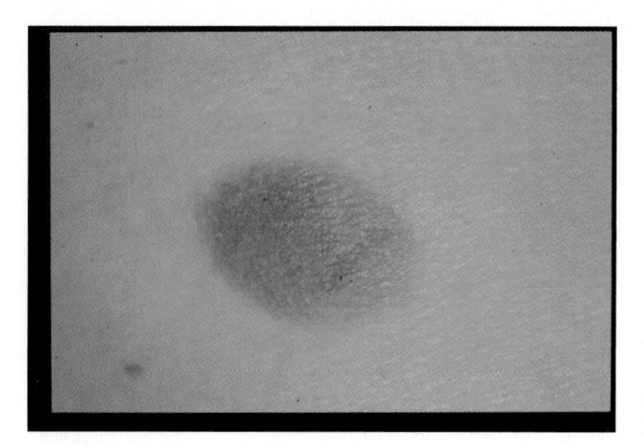

Fig. 15.9. Cutaneous extramedullary hematopoiesis

lineages (Sugimoto et al. 2004). Hernandez and colleagues (1992) have described the occurrence of mixed myeloid (myeloblastic-erythroid-megakaryocytic) or hybrid (myeloid-lymphoid) phenotypes in up to a third of cases, a fact that reflects the pluripotent stem cell origin of the disease. Localized granulocytic sarcomas, or chloromas, can develop in a wide variety of sites, including bone, lymph nodes, and skin and on occasion precede the diagnosis of leukemia.

15.5 Laboratory Features

A normocytic normochromic anemia is characteristic of classic CIMF, as is anisocytosis, poikilocytosis, and teardrop-shaped cells (dacrocytes). The origin of dacrocytes is uncertain but they are thought to be the sine qua non of extramedullary hematopoiesis. Nucleated red cells are present in the peripheral blood of nearly all cases and there is frequently a mild reticulocytosis. The major cause of anemia is ineffective erythropoiesis but other causes may include iron deficiency, red cell sequestration, and hemodilution due to plasma volume expansion as a result of splenomegaly. Hemolysis can be significant and, although frequently direct antiglobulin test (DAT) negative, may be autoimmune in etiology (Bird et al. 1985).

Immunological abnormalities, other than anti-red cell antibodies, are common and include the development of antinuclear and rheumatoid antibodies, lupus-type anticoagulants, antiphospholipid antibodies (Rondeau et al. 1983), hypocomplementemia (Gordon et al. 1981), and increased nodules of lymphoid cells in the bone marrow (Caligaris Cappio et al. 1981). Lewis and Pegrum (1972) described immune complexes on leukocytes while, more recently, antibodies directed against stromal proteins, for example anti-Gal antibodies, have been demonstrated that appear to correlate with disease activity. Interestingly, galactosidic determinants are thought to be expressed by fibroblasts and megakaryocytes in patients with CIMF raising the possibility of an autoimmune pathogenesis (Leoni et al. 1993). A number of these abnormalities are likely to be epiphenomena, resulting from impaired reticulo-endothelial system clearance, but immunological mechanisms have been postulated for the induction and/or maintenance of the disease (Caligaris Cappio et al. 1981); for example, immune complexes could result in platelet activation and additional growth factor release. Interestingly, Gordon and colleagues (1981) noted a correlation between circulating immune complexes and disease activity as manifested by increased transfusion requirements, bone pain, and fever. The immunological hypothesis for myelofibrosis is supported by reports of successful immunosuppressive therapy, including low-dose dexamethasone (Jack et al. 1994), prednisolone (Mesa et al. 2003) and cyclosporin A (Pietrasanta et al. 1994), as well as the reports of myelofibrosis associated with systemic lupus erythematosus (Kaelin and Spivak 1986) and polyarteritis nodosa (Connelly et al. 1982).

15.6 Prognosis

The overall median survival of classical CIMF varies from series to series but is approximately 4 years (Demory et al. 1988; Reilly et al. 1997; Rupoli et al. 1994; Varki et al. 1983), although individual survival may range from 1 to over 30 years. This is considerably lower, however, than the 14-year median survival of age- and sex-matched controls (Rozman et al. 1991). As a result, many groups have used univariate or multivariate analysis to identify clinical and laboratory features that predict survival. Despite the bewildering number of prognostic factors highlighted, most studies agree on the predictive value of anemia (Barosi et al. 1988; Cervantes et al. 1991; Dupriez et al. 1996; Ivanyi et al. 1984; Kreft et al. 2003; Njoku et al. 1983; Reilly et al. 1997; Rupoli et al. 1994; Visani et al. 1990), age at diagnosis (Barosi et al. 1988; Cervantes et al. 1997; Kvasnicka et al. 1977; Reilly et al. 1997; Varki et al. 1983), karyotype (Dupriez et al. 1996; Reilly et al. 1997; Tefferi et al. 2001), and the percentage of immature granulocytes and/or circulating myeloblasts (Barosi et al. 1988; Cervantes et al. 1991; Visani et al. 1990). The data regarding the prognostic value of absolute peripheral blood CD34+ counts, however, are less clear. Several groups, for example, have suggested that, in addition to a possible diagnostic role, elevated CD34+ counts are an important adverse prognostic marker (Barosi et al. 2001; Passamonti et al. 2003; Sagaster et al. 2003). In contrast, Arora and colleagues (2004), although finding that counts above 0.1×10^9/L correlated with shortened survival, noted that this significance was lost on multivariate analysis. Finally, the degree of angiogenesis (Mesa et al. 2000), in contrast to the extent of collagen fibrosis or osteosclerosis (Dupriez et al. 1996; Kvasnicka et al. 1997; Rupoli et al. 1994), has been shown to be a significant and independent risk factor for overall survival.

Two simple and practicable schemas have been reported that allow the identification of patients with limited life expectancy, for whom more aggressive therapeutic approaches might be appropriate (Dupriez et al. 1996; Reilly et al. 1997). The most widely used is the Lille scoring system (Table 15.3) which is based on two adverse prognostic factors, namely hemoglobin <10g/dL and a total white count <4 or $>30\times10^9$/L, and which separates patients into three groups with low (0 factor), intermediate (1 factor), and high risk (2 factors) disease, associated with median survivals of 93, 26, and 13 months, respectively (Dupriez et al. 1996). The Sheffield schema (Table 15.4), by combining age, hemoglobin concentration, and karyotype, identifies patient groups with median survival times that vary from 180 months (good risk) to 16 months (poor risk) (Reilly et al. 1997). However, there are two important caveats that apply to these and many other studies. Firstly, only a few groups have included the full spectrum of the disease, from the early prefibrotic phase to the advanced full-blown osteomyelosclerotic state. This is important as the early prefibrotic stages of CIMF show a more favorable outcome than the advanced stages of disease (Kvasnicka et al. 1997). Secondly, most studies have included very few young patients, a fact that could potentially limit the schema's utility when attempting to identify cases suitable for bone marrow transplantation. This deficiency has been addressed by Cervantes and colleagues (1999), who reported a large collaborative study of 116 patients below the age of 55 years and concluded that, by using a combination of hemoglobin, constitutional symptoms, and percentage of blasts, patients with low- and high-risk disease could be identified. Importantly, the median survival in this cohort was 128 months which is significantly better than that reported for studies of unselected patients.

Table 15.3. The LILLE scoring system

No. of adverse prognostic factors	Risk group	Cases (%)	Median survival (months)
0	Low	47	93
1	Intermediate	45	26
2	High	8	13

Adverse prognostic factors; Hb <10g/dL, WBC <4 or $>30\times10^9$/L. (Reproduced from Dupriez et al. 1997 with permission).

Table 15.4. The SHEFFIELD schema for predicting survival (reproduced from Reilly et al. 1997 with permission)

Age (years)	Hb (g/dl)	Karyotype	Median survival (months) (95% CI)
<68	<10	N	54 (46, 62)
		A	22 (14, 30)
	>10	N	180 (6, 354)
		A	72 (32, 112)
>68	<10	N	44 (31, 57)
		A	16 (5, 27)
	>10	N	70 (61, 79)
		A	78 (26, 130)

Demonstrating median survival times in months with associated 95% confidence intervals in parenthesis;
N, normal; A, abnormal.

15.7 Management

15.7.1 Medical Therapy

15.7.1.1 Cytotoxic Therapy

Cytotoxic chemotherapy has a definite role in the management of CIMF patients. Hydroxyurea, the most widely used agent (Lofvenberg et al. 1990; Manoharan 1991), can reduce the degree of hepatosplenomegaly, decrease or eliminate constitutional symptoms, reduce thrombocytosis and, in some cases, lead to an increase in hemoglobin. Hydroxyurea may also be useful in individuals who develop compensatory hepatic myeloid metaplasia following splenectomy and it has also been shown to improve bone marrow fibrosis (Lofvenberg et al. 1990). The use of busulfan has been reported in the proliferative phase of the disease (Manoharan and Pitney 1984), but the risks of prolonged cytopenias are significant. Responses are often short-lived, lasting a median of only 4.5 months (Silverstein 1975). Low-dose melphalan (starting at 2.5 mg three times a week) may be an alternative option (Petti et al. 2002) but again hematological toxicity is common. 2-chlorodeoxyadenosine (2-CdA) may have a palliative role in controlling the extreme thrombocytosis and leukocytosis, as well as the accelerated hepatomegaly that can occur post splenectomy. Responses were observed in about half of patients and occurred in most cases by the second course (Faoro et al. 2005; Tefferi et al. 1997).

15.7.1.2 Androgens

Anemia, usually normochromic normocytic, is a common problem in CIMF, with 20–25% of presenting cases being symptomatic. Iron deficiency, ineffective hematopoiesis, erythrocytic sequestration, hemodilution secondary to plasma volume expansion, and hemolysis are recognized mechanisms. Patients with normal red cell masses and marked increase in plasma volume have a dilutional form of anemia that does not require treatment. Androgen therapy, including nandrolone, fluoxymesterolone, and oxymetholone, improves marrow function in approximately 40% of patients (Besa et al. 1982; Brubaker et al. 1982; Hast et al. 1978), with optimal responses seen in patients lacking massive splenomegaly and in those with a normal karyotype (Besa et al. 1982). Danazol (400–600 mg/day), a synthetic attenuated androgen, may give similar results with the added benefit of correcting thrombocytopenia and reducing the degree of splenomegaly in some patients (Cervantes et al. 2000, 2005; Levy et al. 1996). Androgen therapy should be continued for a minimum of 6 months and once a response is obtained, it should be reduced to the lowest maintenance dose. Pretreatment variables associated with response to danazol include lack of transfusion requirement and higher hemoglobin concentration at commencement of treatment (Cervantes et al. 2005). Side effects include fluid retention, increased libido, hirsutism, abnormal liver function tests, and hepatic tumors. All treated patients should have regular monitoring of liver function tests and periodic abdominal ultrasound investigation to detect liver tumors. In addition, male patients should be screened for prostate cancer prior to therapy.

15.7.1.3 Erythropoietin

Human recombinant erythropoietin (EPO) has been shown by several groups to be an effective and safe therapy in CIMF, although the number of reported cases remains small (Aloe-Spiriti et al. 1993; Bourantas et al. 1996; Hasselbalch et al. 2002; Tefferi and Silverstein 1994). Hasselbalch et al. (2002), for example, reported that 90% (9 of 10 evaluable cases) attained a favorable response, which was maintained in the majority of patients. Importantly, most responding individuals exhibited inappropriately low serum EPO levels for the degree of anemia. More recently, Cervantes et al. (2004) confirmed these findings and showed that 45% of patients responded favorably to a dose of 10,000 U three times a week. In addition, those with a serum EPO level <125 U/L and those that were transfusion independent had a more favorable outcome. It can be concluded from these studies that EPO is a well-tolerated therapy for the anemia in CIMF but that its use should be restricted to cases with inappropriately low serum EPO levels. It should be noted, however, that the majority of patients have appropriate levels for the degree of anemia (Barosi et al. 1993a). The dose may be doubled if there has been no response after 1–2 months and the treatment discontinued if there has been no response after 3–4 months.

15.7.1.4 Interferon

Parmeggiani et al. (1987) reported the use of α-interferon (α-IFN) for the treatment of painful splenomegaly in CIMF. Splenic pain and pressure symptoms resolved with a decrease in spleen size, although peripheral counts deteriorated. Pegylated IFN, a polyethylene glycol formulation of α-IFN that is administered once a week, is currently undergoing clinical trials in CIMF and may have the advantage of being better tolerated (Verstovsek et al. 2003).

15.7.1.5 Thalidomide

Recently, thalidomide has been advocated as a therapy for controlling angiogenesis in several neoplastic and inflammatory diseases. The marked neo-vascularization that characterizes CIMF bone marrow (Mesa et al. 2000, Reilly et al. 1985b) suggested that thalidomide might be beneficial in this disease and has led to several small studies. A pooled analysis of the latter indicated that thalidomide can ameliorate anemia, thrombocytopenia, and splenomegaly in some cases, but that most patients were intolerant of standard doses (200–800 mg/day), with nearly 50% of cases withdrawing from the studies by the third month (Barosi et al. 2002). As a result, the combination of low-dose thalidomide (50 mg/day) and prednisolone at 0.5 mg/kg/day slowly tapered over the course of 3 months was evaluated and shown to be associated with a higher response rate and lower toxicity (Mesa et al. 2003). A meaningful improvement in anemia was demonstrated in 62% of all patients, while a 70% response rate was obtained for those cases that were transfusion dependent. However, although thrombocytopenia and splenomegaly improved in 75% and 19% of cases, respectively, there was no apparent decrease in extramedullary hematopoiesis or angiogenesis, suggesting that thalidomide's activity may not be due to its antiangiogenic properties. Following the discontinuation of prednisolone, the improvement in anemia and thrombocytopenia was lost in over a third of cases. The role of steroids in this study supports earlier data that indicated the benefit of low-dose dexamethasone (Jack et al. 1994). A recent European study (Marchetti et al. 2004) confirmed the usefulness of single agent low-dose thalidomide (50 mg/day) in a cohort of 63 patients with advanced stage disease and concluded that it was effective especially for transfusion-dependent and/or thrombocytopenic patients and for those requiring control of progressive splenomegaly. A combination of thalidomide and erythropoietin has been shown to correct the anemia in some cases in which both drugs have previously failed as single agents (Visani et al. 2003). Lenalidomide (CC-5013, Revlimid), a more potent drug with less neurotoxicity than thalidomide, has recently been shown to have clinical activity in approximately 20% of patients (Cortes et al. 2005; Tefferi et al. 2005). It should be stressed however, that most patients will become refractory to medical therapies and consequently will require life-long transfusions with resulting iron overload.

15.7.1.6 Experimental Therapy

Etanercept, a recombinant form of the extracellular domain of tissue necrosis factor (TNF) receptor linked to the Fc fragment of human IgG, inhibits TNF-α, a key mediator of malignancy-associated fever, cachexia, and other constitutional symptoms. Two pilot studies have reported its use in CIMF. Steensma and colleagues (2002) observed a 60% reduction in severity of constitutional symptoms, while 20% experienced reduction of splenomegaly and/or improvement of cytopenias. Imatinib mesylate has been evaluated in CIMF on the basis that it inhibits the receptors PDGFR and KIT (Tefferi et al. 2002). However, the drug demonstrated limited efficacy and side effects led to the withdrawal in many patients. R115777, a farnesyl transferase inhibitor, has in vitro antiproliferative activity for CIMF progenitor cells. In a small study, R115777 produced improvement in anemia and splenomegaly in 25% of cases, with responses correlating with high VEGF levels (Cortes et al. 2003). Paradoxically, however, the VEGF tyrosine kinase inhibitor SU5416 possesses minimal therapeutic activity in CIMF (Giles et al. 2003). Studies evaluating the efficacy of new drugs including thalidomide analogues, proteasome inhibitors and VEGF neutralizing antibodies are currently underway.

15.7.2 Surgery and Radiotherapy

15.7.2.1 Splenectomy

The role of splenectomy in the management of myelofibrosis is now fairly well defined (Barosi et al. 1993; Mesa et al. 2004; Tefferi et al. 2000). In contrast to earlier reports, which suggested that the operation be performed in every patient at diagnosis, it is now clear that the procedure should be restricted to carefully selected cases with refractory hemolysis and/or thrombocytopenia, symptomatic splenomegaly, significant splenic infarction, and severe portal hypertension. Splenectomy does not prolong survival and even in the best units is associated with morbidity and mortality rates of approximately 31% and 9%, respectively (Tefferi et al. 2000). The main postoperative complications include bleeding, thromboembolism, subphrenic abscess, and pulmonary atelectasis. In addition, compensatory hepatic myeloid metaplasia leading to rapid hepatic enlargement is an unusual but well-recognized complication, while an unexpectedly high rate of leukemic transformation has been documented (Barosi et al. 1998; López-Guillermo et al. 1991). The explanation for the increased blast transformation is unclear, but it is possible that the procedure could accelerate a pre-existing hyperproliferation state, especially as this complication has not been reported in healthy individuals. A significant postoperative thrombocytosis is observed in approximately 20% of patients and carries an increased thrombotic risk (Barosi et al. 1993a). Once a patient is considered a candidate for splenectomy, an extensive preoperative evaluation is required to determine if the cardiac, hepatic, renal, metabolic, and hemostatic risks are acceptable. The importance of the frequently associated coagulopathy needs to be stressed. Defective platelet aggregation is common and many patients have a prolonged bleeding time. In addition, some cases have laboratory evidence of disseminated intravascular coagulation, which may only become clinically apparent following surgical intervention, while others have a prolonged prothrombin time due to associated liver dysfunction, an isolated factor V deficiency, or the presence of circulating anticoagulants. Surgical expertise is essential, since the operation is often difficult as the spleen may be adherent to adjacent serosal surfaces as well as possessing numerous collateral vessels and dilated spleno-portal arteries and veins. Individuals operated on for portal hypertension and bleeding varices should have dynamic circulatory studies performed during the procedure, since portal hypertension due to splenomegaly is corrected by splenectomy (Silverstein and ReMine 1979), whereas cases secondary to intrahepatic obstruction require a portal-systemic shunt (Tefferi et al. 1994).

15.7.2.2 Radiotherapy

Radiotherapy should be considered as an alternative to splenectomy in those patients who are unfit for surgery. Several studies have reported symptomatic relief, with mild to moderate reduction in spleen size, which lasts for approximately 6 months (Bouabdallah et al. 2000; Elliot et al. 1998). A significant percentage of patients, however, suffer unpredictable, life-threatening cytopenias, resulting in an overall mortality rate of 13%. The transient response, together with the high mortality rate for patients requiring subsequent splenomegaly, suggests that such therapy should not be regarded as an alternative to splenectomy in surgical candidates. Low-dose irradiation, however, remains the treatment of choice for peritoneal and pleural extramedullary hematopoiesis that results in ascites and pleural effusions, respectively (Bartlett et al. 1995; Leinweber et al. 1991), as well as for myeloid metaplasia of vital organs, including the lung, central nervous system, and liver (Price and Bell 1985; Steensma et al. 2002; Tefferi et al. 2001b).

15.7.3 Stem Cell Transplantation

15.7.3.1 Standard Allo-SCT

Currently, allogeneic hematopoietic stem cell transplantation (allo-SCT) is the only curative modality for patients with CIMF. Recently, two large studies have attempted to clarify the issues surrounding patient selection and outcome. Guardiola et al. (1999), in a retrospective multicenter study, reported the results of HLA-identical SCT in 55 patients (median age at transplantation 42 years, range 4–53). The 5-year probability of survival was 47% ± 8% for the overall group, and 54% ± 8% for patients receiving an unmanipulated HLA-matched related transplant. The 1-year probability of transplant-related mortality was 27% ± 6%. Hemoglobin (< 10 g/dL), osteosclerosis, and a high-risk score at the time of transplantation were associated with a worse survival, whereas older age, karyotypic abnormalities, and lack of grade II–IV acute GVHD were associated with treatment failure. Deeg and colleagues (2003) reported the results in 56 patients treated at a single institution with conventional allo-SCT. The median age at transplantation was 43 years (range 10 to 66) with median disease duration of 33 months (range 3 to 312). Fifty-three patients achieved engraftment, while two died from relapse/progressive disease and 18 from other causes. The probability of surviving 3 years was 58%, with patients having lower Lille scores, higher platelet counts, less severe marrow fibrosis, and normal karyotypes doing better than those with more advanced disease. The role of pretransplant splenectomy is unclear. Guardiola and colleagues (1999) reported that although splenectomy was associated with a faster hematopoietic recovery, there was no associated survival benefit. A pragmatic approach, therefore, in view of the mortality and morbidity of splenectomy, would be to restrict the procedure to patients where engraftment might be significantly delayed, for example in cases of osteomyelosclerosis or massive splenomegaly.

15.7.3.2 Reduced Intensity Allo-SCT

Evidence for a graft-versus-myelofibrosis (GvMy) effect has provided the rationale for exploring the role of reduced-intensity, or nonmyeloablative, allo-SCT in CIMF. Guardiola and colleagues (1999), for example, reported that absent or minimal GvHD in the context of conventional allo-SCT correlated with treatment failure, while the infusion of donor lymphocytes in patients failing allo-SCT may lead to disease eradication (Byrne et al. 2000; Cervantes et al. 2000). The initial reports of reduced-intensity allo-SCT were retrospective registry studies with patients receiving a range of conditioning regimes. Nevertheless, encouraging 1-year survival rates of 54% and 90% were reported (Hessling et al. 2002; Rondelli et al. 2003). Recently, the first prospective study using reduced-intensity conditioning has been published (Kröger et al. 2005). This series demonstrated that a busulphan- and fludarabine-based regimen, followed by allo-SCT from either a related or unrelated donor, is a feasible and effective therapeutic option with a low treatment-related mortality. Complete donor chimerism was seen in 95% of cases on day 100 with acute GvHD grades II–IV and III/IV occurring in 48% and 19% of cases respectively, while 55% developed chronic GvHD. The estimated overall and disease-free survival at 3 years was 84%, with no treatment failure, as defined by recurrence or progression of myelofibrosis, being observed after a median follow-up of 22 months. Importantly, despite in vivo T-cell depletion, no relapses were reported. In addition, the results from unrelated donors compared favorably with the outcome of the few cases of unrelated SCT reported using standard conditioning. In the largest series of the latter, for example, seven patients were transplanted from unrelated donors, but only one survived (Guardiola et al. 1999). It should be stressed, however, that the overall experience of reduced-intensity allo-SCT remains limited and crucial questions such as the impact of prior splenectomy, the influence of karyotype and the effect of the degree of fibrosis on outcome, remain unclear. As a result, the use of reduced-intensity conditioning should be restricted to patients aged 45–70 years with high-risk disease.

15.7.3.3 Autologous SCT

The risks of allo-SCT have led clinicians to investigate the palliative option of autologous-SCT, especially for the older patient or for those without a stem cell donor. The feasibility of this approach was demonstrated by Anderson and colleagues (2001) who reported a multicenter retrospective analysis of 21 patients, conditioned using single agent busulphan at a dose of 16 mg/kg. At 2 years the actuarial survival was 61%, with six patients having died of infection, graft failure, or progressive disease. Following transplantation, 15 of 21 patients showed evidence of significant clinical improvement that lasted up to 4 years, including ten of 17 cases with anemia, 7 of 10 patients with symptomatic splenomegaly, and 6 of 8 cases with thrombocytopenia. G-CSF priming was recommended since, although CIMF patients have high circulating CD34+ cell counts, most peripheral CD34+ cells are likely to lack the capacity to maintain long-term hematopoiesis. The mechanism for response is unclear but may include the restoration of intramedullary hematopoiesis as a result of reduced fibrosis, reduced sequestration of nonclonal cells following improvement in the degree of splenomegaly, and the restoration of normal hematopoiesis secondary to a reduction of malignant cells.

References

Abu-Duhier FM, Goodeve AC, Care RS, Gari M, Wilson GA, Peake IR, Reilly JT (2003) Mutational analysis of class III receptor tyrosine kinases (C-KIT, c-FMS, FLT3) in idiopathic myelofibrosis. Br J Haematol 120:464–470

Al-Assar O, Ul-Hassan A, Brown R, Wilson GA, Hammond DW, Reilly JT (2005) Gains on 9p are common genomic aberrations in idiopathic myelofibrosis: a comparative genomic hybridization study. Br J Haematol 129:66–71

Aloe-Spiriti MA, Latagliata R, Avvisati G, Battistel V, Montevusco E, Spadea A,Petti MC (1993) Erythropoietin treatment of idiopathic myelofibrosis. Haematol 78:371–373

Anderson JE, Tefferi A, Craig F, Holmberg L, Chauncey T, Appelbaum FR, Guardiola P, Callander N, Freytes C, Gazitt Y, Razvillas B, Deeg HJ (2001) Myeloablation and autologous peripheral blood stem cell rescue results in hematologic and clinical responses in patients with myelofibrosis. Blood 98:586–593

Andreasson B, Swolin B, Kutti J (2002) Patients with idiopathic myelofibrosis show increased CD34+ cell concentrations in peripheral blood compared to patients with polycythaemia vera and essential thrombocythaemia. Eur J Haematol 68:189–193

Altura RA, Head DR, Wang WC (2000) Long-term survival of infants with idiopathic myelofibrosis. Br J Haematol 109:459–462

Apaja-Sarkkinen M, Autio-Harmainen H, Alavaikko M, Ristelli J, Risteli L (1986) Immunohistochemical study of basement membrane proteins and type III procollagen in myelofibrosis. Br J Haematol 63:571–580

Arora B, Sirhan S, Hoyer JD, Mesa RA and Tefferi A (2004) Peripheral blood CD34 count in myelofibrosis with myeloid metaplasia: a prospective evaluation of prognostic value in 94 patients. Br J Haematol 128:42–48

Ayyildiz O, Isikdogan A, Celik M, Muftuoglu E (2004) Intracranial meningeal extramedullary hematopoiesis inducing serious headache in a patient with idiopathic myelofibrosis. J Pediatr Hematol Oncol 26:28–29

Badon SJ, Ansell J, Smith TW, Coslovsky R, Gill L, Woda BA (1985) Diabetes insipidus caused by extramedullary hematopoiesis. Am J Clin Pathol 83:509–512

Balogh K, O'Hara CJ (1986) Myeloid metaplasia masquerading as a urethral caruncle. J Urol 135:789–790

Barosi G, Berzuini C, Liberato LN, Costa A, Polino G, Ascari E (1988) A prognostic classification of myelofibrosis with myeloid metaplasia. Br J Haematol 70:397–401

Barosi G, Ambrosetti A, Buratti A, Finelli C, Liberato NL, Quaglini S, Ricetti MM, Visani G, Tura S, Ascari E (1993 a) Splenectomy for patients with myelofibrosis with myeloid metaplasia: pretreatment variables and outcome prediction. Leukemia 7:200–206

Barosi G, Liberato LN, Guarnone R (1993 b) Serum erythropoietin in patients with myelofibrosis with myeloid metaplasia. Br J Haematol 83:365–369

Barosi G, Ambrosetti A, Centra A, Falcone A, Finelli C, Foa P, Grossi A, Guarnone R, Rupoli S, Luciano L, Petti MC, Polgliani E, Russo D, Ruggeri M, Quaglini S (1998) Splenectomy and risk of blast transformation in myelofibrosis with myeloid metaplasia. Blood 91:3630–3636

Barosi G, Ambrosetti A, Finelli C, Grossi A, Leoni P, Liberato NL, Petti MC, Pogliani E, Ricetti M, Rupoli S, Visani G, Tura S (1999) The Italian Consenus Conference on Diagnostic Criteria for Myelofibrosis with Myeloid Metaplasia. Br J Haematol 104:730–737

Barosi G, Viarengo G, Pecci A, Rosti V, Piaggio G, Marchette M, Frassoni F (2001) Diagnostic and clinical relevance of the number of circulating CD34(+) cells in myelofibrosis with myeloid metaplasia. Blood 98:3249–3255

Barosi G, Elliot M, Canepa L, Filippo B, Piccaluga PP, Visani G, Marchetti M, Pozzato G, Zorat F, Tefferi A (2002) Thalidomide in myelofibrosis with myeloid metaplasia: a pooled-analysis of individual pateint data from 5 studies. Leuk Lymphoma 43:2301–2307

Bartlett RP, Greipp PR, Tefferi A, Cupps RE, Mullan BP, Trastek VF (1995) Extramedullary hematopoiesis manifesting as a symptomatic pleural effusion. Mayo Clin Proc 70:1161–1164

Baxter EJ, Scott LM, Campbell PJ, East C, Fouroudas N, Swanton S, Vassiliou GS, Bench AJ, Boyd EM, Curtin N, Scott MA, Erber WN, Green AR (2005) Acquired mutation of the tyrosine kinase JAK2 in human myeloproliferative disease. Lancet 365:1054–1061

Bench AJ, Nacheva EP, Champion KM, Green AR (1998) Molecular genetics and cytogenetics of myeloproliferative disorders. Baillières Clin Haematol 11:819–848

Bernabei PA, Arcangeli A, Casini M, Grossi A, Padovani R, Ferrini PR (1986) Platelet-derived growth factor(s) mitogenic activity in patients with myeloproliferative disease. Br J Haematol 63:353–357

Besa, EC, Nowell PC, Geller NL, Gardner FH (1982) Analysis of the androgen response of 23 patients with agnogenic myeloid metaplsia: the value of chromosome studies predicting response and survival. Cancer 49:308–313

Bird GW, Wingham J, Richardson SG (1985) Myelofibrosis, autoimmune haemolytic anaemia and Tn-polyagglutinability. Haematol 18:99–103

Bouabdallah R, Coso D, Gonzague-Casabianca L, Alzieu C, Resbeut M, Gastaut JA (2000). Safety and efficacy of splenic irradiation in the treatment of patients with idiopathic myelofibrosis: a report on 15 patients. Leuk Res 24:491–495

Bourantas KL, Tsiara S, Christou L, Repousis P, Konstantinidou P, Bai M, Seferiadis K (1996) Combination therapy with recombinant human erythropoietin, interferon-α-2b and granulocyte-macrophage colony-stimulating factor in idiopathic myelofibrosis. Acta Haematol 96:79–82

Brogi E, Wu T, Namiki A, Isner JM (1994) Indirect angiogenic cytokines upregulate VEGF and bFGF gene expression in vascular smooth muscle cells whereas hypoxia upregulates VEGF expression only. Circulation 90:649–652

Brubaker LH, Briere J, Laszlo J, Kraut E, Landaw SA, Peterson P, Goldberg J, Donovan P (1982) Treatment of anaemia in myeloproliferative disorders: a randomized study of fluoxymesterone v transfusions only. Arch Intern Med 142:1533–1537

Buhr T, Buesche G, Choritz H, Langer F, Kreipe H (2003) Evolution of myelofibrosis in chronic idiopathic myelofibrosis as evidenced in sequential bone marrow biopsy specimens. Am J Clin Pathol 119:152–158

Buschle M, Janssn JWG, Drexler H, Lyons J, Anger B, Bartram CR (1988). Evidence for pluripotent stem cell origin of idipathic myelofibrosis: clonal analysis of a case characterised by a N-ras gene mutation. Leukemia 2:658–660

Byrne JL, Beshti H, Clark D, Ellis I, Haynes AP, Das-Gupta E, Russell NH (1999) Induction of remission after donor leucocyte infusion for the treatment of relapsed chronic idiopathic myelofibrosis following allogeneic transplantation: evidence for a "graft vs myelofibrosis" effect. Br J Haematol 108:430–433

Caligaris Cappio F, Vigiani R, Novarino A, Camussi G, Campana D, Gavosto F (1981) Idiopathic myelofibrosis:a possible role for immune-complexes in the pathogenesis of bone marrow fibrosis. Br J Haematol 49:17–21

Cameron WR, Ronnert M, Brun A (1981) Extramedullary hematopoiesis of CNS in postpolycythemic myeloid metaplasia. N Eng J Med 305:765

Campbell PJ, Griesshammer M, Dohmer K, Dohner R, Hasselbalch HC, Larsen TS, Pallisgaard N, Giraudier S, Le Bousse-Kerdiles MC, Desterke C, Guerton B, Dupriez B, Bordessoule D, Harrison CN, Green AR, Reilly JT (2006) The V617F mutation in JAK2 is associated with poorer survival in idiopathic myelofibrosis. Blood 107:2098–2100

Carlo-Stella C, Cazzola M, Gasner A, Barosi G, Dezza L, Meloni F, Pedrazzoli P, Hoelzer D, Ascari E (1987) Effects of recombinant alpha and gamma interferons on the in vitro growth of circulating hematopoietic progenitor cells (CFU-GEMM, CFU-Mk, BFU-E, and CFU-GM) from patients with myelofibrosis with myeloid metaplasia. Blood 70:1014–1019

Castro-Malaspina H, Rabellino EM, Yen A, Nachman RL, Moore MAS (1981) Human megakaryocyte stimulation of proliferation of bone marrow fibroblasts. Blood 57:781–787

Cervantes F, Pereira A, Esteve J, Rafel M, Cobo F, Rozman C, Montserrat E (1997) identification of "short-lived" and "long-lived" patients at presentation of idiopathic myelofibrosis. Br J Haematol 97:635–640

Cervantes F, Barosi G, Demory, J-L, Reilly J, Guarone R, Dupriez B, Pereira A, Montserrat E (1998) Myelofibrosis with myeloid metaplasia in young individuals: disease characteristics, prognostic factors and identification of risk groups. Br J Haematol 102:684–690

Cervantes F, Rovira M, Urbano-Ispizua A, Rozman M, Carreras E, Montserrat E (2000) Complete remission of idiopathic myelofibrosis following donor lymphocyte infusion after failure of allogeneic transplantation: demonstration of a graft-versus-myelofibrosis effect. Bone Marrow Transplant 26:697–699

Cervantes F, Hernandez-Boluda JC, Alvarez A, Nadal E, Montserrat E (2002) Danazol treatment of idiopathic myeofibrosis with severe anaemia. Haematol 85:595–599

Cervantes F, Alvarez-Larran A, Hernandez-Boluda JC, Sureda A, Torrebadell M, Montserrat E (2004) Erythropoietin treatment of the anaemia of myelofibrosis with myeloid metaplasia: results in 20 patients and review of literature. Br J Haematol 127:399–403

Cervantes F, Alvarez-Larran A, Domingo A, Arellano-Rodrigo E, Monserrat E (2005) Efficacy and tolerability of danazol as a treatment for the anaemia of myelofibrosis with myeloid metaplasia: long-term results in 30 patients. Br J Haematol 129:771–775

Chaiter Y, Brenner B, Aghai E, Tatarsky I (1992) High incidence of myeloproliferative disorders in Ashkenazi Jews in northern Israel. Leuk Lymphoma 7:251–255

Charbord P (1986) Increased vascularity of bone marrow in myelofibrosis. Br J Haematol 62:595–596

Connelly TJ, Abruzzo JL, Schwab RH (1982) Agnogenic myeloid metaplasia with polyarteritis. Journal of Rheumatology 9:954–956

Cornfield DB, Shipkin P, Alavi A, Becker J, Peyster R (1983). Intracranial myeloid metaplasia: diagnosis by CT and Fe52 scans and treatment by cranial irradiation. Am J Hematol 15:273–278

Cortes J, Albitar M, Thomas D, Giles F, Kurzrock R, Thibault A, Rackoff W, Koller C, O'Brien S, Garcia-Mancro G, Talpaz M, Kantarijian H (2003) Efficacy of the farnesyl tranferase inhibitor R115777 in chronic myeloid leukemia and other hematologic malignancies. Blood 101:1692–1697

Cortes J, Thomas D, Verstovsek S, Giles F, Beran M, Koller C, Kantarjian H (2005) Phase II study of Lenalidomide (CC-5013, Revlimid) for patients (pts) with myelofibrosis (MF) (abstract) 106:114a

Cox MC, Panetta P, Venditti A, Abruzzese E, Del Poeta G, Cantonette M, Amadori S (2001) New reciprocal translocation t(6;10) (q27;q11) associated with idiopathic myelofibrosis. Leuk Res 25:349–351

Craig JIO, Anthony RS, Parker AC (1991) Circulating progenitor cells in myelofibrosis: the effect of recombinant α2b interferon in vivo and in vitro. Br J Haematol 78:155–160

Cunietti E, Gandini R, Marcaro G et al (1981) Defective platelet aggregation and increased platelet turnover in patients with myelofibrosis and other myeloproliferative diseases. Scand J Haematol 26:339–344

Dalley A, Smith JM, Reilly JT, MacNeil S (1996) Investigation of calmodulin and basic fibroblast growth factor (bFGF) in idiopathic myelofibrosis: evidence for a role of extracellular calmodulin in fibroblast proliferation. Br J Haematol 93:856–862

Dameshek W (1951) Some speculations on the myeloproliferative syndromes. Blood 6:372–375

Deeg HJ, Golley TA, Flowers ME, Sale GE, Slattery JT, Anasetti C, Chauncey TR, Doney K, Georges GE, Kiem HP, Martin PJ, Petersdorf EW, Radich J, Sanders JE, Sandmaier BM, Warren EH, Witherspoon RP, Storb R, Appelbaum FR (2003) Allogeneic hematopoietic stem cell transplantation for myelofibrosis. Blood 102:3912–3918

Demory JL, Dupriez B, Fenaux P, Lai JL, Beuscart R, Jouet JP, Deminatti M, Bauters F (1988) Cytogenetic studies and their prognostic significance in agnogenic myeloid metaplasia: a report on 47 cases. Blood 72:855–859

Den Ottolander GJ, Te velde J, Brederoo P, Geraedts JPM, Slee TH, Willemze R, Zwaan FE, Haak HI, Muller HP, Bieger R (1979) Megakaryoblastic leukaemia (acute myelofibrosis): a report of three cases. Br J Haematol 42:9–20

Dingli D, Grand FH, Mahaffey V, Spurbeck J, Ross FM, Reilly JT, Cross NCP, Dewald GW, Tefferi A (2005) Der(6)t(1;6)(q21–23; p21.3): the first specific cytogenetic abnormality in myelofibrosis with myeloid metaplasia. Br J Haematol 130:229–232

Dolan G, Forrest PL, Eastham JM, Reilly JT (1991) Reduced platelet PDGF levels in idiopathic myelofibrosis. Br J Haematol 78:586–588

Donti E, Tabilio A, Bocchini F et al (1990) Partial trisomy 1q in idiopathic myelofibrosis. Leuk Res 14:1035–1040

Dougan LE, Matthews MLV, Armstrong BK (1981) The effect of diagnostic review on the estimated incidence of lymphatic and haematopoietic neoplasms in Western Australia. Cancer 48:866–872

Dupriez B, Morel P, Demory JL, Lai JL, Simon M, Plantier I, Bautiers F (1996) Prognostic factors in agnogenic myeloid metaplasia: a report on 195 cases with a new scoring system. Blood 88:1013–1018

Eastham JM, Reilly JT, MacNeil S (1994) Raised urinary calmodulin levels in idiopathic myelofibrosis: possible implications for the aetiology of fibrosis. Br J Haematol 86:668–670

Elliot MA, Chen MG, Silverstein MN, Tefferi A (1998) Splenic irradiation for symptomatic splenomegaly associated with myelofibrosis with myeloid metaplasia. Br J Haematol 103:505–511

Emadi S, Clay D, Desterke C, Guerton B, Maquarre E, Charpentier A, Jasmin C and Le Bousse-Kerdiles, M-C (2005) IL-8 and its CXCR1 and CXCR2 receptors participate in the control of megakaryocytic proliferation, differentiation, and ploidy in myeloid metaplasia with myelofibrosis. Blood 105:464–473

Faoro LN, Tefferi A, Mesa R (2005) Long-term analysis of the palliative benefit of 2-chlorodeoxyadenosine for myelofibrosis with myeloid mataplasia. Eur J Haematol 74:117–120

Fava RA, Casey TT, Wilcox J, Pelton RW, Moses HL, Nanney LB (1990) Synthesis of transforming growth factor-β1 by megakaryocytes and its localization to megakaryocytes and platelet α-granules. Blood 76:1946–1955

Gaidano G, Guerrasio A, Serra A et al (1993) Mutations in the p53 and ras family genes are associated with tumour progression of bcr/abl negative chronic myeloproliferative disorders. Leukemia 7: 946–953

Garcia S, Miguel A, Linares M, Navarro M, Colomina P (1989) Idiopathic myelofibrosis terminating in erythroleukemia. Am J Hematol 32:70–71

Gay S, Gay RE, Prchal JT (1984) Immunohistological studies of bone marrow collagen. In: Berk P, Castro-Malaspina H, Wasserman LR (eds) Myelofibrosis and the Biology of Connective Tissue. Liss, New York, pp 291–306

Geogii A, Buesche G, Kreft A (1998) The histopathology of chronic myeloproliferative diseases. Baillieres Clin Haematol 11:721–749

Gersuk G, Carmel R, Pattengale PK (1989) Platelet-derived growth factor concentrations in platelet-poor and urine from patients with myeloproliferative disorders. Blood 74:2330–2334

Gibson LE, Dicken CH, Flach DB (1985) Neutrophilic dermatoses and myeloproliferative disease: report of two cases. Mayo Clin Proc 60:735–740

Gilbert HS, Praloran V, Stanley ER (1989) Increased CSF-1 (M-CSF) in myeloproliferative disease: association with myeloid metaplasia and peripheral bone marrow extension. Blood 74:1231–1234

Giles FJ, Cooper MA, Silverman L, Karp JE, Lancet JE, Zangari M, Shami PJ, Khan KD, Hannah AL, Cherrington JM, Thomas DA, Garcia-Manero G, Albitar M, Kantarijian HM, Stopeck AT (2003) Phase II study of SU5416 – a small-molecule, vascular endothelial growth factor tyrosine-kinase receptor inhibitor – in patients with refractory myeloproliferative diseases. Cancer 97:1920–1928

Giraudier S, Chagraoui H, Komura E et al (2002) Overexpression of FKBP51 in idiopathic myelofibrosis regulates the growth factor independence of megakaryocyte progenitors. Blood 100:2932–2940

Gordon BR, Colman M, Kohen P, Day NK (1981) Immunologic abnormalities in myelofibrosis with activation of the complement system. Blood 58:904–910

Guardiola P, Anderson JE, Bandini G, Cervantes F, Runde V, Arcese W, Bacigalupo A, Przepiorka D, O'Donnell MR, Polchi P, Buzyn A, Sutton L, Cazals-Hatem D, Sale G, de Witte T, Deeg HJ, Gluckman E (1999) Allogeneic stem cell transplantation for agnogeneic myeloid metaplasia: a European Group for Blood and Bone Marrow Transplantation, Societé Française de Greffe de Moelle, Gruppo Italiano per il Trapianto del Midollo Osseo, and Fred Hutchinson Cancer Centre Research Center Collaborative Study. Blood 93: 2831–2838

Han ZC, Briere J, Nedellec G, Abgrall JF, Senzebe L, Parent D, Guern G (1988) Characteristics of circulating megakaryocyte progenitor (CFU-MK) in patients with myelofibrosis. Eur J Haematol 40: 130–135

Harmey JH, Dimitriadis E, Kay E, Redmond HP, Bouchier-Hayes D (1998) Regulation of macrophage production of vascular endothelial growth factor (VEGF) by hypoxia and transforming growth fcator β-1. Ann Surg Oncol 5:271–278

Hasselbalch H, Junker P, Lisse I, Bentsen KD, Risteli L, Risteli J (1986) Serum markers for type IV collagen and type III procollagen in the myelofibrosis-osteomeylosclerosis syndrome and other chronic myeloproliferative disorders. Am J Hematol 23:101–111

Hasselbalch HC, Clausen NT, Jensen BA (2002) Successful treatment of anaemia in idiopathic myelofibrosis with recombinant human erythropoietin. Am J Haematol 70:92–99

Hast R, Engstedt L, Jameson S, Killander A, Lundh B, Reizenstein P, Skarberg KO, Uden AM, Wadman B (1978) Oxymethalone treatment in myelofibrosis. Blut 37:12–26

Hernandez JM, San Miguel JF, Gonzalez M et al (1992) Development of acute leukemia after idiopathic myelofibrosis. J Clin Pathol 45:427–430

Hessling J, Kroger N, Werner M, Zabelina T, Hansen A, Kordes U, Ayuk FA, Renges H, Panse J, Erttmann R, Zander AR (2002) Dose-reduced conditioning regimen followed by allogeneic stem cell transplantation in patients with myelofibrosis with myeloid metaplasia. Br J Haematol 119:769–772

Hibbin JA, Njoku OS, Matutes E, Lewis SM, Goldman JM (1984) Myeloid progenitor cells in the circulation of patients with myelofibrosis and other myeloproliferative disorders. Br J Haematol 57:495–503

Horwood E, Dowson H, Gupta R, Kaczmarski R, Williamson M (2003) Myelofibrosis presenting as spinal cord compression. J Clin Pathol 56:154–156

Hu H (1987) Benzene-associated myelofibrosis. Annals of Internal Medicine 106:171–173

Humphrey PA, Vollmer RT (1991) Extramedullary hematopoiesis in the prostate. Am J Surg Pathol 15:486–490

Iványi JL, Mahunka M, Papp A, Kiss A, Telek B (1984) Prognostic significance of bone marrow reticulin fibres in idiopathic myelofibrosis: evaluation of clinicopathological parameters in a scoring system. Haematol 26:75–86

Jack FR, Smith SR, Saunders PWG (1994) Idiopathic myelofibrosis: anaemia can respond to low-dose dexamethasone. Br J Haematol 87:876–884

Jacobson RJ, Salo A, Fialkow PJ (1978) Agnogenic myeloid metaplasia: a clonal proliferation of haematopoietic stem cells with secondary myelofibrosis. Blood 51:189–194

James C, Ugo V, Le Couedic JP, Staerk J, Delmonneau F, Lacout C, Garcon L, Raslova H, Berger R, Bennaceur-Griscelli A, Villeval JL, Constantinescu SN, Casadevall N, Vainchenker W (2005) A unique clonal JAK2 mutation leading to constitutive signalling causes polycythaemia vera. Nature 434:1144–1148

Jantunen E, Hänninen A, Naukkarinen A, Vornanen M, Lahtinen R (1994) Gray platelet syndrome with splenomegaly and signs of extrameduallary hematopoiesis: case report with review of literature. Am J Hematol 46:218–224

Johnson JB, Dalal BI, Israels SJ, Oh S, McMillan E, Begleiter A, Michaud G, Israels LG, Greenberg AH (1995) Deposition of transforming growth factor-β in the marrow in myelofibrosis, and the intracellular localization and secretion of TGF-β by leukemic cells. Am J Clin Pathol 103:574–582

Jones LC, Tefferi A, Idos GE, Kumagai T, Hofman WK, Koeffler HP (2004) RARbeta2 is a candidate suppressor gene in myelofibrosis with myeloid metaplasia. Oncogene 23:7846–7853

Jones LC, Tefferi A, Vuong PT, Desmond JC, Hofmann WK, Koeffler HP (2005) Detection of aberrant gene expression in CD34+ hematopoietic stem cells from patients with agnogenic myeloid metaplasia using oligonucleotide microarrays. Stem Cells 23:631–637

Jowitt SN, Burke DK, Leggat HM, Lewis PS, Cryer RJ (1997) Pleural effusions secondary to extramedullary haematopoiesis in a patients with idiopathic myelofibrosis respondong to pleurodesis and hydroxyurea. Clin Lab Haematol 19:283–285

Kaelin WG, Spivak JL (1986) Systemic lupus erythematosus and myelofibrosis. Am J Med 81:935–938

Kahn A, Bernard JF, Cottreau D, Marie J, Boivin P (1975) Gd(−) Abrami: a deficient G-6PD variant with hemizygous expression in blood cells of a women with primary myelofibrosis. Humangenetik 30:41–46

Katoh O, Kimura A, Kuramoto A (1988) Platelet-derived growth factor is decreased in patients with myeloproliferative disorders. Am J Hematol 27:276–280

Kobayashi S, Teramura M, Hoshino S, Motoji T, Oshimi K, Mizoguchi H (1993) Circulating megakaryocyte progenitors in myeloproliferative disorders are hypersensitive to interleukin-3. Br J Haematol 83:539–544

Komura E, Chagraoui H, de Mas VM, Blanchet B, de Sepulveda P, Larbret F, Larghero J, Tulliez M, Debili N, Vainchenker W, Giraudier S (2003) Spontaneous STAT5 activation induces growth factor independence in idiopathic myelofibrosis: possible relationship with FKBP51 overexpression. Exp Hematol 31:622–630

Komura E, Tonetti C, Penard-Lacronique V, Chagraoui H, Lacout C, Lecouedic JP, Rameau P, Debili N, Vainchenker W, Giraudier S (2005) Role for the nuclear factor kappaB pathway in transforming growth factor-β1 production in idiopathic myelofibrosis: possible relationship with FK506 binding protein 51 overexpression. Cancer Res 65:3281–3289

Kralovics R, Passamonti F, Buser AS, Teo SS, Tiedt R, Passweg JR, Tichelli A, Cazzola M, Skoda RC (2005) A gain-of-function mutation of JAK2 in myeloproliferative disorders. N Eng J Med 352:1779–1790

Kreft A, Weiss M, Wiese B, Choritz H, Buhr T, Busche G, Georgii A (2003) Chronic idiopathic myelofibrosis: prognostic impact of myelofibrosis and clinical parameters on event-free survival in 122 pateints who presented in prefibrotic and fibrotic stages. A retrospective study identifying subgroups of different prognoses by using the RECPAM method. Ann Hematol 82:605–611

Kreipe H, Jaquet K, Felgner J, Radzum HJ, Parwaresch MR (1991) Clonal granulocytes and marrow cells in the cellular phase of agnogenic myeloid metaplasia. Blood 78:1814–1817

Kröger N, Zabelina T, Scheider H, Panse J, Ayuk F, Stute N, Fehse N, Waschke O, Fehse B, Kvasnicka HM, Thiele J, Zander A (2005) Pilot study of reduced-intensity conditioning followed by allogeneic stem cell transplantation from related and unrelated donors in patients with myelofibrosis. Br J Haematol 128:690–697

Kupferschmid JP, Shahian DM, Villanueva AG (1993) Massive hemothorax associated with intrthoraxic extramedullary hematopoiesis involving the pleura. Chest 103:974–975

Kvasnicka HM, Thiele J, Werden C, Zankovich R, Diehl V, Fischer R (1997) Prognostic factors in idiopathic (primary) osteomyelofibrosis. Cancer 80:708–719

Kvasnicka HM, Thiele J, Regn C, Zankovich R, Diehl V, Fischer R (1999) Prognostic impact of apoptosis and proiferation in idiopathic (primary) myelofibrosis. Ann Hematol 78:65–72

Kvasnicka HM, Thiele J, Schroeder M, von Loesch C, Diehl V (2004) Bone marrow angiogenesis – methods of quantification and changes evolving in chronic myeloproliferative disorders. Histol Histopathol 19:1245–1260

Landolfi R, Colosimo C, De Candia E, Castellana MA, De Cristofara R, Trodella L, Leone G (1988) Meningeal hematopoiesis causing exophthalmos and hemiparesis in myelofibrosis: effect of radiotherapy. Cancer 62:2346–2349

Le Bousse-Kerdilés M-C, Chevillard S, Charpentier A, Romquin N, Clay D, Smadja-Jaffe F, Praloran V, Dupriez B, Demory J-L, Jasmin C, Martyré M-C (1996) Differential expression of transforming growth factor-β, basic fibroblast growth factor, and their receptors in $CD34^+$ hematopoietic progenitor cells from patients with myelofibrosis and myeloid metaplasia. Blood 88:4534–4546

Leinweber C, Order SE, Calkins AR (1991) Whole-abdominal irradiation for the management of gastrointestinal and abdominal manifestations of agnogenic myeloid metaplasia. Cancer 68:1251–1254

Leoni P, Ruploi S, Salvi A, Sambo P, Cinciripini A, Gabriella A (1993) Antibodies against terminal galactosyl α(1–3) galactose epitopes in patients with idiopathic myelofibrosis. Br J Haematol 85:313–319

Levine RL, Wadleigh M, Cools J, Ebert BL, Wernig G, Huntly BJP, Boggon TJ, Wlodarska I, Clark JJ, Moore S, Adelsperger J, Koo S, Lee JC, Gabriel S, Mercher T, D'Andrea A, Fröhling S, Döhner K, Marynen P, Vandenberghe P, Mesa RA, Tefferi A, Griffin JD, Eck MJ, Sellers WR, Meyerson M, Golub TR, Lee SJ, Gilliland DG (2005) Activating mutation in the tyrosine kinase JAK2 in polcythemia vera, essential thrombocythemia and myeloid metaplasia with myelofibrosis. Cancer Cell 7:387–397

Levy V, Bourgarit A, Delmer A, Legrand O, Baudard M, Rio B, Zittoun R (1996) Treatment of agnogenic myeloid metaplasia with danazol: a report of four cases. Am J Haematol 53:239–241

Lewis CM, Pegrum GD (1972) Immunocomplexes in myelofibrosis: a possible guide to management. Br J Haematol 39:233–239

Ligumski M, Polliack A, Benbassat J (1979) Metaplasia of the central nervous system in patients with myelofibrosis and agnogenic myeloid metaplasis: report of 3 cases and review of literature. Am J Med Sci 275:99–103

Loewy G, Mathew A, Distenfeld A (1994) Skin manifestations of agnogenic myeloid metaplasia. Am J Hematol 45 167–170

Lofvenberg E, Wahlin A, Roos G, Ost A (1990) Reversal of myelofibrosis by hydroxyurea. Eur J Haematol 44:33–38

López-Guillermo A, Cervantes F, Bruguera M, Pereira A Feliu E, Rozman C (1991) Liver dysfunction following splenectomy in idiopathic myelofibrosis: a study of 10 patients. Acta Haematol 85:184–188

Lundh B, Brandt L, Cronqvist S, Eyrich R (1982) Intracranial myeloid metaplasia in myelofibrosis. Scand J Haematol 28:91–94

Macdonald DHC, Lahiri D, Chase A, Sohal J, Goldman JM, Cross NCP (1999) A case of myelofibrosis with a t(4;13)(q25;q12): evidence for involvement of a second 13q12 locus in chronic myeloproliferative disorders. Br J Haematol 105:771–774

Mackinnon S, McNicol AM, Lee FD, McDonald GA (1986) Myelofibrosis complicated by intestinal extramedullary haematopoiesis and acute bowel obstruction. J Clin Pathol 39:677–679

Manoharan A (1991) Management of myelofibrosis with intermittent hydroxyurea. Br J Haematol 77:252–254

Manoharan A, Pitney WR (1984) Chemotherapy resolves symptoms and reverses marrow fibrosis in myelofibrosis. Scand J Haematol 33:453–459

Marchetti M, Barosi G, Balestri F, Viarengo G, Gentili S, Barulli S, Demory J-L, Ilariucci F, Volpe A, Bordessoule D, Grossi A, Le Bousse-Kerdiles MC, Caenazzo A, Pecci A, Falcone A, Broccia G, Bendotti C, Bauduer F, Buccisano F, Dupriez B (2004) Low-dose thalidomide ameliorates cytopenias and splenomgaly in myelofibrosis with myeloid metaplasia: a phase II trial. J Clin Oncol 22:424–431

Martyré M-C, Magdelenat H, Bryckaert MC, laine-Bidron C, Calvo F (1991) Increased intraplatelet levels of platelet-derived growth factor and transforming growth factor-β in patients with myelofibrosis and myeloid metaplasia. Br J Haematol 77:80–86

Martyré M-C, Le Bousse-Kerdilés M-C, Romquin N, Chevillard S, Praloran V, Demory J-L, Dupriez B (1997) Elevated levels of basic growth factor in megakaryocytes and platelets from patients with idiopathic myelofibrosis. Br J Haematol 97:441–448

Mesa RA, Siverstein MN, Jacobsen SJ, Wollan PC, Tefferi A (1997) Population-based incidence and survival figures in essential thrombocythemia and agnogenic myeloid metaplasia: an Olmstead County Study 1976–1995. Am J Hematol 61:10–15

Mesa MA, Hanson CA, Rajkumar VS, Schroeder G, Tefferi A (2000) Evaluation and clinical correlations of bone marrow angiogenesis in myelofibrosis with myeloid metaplasia. Blood 96:3374–3380

Mesa RA, Steensma DP, Pardanani A, Li, C-Y, Elliot M, Kaufmann SH, Wiseman G, Gray LA, Schroeder G, Reeder T, Zeldis JB, Tefferi A (2003) A phase 2 trial of combination low-dose thalidomide and prednisone for the treatment of myelofibrosis with myeloid metaplasia. Blood 101:2534–2541

Mesa R, Li C-Y, Ketterling RP, Schroeder GS, Knudson RA, Tefferi A (2005) Leukemic transformation in myelofibrosis with myeloid metaplasia: a single-institution experience with 91 cases. Blood 105:973–977

Murate T, Yamashita K, Isogai C, Suzuki H, Ichihara M, Hatano S, Nakahara Y, Kinoshita T, Nagasaka T, Yoshida S, Komatsu N, Miura Y, Hotta T, Fujimoto N, Saito H, Hayakawa T (1997) The production of tissue inhibitors of metalloproteinases (TIMPS) in megakaryopoiesis: possible role of platelet- and megakaryocyte-derived TIMPS in bone marrow fibrosis. Br J Haematol 99:181–189

Nakahata J, Takahashi M, Fuse I, Nakamori Y, Nomoto N, Saitoh H, Tatewaki W, Imanari A, Takeshige T, Koike T (1993) Paroxysmal nocturnal hemoglobinuria with myelofibrosis: progression to acute myeloblastic leukemia. Leuk Lymphoma 12:137–142

Njoku OS, Lewis SM, Catovsky D, Gordon-Smith EC (1983) Anaemia in myelofibrosis: its value in prognosis. Br J Haematol 54:70–89

Novetsky A, Wang JC, Chen C (1997) Plasma VEGF levels in patients with primary myelofibrosis and other myeloproliferative disorders. Blood 90:(abstract)

O'Mahony CA, Albo D, Tuszynski GP, Berger DH (1998) Transforming growth factor-beta 1 inhibits generation of angiostatin by human pancreatic cancer cells. Surgery 124:388–393

Overall CM, Wrana JL, Sodek J (1989) Independent regulation of collagenase, 72 kDa-progelatinase and metalloendoproteinase inhibitor (TIMP) expression in human fibroblasts by transforming growth factor-β. J Biol Chem 264:1860–1869

Passamonti F, Vanelli L, Malabarba L, Rumi E, Pungolino E, Malcovati L, Pascutto C, Morra E, Lazzarino M, Cazzola M (2003) Clinical utility of the absolute number of circulating CD34-positive cells in patients with chronic myeloproliferative disorders. Haematol 88: 1123–1129

Perianin A, Labro-Bryskier MT, Marquetty C et al (1984) Glutathione reductase and nitro-blue tetrazolium reduction deficiencies in neutrophils of patients with primary idiopathic myelofibrosis. Clin Exp Immunol 57:244–248

Petti MC, Latagliata R, Spadea T, Spadea A, Montefusco E, Aloe Spiriti MA, Avvisati G, Breccia M, Pescarmona E, Mandelli F (2002) Melphalan treatment in patients with myelofibrosis with myeloid metaplasia. Br J Haematol 116:576–581

Pietrasanta D, Clavio M, Vallebella E, Beltrami G, Cavaliere M, Gobbi M (1997) Long-lasting effect of cyclosporin-A on anaemia associated with idiopathic myelofibrosis. Haematol 82:458–459

Polliak A, Prokocimer M, Matzner Y (1980) Lymphoblastic leukemic transformation (lymphoblastic crisis) in myelofibrosis and myeloid metaplasia. Am J Hematol 9:211–220

Price F, Bell H (1985) Spinal cord compression due to extramedullary hematopoiesis. Successful treatment in a patient with long standing myelofibrosis. JAMA 253:2876–2877

Rameshwar P, Denny TN, Stein D, Gascon P (1994) Monocyte adhesion in patients with bone marrow fibrosis is required for the production of fibrogenic cytokines. Potential role for interleukin-1 and TGF-β. J Immunol 153:2819–2830

Rameshwar P, Chang VT, Gascon P (1996) Implication of CD44 in adhesion-mediated overproduction of TGF-β and IL-1 in monocytes from patients with bone marrow fibrosis. Br J Haematol 96:22–29

Reeder TL, Bailey RJ, Dewald GW, Tefferi A (2003) Both T and B lymphocytes may be clonally involved in myelofibrosis with myeloid metaplasia. Blood 101:1981–1983

Reilly JT (2005) Cytogenetic and molecular genetic abnormalities in agnogenic myeloid metaplasia. Sem Oncol 32:359–364

Reilly JT, Nash JGR, Mackie MJ, McVerry BA (1985 a) Immuno-enzymatic detection of fibronectin in normal and pathological haematopoietic tissue. Br J Haematol 59:497–504

Reilly JT, Nash JGR, Mackie MJ, McVerry BA (1985 b) Endothelial cell proliferation in myelofibrosis. Br J Haematol 60:625–630

Reilly JT, Nash JGR (1988) Vitronectin (serum spreading factor): its localization in normal and fibrotic tissue. J Clin Pathol 59:1269–1272

Reilly JT, Barnett D, Dolan G, Forrest P, Eastham J, Smith A (1993) Characterization of an acute micromegakaryocytic leukaemia: evidence for the pathogenesis of myelofibrosis. Br J Haematol 83:58–62

Reilly JT, Wilson G, Barnett D, Watmore A, Potter A (1994) Karyotypic and ras gene mutational analysis in idiopathic myelofibrosis. Br J Haematol 88:575–581

Reilly JT, Brindley L, Kay M, Fielding S, Kennedy A, Dolan G, Smith A (1995) Bone marrow and serum connective tissue polypeptides in idiopathic myelofibrosis. Clin Lab Haematol 17:35–39

Reilly JT, Snowden JA, Spearing RL, Fitzgerald PM, Jones N, Watmore A, Potter A (1997) Cytogenetic abnormalities and their prognostic significance in idiopathic myelofibrosis: a study of 106 cases. Br J Haematol 98:96–102

Rege-Cambrin G, Speleman F, Kerim S, Sacravaglio P, Carozzi F, Dal Cin P, Michaux JL, Offner F, Saglio G, Van den Berghe H (1991) Extra translocation +der (1q9p) is a prognostic indicator in myeloproliferative disorders. Leukemia 5:1059–1063

Roberts AB, Sporn MB, Assoian RK, Smith MJ, Roche NS, Wakefiled LM, Heine UI, Liotta LA, Falanga V, Kehrl JH, Fauci AS (1986) Transforming growth factor-β: rapid induction of fibrosis and angiogenesis in vivo and stimuation of collagen formation in vitro. Proc Nat Acad Sci USA 83:4167–4171

Rodríguez JN, Martino ML, Diéguez JC, Prados D (1998) RhuEpo for the treatment of anaemia in myelofibrosis with myeloid metaplasia. Experience in 6 patients and meta-analytical approach. Haematol 83:616–621

Romano M, Viero P, Cortellazzo S, Barbui T, Donati MB, Poggi A (1990) Platelet-derived mitogenic activity and bone marrow fibrosis in myeloproliferative disorders. Haemostasis 20:162–168

Rondeau E, Soal-Celigny P, Dhermy D, Wraclans M, Brousse N, Bernard JF, Boivin P (1983) Immune disorders in agnogenic myeloid metaplasia: relation to fibrosis. Br J Haematol 53:467–475

Rondelli D (2003) Non-myeloablative allogeneic HSCT in high-risk patients with myelofibrosis. Blood 102

Rozman C, Giralt M, Feliu E, Rubio D, Cortes, M-T (1991) Life expectancy of patients with chronic nonleukemic myeloproliferative disorders. Cancer 67:2658–2663

Rupoli S, Da Lio L, Sisti S et al (1994) Primary myelofibrosis: a detailed statistical analysis of the clinicopathological variables influencing survival. Ann Hematol 68:205–212

Sagaster V, Jager E, Weltermann A, Schwarzinger I, Gisslinger H, Lechner K, Geissler K, Oehler L (2003) Circulating hematopoietic progenitor cells predict survival in patients with myelofibrosis and myeloid metaplasia. Hematologica 88:1204–1212

Sacchi S, Curci G, Piccinini L, Messeroti A, Cucci F, Bursi R, Zaniol P, Torrelli V (1986) Platelet alpha-granule release in chronic myeloproliferative disorders with thrombocytosis. J Clin Lab Invest 46:163–166

Schafer AI (1982) Deficiency of platelet lipoxygenase activity in myeloproliferative disorders. N Eng J Med 306:381–386

Schmitt A, Drouin A, Masse JM, Guichard J, Shagraoui H, Cramer EM (2002) Polymorphonuclear neutrophil and megakaryocyte mutual involvement in myelofibrosis pathogenesis. Leuk Lymphoma 43:719–724

Schnuelle P, Waldherr R, Lehmann KJ, Woenckhaus J, Back W, Niemir Z, van der Woude FJ (1999) Idiopathic myelofibrosis with extramedullary hematopoiesis in the kidneys. Clin Nephrol 52:256–262

Shaheen SP, Talwalker SS, Simons R, Yam L (2005) Acute lymphoblastic leukemic transformation in a patient with chronic idiopathic myelofibrosis and paroxysmal nocturnal hemoglobinuria: a case report and review of literature. Arch Pathol Lab Med 129:96–99

Sharma BK, Pounder RE, Cruse JP, Knowles SM, Lewis AA (1986) Extramedullary hematopoiesis in the small bowel. Gut 27:873–875

Silverstein MN (1975) Agnogenic myeloid metaplasia. Publishing Sciences Groups, Massachusetts, p 94–95

Silverstein MN, ReMine WH (1979) Splenectomy in myeloid metaplasia. Blood 53:515–518

Sinclair EJ, Forrest EC, Reilly JT, Watmore AE, Potter AM (2002) Fluorescence in situ hybridization analysis of 25 cases of idiopathic myelofibrosis and two cases of secondary myelofibrosis: monoallelic loss of RB1, D13S319 and D13S25 loci associated with cytogenetic deletion and tranlocation involving 13q14. Br J Haematol 113:365–368

Steensma DP, Hook CC, Stafford SL, Tefferi A (2002) Low-dose, single fraction, whole-lung radiotherapy for pulmonary hypertension associated with myelofibrosis and myeloid metaplasia. Br J Haematol 118:813–816

Strasser-Weippl K, Steurer M, Kees M, Augustin F, Tzankov A, Dirnhofer S, Fiegl M, Gisslinger H, Zojer N, Ludwig H (2005) Chromosome 7 deletions are associated with unfavorable prognosis in myelofibrosis with myeloid metaplasia. Blood 105:4146

Sugimoto N, Ishikawa T, Gotoh S, Shinzato I, Matsusita A, Nagai K, Ohgoh N, Takahashi T (2004) Primary myelofibrosis terminated in basophilic leukemia and successful allogeneic bone marrow transplantation. Int J Hematol 80:183–185

Taksin AL, Couedic JP, Dusanter-Fourt I, Masse A, Giraudier S, Katz A, Wendling F, Vainchenker W, Casadevall N, Debili N (1999) Autonomous megakaryocyte growth in essential thrombocythemia and idiopathic myelofibrosis is not related to a c-mpl mutation or to an autocrine stimulation by Mpl-L. Blood 93:125–139

Tefferi A, Silverstein MN (1994) Recombinant human erythropoietin therapy in patients with myelofibrosis with myeloid metaplasia (letter). Br J Haematol 86:893–896

Tefferi A, Barrett SM, Silverstein MN, Nagorney DM (1994) Outcome of portal-systemic shunt surgery for portal hypertension associated with intrahepatic obstruction in patients with agnogenic myeloid metaplasia. Am J Hematol 46:325–328

Tefferi A, Silverstein MN, Li C-Y (1997) 2-chlorodeoxyadenosine treatment after splenectomy in patients who have myelofibrosis with myeloid metaplasia. Br J Haematol 99:352–357

Tefferi A, Mesa RA, Nagomey DN, Schroeder G, Silverstein MN (2000) Splenectomy in myelofibrosis with myeloid metaplasia: a single-institution experience with 223 patients. Blood 95:2226–2233

Tefferi A, Mesa RA, Schroeder G, Hanson CA, Li CY, Dewald GW (2001 a) Cytogenetic findings and their clinical relevance in myelofibrosis with myeloid metaplasia. Br J Haematol 113:763–771

Tefferi A, Jiménez T, Gray LA, Mesa RA, Chen MG (2001b) Radiation therapy for symptomatic hepatomegaly in myelofibrosis with myeloid metaplasia. Eur J Haematol 66:37–42

Tefferi A, Mesa RA, Hogan WJ, Shaw TA, Reyes GE, Allred JB, Ma CX, Dy GK, Wolanskyj AP, Litzow ML, Steensma DP, Call TG, McClure RF (2005) Lenalidomide (CC-5013) treatment for anemia associated with myelofibrosis with myeloid metaplasia (abstract). Blood 106:726a

Terui T, Niitsu Y, Mahara K, Fugisaki Y, Urushizaki Y, Mogi Y, Kohgo Y, Watanabe N, Ogura M, Saito H (1990) The production of transforming growth factor-β in acute megakaryoblastic leukemia and its possible implications in myelofibrosis. Blood 75:1540–1548

Thiele J, Kvasnicka HM (2002) CD34+ stem cells in chronic myeloproliferative disorders. Histol Histopathol 17:507–521

Thiele J, Kvasnicka HM (2004) Prefibrotic chronic idiopathic myelofibrosis – a diagnostic enigma? Acta Haematol 111:155–159

Thiele J, Kuemmel T, Sander C, Fischer R (1991) Ultrastructure of the bone marrow tissue in so-called primary (idiopathic) myelofibrosis-osteomyelosclerosis (agnogenic myeloid metaplasia). 1. Abnormalities of megakaryopoiesis and thrombocytes. J Submicrosc Cytol Pathol 23:93–107

Thiele J, Kvasnicka HM, Boeltken B, Zankovich R, Diehl V, Fischer R (1999) Initial (prefibrotic) stages of idiopathic (primary) myelofibrosis (IMF) – a clinicopathological study. Leukemia 13:1741–1748

Thiele J, Kvasnicka HM, Zankovich R, Diehl V (2001) Clinical and morphological criteria for the diagnosis of prefibrotic idiopathic (primary) myelofibrosis. Ann Hematol 80:160–165

Thiele J, Imbert M, Pierre R, Vardiman JW, Brunning RD, Flandrin G (2001) Chronic idiopathic myelofibrosis. In: Jaffe ES, Harris NL, Stein H, Vardiman JW (eds) WHO Classification of tumours: tunours of haematopoietic and lymphoid tissues. IARC Press, Lyon, France, pp 35–38

Thiele J, Kvasnicka HM, Schmitt-Gräff A, Diehl V (2003) Dynamics of fibrosis in chronic idiopathic myelofibrosis during therapy: a follow-up study on 309 patients. Leuk Lymphoma 44:549–553

Thorns C, Rohrmoser B, Feller A, Horny HC (2002) Chronic cholecystitis and myeloid metaplasia. Histopathology 41:273–275

Tsurumi S, Nakamura Y, Maki K, Omine M, Fujita K, Okamura T, Niho Y, Hashimoto S, Kanno K, Suzuki K, Hangaishi A, Ogawa S, Hirai H, Mitani K (2002) N-ras and p53 gene mutations in Japanese patients with myeloproliferative disorders. Am J Hematol 71:131–133

Titius BR, Thiele J, Schaefer H, Kreipe H, Fischer R (1994) Ki-S1 and proliferating cell nuclear antigen expression of bone marrow macrophages. Acta Haematol 91:144–149

Tsao M-S (1989) Hepatic sinusoidal fibrosis in agnogenic myeloid metaplasia. Am J Clin Pathol 91:302–305

Tsukamoto N, Morita K, Maehara T, Okamoto K, Sakai H, Karasawa M, Naruse T Omine M (1994) Clonality in chronic myeloproliferative disorders defined by X-chromosome linked probes: demonstration of heterogeneity in lineage involvement. Br J Haematol 86:253–258

Vannucchi AM, Bianchi L, Paoletti F, Di Giacomo V, Migliaccio G, Migliaccio AR (2004) Impaired GATA-1 expression and myelofibrosis in an animal model. Pathol Biol (Paris) 52:275–279

Vannucchi AM, Bianchi L, Paoletti F, Pancrazzi A, Torre E, Nishikawa M, Zingariello M, Di Baldassarre A, Rana RA, Lorenzini R, Alfani E, Migliaccio G, Migliaccio AR (2005) A patho-biological pathway linking thrombopoietin, GATA-1 and TGF-β1 in the development of myelofibrosis. Blood 105:3493–3501

Varki A, Lottenberg R, Griffith R, Reinhard E (1983) The syndrome of idiopathic myelofibrosis: a clinicaopathologic review with emphasis on the prognostic variables predicting survival. Medicine (Baltimore) 62:353–371

Verstovsek S, Lawhorn K, Giles F et al (2003) PEG Intron therapy for patients with myeloproliferative diseases (MPD): interim analysis of phase II study (abstract). Blood 102:919a-920a

Visani G, Finelli C, Castelli U et al (1990) Myelofibrosis with myeloid metaplasia: clinical and haematological parameters predicting survival in a series of 133 patients. Br J Haematol 75:4–9

Visani G, Mele A, Malagola M et al (2003) Sequential combination of thalidomaide and erythropoietin determines transfusion independence and disease control in idiopathic myelofibrosis previously insensitive to both drugs used as single agents. Leukemia 17:1669–1670

Wang JC, Lang HD, Lichter S, Weinstein M, Benn P (1992) Cytogenetic studies of bone marrow fibroblasts cultured from patients with myelofibrosis and myeloid metaplasia. Br J Haematol 80:184–188

Wang JC, Chen C, Lou LH, Mora M (1997) Blood thrombopoietin, IL-6 and IL-11 levels in patients with agnogenic myeloid metaplasia. Leukemia 11:1827–1832

Wang JC, Chen C (1999) p16 gene deletions and point mutations in patients with agnogenic myeloid metaplasia (AMM). Leukemia Res 23:631–635

Wang JC, Hemavathy K, Charles W, Zhang H, Dua PK, Novetsky AD, Chang T, Wong C, Jabara M (2004) Osteosclerosis in idiopathic myelofibrosis is related to the overproduction of osteoprotegerin (OPG). Exp Hematol 32:905–910

Wanless IR, Peterson P, Das A, Boitnott JK, Moore GW, Bernier V (1990) Hepatic vascular disease and portal hypertension in polycythemia vera and agnogenic myeloid metaplasia: a clinicopathological study of 145 patients examined at autopsy. Hepatology 12:1166–1174

Wernig G, Mercher T, Okabe R, Levine RL, Lee BH, Gilliland DG (2006) Expression of Jak2V617F causes a polycythemia vera-like disease with associated myelofibrosis in a murine bone marrow transplant model. Blood 107:4274–4281

Williams ME, Innes DJ, Hutchison WT, Hesse CE (1985) Extramedullary hematopoeiesis: a cause of severe generalised lymphadenopathy in agnogenic myeloid metaplasia. Arch Intern Med 145:1308–1309

Wolf BC, Neiman RS (1987) Hypothesis: splenic filtration and the pathogenesis of extramedullary hematopoiesis in agnogenic myeloid metaplasia. Hematol Pathol 1:77–80

Xu M, Bruno E, Chao J, Huang S, Finazzi G, Fruchtman SM, Popat U, Prchal JT, Barosi G, Hoffman R (2005) The constitutive mobilization of CD34+ cells into the peripheral blood in idiopathic myelofibrosis may be due to the action of a number of proteases. Blood 105:4508–4515

Yan XQ, Lacey D, Hill D, Chen Y, Fletcher F, Hawley RG, McNiece IK (1996) A model of myelofibrosis and osteosclerosis in mice induced by overexpressing thrombopoietin (mpl ligand): reversal of disease by bone marrow transplantation. Blood 88:402–409

Yotsumoto M, Ishida F, Ito T, Ueno M, Kitano K, Kiyosawa K (2003) Idiopathic myelofibrosis with massive ascites. Intern Med 42:525–528

Zanke B, Squire J, Griesser H et al (1994) A hematopoietic protein tyrosine phosphatase (HePTP) gene that is amplified and overexpressed in myeloid malignancies maps to chromosome 1q32.1. Leukemia 8:236–244

Polycythemia Vera – Clinical Aspects

Alison R. Moliterno and Jerry L. Spivak

Contents

Abstract. Polycythemia vera (PV) is an acquired hematopoietic stem cell disorder characterized by the overproduction of red cells, white cells, and platelets in the absence of a defined stimulus. Although involvement of a multipotent hematopoietic progenitor cell is a characteristic of PV, erythrocytosis is the feature that not only sets it apart from its companion myeloproliferative disorders, but also provides insight into its pathogenesis and is related to the major complications of PV, thrombosis, and hemorrhage. The diagnosis of PV requires careful clinical assessment of the myeloproliferative phenotype in the individual patient, and optimal management of PV requires the knowledge of its natural history and complications. This chapter is focused on these concepts and concludes with a strategy for the management of PV.

16.1 Introduction

Polycythemia vera (PV) is an acquired clonal hematopoietic stem cell disorder characterized by the overproduction of morphologically normal red cells, white cells, and platelets in the absence of a definable stimulus and a proclivity to develop extramedullary hematopoiesis. First described in 1892 by the French physician Vaquez (Vaquez 1892), widespread attention to the disorder did not occur until Osler's seminal 1903 publication (Osler 1903). Despite eleven decades since its recognition, years of intense scientific scrutiny and the recent identification of an associated genetic lesion, Vaquez-Osler disease remains a syndromic disorder for which there is no specific diagnostic test and no specific targeted therapy. As such, the diagnosis of PV requires a careful clinical assessment of the individual patient, and optimal management of PV requires the knowledge of its natural history and complications relevant to the individual patient.

16.2 Epidemiology

The incidence of PV is approximately 2/100,000, although estimates from 1/100,000 to greater than 18/100,000 (Johansson et al. 2004; McNally et al. 1997; Ruggeri et al. 2003) have been made depending on the population studied and its age. Rare in children, PV spares no age group amongst adults, with a peak frequency in the fifth decade for females and the sixth decade for males (Berglund and Zettervall 1992; Prochazka and Markowe 1986). There is a slight male predominance in PV, although below the age of 40, PV is more common in females (Fig. 16.1). PV occurs in all ethnic groups but is less common in African-Americans than in Caucasians, and there appears to be an increase in individuals of Ashkenazi descent (Modan et al. 1971). While PV is typically considered an acquired disorder, clustering of PV as well as other myeloproliferative disorders (MPD) within families has been described (Brubaker et al. 1984; Friedland et al. 1981; Gilbert 1998; Manoharan and Garson 1976; Miller et al. 1989; Najean et al. 1998; Ratnoff and Gress 1980), suggesting that there are somatic, heritable factors that increase the risk of developing an MPD.

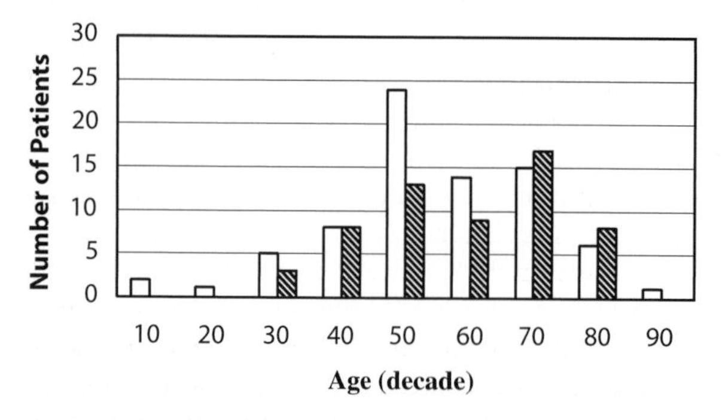

Fig. 16.1. Age at diagnosis of PV in 134 patients cared for at the Center for the Chronic Myeloproliferative Disorders at the Johns Hopkins Hospital. *Open bars* indicate females, *striped bars* indicate males

16.3 Pathogenesis

Hematopoiesis is normally polyclonal, with individual stem cells contributing to hematopoiesis clonally but simultaneously. In PV hematopoiesis is usually monoclonal with the progeny of the transformed pluripotent hematopoietic stem cell supplying the cells of the peripheral blood (Adamson et al. 1976; Levine et al. 2006; Tsukamoto et al. 1994). Although involvement of a multipotent hematopoietic progenitor cell is a characteristic of PV, erythrocytosis is the feature of PV that not only sets it apart from its companion myeloproliferative disorders but also provides insight into its pathogenesis.

16.3.1 Erythropoiesis

The molecular investigation of PV has proceeded in tandem with the technologies available for the study of erythropoiesis. Thus, in the second half of the last century, red cell lifespan was observed not to be prolonged in PV (London et al. 1949), nor was the erythroid pool expanded at the expense of the myeloid progenitor compartment (Eaves et al. 1980). The notion that erythropoiesis in PV was autonomous was supported by the observations of continued erythropoiesis in PV patients despite hyperoxia (Lawrence et al. 1952) or renal failure (Spivak and Cooke 1976), and the extremely low serum erythropoietin levels observed in PV patients as compared to any other form of erythrocytosis (Fig. 16.2). When purified erythropoietin and semisolid culture techniques for the assay of erythroid progenitors became available, the autonomous nature of erythropoiesis in PV was established (Prchal and Axelrad 1974).

The in vitro hypersensitivity of PV erythroid progenitor cells to multiple hematopoietic growth factors led to an examination of hematopoietic growth factor receptor function. Studies of erythropoietin receptor expression and erythropoietin binding in PV erythroid progenitors did not reveal major differences from normal progenitor cells (Broudy et al. 1990; Eaves and Eaves 1978; Means Jr. et al. 1989) nor were there gross rearrangements, amplifications, or functional mutations in the erythropoietin receptor (Hess et al. 1994). Further study into the receptors for IL-3 and stem cell factor revealed no differences in their behaviors in PV as compared to normals (Dai et al. 1991, 1994).

Although a lesion in the erythropoietin receptor could not be implicated in the pathogenesis of PV,

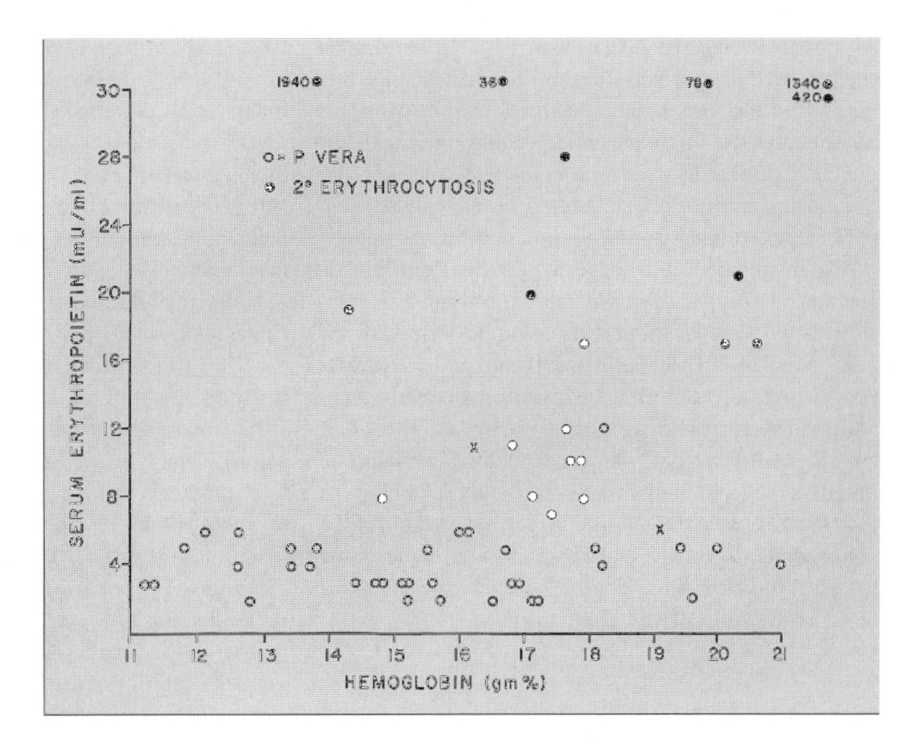

Fig. 16.2. Serum erythropoietin levels in erythrocytosis patients. Erythropoietin levels in polycythemia vera (○), secondary erythrocytosis (●) and spurious erythrocytosis (×)

further observations of PV growth factor receptor biology implicated two other candidate receptors, the IGF-1 receptor and the thrombopoietin receptor (Mpl). PV erythroid progenitor cells were hypersensitive to IGF-1, whereas the IGF-1 receptors in peripheral blood mononuclear cells were reported to be constitutively tyrosine phosphorylated and more sensitive to IGF-1 than normal peripheral blood mononuclear cells (Correa et al. 1994; Mirza et al. 1995). The serum concentration of IGF-1 binding protein-I was also increased in PV patients, and this protein could stimulate erythroid burst formation in vitro (Mirza et al. 1997). Subsequent studies observed increases in IGF-1 binding proteins in PV, but did not replicate the phosphorylation defects and did not identify abnormalities in the sequence of the IGF-1 receptor gene (Michl et al. 2001).

Mpl is an attractive candidate receptor in the pathogenesis of PV as Mpl is expressed in pluripotent hematopoietic progenitors, and its cognate ligand, thrombopoetin, enhanced the survival of these cells (Debili et al. 1995; Ratajczak et al. 1997; Solar et al. 1998). Excessive thrombopoietin exposure in mice produced granulocytosis, thrombocytosis, osteomyelofibrosis, and extramedullary hematopoiesis, recapitulating many features of the myeloproliferative phenotype (Ulich et al. 1996; Villeval et al. 1997). Importantly, the myeloproliferative leukemia retrovirus (MPLV), which encoded a truncated form of Mpl, induced a syndrome in mice mimicking PV (Wendling et al. 1986), whereas hematopoietic progenitors infected with MPLV were growth-factor independent in vitro and capable of terminal differentiation in the absence of growth factors (Souyri et al. 1990).

In contrast to the erythropoietin receptor in PV, in which there were no changes in expression and ligand binding, Mpl protein expression was markedly decreased in PV platelets and megakaryocytes, and was associated with markedly reduced thrombopoietin-induced signal transduction in platelets (Moliterno et al. 1998). The basis for the loss of Mpl protein expression was due to impaired posttranslational processing resulting in loss of glycosylation and retention in the Golgi complex, and associated with reduced plasma membrane expression (Moliterno and Spivak 1999). This defect was observed in most PV patients and not at all in secondary causes of erythrocytosis or thrombocytosis (Elliot et al. 2002; Horikawa et al. 1997). Furthermore, the extent of impaired Mpl expression correlated with disease duration and the extent of extramedullary hematopoiesis (Moliterno and Spivak 1999), and was not a consequence of platelet, white cell or red cell count, or therapy, suggesting that loss of Mpl expression tracked with disease presence and activity.

Loss of Mpl expression and signal transduction was an unexpected and counterintuitive finding in a disorder characterized by exuberant hematopoiesis. How loss of cytokine receptor cell surface expression could be associated with diseases of myeloproliferation was not immediately apparent, but suggested that loss of Mpl surface expression per se might relieve a negative regulatory role of Mpl. Further evidence supporting this contention include an Mpl polymorphism that disrupts Mpl processing and cell surface expression that associates with a myeloproliferative phenotype (Moliterno et al. 2004), constitutive growth induced by disruption of the distal N-terminal domain of Mpl (Sabath et al. 1999), and extensive studies in Mpl knockout mice, which under a variety of conditions, develop marked uncontrolled myeloproliferation (Carpinelli et al. 2004; Levin et al. 2001; Metcalf et al. 2005).

16.3.2 Signal Transduction

While the discovery of constitutive tyrosine kinase activity in some myeloproliferative disorders (Cools et al. 2003; Cross and Reiter 2002) gave hope to the possibility that such a molecular lesion may be present in PV, direct evidence for constitutive tyrosine kinase activity in PV had been meager, particularly considering the presence of growth factor hypersensitivity. Indirect evidence of enhanced kinase activity included the reports that inhibitors of JAK2, PIK3, or Src abolished PV erythropoietin-independent colony (EEC) formation in vitro (Roder et al. 2001), that a higher degree of PKC inhibition was required to abolish PV EEC than erythropoietin-stimulated erythroid colony formation (Kawada et al. 1997), and in vitro orthovanadate exposure did not enhance PV erythroid cell proliferation or tyrosine phosphorylation in contrast to normal (Dai et al. 1997).

The observations that endogenous erythroid colony growth in PV progenitors was suppressed by inhibitors of JAK2 kinase led to sequencing of the JAK2 gene and the discovery of a point mutation (V617F) in the JAK2 pseudokinase domain (James et al. 2005; Ugo et al. 2004). This observation was simultaneously reported by other groups (Baxter et al. 2005; Jones et al. 2005; Kralovics et al. 2005; Levine et al. 2005; Zhao et al. 2005) as part of large scale sequencing projects. JAK2 V617F was found in approximately 90% of patients with PV and about 50% of patients with idiopathic myelofibrosis (IMF) or essential thrombocythemia (ET) (Vizmanos et al. 2006; see also Chaps. 15 Chronic Idiopathic Myelofibrosis and 18 Essential Thrombocythemia). The biochemical effect of JAK2V617F in vitro appears to result in constitutive phosphorylation of JAK2 and growth factor-independent cell proliferation, presumably due to loss of autoinhibition that the pseudokinase domain of JAK2 normally provides (Saharinen et al. 2003) (see also Chap. 16).

JAK2 V617F provided a biochemical explanation for many of the features of PV. A constitutively-activated JAK2 could account for EPO-independent PV erythroid colony formation, hypersensitivity to EPO and other hematopoietic growth factors, the observed resistance to apoptosis of PV erythroid progenitor cells in vitro in the absence of EPO, and the increase in their Bcl-xL expression. Importantly, JAK2 is not merely the cognate signaling tyrosine kinase for Mpl and the EPO receptor; it is also the chaperone responsible for transporting both out of the Golgi (Huang et al. 2001; Royer et al. 2005). While the number of EPO receptors on PV erythroid cells is normal (Means, Jr. et al. 1989), the EPO receptor has only one N-linked glycosylation site, which is dispensable for its function (Nagao et al. 1995), while Mpl with its reduplicated extracellular domain has four N-linked glycosylation sites. A JAK2 abnormality could account for the impaired Mpl processing seen in PV as well as the other chronic myeloproliferative disorders; alternatively, improperly processed Mpl could retain JAK2 in the Golgi. Inappropriate cellular localization of JAK2 could result in aberrant JAK2 signaling much like the aberrant Bcr-Abl cytoplasmic signaling in chronic myelogenous leukemia (Wetzler et al. 1993).

Given the indolent pace of PV and the genomic stability of the disease clone over decades, JAK2 V617F may not exert its oncogenic effect via a high grade constitutive process in a manner like Bcr-Abl in CML, but rather via the sum of effects including both positive, constitutive signaling and loss of negative regulation of signal transduction. Indeed, the fact that JAK2 V617F has been associated not only with PV, IMF, and ET phenotypes but also with chronic neutrophilic leukemia, chronic myelomonocytic leukemia and sideroblastic anemia (Steensma et al. 2005), indicate that important host and/or other genetic lesions in addition to JAK2 V617F genotype are required to generate unique disease phenotypes (Fig. 16.3). Future challenges will be to identify the contributing genetic and epigenetic factors

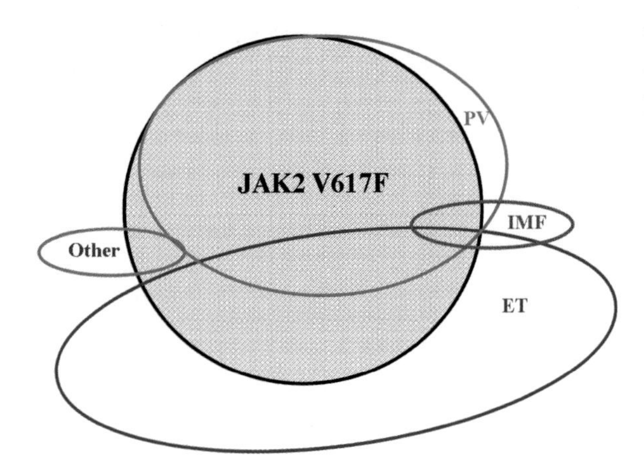

Fig. 16.3. Prevalence of JAK2 V617F in myeloproliferative disorders. All JAK2 V617F positive patients are indicated by the *shaded circle*. The clinical myeloproliferative disorders associated with JAK2 V617F are represented by the *open circles* and the approximate percentage of JAK2 V617F-positive patients within the clinical classifications are indicated by the *shaded area* within the *circles*

responsible for extending or limiting the disease phenotypes associated with JAK2 V617F, and to identify key signaling pathways critical to the development of a PV phenotype.

16.4 The Differential Diagnosis of PV

Osler was not the first to describe PV but he was the first to recognize its phenotypic mimicry and the first to develop diagnostic criteria for it (Osler 1903). These criteria have been subsequently supplemented by a number of groups but at their core, they have not been significantly improved. Table 16.1 compares Osler's 1908 diagnostic criteria with the 1967 criteria of the Polycythemia Vera Study Group (PVSG) (Wasserman 1971) and the 2000 criteria of the World Heath Organization (WHO) (Johansson et al. 2005). Surprisingly, Osler did not consider the leukocyte count to be of particular diagnostic significance and, of course, platelet physiology as well as the platelet's clinical significance was not well understood in his era. The PVSG criteria were developed to ensure diagnostic uniformity and to avoid misdiagnosis for clinical trial purposes; they also reflect the practice environment of the time since many of the tests subsequently proposed for diagnostic purposes, such as those in the WHO criteria, were not available in 1967. Recognizing what is unique about PV is central to establishing its diagnosis. The reason for this should be clear from Table 16.2, which lists the features of PV that it shares in common with its companion myeloproliferative disorders, IMF and ET, and those that are unique to each disorder. PV is easy to recognize when it presents with extreme trilineage hematopoietic cell hyperplasia. However, this clinical presentation occurs only in a minority of patients and it is more often the case that the disorder presents with features mimicking IMF and ET. Thus, PV can present with myelofibrosis and splenomegaly, as isolated thrombocytosis, or, rarely, with isolated leukocytosis. Therefore, the only way to determine if the blood abnormalities are actually caused by PV is to establish that the red cell mass is elevated.

While it may seem intuitive that a high hemoglobin or hematocrit should be able to distinguish PV from its companion myeloproliferative disorders, unfortunately in reality the situation is not that simple. Unless the hemoglobin level is ≥20 g/dl in a man or ≥17 g/dl in a woman (hematocrit ≥60% in a man or ≥50% in a woman), it is not possible to be certain that an absolute elevation of the red cell mass is present (Pearson et al. 1984). This is because normally there is no fixed relationship between the red cell mass and the plasma volume, nor is there a linear relationship between the hematocrit and the red cell mass (Bentley and Lewis 1976) (Fig. 16.4 and Table 16.3). Consequently, the measured hemoglobin or hematocrit level in a peripheral blood sample could reflect either a true increase in the red cell mass or simply a decrease in the plasma volume. Despite this fact and the previously documented hemoglobin and hematocrit limits cited above, the WHO has stipulated hemoglobin levels (>18.5 g/dl in men and >16.5 g/dl in women) that it considers diagnostic for the presence of absolute erythrocytosis. Indeed, when the hemoglobin levels recommended by the WHO were subjected to scrutiny, they were found to miss the diagnosis of PV in over 60% of patients who were positively identified using a direct red cell mass determination, while at the same time falsely diagnosing the disorder in up to 35% of patients who actually had a contracted plasma volume syndrome and a normal red cell mass (Johansson et al. 2005).

It was recognized over 80 years ago that a hemoglobin or hematocrit determination on blood taken from a peripheral artery or vein did not reflect the total body hemoglobin concentration or hematocrit level (Smith et al. 1921). This is because as blood flows through a vessel, red cells occupy the center of the vessel while the plasma, white cells, and platelets occupy its periphery

Table 16.1. The diagnosis of polycythemia vera

1903	1971	2001
Erythrocytosis	Elevated red cell mass	A1: Elevated red cell mass
Chronic cyanosis	Normal O2 saturation	A2: No cause of secondary erythrocytosis
Splenomegaly	Splenomegaly	A3: Splenomegaly
	Plus any two below if no splenomegaly:	A4: Clonal cytogenetic defect
	Leukocytosis	A5: Endogenous erythroid colony formation
	Thrombocytosis	B1: Thrombocytosis
	LAP > 100	B2: Leukocytosis
	Elevated B12 or B12 binding capacity	B3: Bone marrow biopsy with panmyelosis
		B4: Low EPO level
		PV if A1, A2 and any other A, or any two B criteria

Table 16.2. Features common to the chronic myeloproliferative disorders

Involvement of a multipotent hematopoietic progenitor cell
Dominance of the abnormal clone over normal clones
Abnormalities of chromosomes 1, 8, 9, 13, and 20
Marrow hypercellularity and megakaryocyte dysplasia
Growth factor-independent colony formation
Overproduction of one or more of the formed elements of the blood
Thrombosis and hemorrhage
Myelofibrosis
Extramedullary hematopoiesis
Transformation to acute leukemia
Expression of JAK2 V617F, overexpression of PRV-1, impaired expression of Mpl

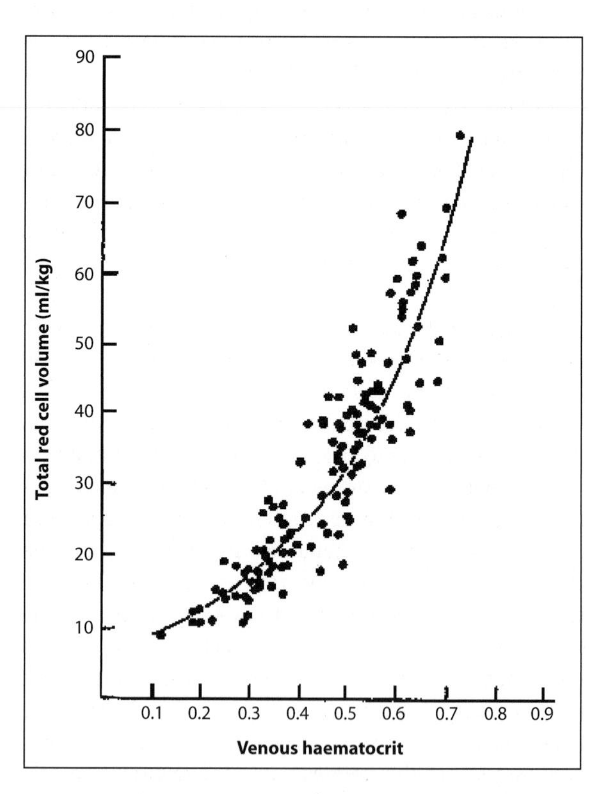

Fig. 16.4. Relationship between the venous hematocrit and the red cell mass (Bentley & Lewis 1976)

where they are subject to friction exerted by the vessel walls. In smaller vessels, this friction is magnified such that the red cells flow much faster than the plasma. As a consequence, at any given time, the small vessels of the body, which comprise the bulk of the vascular space, contain more plasma than red cells (Fahraeus and Lindqvuist 1931). Thus, the hematocrit may be as low as 15% in the kidneys and 18% in the brain, while it is 41% in the liver and 82% in the spleen (Ebert and Stead 1941). Taken as a whole, the total body hematocrit under normal circumstances is approximately 10% less than the measured hematocrit in a peripheral vein or artery.

To determine the red cell mass, a measured aliquot of the patient's red cells is labeled with ^{51}Cr and reinfused into the patient. An aliquot of patient plasma containing a known amount of ^{131}I-labelled albumin is also

Table 16.3. Red cell mass and plasma volume measurements in the evaluation of suspected erythrocytosis

	A. Androgen therapy 52-year-old male, HCT=56%, S=2.15		B. Chronic renal disease 37-year-old female, HCT=47%, S=1.99		C. Polycythemia Vera 55-year-old female, HCT=46%, S=1.41	
	Expected*	Observed	Expected*	Observed	Expected*	Observed
RCM	2370	2661	1675	1976	1209	1640
PV	3393	1824	2776	2230	1967	2169
TBV	5763	4485	4451	4206	3176	3809

* The expected values were derived from the formulas in Br J Haematol 89:748, 1995. Patient A illustrates the profound plasma volume contraction and minimal erythrocytosis that can occur with androgen administration. Patient B illustrates the secondary erythrocytosis associated with renal cysts in a patient with end stage renal disease with elevation of the red cell mass (RCM) and contraction of the plasma volume (PV). Patient C illustrates the plasma volume expansion occurring in polycythemia vera that masks the increase in the RCM. TBV, total blood volume; S, body surface area.

reinfused. After the infusions, samples of whole blood are taken over a 90-min period to insure adequate mixing (Pearson et al. 1995), then the red cell mass and plasma volume are determined by the isotope dilution principle. Contrary to recent contentions, the test is very precise and has a false positive rate of ~1% and published, gender-specific formulas are available that account for the effects of weight (Pearson et al. 1995; Wright et al. 1975). Importantly, as shown in Table 16.3, dividing the total body hematocrit calculated from the measured red cell mass and plasma volume by the measured venous hematocrit shows that normally the total body hematocrit is about 10% less than the venous hematocrit. This difference between the two, which reflects the greater proportion of plasma in the small vessels, has been designated *f*. Theoretically, if *f* was always constant, it would not be necessary to measure the red cell mass as one could simply calculate it using *f* and the measured plasma volume. Unfortunately, *f* has a wide variation that is magnified by disease and also by the presence of splenomegaly, which increases *f* to greater than unity (Rothschild et al. 1954). Thus, it should not be surprising that, although attempts have been made to estimate the red cell mass based on numerical formulas using *f*, the hematocrit and a plasma volume determination, when compared to direct red cell mass measurement, none have been sufficiently accurate for clinical use (Balga et al. 2000).

Unfortunately, while it would thus seem to be a simple matter to distinguish PV from IMF or ET by performing a red cell mass and plasma volume determination, the situation is also complicated by the many other disorders that cause erythrocytosis (Table 16.4). The list of disorders causing erythrocytosis is, indeed, daunting, because not only are the diagnostic tests that identify certain disorders such as Chuvash erythrocytosis or erythropoietin receptor mutations not widely available, but also because PV can present as isolated erythrocytosis. To address this dilemma, a diagnostic algorithm for the evaluation of suspected erythrocytosis is presented in Fig. 16.5. It is important to emphasize that this approach is not designed to determine whether the patient specifically has PV but whether, according to physiologic principles, erythrocytosis is present and why.

When confronted with a high hemoglobin or hematocrit level the first issue is to determine its duration. Obviously, a temporal change in these values suggests an acquired as opposed to a constitutional disorder. The second issue is to remember that secondary forms of erythrocytosis are more common than PV. Thus, the use of inappropriate surrogate tests such as a bone marrow examination cannot be justified from either an economic or clinical perspective. The algorithm in Fig. 16.5 is designed with this fact in mind and will separate patients into three groups: those with normal values (usually at the upper limit of normal for the red cell mass and the lower limit of normal for the plasma volume), those with a plasma volume contraction syndrome, and those with an absolute elevation of the red cell mass.

Once the presence of an elevated red cell mass is established, the cause must be sought. Thus, normal arterial oxygen saturation will separate patients who are hypoxic at ambient oxygen tensions from those who are not. However, it is important to emphasize that normal arterial oxygen saturation does not exclude the

Table 16.4. Causes of erythrocytosis

Causes of erythrocytosis
Relative Erythrocytosis
Hemoconcentration secondary to dehydration, androgens or tobacco use
Absolute erythrocytosis
Hypoxia
Carbon monoxide intoxication
High affinity hemoglobin
High altitude
Pulmonary disease
Right to left shunts
Sleep apnea syndrome
Neurologic disease
Renal disease
Renal artery stenosis
Focal sclerosing or membranous glomerulonephritis
Renal transplantation
Tumors
Hypernephroma
Hepatoma
Cerebellar hemangioblastoma
Uterine fibroma
Adrenal tumors
Meningioma
Pheochromocytoma
Drugs
Androgens
Recombinant erythropoietin
Familial (with normal hemoglobin function)
Polycythemia vera

presence of a high affinity hemoglobin, chronic carbon monoxide intoxication, or intermittent causes of hypoxia such as sleep apnea. The next test should be an assay for the JAK2 V617F mutation. Its presence, in association with an elevated red cell mass determination, assures the diagnosis of PV; the corollary, however, is not true. A negative assay for JAK2 V617F does not exclude the diagnosis of PV, nor can its presence in the absence of a demonstrated increase in the red cell mass confirm the presence of PV.

It is when JAK2 V617F is absent that other diagnostic criteria must be explored and if the patient fulfills the PVSG criteria, the diagnosis is assured. An elevated erythropoietin level excludes PV as a cause of erythrocytosis; a normal or low level, however, is not unequivocally diagnostic for the disease (Fig. 16.2). The erythropoietin level can be low in normal individuals and normal in patients with secondary forms of erythrocytosis. This is because the erythrocytosis may compensate for tissue hypoxia, because hyperviscosity reduces erythropoietin production and because the normal range for plasma erythropoietin is wide and a doubling within the normal range could increase erythropoiesis substantially but not be recognized as abnormal.

Because of this, a number of other tests such as endogenous erythroid colony formation, cytogenetic abnormalities, bone marrow morphology, CT or ultrasound for splenic enlargement, and platelet Mpl or granulocyte PRV-1 mRNA assays have been recommended. None of these, however, can be endorsed. While endogenous erythroid colony formation is a feature of PV, this test is not standardized, not available clinically, and a negative test does not exclude PV as a cause for erythrocytosis (Zwicky et al. 2002). Cytogenetic abnormalities are present in less than 30% of patients with PV at the time of diagnosis, none are specific for the disease and a bone marrow aspirate is required for this assay. Bone marrow morphology, of course, is obviously not a surrogate for a red cell mass determination and marrow morphology can be normal or even if abnormal, will not distinguish PV from IMF or ET. This also raises the issue of test utilization since many more patients will have a benign cause for erythrocytosis than will have PV and thus the diagnostic yield with respect to cytogenetic abnormalities will be very low and not cost-effective. Radiographic studies, except in the morbidly obese, should also not be used to establish the presence of splenomegaly since there are no weight and gender-based criteria to define splenomegaly in this situation if the spleen cannot be palpated.

In summary, as indicated above, establishing a diagnosis of PV is not a simple task and in some patients, particularly those with isolated erythrocytosis for which no other etiology can be established, observation alone may be the only way to determine if PV is the cause. As a corollary, since PV can present with myelofibrosis or isolated thrombocytosis, it is important to periodically re-evaluate patients with these abnormalities to ensure that their disease has not evolved further

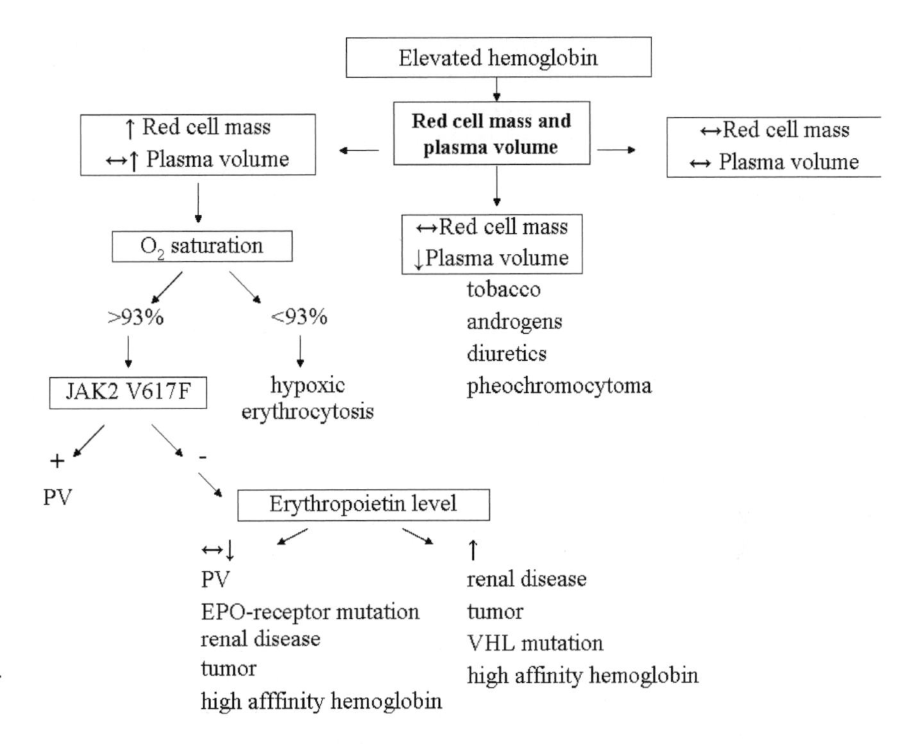

Fig. 16.5. Diagnostic algorithm for polycythemia vera and other forms of erythrocytosis

(Janssen et al. 1990; Jantunen et al. 1999). It is also clear that reliance on a specific hemoglobin or hematocrit level is unacceptable for establishing the presence of PV. In the appropriate clinical situation, if PV is a diagnostic consideration, a red cell mass and plasma volume determination are mandatory. These tests have the advantage of not only establishing or excluding this diagnosis, they also provide an indication of how much blood must be removed to alleviate the erythrocytosis and avoid thrombotic or hemorrhagic complications.

16.5 The Clinical Manifestations of PV

16.5.1 Symptoms

As listed in Table 16.5, the presenting symptoms of PV are both nonspecific and nondiagnostic. In general, they reflect the hyperviscosity imposed by the elevated red cell mass with the most notable effects of the circulatory stasis being evident in the central nervous system. Aquagenic pruritus, which afflicts approximately 30% of PV patients, is the symptom most specific for the disease, although it may occur in other situations as well (Steinman and Greaves 1985). Erythromelalgia, manifest as either burning or pain in the extremities, or its equivalent, ocular migraine, is another unique

Table 16.5. Presenting symptoms in PV (From Spivak JL. Myeloproliferative disorders. In: Handin RI, ed. Blood. Philadelphia: Lippincott Williams & Wilkins, 2003, with permission)

	Percentage (%)	Range
Weakness or fatigue	51	31–66
Headache	50	31–90
Dizziness or vertigo	48	28–70
Bleeding or bruising	34	30–40
Dyspnea	31	17–40
Abdominal pain	30	23–50
Visual symptoms	29	7–37
Paresthesias or extremity pain	27	13–60
Pruritus	27	10–50
Thrombosis	26	17–45
Dyspepsia	13	8–19

symptom complex that should suggest the presence of PV or its companion myeloproliferative disorder, ET. In an era of improved access to medical care, it is important to remember that PV patients are being recognized much earlier in the course of the disease, often when they are still asymptomatic.

16.5.2 Signs

What is true for symptoms is also true for the signs of PV, which is now frequently recognized when a routine complete blood count is obtained in an asymptomatic patient. Unfortunately, as shown in Table 16.6, more often than not simultaneous elevation of the red cell, white cell, and platelet counts is not found. Of course, as observed by Osler and endorsed by the PVSG, some patients can present with erythrocytosis and splenomegaly alone (Osler 1903). Because of a propensity to hemorrhage, particularly in the gastrointestinal tract, PV patients can present with a microcytosis. Microcytic erythrocytosis is an important diagnostic clue but can be seen with other forms of erythrocytosis and in thalassemia trait; in the latter situation in the absence of iron deficiency, however, the red cell distribution width (RDW) will be normal (Bessman 1977). PV is a hypercoagulable state and thus, the disorder needs to be considered with any unexplained episode of thrombosis, and particularly intra-abdominal venous thrombosis, since PV is the commonest cause of hepatic vein thrombosis in the Western hemisphere (Parker 1959). In young women, hepatic vein thrombosis is a frequent presenting manifestation (Valla et al. 1985).

Table 16.6. Laboratory abnormalities in PV (From Spivak JL. Myeloproliferative disorders. In: Handin RI, ed. Blood. Philadelphia: Lippincott Williams & Wilkins, 2003, with permission)

	Percentage (%)	Range
Erythrocytosis	91	88–99
Leukocytosis	67	43–84
Thrombocytosis	52	40–63
Reticulocytosis	35	6–54
Elevated Leukocyte Alkaline Phosphatase	81	63–100

Plethora, particularly of the face, conjunctiva, mucous membranes, and hands can be striking and hypertension is another sign of the expanded red cell mass. Easy bruising, epistaxis, or gingival bleeding occur as a consequence of circulatory stasis, or of acquired type IIa von Willebrand's disease, if the platelet count is in excess of 1,000,000/µl. Splenomegaly is the most common physical finding other than plethora and is usually modest in extent. Hepatomegaly is much less common and, with the exception of hepatic vein thrombosis, is not seen in the absence of splenomegaly. Gout or renal stones are rarely presenting manifestations of the disease.

16.6 The Consequences of PV

The consequences of PV are listed in Table 16.7. Given the increasing burden of hematopoietic progenitor cells and their progeny, the complications of PV are diverse and usually the result of cell accumulation, cellular metabolism, or cellular transformation.

Thrombotic and hemorrhagic events are the most common and frequent severe complications of PV. Historically, thrombosis was the presenting feature in PV in up to 49% of patients, while there was a 40% incidence of thrombosis during the course of the illness (Spivak 2002). Not surprisingly, thrombotic events tended to reoccur in patients who previously had a thrombotic event. Importantly, several studies have emphasized a high frequency of vascular accidents in patients several years before the diagnosis of PV was first made (Anger

Table 16.7. The consequences of polycythemia vera

Consequence	Cause
Thrombosis, hemorrhage, hypertension	Elevated red cell mass, decreased vWF multimers
Organomegaly	Extramedullary hematopoiesis or elevated red cell mass
Pruritis, acid-peptic disease	Inflammatory mediators
Erythromelalgia	Thrombocytosis
Hyperuricemia, gout, renal stones	Increased cell turnover
Myelofibrosis	Reaction to the neoplastic clone
Acute leukemia	Therapy-induced or clonal evolution

et al. 1989; Gruppo Italiano Studio Policitemia 1995). Thrombosis also accounted for up to 40% of deaths. Arterial thrombosis was more common than venous thrombosis with myocardial infarction and stroke being the most frequent events. Remarkably, although PV is the commonest cause of intra-abdominal venous thrombosis (Najean et al. 1987; Parker 1959), peripheral venous thrombosis was the commonest site for venous thrombosis in several large series (Gruppo Italiano Studio Policitemia 1995; Landolfi et al. 2004).

The incidence of hemorrhage is less common than thrombosis, occurring in approximately 20% of patients and involving the gastrointestinal tract or the central nervous system. However, it is fatal in less than 10% of patients (Wehmeier et al. 1991). Bleeding in PV has two major mechanisms: vascular stasis with endothelial cell damage due to hyperviscosity, and the development of acquired type IIa von Willebrand disease. The contribution of an elevated red cell mass to a hemorrhagic diathesis is well illustrated in mice genetically engineered to overproduce erythrocytes, in whom death occurred as a consequence of disseminated hemorrhage (Shibata et al. 2003). It is of further interest to note that many of the patients initially described as having "hemorrhagic thrombocytosis" actually had PV (Ozer et al. 1960). This is a reflection of the role of the platelets in contributing to the hemorrhagic diathesis of PV. As the platelet count increases, the concentration of high molecular weight von Willebrand multimers decreases (Budde et al. 1993), presumably due to platelet binding and proteolysis (van Genderen et al. 1996).

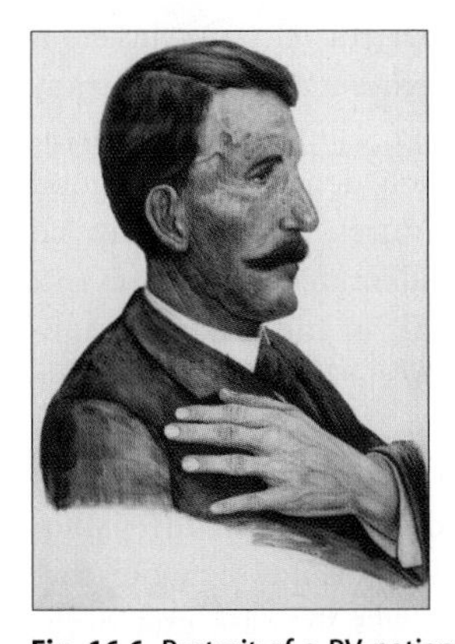

Fig. 16.6. Portrait of a PV patient of William Osler, circa 1915. The plethora and engorgement of blood vessels are evident in this gentleman with an expanded red cell mass and systolic hypertension

Systolic hypertension is another feature of red cell mass expansion in PV but a feature that is more common to early descriptions of the disease when patients presented later in the course of the disease (Fig. 16.6). Initially, in PV, as the red cell mass increases, the plasma volume also increases, in contrast to secondary forms of erythrocytosis where there is plasma volume contraction in an attempt to maintain a normal blood volume. With expansion of the blood volume, there is initially a reduction in peripheral vascular resistance but eventually, with continued distention of the vascular system, hypertension ensues.

Platelet activation in PV causes a variety of occlusive or vasospastic syndromes including erythromelalgia, transient ischemic attacks, and ocular migraine. The frequency of these complications varies and in one recent large series in which many patients were pretreated to lower the leukocyte and platelet counts and their activation, erythromelalgia occurred in only 5% (Landolfi et al. 2004). Erythromelalgia is a peculiar syndrome characterized by erythema, warmth, and burning pain primarily in the feet but also in the hands that is aggravated by heat, positional dependency, and exercise and relieved by elevation or cooling of the affected extremities (Kurzrock and Cohen 1989). Erythromelalgia can be idiopathic, or due to conditions affecting the peripheral vessels or their enervation. However, it is most often seen in the chronic myeloproliferative diseases, PV and ET (Kalgaard et al. 1997), where it is caused by platelet aggregation and platelet-endothelial cell interactions that result in swelling and occlusion of arterioles that can be transient or permanent (Michiels 1997), with acrocyanosis and ulceration or necrosis of affected digits with preservation of peripheral pulses. Ocular migraine, which is characterized by scintillating scotomata, dizziness, headache, transient ischemic attacks, and cortical blindness, is essentially the central nervous system equivalent of erythromelalgia. Importantly, these syndromes, while alarming, rarely leave permanent sequelae. The etiology undoubtedly involves both platelet number and platelet activation since a reduction in either alleviates symptoms and aborts the syndrome. The role of platelet activation is implicated by the increase in urinary excretion of the platelet arachidonic acid metabolite thromboxane B_2, associated with symptoms, histologic evidence of arteriolar thrombi, and aborting of the attack by cyclo-oxygenase inhibitors such as aspirin or indomethacin or reducing platelet number (Michiels et al. 1985). Indeed, alleviation of symptoms with a single aspirin tablet is pathognomonic for erythromelalgia.

Acid-peptic disease is claimed to occur with a greater frequency in PV than in the general population but the observations upon which this claim is based are primarily from older studies. A specific blood group relationship was not observed (Perkins et al. 1964) and the role if any of *H. pylori* is unknown, as is the role of promiscuous histamine (Westin et al. 1975) or cytokine release (Gilbert et al. 1966). A relationship to circulatory stasis and vasoconstriction due to nitric oxide scavenging by hemoglobin also need to be considered when the red cell mass has not been controlled (Huang et al. 2005). Hyperuricemia in PV is due to the excessive turnover of blood cells, not altered urate metabolism (Yu et al. 1956), but the development of secondary gout or uric acid stones are uncommon in the absence of cytoreductive therapy.

Pruritus, usually aquagenic in nature and, like erythromelalgia, a not infrequent presenting manifestation of PV whose diagnostic significance is commonly overlooked initially, occurs in about 30% of patients. For some, the pruritus is a minor annoyance but for other patients it is an exquisite form of pain that prevents them from conducting their normal activities. The mechanism for pruritus in PV has been a matter of debate. Evidence for (Jackson et al. 1987) and against (Buchanan et al. 1994) a role for increased cutaneous mast cell activity has been obtained and roles for histamine (Westin et al. 1975), iron deficiency (Salem et al. 1982), and platelets have been proposed. Vascular stasis is undoubtedly involved since phlebotomy alleviates the pruritus in some patients. Indeed, it appears safe to say that the mechanisms for pruritus in PV are probably multiple, but why not all patients are affected is unknown.

Organomegaly, with its attendant mechanical problems including portal hypertension, is due initially to engorgement of the spleen with blood in untreated patients but with time, in some patients more than others, the enlargement of the spleen and liver is due to extramedullary hematopoiesis as discussed above. In addition to its space-occupying effects, splenic enlargement leads to an increase in splanchnic blood flow to a degree that portal hypertension ensues (Rosenbaum et al. 1966) and in some patients esophageal varices develop, often complicated by hemorrhage. Thrombosis of the hepatic vein can also lead to portal hypertension, and splenic vein thrombosis can lead to gastric varices. Hepatomegaly is common with hepatic vein thrombosis and also after splenectomy as the liver becomes a major site of extramedullary hematopoiesis (Towell and Levine 1987).

As discussed above, much has been written about the development of myelofibrosis in PV and the spent or postpolycythemic myeloid metaplasia phase of the disease. Myelofibrosis, of course, is a reactive process and poses no impediment to marrow cell function. Myeloid metaplasia also does not represent a failure of bone marrow function either, since there is no correlation between its presence and bone marrow failure. Confusion has arisen with respect to these processes, because a distinction was never made between the bone marrow failure state caused by the use of alkylating agents and the natural course of PV. Bone marrow failure is an expected consequence of the use of alkylating agents, while the frequency with which bone marrow failure occurs in PV in their absence is still unknown.

16.7 The Management of PV

16.7.1 A Strategy for the Treatment of PV

Any discussion of the treatment of PV must first acknowledge some disturbing shortcomings with respect to our knowledge about this disorder. First, since a specific clonal marker for the disease is lacking, we do not know whether what has been clinically defined as PV represents a single disease or a group of related disorders. Indeed, given variable natural history of PV and the epidemiology of the JAK2 V617F mutation, the latter is a likely possibility. Second, prior to the discovery of JAK2 V617F and lacking a specific clonal marker, it was not possible to decide whether a particular therapy was curative or merely palliative. Third, while the natural history of PV is not completely defined, there is good evidence that disease tempo varies. Unfortunately, no laboratory markers have been identified that permit risk stratification with respect to this or the known complications of the disorder. Fourth, current concepts of the treatment of PV are based on flawed natural history studies and clinical trials in which there was treatment bias based on a total misunderstanding of the pathophysiology of the disease. Fifth, PV is now being discovered earlier in its course than was the case previously, but no attempt has yet been made to redefine treatment goals in light of this. Finally, with respect to this latter situation, current estimates of longevity in PV are based on studies of patient populations diagnosed years ago and treated with drug regimens that are no longer considered safe (Gruppo Italiano Studio Policitemia 1995; Passamonti et al. 2004).

16.7.2 Phlebotomy

As discussed earlier, expansion of the red cell mass in PV, in contrast to other forms of erythrocytosis, is associated with either no change or an increase in the plasma volume (Table 16.3). This results initially in a fall in blood vessel dilatation and a decline in peripheral vascular resistance, but with time peripheral vascular resistance increases as blood vessels are distended to the extent possible. This was probably best described by Weber in 1908, who noted, "In every case examined after death the distention of the visceral vessels has been very striking, the mesenteric vessels presenting sometimes the appearance of having been forcibly injected for purposes of anatomical dissection" (Weber 1908). There are several important issues involved here. First, the hematocrit is the principle determinant of blood viscosity but as discussed above, it is not possible to estimate the extent of red cell mass expansion from the peripheral blood hematocrit. Second, blood viscosity is an exponential function of the hematocrit, and red cell aggregation also increases as the hematocrit rises (Wells and Merrill 1962). In addition to vessel wall distention and endothelial cell injury, the increased number of red cells forces leukocytes and platelets against the vascular endothelium and against each other, where cell-cell interactions can lead to activation of coagulation.

Phlebotomy is a global antidote for these problems (Table 16.7) and also relieves the symptomatology associated with impaired cerebral blood flow (Thomas et al. 1977). The initial red cell mass determination permits an assessment of the amount of blood that needs to be removed, and target hematocrits of <45% in men and <42% in woman should be the goal. Current data suggests that the rate of thrombosis is negligible at these gender-specific hematocrits (Pearson and Weatherly-Mein 1978) and cerebral blood flow is normalized. This approach will alleviate the symptoms of headache, confusion, tinnitus, dizziness, and epistaxis and sometimes even alleviate itching. Phlebotomy also quickly improves blood viscosity by expanding the plasma volume. Contrary to common intuition, phlebotomy does not provoke thrombocytosis (Messinezy et al. 1985). Although most patients tolerate rapid lowering of the red cell mass, in some elderly patients there may be vasomotor instability initially (Kiraly et al. 1976); in this situation, removal of smaller amounts of blood (250 ml) and replacement with crystalloid is prudent. Phlebotomy also has the useful effect of restoring balance to the coagulation system and restoring platelet function to normal (Wehmeier et al. 1990).

The goal of phlebotomy is twofold: first, to restore the red cell mass to normal to prevent thrombosis or hemorrhage and to alleviate symptoms and second, to develop a state of iron deficiency to prevent a rapid recurrence of red cell mass expansion. Iron absorption is maximal in PV (Finch et al. 1950), and once a state of iron deficiency is created, it will take approximately 3 months for iron balance to be restored and for phlebotomy to become necessary again. Not only will the interval for phlebotomy be increased but its frequency will also decline unless an additional source of iron is introduced. Iron deficiency in the adult in the absence of anemia does not impair aerobic performance (Rector et al. 1982) but may induce pica, usually in the form of ice craving (pagophagia). It is also worth emphasizing the benefits of phlebotomy are immediate, while attempts to lower the red cell mass with chemotherapy not only take time, they are also often unsuccessful (Gruppo Italiano Studio Policitemia 1995; Najean and Rain 1997).

16.7.3 Management of Leukocytosis and Thrombocytosis

Leukocytosis is rarely extreme in PV but patients may become symptomatic if the leukocyte count exceeds 50,000/μl, possibly from either cytokine release or small vessel stasis of immature leukocytes in the lungs or elsewhere. Leukocytosis may also be associated with hyperuricemia and this will require therapy if the uric acid exceeds 10 mg% or when chemotherapy is contemplated.

Asymptomatic thrombocytosis in PV ordinarily requires no treatment. Exceptions to this rule would be patients with conditions predisposing to thrombosis such as coronary artery disease, peripheral vascular disease, diabetes mellitus, hypertension, tobacco abuse, or a history of prior thrombosis. In a number of studies, myeloproliferative disease patients over age 65 also appeared to be more vulnerable to thrombosis than their younger counterparts without cardiovascular risk factors (Barbui and Finazzi 1997; Cortelazzo et al. 1995). Erythromelalgia or ocular migraines do dictate treatment to inhibit platelet function or reduce platelet number. Aspirin (or ibuprofen) is the simplest and quickest treatment for erythromelalgia, but the remedy is temporary and not always completely effective. Both aspirin and ibuprofen can also promote bleeding and are contraindicated when the platelet count is sufficiently high to cause a reduction in von Willebrand multimers and a prolongation of the ristocetin cofactor assay. This usually occurs when the platelet count exceeds 1,000,000/μl. In this instance, a reduction in platelet number will be necessary to control symptoms.

There are three choices of therapy for thrombocytosis when either aspirin or ibuprofen is not sufficient: hydroxyurea, interferon alpha, or the imidazolequinazoline derivative, anagrelide. Hydroxyurea has been the drug of choice because it is easy to administer, has a low incidence of side effects, and was shown to be superior to aspirin in controlling microvascular thrombosis in ET (Cortelazzo et al. 1995). The recent ECLAP study also suggested that hydroxyurea was not leukemogenic (Landolfi et al. 2003). However, that study, like others before it, lacked a sufficient duration of observation to solidify this contention. It also needs to be emphasized that all major studies of the treatment of thrombocytosis have been conducted in ET and the extent to which the results can be extrapolated to PV is unknown. Therefore, the choice of therapy in this instance should be based on a physician-patient dialogue concerning the pros and cons of the available treatment options. It is the authors' preference to use anagrelide or interferon alpha in younger patients while reserving hydroxyurea therapy for patient's intolerant to these agents or with known cardiovascular risk factors.

The extent to which the platelet count should be reduced is also a matter of debate. Anecdotal studies replete with reportorial bias suggest that the platelet count should be normalized (Regev et al. 1997), despite the fact that the platelets themselves will not be functionally normal, nor is there any data to suggest that a normal platelet count would be protective. Tailoring treatment to the individual patient appears logical. Thus, when there are cardiovascular risk factors or a prior history of thrombosis, lowering the platelet count to 500,000/l or less would be prudent; when no such risk factors exist, lowering the platelet count to achieve alleviation of symptoms or correction of a coagulopathy should be sufficient. Plateletpheresis has a very limited role in the management of thrombocytosis because it is not only inefficient when the platelet count is very high but its effect is also transient. Additionally, combination therapy such as aspirin and interferon alpha or aspirin and hydroxyurea may be useful but there is an increased risk of bleeding when aspirin is coupled with anagrelide (Harrison et al. 2005). Finally, since interferon alpha is not mutagenic and hydroxyurea appears to be, it seems more prudent to use hydroxyurea intermittently whenever possible.

16.7.4 Pruritus

Pruritus, usually aquagenic in origin, afflicts approximately 30% of PV patients. The symptoms may be mild and transient but in some patients the itching, stinging, or burning sensation provoked by water contact or even a humid environment can be unbearable. Since the mechanism is unknown, treatment has been empirical. In some patients, phlebotomy brings relief; in others a change in bathing habits or the use of a long-acting antihistamine is effective, but determining which one is often a matter of trial and error. Success has been claimed for serotonin antagonists (Wasserman 1976), antidepressants (Diehn and Tefferi 2001), danazol (Kolodny 1996), and iron repletion (Salem et al. 1982) but these claims are all anecdotal. Psoralen and ultraviolet A light therapy is an effective, if inconvenient and temporary remedy, but has its own toxicities such as skin hyperpigmentation and burns (Morison and Nesbitt 1993); ultraviolet B has its proponents as well (Baldo et al. 2002). Interferon alpha has a success rate of approximately 60% (Finelli et al. 1993) and a response can be seen in several weeks. Leukocyte reduction with hydroxyurea is also effective.

16.7.5 Extramedullary Hematopoiesis

Control of extramedullary hematopoiesis in PV and, in particular, the splenomegaly that is its most common and prominent manifestation is the most difficult therapeutic challenge in this disorder. Initially, splenomegaly may respond to phlebotomy therapy but as the disease progresses, splenic enlargement is due to hematopoietic progenitor cell proliferation. There are currently four approaches for controlling splenomegaly due to extramedullary hematopoiesis: chemotherapy, radiotherapy, biologic response modifiers, and splenectomy. Alkylating agents such as busulphan were once the mainstay of therapy for this purpose in PV. However, these agents are not only leukemogenic but also can cause severe cytopenias and chronic bone marrow failure. Hydroxyurea is modestly effective in controlling splenomegaly but is leukemogenic when given in combination with an alkylating agent or even after one. Imatinib mesylate has also been used successfully to control splenomegaly in PV (Jones and Dickinson 2003; Silver 2003), but the response rate varies and the reasons for this are unknown. Splenic irradiation can be an effective temporizing remedy but has the risk of depressing bone marrow function because the effective dose is not predictable (Elliott et al. 1998). Furthermore, the adhesions that develop can make subsequent splenectomy difficult and hazardous. The reduction in spleen size is also temporary, although the treatment can be repeated successfully. Interferon alpha can reduce spleen size in approximately 60% of patients and while the effect is temporary if the interferon is discontinued, it can be reinstituted as needed (Lengfelder et al. 2000; Silver 1997). Thalidomide is another biologic response modifier that has been used successfully to reduce splenomegaly in patients with idiopathic myelofibrosis (Mesa et al. 2003). Whether it is effective in PV is not known.

Splenectomy, while providing a definitive solution to the problem, has the disadvantages of the obligate morbidity and mortality associated with any major abdominal surgery, in addition to the particular risks in removing a massive spleen, the most important of which are hemorrhage and thrombosis. The risk of hemorrhage is increased if the red cell mass is not controlled, if there is extreme thrombocytosis with the development of acquired von Willebrand disease, and if there are significant adhesions due to splenic infarction or prior irradiation. Splenic, mesenteric, or portal vein thrombosis occurs in approximately 6–7% of patients postsplenectomy and is not correlated with the degree of thrombocytosis (Broe et al. 1981). Generally, this complication occurs within a month of surgery, and may be asymptomatic and difficult to detect by ultrasound in the immediate postoperative period (Chaffanjon et al. 1998). It is imperative that the patient's nutritional status be satisfactory before surgery and this may require parenteral hyperalimentation.

Evaluation for portal hypertension should also be performed before surgery since splenectomy alone will not resolve this problem if varices are present. Postsplenectomy, hepatic enlargement is not uncommon and has been observed occasionally to be fulminant with a fatal outcome (Towell and Levine 1987). Control of hepatomegaly in this situation can be difficult and there is not adequate experience with any remedy for guidance; irradiation is a temporary and toxic approach while 2-chlorodeoxyadenosine has been effective at the risk of severe myelosuppression (Tefferi et al. 1997). Low dose cyclophosphamide has also been anecdotally effective. Postsplenectomy leukocytosis and thrombocytosis are expected complications that may require chemotherapy (Schilling 1980).

16.7.6 Hepatic Vein Thrombosis

Hepatic vein thrombosis is an uncommon but frequently catastrophic manifestation of PV. Since PV is the commonest cause of hepatic vein thrombosis, this diagnosis always needs to be considered when hepatic vein thrombosis is encountered, even if the hematocrit is normal, since this may be due to an expanded plasma volume (Lamy et al. 1997). Hepatic vein thrombosis is a medical emergency that needs to be recognized promptly to relieve liver congestion and reduce portal venous pressure. If the thrombosis is acute, thrombolytic therapy, which may require a supplemental supply of plasminogen in the form of fresh frozen plasma, may be effective. Otherwise, anticoagulation, stenting, or a transjugular intrahepatic portosystemic shunt (TIPS) procedure should be instituted promptly together with hematocrit reduction if it is elevated or even normal.

16.7.7 Pregnancy

Pregnancy is not an uncommon issue in PV given that among patients below the age of 40, PV is predominantly a disease of women. Unfortunately, published experience is limited (Ferguson et al. 1983) and this, coupled with lack of understanding of the pathophysiology of PV, has led many physicians to advise against conception for these patients. However, the major risks of PV are not different in pregnancy than they are in its absence and the most important of these is thrombosis. The particular risk in this regard in pregnancy is the expansion of the plasma volume that normally accompanies this condition. Plasma volume expansion only further serves to mask the expanded red cell mass of PV and creates a false appearance of normalcy. Stated differently, a normal hematocrit in a pregnant PV patient is evidence for an expanded red cell mass and an invitation for placental insufficiency or a thrombotic event. Therefore, PV patients who wish to become pregnant should have their hematocrit maintained no higher than 36% and once pregnant, the hematocrit should not be allowed to rise above 33%. There should be no concern in this regard with respect to the fetal iron supply but folic acid supplementation is mandatory. It is expected that a high platelet count will fall during pregnancy (Turhan et al. 1988) and von Willebrand factor will rise physiologically. Splenomegaly can be controlled before pregnancy or safely during it with interferon alpha; hydroxyurea and anagrelide are contraindicated. There is no evidence for or against the use of aspirin but it did not influence the outcome of pregnancy in ET (Elliott and Tefferi 2003).

References

Adamson JW, Fialkow PJ, Murphy S, Prchal JF, Steinmann L (1976) Polycythemia vera: stem-cell and probable clonal origin of the disease. N Engl J Med, 295:913–916

Alfaham MA, Ferguson SD, Sihra B, Davies J (1987) The idiopathic hypereosinophilic syndrome. Arch Dis Child 62:601–613

Anger B, Haug U, Seidler R, Heimpel H (1989) Polycythemia vera. A clinical study of 141 patients. Blut, 59:493–500

Baldo A, Sammarco E, Plaitano R, Martinelli V, Monfrecola (2002) Narrowband (TL-01) ultraviolet B phototherapy for pruritus in polycythaemia vera 1. Br J Dermatol 147:979–981

Balga I, Solenthaler M, Furlan M (2000) Should whole-body red cell mass be measured or calculated? Blood Cells Mol Dis 26:25–31

Barbui T, Finazzi G (1997) Risk factors and prevention of vascular complications in polycythemia vera. Semin Thromb Hemost 23:455–461

Baxter EJ, Scott LM, Campbell PJ, East C, Fourouclas N, Swanton S, Vassiliou GS, Bench AJ, Boyd EM, Curtin N, Scott MA, Erber WN, Green AR (2005) Acquired mutation of the tyrosine kinase JAK2 in human myeloproliferative disorders. Lancet 365:1054–1061

Bentley SA, Lewis SM (1976) The relationship between total red cell volume, plasma volume and venous haematocrit. Br J Haematol 33:301–307

Berglund S, Zettervall O (1992) Incidence of polycythemia vera in a defined population. Eur J Haematol 48:20–26

Bessman DJ (1977) Microcytic polycythemia: frequency of nonthalassemic causes. JAMA 238:2391–2392

Broe PJ, Conley CL, Cameron JL (1981) Thrombosis of the portal vein following splenectomy for myeloid metaplasia. Surg Gynecol Obstet 152:488–492

Broudy VC, Kin N, Papayannopoulou T (1990) Erythropoietin receptors in polycythemia vera. Exp Hematol 18:576

Brubaker LH, Wasserman LR, Goldberg JD, Pisciotta AV, McIntyre OR, Kaplan ME, Modan B, Flannery J, Harp R (1984) Increased prevalence of polycythemia vera in parents of patients on polycythemia vera study group protocols. Am J Hematol 16:367–373

Buchanan JG, Ameratunga RV, Hawkins RC (1994) Polycythemia vera and water-induced pruritus: evidence against mast cell involvement. Pathology 26:43–45

Budde U, Scharf RE, Franke P, Hartmann-Budde K, Dent J, Ruggeri ZM (1993) Elevated platelet count as a cause of abnormal von Willebrand factor multimer distribution in plasma. Blood 82: 1749–1757

Carpinelli MR, Hilton DJ, Metcalf D, Antonchuk JL, Hyland CD, Mifsud SL, Di Rago L, Hilton AA, Willson TA, Roberts AW, Ramsay RG, Nicola NA, Alexander WS (2004) Suppressor screen in Mpl-/- mice: c-Myb mutation causes supraphysiological production of platelets in the absence of thrombopoietin signaling. Proc Natl Acad Sci USA 101:6553–6558

Chaffanjon PC, Brichon PY, Ranchoup Y, Gressin R, Sotto JJ (1998) Portal vein thrombosis following splenectomy for hematologic disease: prospective study with Doppler color flow imaging. World J Surg 22:1082–1086

Cools J, DeAngelo DJ, Gotlib J, Stover EH, Legare RD, Cortes J, Kutok J, Clark J, Galinsky I, Griffin JD et al (2003) A tyrosine kinase created by fusion of the PDGFRA and FIP1L1 genes as a therapeutic target of imatinib in idiopathic hypereosinophilic syndrome. N Engl J Med 348:1201–1214

Correa PN, Eskinazi D, Axelrad AA (1994) Circulating erythroid progenitors in polycythemia vera are hypersensitive to insulin-like growth factor-1 in vitro: studies in an improved serum-free medium. Blood 83:99–112

Cortelazzo S, Finazzi G, Ruggeri M, Vestri O, Galli M, Rodeghiero F, Barbui T (1995) Hydroxyurea for patients with essential thrombocythemia and a high risk of thrombosis. N Engl J Med 332:1132–1136

Cross NC, Reiter A (2002) Tyrosine kinase fusion genes in chronic myeloproliferative diseases. Leukemia 16:1207–1212

Dai CH, Krantz S, Means RT, Hom ST, Gilbert HS (1991) Polycythemia vera erythroid burst-forming units-erythroid are hypersensitive to interleukin-3. J Clin Invest 87:391

Dai CH, Krantz SB, Green WF, Gilbert HS (1994) Polycythaemia vera. III. Burst-forming units-erythroid (BFU-E) response to stem cell factor and c-kit receptor expression. Br J Haematol 86:12–21

Dai CH, Krantz SB, Sawyer ST (1997) Polycythemia vera. V. Enhanced proliferation and phosphorylation due to vanadate are diminished in polycythemia vera erythroid progenitor cells: a possible defect of phosphatase activity in polycythemia vera. Blood 89:3574–3581

Debili N, Wendling F, Cosman D, Titeux M, Florindo C, Dusanter-Fourt I, Schooley K, Methia N, Charon M, Nador R (1995) The Mpl receptor is expressed in the megakaryocytic lineage from late progenitors to platelets. Blood 85:391–401

Diehn F, Tefferi A (2001) Pruritus in polycythaemia vera: prevalence, laboratory correlates and management. Br J Haematol 115:619–621

Eaves AC, Henkelman DH, Eaves CJ (1980) Abnormal erythropoiesis in the myeloproliferative disorders: an analysis of underlying cellular and humoral mechanisms. Exp Hematol 8:235–247

Eaves CJ, Eaves AC (1978) Erythropoietin (Ep) dose-response curves for three classes of erythroid progenitors in normal human marrow and in patients with polycythemia vera. Blood 52:1196–1210

Ebert R, Stead EA (1941) Demonstration that the cell plasma ratio of blood contained in minute vessels is lower than that of venous blood. J Clin Invest 20:317–321

Elliott MA, Tefferi A (2003) Thrombocythaemia and pregnancy. Best Pract Res Clin Haematol 16:227–242

Elliott MA, Chen MG, Silverstein MN, Tefferi A (1998) Splenic irradiation for symptomatic splenomegaly associated with myelofibrosis with myeloid metaplasia. Br J Haematol 103:505–511

Elliot MA, Yoon SY, Kao P, Li CY, Tefferi A (2002) Simultaneous measurement of serum thrombopoietin and expression of megakaryocyte c-Mpl with clinical and laboratory correlates for myelofibrosis with myeloid metaplasia. Eur J Haematol 68:175–179

Fahraeus R, Lindqvuist T (1931) The viscosity of the blood in narrow capillary tubes. Am J Physiol 96:562–568

Ferguson JE, Ueland K, Aronson WJ (1983) Polycythemia rubra vera and pregnancy. Obstet Gynecol, 62:16 s–20 s

Finch S, Haskins D, Finch CA (1950) Iron metabolism hematopoiesis following phlebotomy iron as a limiting factor. J Clin Invest 8: 1078–1086

Finelli C, Gugliotta L, Gamberi B, Vianelli N, Visani G, Tura S (1993) Relief of intractable pruritus in polycythemia vera with recombinant interferon alfa. Am J Hematol 43:316–318

Friedland ML, Wittels EG, Robinson RJ (1981) Polycythemia vera in identical twins. Am J Hematol 10:101–103

Gilbert HS (1998) Familial myeloproliferative disease. Baillieres Clin Haematol 11:849–858

Gilbert HS, Warner RR, Wasserman LR (1966) A study of histamine in myeloproliferative disease. Blood 28:795–806

Gruppo Italiano Studio Policitemia (1995) Polycythemia vera: the natural history of 1213 patients followed for 20 years. Ann Intern Med 123:656–664

Harrison CN, Campbell PJ, Buck G, Wheatley K, East CL, Bareford D, Wilkins BS, van der Walt JD, Reilly JT, Grigg AP, Revell P, Woodcock BE, Green AR (2005) Hydroxyurea compared with anagrelide in high-risk essential thrombocythemia. N Engl J Med 353:33–45

Hess G, Rose P, Gamm H, Papadileris S, Huber C, Seliger B (1994) Molecular analysis of the erythropoietin receptor system in patients with polycythaemia vera. Br J Haematol 88:794–802

Horikawa Y, Matsumura I, Hashimoto K, Shiraga M, Kosugi S, Tadokoro S, Kato T, Miyazaki H, Tomiyama Y, Kurata Y, Matsuzawa Y, Kanakura Y (1997) Markedly reduced expression of platelet c-mpl receptor in essential thrombocythemia. Blood 90:4031–4038

Huang LJ, Constantinescu SN, Lodish HF (2001) The N-terminal domain of Janus kinase 2 is required for Golgi processing and cell surface expression of erythropoietin receptor. Mol Cell 8:1327–1338

Huang Z, Shiva S, Kim-Shapiro DB, Patel RP, Ringwood LA, Irby CE, Huang KT, Ho C, Hogg N, Schechter AN, Gladwin MT (2005) Enzymatic function of hemoglobin as a nitrite reductase that produces NO under allosteric control. J Clin Invest 115:2099–2107

Jackson N, Burt D, Crocker J, Boughton B (1987) Skin mast cells in polycythaemia vera: relationship to the pathogenesis and treatment of pruritus. Br J Dermatol 116:21–29

James C, Ugo V, Le Couedic JP, Staerk J, Delhommeau F, Lacout C, Garcon L, Raslova H, Berger R, Bennaceur-Griscelli A, Villeval JL, Constantinescu SN, Casadevall N, Vainchenker W (2005) A unique clonal JAK2 mutation leading to constitutive signalling causes polycythaemia vera. Nature 434:1144–1148

Janssen JW, Anger BR, Drexler HG, Bartram CR, Heimpel H (1990) Essential thrombocythemia in two sisters originating from different stem cell levels. Blood 75:1633–1636

Jantunen R, Juvonen E, Ikkala E, Oksanen K, Anttila P, Ruutu T (1999) Development of erythrocytosis in the course of essential thrombocythemia. Ann Hematol 78:219–222

Johansson P, Kutti J, Andreasson B, Safai-Kutti S, Vilen L, Wedel H, Ridell B (2004) Trends in the incidence of chronic Philadelphia chromosome negative (Ph-) myeloproliferative disorders in the city of Goteborg, Sweden, during 1983–99. J Intern Med 256:161–165

Johansson PL, Safai-Kutti S, Kutti J (2005) An elevated venous haemoglobin concentration cannot be used as a surrogate marker for absolute erythrocytosis: a study of patients with polycythaemia vera and apparent polycythaemia. Br J Haematol 129:701–705

Jones AV, Kreil S, Zoi K, Waghorn K, Curtis C, Zhang L, Score J, Seear R, Chase AJ, Grand FH, White H, Zoi C, Loukopoulos D, Terpos E, Vervessou EC, Schultheis B, Emig M, Ernst T, Lengfelder E, Hehlmann R, Hochhaus A, Oscier D, Silver RT, Reiter A, Cross NC (2005) Widespread occurrence of the JAK2 V617F mutation in chronic myeloproliferative disorders. Blood 106:2162–2168

Jones CM, Dickinson TM (2003) Polycythemia vera responds to imatinib mesylate. Am J Med Sci 325:149–152

Kalgaard OM, Seem E, Kvernebo K (1997) Erythromelalgia: a clinical study of 87 cases. J Intern Med 242:191–197

Kawada E, Tamura J, Kubota K, Murakami H, Naruse T, Tsuchiya J (1997) Possible involvement of protein kinase C in the aberrant regulation of erythropoiesis in polycythemia vera. Leuk Res 21:101–105

Kiraly JF, Feldmann JE, Wheby MS (1976) Hazards of phlebotomy in polycythemic patients with cardiovascular disease. JAMA 236: 2080–2081

Kolodny L (1996) Danazole is Safe and Effective in Relieving Refractory Pruritus in Patients with Myeloproliferative Disorders and other Diseases. Am J Hematol 51:112–116

Kralovics R, Passamonti F, Buser AS, Teo SS, Tiedt R, Passweg JR, Tichelli A, Cazzola M, Skoda RC (2005) A gain-of-function mutation of JAK2 in myeloproliferative disorders. N Engl J Med 352:1779–1790

Kurzrock R, Cohen PR (1989) Erythromelalgia and myeloproliferative disorders. Arch Intern Med, 149:105–109

Lamy T, Devillers A, Bernard M, Moisan A, Grulois I, Drenou B, Amiot L, Fauchet R, Le Prise PY (1997) Inapparent polycythemia vera: an unrecognized diagnosis. Am J Med 102:14–20

Landolfi R, Marchioli R, Kutti J, Gisslinger B, Tognoni G (2003) Efficacy and safety of low dose aspirin in polycythemia vera (ECLAP Study). Blood 102:5 a

Landolfi R, Marchioli R, Kutti J, Gisslinger H, Tognoni G, Patrono C, Barbui T (2004) Efficacy and safety of low-dose aspirin in polycythemia vera. N Engl J Med 350:114–124

Lawrence JH, Elmlinger PJ, Fulton G (1952) Oxygen and the control of red cell production in primary and secondary polycythemia: effects on iron turnover pattern with Fe^{59} as a tracer. Cardiologia, 21:346

Lengfelder E, Berger U, Hehlmann R (2000) Interferon in the treatment of polycythemia vera. Ann Hematol 79:103–109

Levin J, Cocault L, Demerens C, Challier C, Pauchard M, Caen J, Souyri M (2001) Thrombocytopenic c-mpl(–/–) mice can produce a normal level of platelets after administration of 5-fluorouracil: the effect of age on the response. Blood 98:1019–1027

Levine RL, Wadleigh M, Cools J, Ebert BL, Wernig G, Huntly BJ, Boggon TJ, Wlodarska I, Clark JJ, Moore S, Adelsperger J, Koo S, Lee JC, Gabriel S, Mercher T, D'Andrea A, Frohling S, Dohner K, Marynen P, Vandenberghe P, Mesa RA, Tefferi A, Griffin JD, Eck MJ, Sellers WR, Meyerson M, Golub TR, Lee SJ, Gilliland DG (2005) Activating mutation in the tyrosine kinase JAK2 in polycythemia vera, essential thrombocythemia, and myeloid metaplasia with myelofibrosis. Cancer Cell 7:387–397

Levine RL, Belisle C, Wadleigh M, Zahrieh D, Lee S, Chagnon P, Gilliland DG, Busque L (2006) X-inactivation based clonality analysis and quantitative JAK2V617F assessment reveals a strong association between clonality and JAK2V617F in PV but not ET/MMM, and identifies a subset of JAK2V617F negative ET and MMM patients with clonal hematopoiesis. Blood 107:4139–4141

London IM, Shemin D, West R, Rittenberg D (1949) Heme synthesis and red blood cell dynamics in normal humans and in subjects with polycythemia vera, sickle -cell anemia, and pernicious anemia. J Biol Chem 179:463–484

Manoharan A, Garson OM (1976) Familial polycythaemia vera: a study of 3 sisters. Scand J Haemat 17:10–16

McNally RJ, Rowland D, Roman E, Cartwright RA (1997) Age and sex distributions of hematological malignancies in the UK. Hematol Oncol 15:173–189

Means Jr RT, Krantz SB, Sawyer ST, Gilbert HS (1989) Erythropoietin receptors in polycythemia vera. J Clin Invest 84:1340–1344

Mesa RA, Steensma DP, Pardanani A, Li CY, Elliott M, Kaufmann SH, Wiseman G, Gray LA, Schroeder G, Reeder T, Zeldis JB, Tefferi A (2003) A phase 2 trial of combination low-dose thalidomide and prednisone for the treatment of myelofibrosis with myeloid metaplasia. Blood 101:2534–2541

Messinezy M, Pearson TC, Prochazka A, Wetherley-Mein G (1985) Treatment of primary proliferative polycythaemia by venesection and low dose busulphan: retrospective study from one centre. Br J Haematol 61:657–666

Metcalf D, Carpinelli MR, Hyland C, Mifsud S, Dirago L, Nicola NA, Hilton DJ, Alexander WS (2005) Anomalous megakaryocytopoiesis in mice with mutations in the c-Myb gene. Blood 105:3480–3487

Michiels JJ (1997) Erythromelalgia and vascular complications in polycythemia vera. Semin Thromb Hemost 23:441–454

Michiels JJ, Abels J, Steketee J, van Vliet HH, Vuzevski VD (1985) Erythromelalgia caused by platelet-mediated arteriolar inflammation and thrombosis in thrombocythemia. Ann Intern Med 102:466–471

Michl P, Spoettl G, Engelhardt D, Weber MM (2001) Alterations of the insulin-like growth factor system in patients with polycythemia vera. Mol Cell Endocrinol 181:189–197

Miller RL, Purvis JD, III, Weick JK (1989) Familial polycythemia vera. Cleve Clin J Med 56:813–818

Mirza AM, Correa PN, Axelrad AA (1995) Increased basal and induced tyrosine phosphorylation of the insulin-like growth factor I receptor beta subunit in circulating mononuclear cells of patients with polycythemia vera. Blood 86:877–882

Mirza AM, Ezzat S, Axelrad AA (1997) Insulin-like growth factor binding protein-1 is elevated in patients with polycythemia vera and stimulates erythroid burst formation in vitro. Blood, 89:1862–1869

Modan B, Kallner H, Zemer D, Yoran C (1971) A note on the increased risk of polycythemia vera in Jews. Blood 37:172–176

Moliterno AR, Spivak JL (1999) Posttranslational processing of the thrombopoietin receptor is impaired in polycythemia vera. Blood 94:2555–2561

Moliterno AR, Hankins WD, Spivak JL (1998) Impaired expression of the thrombopoietin receptor by platelets from patients with polycythemia vera. N Engl J Med 338:572–580

Moliterno AR, Williams DM, Gutierrez-Alamillo LI, Salvatori R, Ingersoll RG, Spivak JL (2004) Mpl Baltimore: a thrombopoietin receptor polymorphism associated with thrombocytosis. Proc Natl Acad Sci USA 101:11444–11447

Morison WL, Nesbitt JA (1993) Oral psoralen photochemotherapy (PUVA) for pruritus associated with polycythemia vera and myelofibrosis. Am J Hematol 42:409–410

Nagao M, Morishita E, Hanai Y, Kobayashi K, Sasaki R (1995) N-glycosylation-defective receptor for erythropoietin can transduce the ligand-induced cell proliferation signal. FEBS Lett 373:225–228

Najean Y, Rain J (1997) Treatment of polycythemia vera: The use of hydroxyurea and pipobroman in 292 patients under the age of 65 years. Blood 90:3370–3377

Najean Y, Mugnier P, Dresch C, Rain JD (1987) Polycythaemia vera in young people: an analysis of 58 cases diagnosed before 40 years. Br J Haematol, 67:285–291

Najean Y, Rain JD, Billotey C (1998) Epidemiological data in polycythaemia vera: a study of 842 cases. Hematol Cell Ther 40:159–165

Osler W (1903) Chronic Cyanosis, with polycythemia and enlarged spleen: a new clinical entity. Am J Med Sci 126:176–201

Ozer F, Truax W, Miesch D, Levin W (1960) Primary hemorrhagic thrombocythemia. Am J Med 28:807–823

Parker RG (1959) Occlusion of the hepatic veins in man. Med 38:369–402

Passamonti F, Rumi E, Pungolino E, Malabarba L, Bertazzoni P, Valentini M, Orlandi E, Arcaini L, Brusamolino E, Pascutto C, Cazzola M, Morra E, Lazzarino M (2004) Life expectancy and prognostic factors for survival in patients with polycythemia vera and essential thrombocythemia. Am J Med 117:755–761

Pearson TC, Weatherly-Mein G (1978) Vascular occlusive episodes and venous haematocrit in primary proliferative polycythaemia. Lancet 2:1219–1221

Pearson TC, Botterill CA, Glass UH, Wetherley-Mein G (1984) Interpretation of measured red cell mass and plasma volume in males with elevated venous PCV values. Scand J Haematol 33:68–74

Pearson TC, Guthrie DL, Simpson J, Chinn S, Barosi G, Ferrant A, Lewis SM, Najean Y (1995) Interpretation of measured red cell mass and plasma volume in adults: Expert Panel on Radionuclides of the International Council for Standardization in Haematology. Br J Haematol 89:748–756

Perkins J, Israels MCG, Wilkinson JF (1964) Polycythemia vera: clinical studies on a series of 127 patients managed without radiation therapy. Q J Med 33:499–518

Prchal JF, Axelrad AA (1974) Letter: Bone-marrow responses in polycythemia vera. N Engl J Med 290:1382

Prochazka AV, Markowe HL (1986) The epidemiology of polycythaemia rubra vera in England and Wales 1968–1982. Br J Cancer 53:59–64

Ratajczak MZ, Ratajczak J, Marlicz W, Pletcher CH, Machalinski B, Moore J, Hung H, Gerwirtz AM (1997) Recombinant human thrombopoietin (TPO) stimulates erythropoiesis by inhibiting erythroid progenitor cell apoptosis. Br J Haematol 98:8–17

Ratnoff WD, Gress RE (1980) The familial occurrence of polycythemia vera: report of a father and son, with consideration of the possible etiologic role of exposure to organic solvents, including tetrachloroethylene. Blood 56:233–236

Rector WG, Fortuin NJ, Conley CL (1982) Non-hematologic effects of chronic iron deficiency. A study of patients with polycythemia vera treated solely with venesections. Medicine (Baltimore) 61:382–389

Regev A, Stark P, Blickstein D, Lahav M (1997) Thrombotic complications in essential thrombocythemia with relatively low platelet counts. Am J Hematol, 56:168–172

Roder S, Steimle C, Meinhardt G, Pahl HL (2001) STAT3 is constitutively active in some patients with Polycythemia rubra vera. Exp Hematol 29:694–702

Rosenbaum DL, Murphy GW, Swisher SN (1966) Hemodynamic studies of the portal circulation in myeloid metaplasia. Am J Med 41:360–368

Rothschild MA, Bauman A, Yalow RS, Berson S (1954) Effect of splenomegaly on blood volume. J Appl Physiol 6:701–706

Royer Y, Staerk J, Costuleanu M, Courtoy PJ, Constantinescu SN (2005) Janus kinases affect thrombopoietin receptor cell surface localization and stability. J Biol Chem 280:27251–27261

Ruggeri M, Tosetto A, Frezzato M, Rodeghiero F (2003) The rate of progression to polycythemia vera or essential thrombocythemia in patients with erythrocytosis or thrombocytosis. Ann Intern Med 139:470–475

Sabath DF, Kaushansky K, Broudy VC (1999) Deletion of the extracellular membrane-distal cytokine receptor homology module of Mpl results in constitutive cell growth and loss of thrombopoietin binding. Blood 94:365–367

Saharinen P, Vihinen M, Silvennoinen O (2003) Autoinhibition of Jak2 tyrosine kinase is dependent on specific regions in its pseudokinase domain. Mol Biol Cell 14:1448–1459

Salem HH, Van der Weyden MB, Young IF, Wiley JS (1982) Pruritus and severe iron deficiency in polycythaemia vera. Br Med J (Clin Res Ed), 285:91–92

Schilling RF (1980) Platelet millionaires. Lancet 2:372–373

Shibata J, Hasegawa J, Siemens HJ, Wolber E, Dibbelt L, Li D, Katschinski DM, Fandrey J, Jelkmann W, Gassmann M, Wenger RH, Wagner KF (2003) Hemostasis and coagulation at a hematocrit level of 0.85: functional consequences of erythrocytosis. Blood 101: 4416–4422

Silver RT (1997) Interferon alfa: effects of long-term treatment for polycythemia vera. Semin Hematol 34:40–50

Silver RT (2003) Imatinib mesylate (Gleevec) reduces phlebotomy requirements in polycythemia vera. Leukemia 17:1186–1187

Smith HP, Arnold HR, Whipple GH (1921) Comparative values of welcker, carbon monoxide and dye methods for blood volume determinations. accurate estimation of absolute blood volume. Am J Physiol 56:336–360

Solar GP, Kerr WG, Zeigler FC, Hess D, Donahue C, de Sauvage FJ, Eaton DL (1998) Role of c-mpl in early hematopoiesis. Blood 92:4–10

Souyri M, Vigon I, Penciolelli JF, Heard JM, Tambourin P, Wendling F (1990) A putative truncated cytokine receptor gene transduced by the myeloproliferative leukemia virus immortalizes hematopoietic progenitors. Cell 63:1137–1147

Spivak JL (2002) Polycythemia vera: myths, mechanisms, and management. Blood 100:4272–4290

Spivak JL, Cooke CR (1976) Polycythemia vera in an anephric man. Am J Med Sci 272:339–344

Steensma DP, Dewald GW, Lasho TL, Powell HL, McClure RF, Levine RL, Gilliland DG, Tefferi A (2005) The JAK2 V617F activating tyrosine kinase mutation is an infrequent event in both "atypical" myeloproliferative disorders and myelodysplastic syndromes. Blood 106: 1207–1209

Steinman HK, Greaves MW (1985) Aquagenic pruritus. J Am Acad Dermatol 13:91–96

Tefferi A, Silverstein MN, Li CY (1997) 2-Chlorodeoxyadenosine treatment after splenectomy in patients who have myelofibrosis with myeloid metaplasia. Br J Haematol 99:352–357

Thomas DJ, du Boulay GH, Marshall J, Pearson TC, Ross Russell RW, Symon L, Wetherley-Mein G, Zilkha E (1977) Cerebral blood-flow in polycythaemia. Lancet 2:161–163

Towell BL, Levine SP (1987) Massive hepatomegaly following splenectomy for myeloid metaplasia. Case report and review of the literature. Am J Med 82:371–375

Tsukamoto N, Morita K, Maehara T, Okamoto K, Sakai H, Karasawa M, Naruse T, Omine M (1994) Clonality in chronic myeloproliferative disorders defined by X-chromosome linked probes: demonstration of heterogeneity in lineage involvement. Br J Haematol 86: 253–258

Turhan AG, Humphries RK, Cashman JD, Cuthbert DA, Eaves CJ, Eaves AC (1988) Transient suppression of clonal hemopoiesis associated with pregnancy in a patient with a myeloproliferative disorder. J Clin Invest 81:1999–2003

Ugo V, Marzac C, Teyssandier I, Larbret F, Lecluse Y, Debili N, Vainchenker W, Casadevall N (2004) Multiple signaling pathways are involved in erythropoietin-independent differentiation of erythroid progenitors in polycythemia vera. Exp Hematol 32:179–187

Ulich TR, del Castillo J, Senaldi G, Kinstler O, Yin S, Kaufman S, Tarpley J, Choi E, Kirley T, Hunt P, Sheridan WP (1996) Systemic hematologic effects of PEG-rHuMGDF-induced megakaryocyte hyperplasia in mice. Blood 87:5006–5015

Valla D, Casadevall N, Lacombe C, Varet B, Goldwasser E, Franco D, Maillard JN, Pariente EA, Leporrier M, Rueff B (1985) Primary myeloproliferative disorder and hepatic vein thrombosis. A prospective study of erythroid colony formation in vitro in 20 patients with Budd-Chiari syndrome. Ann Intern Med 103:329–334

van Genderen PJ, Budde U, Michiels JJ, van Strik R, van Vliet HH (1996) The reduction of large von Willebrand factor multimers in plasma in essential thrombocythaemia is related to the platelet count. Br J Haematol 93:962–965

Vaquez H (1892) Sur une forme speciale de cyanose s'accompagnant d' hyperglobulie excessive et peristante. C R Soc Biol (Paris) 44: 384–388

Villeval JL, Cohen-Solal K, Tulliez M, Giraudier S, Guichard J, Burstein SA, Cramer EM, Vainchenker W, Wendling F (1997) High thrombopoietin production by hematopoietic cells induces a fatal myeloproliferative syndrome in mice. Blood 90:4369–4383

Vizmanos JL, Ormazabal C, Larrayoz MJ, Cross NC, Calasanz MJ (2006) JAK2 V617F mutation in classic chronic myeloproliferative diseases: a report on a series of 349 patients. Leukemia, 20:534–535

Wasserman L (1971) The management of polycythemia vera. Br J Haematol 21:371–376

Wasserman LR (1976) The treatment of polycythemia vera. Semin Hematol 13:57–78

Weber FP (1908) Polycythaemia, erythrocytosis and erythraemia. Q J Med 2:85–134

Wehmeier A, Fricke S, Scharf RE, Schneider W (1990) A prospective study of haemostatic parameters in relation to the clinical course of myeloproliferative disorders. Eur J Haematol 45:191–197

Wehmeier A, Daum I, Jamin H, Schneider W (1991) Incidence and clinical risk factors for bleeding and thrombotic complications in myeloproliferative disorders. A retrospective analysis of 260 patients. Ann Hematol 63:101–106

Wells RE, Merrill EW (1962) Influence of flow properties of blood upon viscosity-hematocrit relationship. J Clin Invest, 41:1591–1598

Wendling F, Varlet P, Charon M, Tambourin P (1986) MPLV: a retrovirus complex inducing an acute myeloproliferative leukemic disorder in adult mice. Virology 149:242–246

Westin J, Granerus G, Weinfeld A, Wetterquist H (1975) Histamine metabolism in polycythaemia vera. Scand J Haematol 15:45–57

Wetzler M, Talpaz M, Van Etten RA, Hirsh-Ginsberg C, Beran M, Kurzrock R (1993) Subcellular localization of Bcr, Abl, and Bcr-Abl proteins in normal and leukemic cells and correlation of expression with myeloid differentiation. J Clin Invest 92:1925–1939

Wright RR, Tono M, Pollycove M (1975) Blood volume. Semin Nucl Med 5:63–78

Yu TF, Weissmann B, Sharney L, Kupfer S, Gutman AB (1956) On the biosynthesis of uric acid from glycine-N in primary and secondary polcythemia. Am J Med 6:901–917

Zhao R, Xing S, Li Z, Fu X, Li Q, Krantz SB, Zhao ZJ (2005) Identification of an acquired JAK2 mutation in polycythemia vera, J Biol Chem, 280:22788–22692

Zwicky C, Theiler L, Zbaren K, Ischi E, Tobler A (2002) The predictive value of clonogenic stem cell assays for the diagnosis of polycythaemia vera. Br J Haematol 117:598–604

Polycythemia Vera and Other Polycythemic Disorders – Biological Aspects

Sonny O. Ang and Josef T. Prchal

Contents

Abstract. Myeloproliferative disorders (MPD) constitute a subset of hematological malignancies characterized by a stem cell-originated clonal proliferation of aberrant myeloid cells, one of which is polycythemia vera (PV). PV is the most common myeloproliferative disorder with an annual incidence of at least 23 cases per million in North America and Western Europe. PV patients suffer high risk of thrombotic and hemorrhagic complications and propensity to clonal evolution to acute leukemia and myelodysplastic syndrome. Current treatment involves reduction of whole blood erythrocytosis by phlebotomy to reduce blood viscosity and use of myelosuppressive therapy. On average, after 10 years of treatment, a significant portion of PV patients (5–15%) progress to postpolycythemic myeloid metaplasia and/or leukemia; the majority of these patients (70%) die within 3 years. Distinguishing PV from other polycythemic disorders can be very challenging and in this chapter PV will be discussed in the context of other polycythemic disorders. Recent research breakthroughs in the understanding of its molecular basis have improved our understanding of PV pathophysiology and open the possible vista of specific pharmaceutical intervention.

17.1 Introduction

Polycythemia means "too many cells in the blood" derived from the Greek for "many," "cells," and "blood." Another term, erythrocytosis, derived from the Greek for "red" and "cells," is also frequently used. For historical purposes, the two terms are loosely equivalent and no consensus on which term to use has been achieved. Because erythrocyte is the most abundant cell type, polycythemia actually means "too many red blood cells."

True polycythemia is defined as an elevated erythrocyte mass in excess of 32 mL/kg for males and 28 mL/kg for females (Berlin 1975). Relative polycythemia can result from a decrease of plasma volume instead of an actual increase of erythrocyte mass and will not be discussed here.

17.2 Classifications of Polycythemia

Polycythemias can be classified according to their cellular and molecular basis (Prchal 2001b). Primary polycythemias are caused by inherited or acquired genetic defects affecting the primary cells (hematopoietic progenitors), leading to dysregulated proliferation. Biochemical parameters associated with this condition include:

1. Decreased or a low normal serum erythropoietin (Epo) levels, and
2. Excessive erythroid proliferation in response to cytokines [e.g., Epo, Insulin-like growth factor 1 (IGF-1)] (Prchal 2001b).

Clinical entities comprising primary polycythemias include:

1. Polycythemia vera (PV), a clonal precursor to malignant development,
2. Primary familial congenital polycythemia (PFCP),
3. Chuvash polycythemia (with features of both primary and secondary polycythemia).

Secondary polycythemias are caused by extrinsic factors such as elevated or inappropriately normal serum levels of Epo, IGF-1 or cobalt (Jacobson et al. 2000). These extrinsic factors (e.g., Epo) overstimulate erythropoiesis in the bone marrow in excess of the physiological needs "*inappropriate polycythemias*," or appropriately respond to hypoxic stimulus "*appropriate polycythemia*." Elevated hematocrit in turn leads to increased viscosity and at extreme ranges of elevation to decreases in tissue oxygen delivery (Prchal 1995). Biochemical parameters associated with this condition are:

1. Elevated (or inappropriately normal for elevated red cell mass) circulating Epo levels, and
2. Normal erythroid response to cytokines (Prchal 2001b).

Based on physiological requirements, secondary polycythemias can present as (Prchal and Prchal 1999):

1. Physiologically *appropriate* elevation of Epo in response to tissue hypoxia (polycythemias of high altitude, chronic mountain sickness, chronic pulmonary disease, cyanotic heart disease, hemoglobin variant with abnormal oxygen affinity, 2,3-diphosphoglycerate (DPG) deficiency, and methemoglobinemia).
2. Physiologically *inappropriate* Epo production in the absence of tissue hypoxia (paraneoplastic Epo production, renal cysts, liver tumors, pheochromocytoma, post kidney transplant polycythemias, and drug-induced polycythemia such as seen in Epo doping).

17.2.1 Genetics of Polycythemia

Most polycythemias are acquired, but both primary and secondary polycythemias may be inherited (Prchal 2003). There are dominant and recessive forms of inherited polycythemias. Polycythemia can also be associated with genetic syndromes such as von Hippel Landau syndrome, hereditary hemorrhagic telangiectasia, glycogen storage disease type VII (also known as Tarui disease), fibrocystic pulmonary dysplasia, and hypokalemic alkalosis with hypercalciuria [also known as Bartter syndrome (Erkelens et al. 1973)]. Nonsyndromic polycythemias include PV, PFCP, and Chuvash polycythemia.

17.3 Etiology

Understanding the etiology of polycythemias is a vital first step in elucidating the molecular basis for a particular polycythemia and should be the fulcrum for differentiating PV from other polycythemic states. The primary molecular defect or defects responsible for PV have not been elucidated until recently, and we submit are still not entirely clear at this date, making both the diagnosis and treatment options of PV controversial. Development of an accurate diagnostic test, targeted therapy, and eventual cure of this disorder will become possible when both the primary event, as well as contributory germ line and somatic mutations that cause PV, are identified. In contrast, the molecular defects of two primary inherited polycythemic disorders (PFCP and Chuvash polycythemia) have been elucidated. Central to our understanding polycythemias is our understanding of cellular responses to hypoxia as it relates to *EPO* regulation and Epo signaling; perturbation of these physiological mechanisms results in appropriate (polycythemia of high altitude or due to mutant hemoglobins with high O_2 affinity), as well as inappropriate polycythemias (Chuvash polycythemia due to dysregulation of hypoxia sensing, polycythemias due to Epo-producing tumors, and PV wherein there is the unhinged post *EPO* receptor signaling from Epo).

17.3.1 Cellular Responses to Hypoxia

Erythropoiesis, the process of making red blood cells, is tightly regulated to provide an adequate supply of oxygen to meet the demands of tissue metabolism. Perturbation in oxygen-carrying capacity (e.g., mutated hemoglobin) or in the cardiovascular delivery system (right to left cardiac shunts) affects the homeostasis and often results in pathological states such as polycythemia.

The prime regulator of erythropoiesis is a potent cytokine, Epo, which is produced mainly in the kidneys and to lesser degree in the liver (Eckardt et al. 1992). It binds to its receptor (erythropoietin receptor, EpoR), changing the conformation of EpoR homodimers (Constantinescu et al. 2001) and thereby initiates a cascade of events mediated via the JAK2/STAT pathway resulting in proliferation, differentiation (Koury et al. 1990), and antiapoptotic signals in erythroid cells.

Epo, present at very low concentrations in the blood, is not stored and is produced continuously (Prchal 1995). Under decreased oxygen tension, Epo production in the kidney (Koury et al. 1990) and liver increases. Enhanced erythropoiesis results in an increase in red cell mass that may relieve the hypoxic stress, completing a negative feedback loop (Fig. 17.1).

Analysis of hypoxia-inducible *cis*-acting sequences in the 3′-flanking region of the *EPO* gene led to the discovery of a transcriptional hypoxia response element (HRE), a 50 base pair (bp) sequence (Beck et al. 1991; Semenza et al. 1991) with DNA-binding sites for the transcription factor HIF-1, a ubiquitously expressed

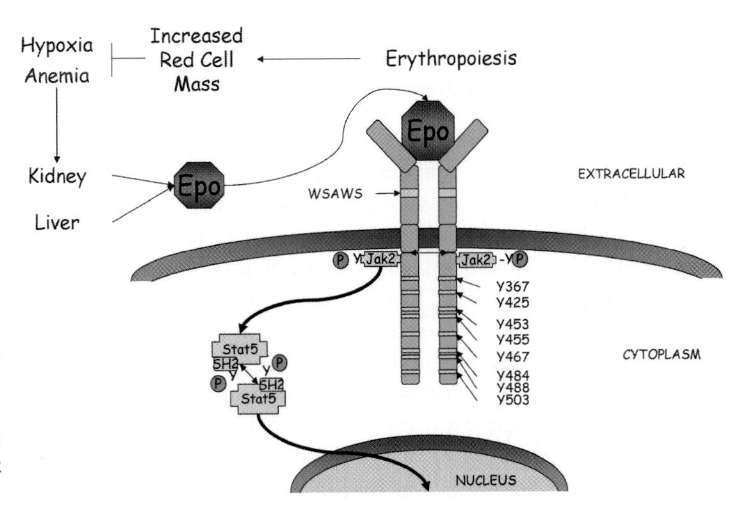

Fig. 17.1. Epo–Epo receptor signaling pathway. Epo is not stored and is produced continuously. Under decreased oxygen tension, Epo production in kidney and liver increases. Enhanced erythropoiesis results in an increase in red cell mass that relieves the hypoxic stress, completing a negative feedback loop

transcription factor. HIF-1 plays a pivotal role in the chain of reaction starting with oxygen sensing and gene transcription and resulting in physiological adaptation to hypoxia in vivo. Target genes regulated by HIF-1 (Semenza 1999) include those involved in glucose/energy metabolism (Carmeliet et al. 1998; Dietrich et al. 1993; Iyer et al. 1998; Ryan et al. 1998; Wood et al. 1998), cell proliferation/viability (Bruick 2000; Caniggia et al. 2000; Carmeliet et al. 1998; Feldser et al. 1999; Tazuke et al. 1998), erythropoiesis/iron metabolism (Jiang et al. 1996; Lok et al. 1999; Mukhopadhyay et al. 2000; Rolfs et al. 1997; Semenza et al. 1992; Tacchini et al. 1999), vascular development/remodeling (Carmeliet et al. 1998; Cormier-Regard et al. 1998; Eckhart et al. 1997; Gerber et al. 1997; Hu et al. 1998; Iyer et al. 1998; Kietzmann et al. 1999; Ryan et al. 1998), vasodilation (Lee et al. 1997; Palmer et al. 1998), and other functions (Bhattacharya et al. 1999; Takahashi et al. 2000; Wykoff et al. 2000).

At the molecular level, oxygen homeostasis is primarily modulated by HIF-1. It is expressed in all cells tested thus far (Semenza 2000a) with the highest levels of expression in the kidney and heart (Hogenesch et al. 1997). Reporter assays using the Epo HRE were shown to be functional in a wide variety of cells including those that do not express *EPO* (Beck et al. 1993; Maxwell et al. 1993; Wang et al. 1993), suggesting that the HRE is part of a conserved oxygen-sensing pathway in mammalian cells. This pathway is critical in many physiological events arising from hypoxic stress, including vasculogenesis, which is required for proper embryonic development and tumor formation (Bunn et al. 1996; Semenza 2000b, c).

17.3.2 Interplay of HIF-VHL in Gene Regulation and Oxygen Sensing

HIF-1 is a heterodimeric complex composed of α and β subunits. The α subunit is exquisitely regulated in an oxygen-dependent manner at the posttranslational level (Ema et al. 1999; Jiang et al. 1997; Gradin et al. 1996; Huang et al. 1996; Kallio et al. 1998; Pugh et al. 1997; Semenza 2000a), whereas expression of the β subunit is constitutive. HIF-1α is stable under hypoxic conditions but is targeted for polyubiquitination and proteasomal degradation under normoxic conditions, resulting in one of the shortest half-lives of any protein (Wang et al. 1995; Yu et al. 1998). The von Hippel Lindau tumor suppressor protein (pVHL) serves as the recognition component of an E3 ubiquitin ligase complex to ubiquitinate HIF-1α (Cockman et al. 2000; Maxwell et al. 1999; Ohh et al. 2000; Tanimoto et al. 2000). Oxygen- and iron-dependent prolyl hydroxylations of HIF-1α are required before being targeted by VHL (Epstein et al. 2001; Ivan et al. 2001; Jaakkola et al. 2001; Maxwell et al. 1999;) for ubiquitination and subsequent degradation by the 26S proteosome. Three prolyl hydroxylases (PHDs; PHD1-3) were identified as putative dioxygenases (Epstein et al. 2001) for the modification of HIF-1α. Hypoxia, iron chelators, and cobaltous ions exert similar effects on these enzymes, raising the possibility that the PHDs (PHD1-3) and their interacting proteins and other components could function as oxygen sensors. This finding provides a mechanistic link to the observation that iron chelators and transition metals (cobalt, nickel) can mimic the effects of hypoxia in stabilizing HIF-1α. Because proline hydroxylation requires molecular oxygen and iron, this protein modification may play a key role in mammalian oxygen sensing (Ivan et al. 2001). An absolute requirement for dioxygen as a cosubstrate and iron as a cofactor also suggests that the PHDs may function directly as cellular oxygen sensors. In addition, HIF-1α function is also regulated by redox-dependent asparaginyl hydroxylation (Lando et al. 2002). Immunoblot analysis showed that asparaginyl hydroxylation blocked the interaction of HIF-1α with p300/CBP, a transcription activator involved in HIF-1-regulated gene expression. These findings established a molecular framework to account for the redox-sensitive nature of HIF-1 protein stability and transactivation. Cells lacking a normal ubiquitin-proteasome machinery (Huang et al. 1998; Salceda et al. 1997) or pVHL (Maxwell et al. 1999) express HIF-1α at constitutively high levels. Reintroduction of VHL into these cells restored their hypoxia-inducibility. Thus, dysregulation in the HIF-VHL pathway may cause upregulation of genes such as *EPO* and result in polycythemia. Indeed, conditional VHL knock-out mice with gene deletion in the liver (Haase et al. 2001) have polycythemia with upregulation of hypoxia-regulated genes including *EPO*.

17.3.3 Chuvash Polycythemia

Chuvash polycythemia is the only documented endemic congenital polycythemia. Chuvash polycythemia is an autosomal recessive disorder caused by a defect in the oxygen-sensing pathway (Ang et al. 2002b). First reported in the early 1970s (Polyakova 1974), these patients show signs of plethora, and most complained of fatigue and headaches (Polyakova 1974, 1977; Sergeyeva et al. 1997). Linkage to the *EPO* and *EPOR* gene loci (Sergeyeva et al. 1997) was ruled out. Exploiting a presumed founder effect in the isolated Chuvash population (Polyakova 1974, 1977; Sergeyeva et al. 1997), a whole-genome screen revealed a candidate region on chromosome 3p25 (Ang et al. 2002b). Subsequently, we demonstrated homozygosity for an R200W missense mutation of the *VHL* gene (*VHL 598C*→T) as the molecular basis of Chuvash polycythemia (Ang et al. 2002b). The resultant attenuation of VHL function in Chuvash polycythemia perturbs the degradation of HIF-1*α*, resulting in accumulation of HIF-1*α* and consequent upregulation of downstream target genes including erythropoietin (*EPO*), *GLUT1*, and vascular endothelial growth factor (*VEGF*) (Ang et al. 2002a, b).

Chuvash polycythemia has features of both primary and secondary polycythemias (Ang et al. 2002a, b) since the erythroid progenitors of CP patients are hypersensitive in vitro to extrinsic Epo while some patients have elevated serum Epo levels. Epo levels, the principal determinant of hemoglobin concentration, are not elevated above the normal range in all Chuvash patients; however, Epo levels are inappropriately high relative to the elevated hemoglobin concentrations in almost all patients (Ang et al. 2002b).

The Chuvash polycythemia mutation has been found in non-Chuvash populations and with patients harboring compound heterozygous VHL mutations (Gordeuk et al. 2005). Using samples from Chuvash, Southeast Asian, Caucasian, Hispanic, and African-American subjects harboring the *VHL 598C*→T mutation (Liu et al. 2004), haplotype analysis of the VHL locus suggested emergence of a single mutational event between 12,000 and 51,000 years ago. However, a Turkish polycythemic family with a *VHL 598C*→T mutation seems to have acquired the lesion independently (Cario et al. 2005). Recently another endemic enclave was discovered in the Southern Italian island of Ischia, where the gene frequency of this VHL mutation (0.07) exceeds even that reported among the Chuvash population (Perrotta et al. 2006); interestingly, the *VHL 598C*→T mutation in this Italian isolate is present also on the common Chuvash polycythemia haplotype.

Since Chuvash homozygotes usually do not survive beyond the age of 40 (Polyakova 1977) due to increased lethal thrombotic and hemorrhagic vascular complications (Gordeuk et al. 2004), negative selection pressure for the mutant allele is expected. Consequently, the retention and propagation of the *VHL 598C*→T mutant allele suggests a survival advantage for heterozygotes. Such an advantage might involve subtle improvement in iron metabolism, erythropoiesis, protection against preeclampsia (via HIF-1-mediated regulation of VEGF) (Luttun et al. 2003), or protection against bacterial infections (via hypoxia-mediated bactericidal activity in neutrophils (Cramer et al. 2003).

17.3.4 Primary Familial and Congenital Polycythemia (PFCP)

PFCP is inherited in an autosomal dominant fashion (Prchal 2003), with clinically benign manifestations. There is no bleeding tendency and no splenomegaly with typically normal development in the childhood. PFCP patients are not known to progress to leukemia (Prchal 1995). Nevertheless, PFCP can lead to increased cardiovascular disease. Clinical features of PFCP are evaluated as isolated erythrocytosis with no leukocytosis or thrombocytosis and normal vitamin B_{12} levels. The hemoglobin-oxygen dissociation curve (P50) is normal in PFCP, whereas serum Epo levels are always low.

PFCP has been linked to mutations in the *EPOR* gene. The cytoplasmic domain of EpoR contains both a positive and a negative growth-regulatory domain. Upon binding Epo, EpoR changes the conformation of the homodimers and is phosphorylated by Janus 2 tyrosine kinase (JAK2) (Miura et al. 1991), which binds to the positive growth-regulatory domain, initiating a cascade of proliferative signals.

The cytoplasmic negative regulatory region is necessary for downregulation of the transduced signal. A hematopoietic cell phosphatase (also known as SHP-1), a negative regulator of EpoR signal transduction (Klingmuller et al. 1995), binds to this region (docking at residue Tyr430 of human EpoR) to dephosphorylate the residues phosphorylated by Jak2. The dephosphorylation is necessary and sufficient to terminate the proliferative signal. In addition, another negative regulator (Masuhara et al. 1997), cytokine-inducible SH2 protein 3 (CIS-3, also known as suppressor of cytokine signaling 3 (SOCS3) (Starr et al. 1997) and STAT-induced STAT inhibitor 3 (SSI3) (Minamoto et al. 1997), also binds to the negative regulatory region, silencing the proliferative signal (Masuhara et al. 1997; Sasaki et al. 2000; Yoshimura et al. 1995). CIS-3 is an SH2-containing protein that binds to the activation loop of Janus kinases, inhibiting kinase activity and thereby suppressing cytokine signaling. During embryonic development, CIS-3 is highly expressed in erythroid cells and is Epo independent. Transgene-mediated expression in mice blocked fetal erythropoiesis, resulting in embryonic lethality (Marine et al. 1999). Homozygous inactivation of the *Cis-3* gene in mice resulted in embryonic lethality at 12–16 days, accompanied by marked polycythemia (Roberts et al. 2001). Moreover, the in vitro proliferative capacity of erythroid progenitors was greatly increased. *Cis-3*-deficient fetal liver stem cells could reconstitute hematopoiesis in lethally irradiated adults, indicating that its absence does not disturb bone marrow erythropoiesis. As a whole, these results demonstrated that *CIS-3* is critical in negatively regulating fetal liver hematopoiesis.

Loss of the negative regulatory domain (e.g., by truncation due to nonsense mutation) in effect causes apparent excessive (Fisher et al. 1994) activation of EpoR. *EPOR* gene mutations associated with PFCP invariably truncate the cytoplasmic carboxyl terminus of the protein (Arcasoy et al. 1997; de la Chapelle et al. 1993a, b; Furukawa et al. 1997; Kralovics et al. 1997a, 1998, 2001; Le Couedic et al. 1996; Percy et al. 1998; Sokol et al. 1994, 1995; Watowich et al. 1999). Receptor lacking carboxyl terminal tyrosine residues (eight in normal human EpoR) cannot be deactivated after ligand binding-induced activation. Truncation of EpoR due to mutations leads to a lack of signal termination, causing enhanced proliferation in erythroid progenitor cells leading to polycythemia (Kralovics et al. 2001). A mouse model of polycythemia bearing a normal human *EPOR* and a mutation identified in a PFCP patient was created (Divoky et al. 2001), with the mice showing the expected phenotype. The gain-of-function mutations primarily affect erythroid cells, but *EPOR* is also expressed in endothelial cells and the brain. The mouse model in combination with tissue-specific *cre* expression will be useful for further molecular characterization of the disease, as well as delineating the functions of EpoR in other tissues. The role of EpoR in erythropoiesis is crucial because *EPOR* knock-out mice do not develop fetal and adult mature erythrocytes (Wu et al. 1995).

In contrast to the EpoR C-terminal truncations in PFCP which render the receptor hyper-responsive to Epo, a point mutation (R129C) in the exoplasmic domain causes constitutive EpoR homodimerization and activation in the absence of its cognate ligand. This altered EpoR conformation induces Epo-independent proliferation and tumorigenesis in mice, reminiscent of the association between the wild-type EpoR and gp55 (the glycoprotein from the Friend virus) which results in Epo-independent activation (Yoshimura et al. 1990; Youssoufian et al. 1993).

Many PFCP patients have mutations in their *EPOR* gene, whereas some have no identifiable mutation thus far (Kralovics et al. 2001). Therefore, it is certain that PFCP can be due to mutations in other genes along the Epo-EpoR signaling pathway.

17.3.5 Polycythemia as a Result of Hemoglobinopathies

Familial erythrocytosis can be caused by presence of high-affinity hemoglobin. Hemoglobin, the primary transporter of oxygen in blood, is composed of an $\alpha 2/\beta 2$ allosteric tetramer. Conformational oscillations of the quarternary complex between tense (fully deoxygenated) and relaxed (fully oxygenated) states coincide with binding and releasing of oxygen (Prchal 1999).

More than 100 mutations causing an increase in oxygen affinity in hemoglobin have been described (Prchal 2001a). Increased oxygen affinity decreases oxygen release to the tissues, causing tissue hypoxia. The hypoxia results in a physiologically appropriate increased Epo production and polycythemia. Patients inheriting these hemoglobin mutations are generally asymptomatic because compensatory polycythemia ensures normal tissue oxygenation. Although some patients complain of headache and nose bleeds, no severe complication (including splenomegaly) accompanies the presentation of polycythemia. Thus, this type of familial erythrocytosis is considered clinically benign.

Hemoglobin variants may be electrophoretically silent, so evaluation of hemoglobin oxygen dissociation kinetics is the best initial screen (Kralovics et al. 2000). Many high oxygen affinity mutants are located in the $\alpha 2/\beta 2$ interface. Some mutations interfere with tense/relaxed conformation shift or the binding of 2,3-biphosphoglycerate (2,3BPG, also known as DPG; see below), whereas others introduce structural perturbation affecting the binding of heme at the carboxyl terminus of the globin subunits (Kralovics et al. 2000). Both human globin α gene (HBA) (Charache et al.

1966; Clegg et al. 1966; Harano et al. 1983, 1996; Moo-Penn et al. 1987; Wajcman et al. 1994; Williamson et al. 1992) and β gene (HBB) (Bento et al. 2000; Carbone et al. 1999; Hoyer et al. 1998; Kiger et al. 1996; Novy et al. 1967; Perutz et al. 1984; Rahbar et al. 1983, 1985; Schneider et al. 1979; Wajcman et al. 1999; Weatherall et al. 1977; Williamson et al. 1994) loci have mutations associated with polycythemia. Those inheriting α globin variants have elevated hemoglobin at birth, whereas those with β globin variants develop polycythemia later on in life (Prchal and Prchal 1999).

Mutations in other globin loci can also cause polycythemia, including the globin $\alpha 2$ locus (Reed et al. 1974) and the globin δ locus, which determines the δ, or non-β, chain of hemoglobin: A(2) (α-2/δ-2) (Salkie et al. 1982). There is immense instructive value in these mutant proteins because these naturally occurring genetic lesions provide significant insight into the inner workings of hemoglobin.

Hemoglobin is functionally regulated by 2,3BPG. 2,3BPG is abundant in red blood cells, where it associates with the deoxygenated hemoglobin tetramers and decreases their oxygen affinity, shifting the oxygen dissociation curve to the right. Loss of this function due to 2,3BPG deficiency decreases tissue release of oxygen and results in physiologically appropriate increase in Epo levels. The glycolytic enzyme 2,3BPG mutase modulates the level of 2,3BPG. Both hemolytic anemia and polycythemia have been observed with deficiency of 2,3BPG mutase (Scott et al. 1982). Deficiency in other glycolytic enzymes [e.g., pyruvate kinase (Rosa et al. 1981)] in the erythrocyte may also be associated with extremely rare cases of polycythemia.

Methemoglobin in health constitutes only a small proportion of hemoglobin (approximately 1%). In methemoglobin the iron in the heme ring is irreversibly locked in the Fe^{3+} (ferric state, ferriheme) instead of the normal Fe^{2+} (ferrous state, ferroheme). Oxygen binds reversibly to the ferrous form in deoxyhemoglobin but not to the ferric methemoglobin. When the iron is oxidized, methemoglobin can no longer carry oxygen. In addition, ferrihemes cause allosteric conformational changes, left shifting the dissociation curve of remaining deoxyhemoglobin subunits by increasing the oxygen affinity of the $\alpha 2/\beta 2$ hemoglobin tetrameric complex (Kralovics et al. 2000). This decreases oxygen release into the tissues.

Acute acquired increase of methemoglobin in the blood leads to a hypoxic state and even death. In contrast, most inherited methemoglobinemias generally are asymptomatic but are associated with cyanosis, and compensatory polycythemia may result. Three inherited causes of methemoglobinemia have been identified, dominantly inherited globin mutations (hemoglobin Ms), recessively inherited cytochrome b5 reductase deficiency, and extremely rare cytochrome b5 deficiency (Prchal 1995). Cytochrome b5 reductase deficiency exists in two forms: the more common type 1 causes asymptomatic cyanosis due to the isolated erythrocyte defect, while type 2 is due to the generalized enzyme defect in all cells and invariably causes fatality in infancy (Prchal and Gregg 2005).

17.3.6 Other Causes of Polycythemia

Polycythemias can also result from causes other than the ones mentioned above. Hypoxia is the sine qua non of high altitude. Compensatory polycythemias of high altitude and chronic mountain sickness are consequences of physiological adaptation to living at high altitudes; however, there are considerable genetically determined differences in the human population in polycythemic responses to high altitude exposure (Prchal and Beutler 2005).

In acquired and congenital cardiopulmonary diseases, severe oxygen deprivation may result due to inadequate delivery of oxygen. Upregulation of erythropoiesis to boost the oxygen-carrying capacity may result in polycythemia.

In paraneoplastic development such as renal cysts [the majority of Epo is produced in the adult kidney (Eckardt et al. 1992)], liver tumors [liver contributes Epo in adult humans (Eckardt et al. 1992)], pheochromocytoma (adrenal glands produce catecholamines that may affect Epo production), dysregulation of Epo production can result in polycythemia. Additionally, polycythemia can also occur after kidney transplant or can be induced by drugs (Prchal 2001a). The exact mechanisms are unknown, although IGF-1 is known to play a role in regulating erythropoiesis in patients with end-stage renal disease who lack the usual anemia (Shih et al. 1999) and is also involved in the relatively common erythrocytosis of postrenal transplantation where the major mechanism appears to be angiotensin II related (Mrug et al. 1997, 2004).

17.4 Polycythemia Vera

Polycythemia vera (PV), the most common primary polycythemia, is initiated by somatic change in a single hematopoietic stem cell resulting in a clonal myeloproliferative disorder. Recent data from Sweden indicate that PV is the most common myeloproliferative disorder (Kutti et al. 2001). The estimated annual incidence in North America and Western Europe is 23 cases per million individuals (Prchal 1995). Typically an adult onset disease that manifests in the 5th and 6th decades of life, PV has a median age at onset of 60 years (Kralovics et al. 2000). It is usually sporadic but congenital and dominant pedigrees have been reported. (Kralovics et al. 2000). Familial cases are very rare; they generally have incomplete penetrance and are typically acquired and develop in older age (Kralovics et al. 2003b).

Symptoms are variable (Kralovics et al. 2000; Prchal 1995) with many patients complaining of headache, night sweats, difficult-to-control pruritus, dizziness, vertigo, visual disturbances, and weight loss. Plethoric complexion, hepatomegaly (40–50% of patients) and progressive splenomegaly (75% of patients) are the most prominent physical findings. Some patients suffer from ruddy cyanosis.

The characteristic trilineage defect is often evident in laboratory findings of erythrocytosis, thrombocytosis, and leukocytosis in addition to elevated red cell mass and frequent hyperuricemia. PV patients suffer very high risks of thrombotic and hemorrhagic complications that may be reduced by treatment. The propensity for thrombosis and hemorrhage is often attributed to elevated blood viscosity as a result of erythrocytosis. As many as 30–40% of patients die of thrombotic events. While most of these are cerebrovascular, cardiovascular, and peripheral vascular thromboses, other atypical vascular beds, e.g., portal, hepatic, splenic, and mesenteric sites may be involved and may affect both venous and arterial vasculature (Landolfi et al. 2004). Although rare, a typical complication in PV patients is Budd-Chiari syndrome, which is characterized by obstruction and occlusion of the suprahepatic veins. Approximately 10% of Budd-Chiari syndrome cases are reported to occur in conjunction with PV; Budd-Chiari syndrome is frequently a presenting symptom of PV and substantial proportion of these patients do not have elevated hematocrit at the time of this often catastrophic event (Gregg et al. 2005; Prchal and Beutler 2005).

Current treatment for PV involves reduction of whole blood erythrocytosis by phlebotomy to reduce blood viscosity and to keep fatal thrombotic and hemorrhagic events in check. PV patients with hematocrits of 53–62% have reduced cerebral blood flow. In addition, the seminal studies of Pearson and colleagues showed that the hematocrit is directly correlated with thrombotic events in PV patients (Pearson 1997; Pearson et al. 1978). Phlebotomy improves cerebral blood flow thus there is an assumption that there would be a concomitant decrease in thromboses. Hence, phlebotomy is assumed by many to be valuable therapeutic management option for PV; however, in the original first randomized control trial (PVSG) phlebotomy therapy was associated with more thrombotic complications than myelosuppressive alternatives. However, treatment with ^{32}P and alkylating agents that were employed by the Polycythemia Vera Study Group (PVSG) were associated with increased risk of transformation to acute leukemia or myelodysplastic syndrome. Hydroxycarbamine (hydroxyurea), a cytoreductive agent, has been successfully used in PV resulting in significant reduction in thrombotic/hemorrhagic episodes with anticipated, but yet no demonstrated increase in leukemogenicity.

About 5–15% of PV patients progress to postpolycythemic myeloid metaplasia (also known as spent phase) after an average of 10 years of treatment. The clonal evolution leading to a PV spent phase is characterized by massive splenomegaly, tear-drop-shaped red cells (dacrocytes), bone marrow fibrosis, leukoerythroblastic peripheral blood smear, and a normal or decreasing red cell mass (anemia). The majority of patients (70%) die within 3 years of the onset of myeloid metaplasia, often because this phase heralds leukemic transformation (Fruchtman 2004).

Recent research breakthroughs have presented a glimpse into the possible molecular mechanism behind the pathogenesis of PV (Baxter et al. 2005; James et al. 2005; Kralovics et al. 2005; Levine et al. 2005b). Various research groups have independently identified and verified an invariant mutation in the *JAK2* kinase gene product in PV; however, this mutation is also found in essential thrombocytosis and idiopathic myelofibrosis (myelofibrosis with myeloid metaplasia). This allows for more accurate molecular classification of the disease while opening up the possibility of specific targeted pharmacological intervention.

Table 17.1. Clinical criteria for diagnosis of polycythemia

Category A	Category B
1. Increased red cell mass	1. Thrombocytosis >400,000
2. Arterial O_2 saturation >92%	2. Leukocytosis >12,000
3. Splenomegaly	3. Elevated vitamin B_{12} or unbound B_{12} binding capacity

17.4.1 Clinical Evaluation of Polycythemia Vera

Clinical evaluations and diagnosis of PV involve laboratory studies to determine the hematocrit level (elevated), as well as the presence of leukocytosis (60–70%) and thrombocytosis (50%). Bone marrow biopsies are performed to detect hypercellularity, erythroid hyperplasia, and increased megakaryocytes (Thiele et al. 2001, 2005). A positive diagnosis for PV as defined by PVSG: as presence of all conditions in category A (Table 17.1), as presence of condition 1 of category A and two conditions from category B, or as two conditions of category A and two from category B.

However, the World Health Organization has also issued other diagnostic criteria that are also used by many (Michiels et al. 2002).

PV is caused by clonal expansion of all myeloid lineages (Kralovics et al. 2000). The primary molecular pathogenesis of PV is largely unknown. In vitro clonogenic assays show hypersensitivity of erythroid progenitors to cytokines. Progenitor cells from PV patients are Epo independent (Prchal and Axelrad 1974) and hypersensitive to IGF-1 (Prchal 1995), a cytokine that can substitute for Epo in normal erythropoiesis (Prchal 2001a). Anephric patients with undetectable Epo and normal hematocrits can have elevated IGF-1 levels (Brox et al. 1989).

Clonal expansion of myeloid lineages is sometimes associated with cytogenetic abnormalities, including a loss of heterozygosity (LOH) at chromosome 9p (Kralovics et al. 2002).

17.4.2 Laboratory Parameters for Differential Diagnosis of Polycythemia Vera

Various laboratory analyses are available to aid the proper diagnosis of PV. The value of quantitation of neutrophil PRV-1 mRNA, in vitro assays of erythroid progenitor cells, serum erythropoietin levels, c-mpl quantitation, and X-chromosome-based polymorphism clonality assays in female subjects is discussed below.

17.4.2.1 Differential Expression of PRV-1

By using a technique known as subtractive hybridization, Pahl's laboratory hunted for genes that are differentially expressed by the clonal PV neutrophils compared with neutrophils from normal individuals (Temerinac et al. 2000). Their efforts resulted in the discovery of an upregulated transcript they termed PRV-1 (which was previously and independently identified by others as CD177 antigen on normal neutrophils). PRV-1 mRNA was reported to be upregulated only in PV granulocytes but not in their progenitors (Klippel et al. 2002). There is no detectable difference in the gene product (protein) between normal and PV cells. While the normal function of PRV-1 in hematopoiesis is still not clear, the differential expression of this gene could be a useful parameter for diagnostic purposes. Nevertheless, quantitation of PRV-1 mRNA levels does not reliably discriminate PV from congenital polycythemias and various disorders with thrombocytoses (Kralovics et al. 2003a; Liu et al. 2003; Tefferi et al. 2004).

17.4.2.2 Endogenous Erythroid Colonies (EEC)

The most specific test for PV is the detection of endogenous erythroid colonies (EEC) in cultures of bone marrow or more conveniently from peripheral blood cells (Fig. 17.2). Thus, erythroid progenitor cells form colonies of easily distinguishable hemoglobinized cells without any added Epo (Kralovics et al. 2003a; Liu et al. 2003; Prchal and Axelrad 1974; Weinberg 1997). Although the in vitro culture assays of erythroid progenitors are very laborious, expensive, and not easy to standardize, the formation of EEC is useful to distinguish PV from secondary polycythemias. Importantly, the presence of EECs is indicative of abnormal growth of hematopoietic progenitors. This in turn points to possible defects in cytokine receptor signaling pathways. Indeed, 30% of PV patients have constitutively activated STAT3 protein (Roder et al. 2001). Erythroid differentiation in PV can be blocked by inhibitors of JAK2, phosphatidylinositol 3′ kinase, or kinases of the Src family (Ugo et al. 2004). Patients with PV reportedly respond to administration of imatinib mesylate, the agent

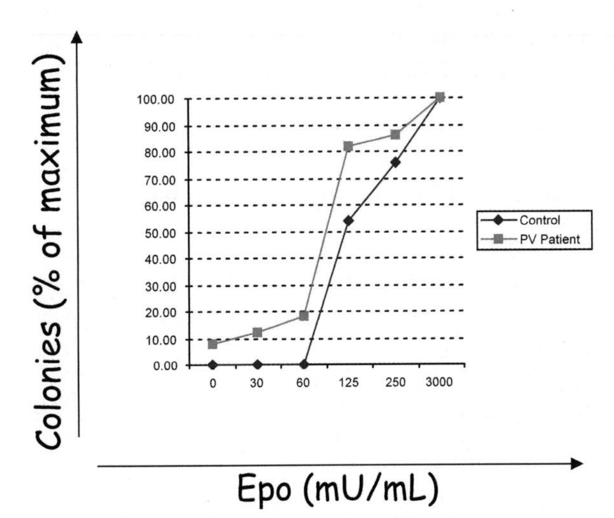

Fig. 17.2. EEC assay. Endogenous Erythroid Colonies (EEC) assay in cultures of bone marrow or peripheral blood cells. Erythroid progenitor cells from PV patient form Epo-independent colonies

that inhibits the BCR-ABL tyrosine kinase in CML (Silver 2003; Spivak et al. 2004). Taken together, the involvement of a kinase in the pathogenesis of PV can be inferred and this realization led to the recent finding of the somatic mutation in JAK2 that explains many of the observed in vitro PV characteristics.

17.4.2.3 Serum Erythropoietin Levels

Serum Epo levels in PV patients were reported to be below the normal reference range (Birgegard et al. 1992; Messinezy et al. 2002; Mossuz et al. 2004). While an elevated or midrange Epo level generally excludes the diagnosis of PV, a low Epo level is not specific for PV since patients with PFCP also have similarly low or even lower Epo levels (Prchal 2003).

17.4.2.4 Quantitation of Mpl (Thrombopoietin Receptor)

Being a trilineage defect, thrombocytosis is a common feature of PV along with erythrocytosis. Platelet production is regulated mainly via the thrombopoietin-thrombopoietin receptor signaling pathway. Completing the feedback loop, the thrombopoietin receptor on platelets is the major regulator of circulating thrombopoietin. It was therefore of particular interest when the expression of the thrombopoietin receptor was reported to be downregulated in PV (Moliterno et al. 1998). This finding could provide a plausible explanation for the increased platelet production in PV patients and thus had the potential to provide a good diagnostic marker. Unfortunately, the assay is not specific for PV (Kralovics et al. 2003a). Decrease in the level of the thrombopoietin receptor protein in platelets can be detected in both PV and essential thrombocythemia (Kralovics et al. 2003a; Moliterno et al. 1998).

17.4.2.5 Clonality Markers

PV is initiated by the transformation of a single hematopoietic stem cell into a cell with selective growth advantage. Because of this proliferative advantage intrinsic to the progenitor cell, the offspring of this mutated cell eventually overwhelm the hematopoietic system and become the predominant source of myeloid precursors. This is supported by evidence from clonality assays based on random X-chromosome inactivation.

Clonality studies have provided crucial evidence for our understanding of the hierarchical nature of hematopoiesis and leukemic progression. Current evidence indicates that all malignant processes and many premalignant disorders are clonal (Beutler et al. 1967; Knudson et al. 1972).

Clonality assays are based on random X-chromosome inactivation. Detection of clonality are based on three methodological principles:

1. Detection of protein polymorphisms of X-chromosome-encoded genes (Beutler et al. 1967);
2. Detection of methylation differences between an active and an inactivated X-chromosome (Vogelstein et al. 1985) [e.g., HUMARA assay being most informative (Mitterbauer et al. 1999)];
3. Discrimination of an active from an inactivated X chromosome by the transcript(s) of the gene(s) located on the active X-chromosome (Curnutte et al. 1992; Prchal and Guan; Prchal et al. 1993).

Detailed analysis of approximately one hundred female PV patients using this method showed that their reticulocytes, platelets, and granulocytes were always clonal (Liu et al. 2003), while PV T and NK lymphocytes are always polyclonal. On the other hand, B lymphocytes from PV patients run the gamut from being clonal to showing a skewed X-chromosome usage ratio resembling that seen in myeloid cells (Gregg et al. 1996; Phelan, II et al. 2001; Prchal and Guan 1993; Prchal et al. 1993). The experience of our group and others (Liu et al. 2003) is in contrast to other reports of polyclonal hematopoiesis in myeloproliferative disorders, but genomic DNA methylation-based clonality assays were used in these reports for assessment of clonality (Mitterbauer et al. 1999) and the data may not be comparable with the approach used here which we believe may have a sounder biological basis. In our hands the only exceptions were detected in a few patients who had clearly reverted to polyclonal from previously documented clonal hematopoiesis after treatment with interferon alpha (Liu et al. 2003).

Transcriptionally based clonality assays can be performed with relative ease on circulating myeloid cells in females. Nevertheless, the X-chromosome-inactivation-based analysis is not informative for every female. In addition, the normal skewing in X-chromosome allelic expression if often misinterpreted as evidence of clonality (Prchal et al. 1996). The potentially clonal myeloid cells should always be compared with the polyclonal T lymphocyte control cells from the same patient (Liu et al. 2003; Prchal and Guan 1993; Prchal et al. 1993, 1996).

17.5 Strategies for Identifying the Molecular Basis of Polycythemia Vera

Several different strategies have been employed to identify the primary molecular defect of PV. While some advances have been made, various detours along the way have led to dead ends, including claims of locating the PV somatic mutation at chromosome 20q, focusing on bcl-xL upregulation, c-mpl downregulation, and quantification of the *PRV-1* gene transcript, among others. Dissection of the erythropoietic process starting with Epo signal transduction has also received intense study and has yielded significant insights. Thus, the focus had been on hematopoietic cell phosphatase (SHP1) or on abnormal tyrosine kinases activated in the cytokine signaling pathway such as JAK2 (James et al. 2005; Ugo et al. 2004). Integration of all this historical information is helpful to understand and to dissect the complexity of the pathogenesis of PV. This underscores the likely involvement of multiple genetic events in the initiation of PV.

A simple and definitive diagnostic laboratory test for PV would be highly valuable but until recently none has existed. The validation of JAK2 mutation (see below) as a specific diagnostic test for PV awaits clinical verification.

17.5.1 Chromosomal and Cytogenetic Abnormalities

Unlike acute leukemias, only 10–15% of PV patients have chromosomal abnormalities making the genetic element difficult to localize by this approach. The most common single abnormality is the deletion in chromosome 20q (Bench et al. 2000). A group at Cambridge found anomalies on the long arm of chromosome 20 (20q) (Bench et al. 1998). Their most recent findings (Li et al. 2004) pointed to a genetic locus in the deleted region which undergoes as yet unrecognized imprinting. Unfortunately, these loci cannot be definitively linked to PV by segregation studies, thus their value to the elucidation of the PV defect is uncertain at this point and likely limited. Another group (Najfeld et al. 2002) detected variable lesions in the short arm of chromosome 9 (9p) in about one third of PV patients. Other reports, however, postulated that the gene amplification on chromosome 9p likely plays a crucial role in the pathogenesis of PV (Chen et al. 1998; Kralovics et al. 2002).

17.5.2 Functional Cloning

The basis for functional cloning is the assumption that the PV phenotype is caused by a dominant defective genetic element expressed in hematopoietic progenitor cells. This element could take the form of a mutated or overexpressed mRNA transcript. While the in vitro Epo independence was reproduced by transfection of normal stem cells by PV expression library, no consistent gene defects were identified (Kralovics et al. 1995).

17.5.3 Familial Polycythemia Vera

Analysis of familial PV can facilitate the search for the PV molecular defect. Familial PV is extremely rare with only a few documented cases. Using a genetic approach to identify the PV-causing gene in these families, we (Kralovics et al. 2003b) found that the familial predisposition to PV follows an autosomal dominant inheritance pattern with incomplete penetrance. All female family members with PV who were informative for a transcriptional clonality assay had clonal hematopoiesis. This underscores the fact that the disorder is acquired and not congenital. The genetic analyses positively excluded previously proposed candidate disease loci including the 9p LOH locus described below.

17.5.4 Genome Wide Search for Polycythemia Vera Mutation-9p LOH

By analyzing polymorphisms to differentiate DNA alleles in clonal granulocytes and polyclonal T lymphocytes (or fibroblasts) from the same PV patient, important insights were obtained. This technique was used to search for loss-of-heterozygosity (LOH) regions in the clonal cells. By screening the whole genome, LOH of chromosome 9p was detected in the absence of discernible cytogenetic anomalies. About one third of PV patients have LOH mediated by a mitotic crossover mechanism (Kralovics et al. 2002) on chromosome 9p.

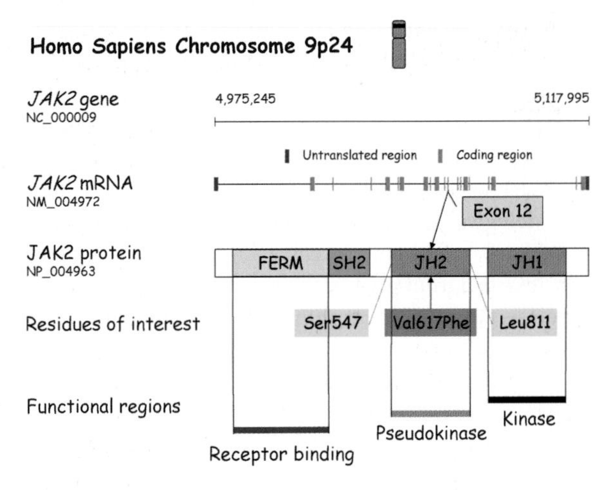

Fig. 17.3. Janus kinase 2 gene and protein structure and functional regions. Diagrammatic representation of the Janus Kinase 2 gene and protein structures are shown along with the FERM, SH2, JH2, and JH1 domains. The Val617Phe mutation is located in the JH2 pseudokinase domain. FERM, band 4.1(f), ezrin, radixin, and moesin; SH2, SRC homology 2; JH2, Janus kinase homology region 2; JH1, Janus kinase homology region 1

17.5.5 Janus Kinase 2 (Jak2) Mutation and Polycythemia Vera

The loss of heterozygosity (LOH) on chromosome 9p (Kralovics et al. 2002) suggested that this region harbors a mutation that contributes to clonal expansion of hematopoietic cells in PV. This region contains dozens of genes including an attractive candidate gene, JAK2 kinase (Pritchard et al. 1992; Ugo et al. 2004).

Jak2 is a member of the Janus kinase (Jak) family (JAK1, JAK2, JAK3, and TYK2) of protein tyrosine kinases (PTKs) involved in cytokine receptor signaling. Each family member has a kinase domain (JAK homology 1, or JH1) as well as a second pseudokinase domain with regulatory function immediately N-terminal to the PTK domain (JAK homology 2, or JH2). The presence of these two similar but functionally divergent domains was reminiscent of the Roman god Janus who could look simultaneously in two directions, hence the name (Fig. 17.3).

Jak2 is an important component of the Epo–Epo receptor signaling pathway. In addition to its kinase activity required for cytokine receptor signaling, Jak2 is also an essential subunit required for surface expression of cytokine receptors. Specifically, residues 32 to 58 of the JH7 N-terminal domain bind to EpoR in the endoplasmic reticulum and promote its cell surface expression (Huang et al. 2001).

Numerous cellular aspects of lymphoid and myeloid cell function are controlled by cytokines, all of which signal through a related and specific set of receptors. All these receptors are associated with one or more members of the Janus kinase family of kinases (Ihle 1995). These kinases phosphorylate various proteins along the signaling pathway and proteins in a unique family of transcription factors known as the signal transducers and activators of transcription, or STATs. The cytokine receptors included those for interleukin-3, interleukin-6, and Epo. Northern blot analysis detected expression of Jak2 in all tissues tested, except heart and skeletal muscle, with the highest expression detected in spleen, peripheral blood leukocytes, and testis. JAK2 can phosphorylate STAT1, STAT2, STAT3, STAT4, and STAT5, but not STAT6 (Saltzman et al. 1998). STAT5 in particular is important in Epo–EpoR signaling. It is activated in a broad spectrum of human hematological malignancies. Schwaller and colleagues showed that activation of STAT5 is necessary for the myelo- and lymphoproliferative disease induced by the TEL/JAK2 fusion gene (Schwaller et al. 2000).

Jak2-deficient mice are embryonic lethal due to the absence of definitive erythropoiesis and die around day 12.5 postcoitum (Neubauer et al. 1998; Parganas et al. 1998). Compared to Epo receptor-deficient mice, the phenotype of Jak2 deficiency was more severe. Fetal liver myeloid progenitors failed to respond to Epo, thrombopoietin, interleukin-3, or granulocyte/macrophage colony-stimulating factor. This is in contrast to the response to granulocyte-specific colony-stimulating factor, which was unaffected. It thus plays a pivotal and nonredundant role in the signal transduction of a specific group of cytokine receptors in hematopoiesis (Parganas et al. 1998).

Since PV has an intrinsic stem cell defect with dysregulation in granulopoiesis and thrombopoiesis, and the PV clone includes a variable proportion of B and T cells (Prchal 2005), searching for a functional defect in JAK2 was deemed by many in the field to be somewhat naïve. Nevertheless, Vainchenker's group (James et al. 2005; Ugo et al. 2004) was richly rewarded for focusing on JAK2. They found that the majority of PV patients (40 out of 45 patients or 88%) have a single nucleotide mutation (V617F) in the *JAK2* gene, a tyrosine kinase that is normally activated via the Epo–Epo receptor pathway in erythropoiesis (James et al. 2005). Remarkably, the presence of this mutation in most PV patients has been confirmed by several articles published in rapid succession (Baxter et al. 2005; Kralovics et al. 2005; Levine et al. 2005b; Zhao et al. 2005). Although these groups found exactly the same mutation, the logic and experimental approach were different and unique. Kralovics et al. started with prior observation that some PV patients had a loss of heterozygosity at chromosome 9p, which encompassed the JAK2 gene, leading them to search for mutations in JAK2 (Kralovics et al. 2002, 2005). The French group (James et al. 2005) previously observed inhibited endogenous erythroid colony formation in the presence of JAK2 inhibitors (Ugo et al. 2004). The Boston group were fishing for mutations in tyrosine kinases using samples from patients with myeloproliferative disorders with a high-throughput method that detected the JAK2 mutation (Levine et al. 2005b). The Cambridge group decided to focus on JAK2 after considering its pivotal role in signal transduction involving multiple cytokine receptors (Baxter et al. 2005).

The Cambridge, Basel, and Boston groups also found that 97% (71 of 73), 65% (83 of 128), and 74% (121 of 164) of their patients with PV, respectively, carried the same invariant and recurrent V617F mutation. (Baxter et al. 2005; Kralovics et al. 2005; Levine et al. 2005).

This single lesion alone can recapitulate many properties of native PV erythroid progenitors, including Epo independence as well as hypersensitivity of PV erythroid colonies. The V617F mutation was predicted to dysregulate kinase activity by disrupting the JH2 inhibitory regulation of JAK2, allowing the enzyme to be con-

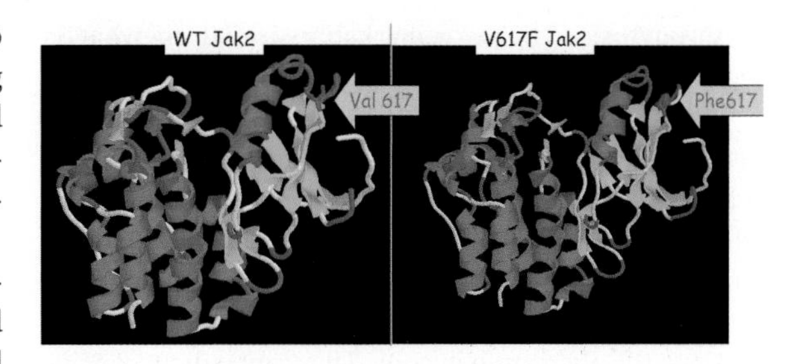

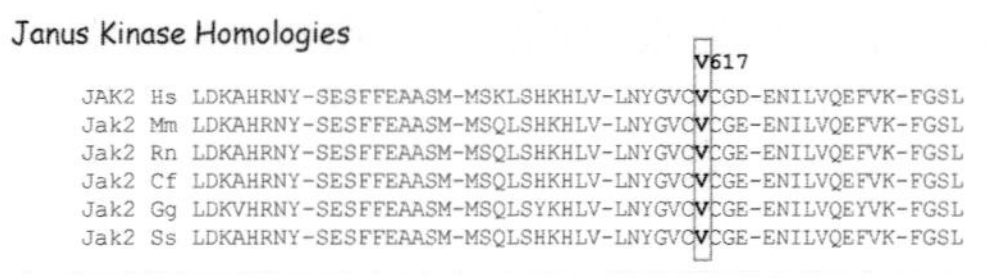

Fig. 17.4. Molecular model of Jak2 JH2 domain structure. An energy-minimized model of the Jak2 JH2 domain was constructed using the SwissModel automated structure modeling program [Schwede, T., Kopp, J., Guex, N., and Peitsch, M.C. (2003). SWISS-MODEL: An automated protein homology-modeling server. Nucleic Acids Res. 31, 3381–3385]. The amino acid sequence for residues Ser547 to Leu811 of the Jak2 JH2 domain was submitted to the SwissModel protein modeling server (http://swissmodel.expasy.org) using the crystallographic structure for Bruton's tyrosine kinase (Protein Data Bank http://www.pdb.org accession code 1K2P) as a three-dimensional template [Mao, C., Zhou, M., and Uckun, F.M. (2001). Crystal structure of Bruton's tyrosine kinase domain suggests a novel pathway for activation and provides insights into the molecular basis of X-linked agammaglobulinemia. J. Biol. Chem. 276, 41435–41443]. The larger, mainly alpha-helical C-globule and the smaller N-globule composed mostly of beta-sheets along with Val617 (in *red*) is shown. The figure was made using the RasMol program. A sequence alignment of part of the JH2 domain is shown below with residue 617 highlighted in red. Hs, Homo sapiens (human); Mm, Mus musculus (mouse); Rn, Rattus norvegicus (rat); Cf, Canis familiaris (dog); Gg, Gallus gallus (chicken); Ss, Sus scrofa (pig)

stitutively activated (Fig. 17.4). The mutant Jak2 was shown to promote constitutive tyrosine phosphorylation activity (Baxter et al. 2005; Kralovics et al. 2005), which could then bind to a receptor and recruit STATs in the complete absence or in the presence of trace amounts of hematopoietic growth factors. The Cambridge group also showed that all PV patients with the mutation had cells that formed in vitro erythroid colonies in the absence of erythropoietin (Baxter et al. 2005). This nicely explains the long-standing observation of in vitro cytokine hypersensitivity.

The Paris group provided most direct evidence connecting this Jak2 mutation to the PV phenotype (James et al. 2005). When they retrovirally transduced the mutant gene into murine bone marrow cells, the transplanted mice exhibited a clinical phenotype including erythrocytosis. This is remarkably similar to what is seen in a typical patient (James et al. 2005).

Given that most PV patients examined so far are heterozygous and have only one mutated *JAK2* allele, such a mutant should be a "*dominant*" with overriding effects on a normal *JAK2* allele. Surprisingly, the simultaneous introduction of mutant and wild-type *JAK2* genes into reporter cells (James et al. 2005) did not reproduce the aberrant behavior. This contradicts conclusion of a "dominant" mutation by other investigators (Kralovics et al. 2005; Levine et al. 2005b) who utilized a different experimental approach. Kralovics et al. (Kralovics et al. 2005) identified the V617F mutation in all 51 patients with LOH of chromosome 9p. For patients without 9p LOH, 66 out of 193 were heterozygous for V617F and 127 did not have the mutation.

Interestingly, a subset (30%) of PV patients are homozygous and thus have the same mutation in both *JAK2* alleles (Kralovics et al. 2002). As a result of mitotic recombination or a phenomenon known as uniparental disomy, the loss of heterozygosity in most cases is caused by duplication of a portion of the chromosome 9p bearing the mutated *JAK2* (Kralovics et al. 2002) in a multipotent progenitor capable of giving rise to erythroid and myeloid cells. Although identification of the *JAK2* mutation solved many mysteries, it raised many more provocative questions. For one, a significant proportion of patients with idiopathic myelofibrosis (IMF) and essential thrombocythemia (ET) were also reported to harbor this mutation. From recent publications, the incidence of *JAK2* mutations reported ranged from 74 to 97% in PV, 35 to 50% in IMF, and 33 to 57% in ET. Baxter et al. determined that 29 (57%) of 51 patients with essential thrombocythemia, and 8 (50%) of 16 patients with idiopathic myelofibrosis had a G-to-T transversion in exon 12 of the *JAK2* gene, (V617F) in the negative regulatory JH2 domain (Baxter et al. 2005). Kralovics et al. detected the V617F mutation at a frequency of 57% (13 of 23) among patients with idiopathic myelofibrosis, and 23% (21 of 93) among patients with essential thrombocythemia (Kralovics et al. 2005). Finally, Jak2 V617F was also identified in 32% (37 of 115) ET and 35% (16 of 46) MMM patients by the Boston group (Levine et al. 2005b) (Table 17.2). How does the same exact acquired mutation cause three distinct clinical entities? Could these patients with *JAK2* mutations exhibit a variant form of PV, or early or late (spent) phases of PV? Are there other mutations acting in concert with the mutant *JAK2*? Are other genetic abnormalities present before or

Table 17.2. Human hematologic malignancies with dysregulated protein kinases

Malignancy	Protein kinase
ALCL	ALK-1
ALL	BCR-ABL
	FLT3
	TEL-ABL
	TEL-JAK2
AML	BCR-ABL
	FMS
	KIT
	FLT3
	PDGFRβ
	TEL-ABL
AML/MPD	FGFR
CEL	PDGFRα
CML	BCR-ABL
Atypical CML	TEL-ABL
	TEL-JAK2
CMML	FMS
	PDGFRβ
HES	PDGFRα
	PDGFRβ
MDS	FMS
	FLT3
PV/ET/IMF	JAK2
SMCD	KIT
	PDGFRα

ALL, acute lymphoblastic leukemia; ALCL, anaplastic large cell lymphoma; AML, acute myeloid leukemia; CEL, chronic eosinophilic leukemia; CML, chronic myelogenous leukemia; CMML, chronic myelomonocytic leukemia; ET, essential thrombocythemia; IMF, idiopathic myelofibrosis; HES, hypereosinophilic syndrome; MDS, myelodysplastic syndrome; MPD, myeloproliferative disorder; PV, polycythemia vera; SMCD, systemic mast cell disease/systemic mastocytosis; ALK-1, anaplastic lymphoma kinase-1; BCR-ABL, breakpoint cluster region/v-abl abelson murine leukemia viral oncogene homolog; fms, mcdonough feline sarcoma viral (v-fms) oncogene homolog; (colony stimulating factor 1 receptor); KIT, v-kit Hardy-Zuckerman 4 feline sarcoma viral oncogene homolog; (stem cell factor receptor); FGFR, fibroblast growth factor receptor; FLT3, Fms-related tyrosine kinase 3; JAK2, janus kinase 2; PDGFRα, platelet derived growth factor receptor alpha; PDGFRβ, platelet derived growth factor receptor beta; TEL-ABL, ETS variant gene 6 (TEL oncogene) – ABL fusion protein; TEL-JAK2, TEL-Janus kinase 2 fusion protein after the acquisition of the *JAK2* mutation? What makes a relatively benign condition (PV) progress to acute leukemia in some, but not all, cases? These and many other questions will make for exciting explorations in ongoing investigations.

Are there some other somatic changes necessary for the development of diverse phenotypes of multiple hematopoietic disorders? Interestingly, patients with the V617F mutation had the disease longer with a corresponding higher rate of hemorrhagic, thrombotic, and fibrotic complications (Kralovics et al. 2005) compared to patients with wild-type *JAK2*. In addition, patients homozygous for the V617F mutation also had the disease longer those who were heterozygous. The temporal lag could be due to the progressive or step-wise acquisition of homozygosity (Kralovics et al. 2005). The allelic ratio of *JAK2* V617F is highly correlated with clonality for PV but not for ET or MMM, which suggests that the V617F mutation may be sufficient for the development of PV, but additional genetic events may be necessary in ET and MMM (Levine et al. 2006). Patients with idiopathic myelofibrosis carrying the V617F mutation had higher neutrophil and white cell counts compared to noncarriers (Campbell et al. 2006). Patients positive for V617F were also less likely to require blood transfusion but had poorer overall survival (Campbell et al. 2006).

Secondly, more recent data suggest that *JAK2* mutations may not be the specific lesion for PV. A Mayo clinic study reported that 5% of 101 patients with myelodysplastic syndrome have this mutation (Steensma et al. 2005). In addition, some patients with chronic myelomonocytic and neutrophilic leukemias also harbor the same mutation (Steensma et al. 2005). Another report by the M.D. Anderson group in Houston which analyzed 325 patients with various hematological malignancies, confirmed the Mayo clinic findings in myelodysplastic syndrome and chronic myelomonocytic and neutrophilic leukemias. They documented the same *JAK2* V617F mutation in 25% of patients with Ph-negative chronic myelogenous leukemia and 18% of patients with megakaryocytic leukemia, but only in 5/10 acute myeloid leukemia patients with an antecedent PV (Jelinek et al. 2005). In another study, a survey of 480 MPD patients, Jones et al. found that 20% of atypical MPD, 2% of idiopathic hypereosinophilic syndrome, 81% of PV 58/72 (81%), 41% of essential thrombocythemia, and 43% of idiopathic myelofibrosis patient samples were positive for the JAK2 V617F mutation (Jones et al. 2005). None of their patients with systemic mastocytosis, chronic or acute myeloid leukemia, secondary erythrocytosis or normal controls carry the mutation. Interestingly, although they detected homozygosity for V617F in 43% of mutant samples, homozygous ET samples were less common compared to other MPD subtypes. PRV-1 expression levels were significantly higher in cases with the V617F mutation compared to those without. The *JAK2* V617F allele was also found in acute and chronic myeloid malignancies (Lee et al. 2006; Levine et al. 2005a) but not in lymphoid malignancies (Levine et al. 2005a).

Table 17.3. Frequency of JAK2 V617F mutation in myeloproliferative disorders

Group principal investigator	PV	ET	IMF
Anthony R Green	97%	57%	50%
(Lancet **365**:9464, 2005)	71 of 73 patients	29 of 51 patients	8 of 16 patients
D Gary Gilliland	74%	33%	35%
(Cancer Cell **7**:387, 2005)	121 of 164 patients	37 of 115 patients	16 of 46 patients
William Vainchenker	89%	43%	43%
(Nature **434**:1144, 2005)	40 of 45 patients	9 of 21 patients	3 of 7 patients
Radek Skoda	65%	23%	57%
(NEJM **352**:17, 2005)	83 of 128 patients	21 of 93 patients	12 of 23 patients
Cumulative	77%	34%	42%
	315 of 410 patients	96 of 280 patients	39 of 92 patients

ET, essential thrombocythemia; IMF, idiopathic myelofibrosis; PV, polycythemia vera; NEJM, New England Journal of Medicine

Finally, while we can account for the effects of mutated *JAK2* on erythropoiesis, how do we ascribe its functions in myeloid, megakaryocytic, and pluripotent stem cells? Although majority T lymphocytes do not harbor the V617F *JAK2* mutation (Kralovics et al. 2005), it is still clear that the initiating mutation occurs in hematopoietic stem cells (Kralovics et al. 2002). The lesion may not be compatible with lymphocyte differentiation and hence selected against. Conditional knock-in mice harboring the *V617F JAK2* mutation may help to resolve this issue as well as ongoing studies in Vainchenker's group of longitudinal follow-up of their *V617F JAK2* mouse (James et al. 2005). Are there some other genetic events essential for creating the full PV phenotype? What is the primary PV lesion? These and other questions will be answered in future experiments. Nevertheless, this is clearly the most important discovery as yet in our understanding of PV pathogenesis. PV and maybe IMF and ET have now joined the ranks of hematological disorders with dysregulated protein kinases (Table 17.3).

17.6 Treatment Options

Although there is currently no cure for PV, phlebotomy is helpful as a treatment option in preventing hemodynamic and rheologic complications (Wagner et al. 2001), the exact level of hematocrit has not been determined, and it is likely that factors other than elevated hematocrit are equally or more important in thrombophilic risk of PV (Prchal and Beutler 2005).

Elucidation of the *JAK2* V617F mutation as a causative constituent of the PV phenotype will have a fundamental impact on the diagnosis of myeloproliferative disorders. At the very least, a new molecular classification can be established. It will also provide an obvious target for rational drug design in the treatment of PV. Hopefully, a pharmacological inhibitor can be found which could replicate the success of imatinib mesylate in the treatment of CML, to the benefit of PV patients.

17.7 Conclusion

Growing evidence and research data strongly suggest the involvement of multiple genetic loci in initiating the PV phenotype. Elucidation of the molecular basis of PV will therefore entail a multipronged strategy to delineate these genetic lesions. Because PV is a relatively rare disease, close collaboration of multiple clinical research centers coupled with close interaction with laboratory scientists will lead to accelerated progress in unraveling the mechanism(s) underlying PV. The feasibility of such a collaboration was aptly demonstrated by a recent publication "The European Collaboration on Low-dose Aspirin in Polycythemia Vera (ECLAP)" which involved the participation of over 1600 patients (Landolfi et al. 2004).

References

Ang SO, Chen H, Gordeuk VR, Sergueeva AI, Polyakova LA, Miasnikova GY, Kralovics R, Stockton DW, Prchal JT (2002a) Endemic polycythemia in Russia: mutation in the VHL gene. Blood Cells Mol Dis 28:57–62

Ang SO, Chen H, Hirota K, Gordeuk VR, Jelinek J, Guan Y, Liu E, Sergueeva AI, Miasnikova GY, Mole D, Maxwell PH, Stockton DW, Semenza GL, Prchal JT (2002b) Disruption of oxygen homeostasis underlies congenital Chuvash polycythemia. Nat Genet 32:614–621. Epub 2002 Nov 4

Arcasoy MO, Degar BA, Harris KW, Forget BG (1997) Familial erythrocytosis associated with a short deletion in the erythropoietin receptor gene. Blood 89:4628–4635

Baxter EJ, Scott LM, Campbell PJ, East C, Fourouclas N, Swanton S, Vassiliou GS, Bench AJ, Boyd EM, Curtin N, Scott MA, Erber WN, Green AR (2005) Acquired mutation of the tyrosine kinase JAK2 in human myeloproliferative disorders. Lancet 365:1054–1061

Beck I, Ramirez S, Weinmann R, Caro J (1991) Enhancer element at the 3′-flanking region controls transcriptional response to hypoxia in the human erythropoietin gene. J Biol Chem 266:15563–15566

Beck I, Weinmann R, Caro J (1993) Characterization of hypoxia-responsive enhancer in the human erythropoietin gene shows presence of hypoxia-inducible 120-Kd nuclear DNA binding protein in erythropoietin-producing and nonproducing cells. Blood 82:704–711

Bench AJ, Nacheva EP, Champion KM, Green AR (1998) Molecular genetics and cytogenetics of myeloproliferative disorders. Baillieres Clin Haematol 11:819–848

Bench AJ, Nacheva EP, Hood TL, Holden JL, French L, Swanton S, Champion KM, Li J, Whittaker P, Stavrides G, Hunt AR, Huntly BJ, Campbell LJ, Bentley DR, Deloukas P, Green AR (2000) Chromosome 20 deletions in myeloid malignancies: reduction of the common deleted region, generation of a PAC/BAC contig and identification of candidate genes. UK Cancer Cytogenetics Group (UKCCG). Oncogene 19:3902–3913

Bento MC, Ribeiro ML, Cunha E, Rebelo U, Granjo E, Granado C, Tamagnini GP (2000) Hb Vila Real [beta36(C2)Pro → His]: a newly discovered high oxygen affinity variant. Hemoglobin 24:59–63

Berlin NI (1975) Diagnosis and classification of the polycythemias. Sem Hematol 12:339–351

Beutler E, Collins Z, Irwin LE (1967) Value of genetic variants of glucose-6-phosphate dehydrogenase in tracing the origin of malignant tumors. N Eng J Med 276:389–391

Bhattacharya S, Michels CL, Leung MK, Arany ZP, Kung AL, Livingston DM (1999) Functional role of p35srj, a novel p300/CBP binding protein, during transactivation by HIF-1. Genes Dev 13:64–75

Birgegard G, Wide L (1992) Serum erythropoietin in the diagnosis of polycythaemia ad after phlebotomy treatment. Br J Haematol 81:603–606

Brox AG, Congote LF, Fafard J, Fauser AA (1989) Identification and characterization of an 8-kd peptide stimulating late erythropoiesis. Exp Hematol 17:769–773

Bruick RK (2000) Expression of the gene encoding the proapoptotic Nip3 protein is induced by hypoxia. Proc Nat Acad Sci USA 97:9082–9087

Bunn HF, Poyton RO (1996) Oxygen sensing and molecular adaptation to hypoxia. Physiol Rev 76:839–885

Campbell PJ, Griesshammer M, Dohner K, Dohner H, Kusec R, Hasselbalch HC, Larsen TS, Pallisgaard N, Giraudier S, Le Bousse-Kerdiles MC, Desterke C, Guerton B, Dupriez B, Bordessoule D, Fenaux P, Kiladjian JJ, Viallard JF, Briere J, Harrison CN, Green AR, Reilly JT (2006) V617F mutation in JAK2 is associated with poorer survival in idiopathic myelofibrosis. Blood 107:2098–2100

Caniggia I, Mostachfi H, Winter J, Gassmann M, Lye SJ, Kuliszewski M, Post M (2000) Hypoxia-inducible factor-1 mediates the biological effects of oxygen on human trophoblast differentiation through TGFbeta(3). J Clin Invest 105:577–587

Carbone V, Salzano A M, Pagano L, Viola A, Buffardi S, De Rosa C, Pucci P (1999) Hb Rainier [beta145(HC2)Tyr → Cys] in Italy. Characterization of the amino acid substitution and the DNA mutation. Hemoglobin 23:111–124

Cario H, Schwarz K, Jorch N, Kyank U, Petrides PE, Schneider DT, Uhle R, Debatin KM, Kohne E (2005) Mutations in the von Hippel-Lindau (VHL) tumor suppressor gene and VHL-haplotype analysis in patients with presumable congenital erythrocytosis. Haematologica 90:19–24

Carmeliet P, Dor Y, Herbert JM, Fukumura D, Brusselmans K, Dewerchin M, Neeman M, Bono F, Abramovitch R, Maxwell P, Koch CJ, Ratcliffe P, Moons L, Jain RK, Collen D, Keshert E (1998) Role of HIF-1alpha in hypoxia-mediated apoptosis, cell proliferation and tumour angiogenesis. Nature 394:485–490

Charache S, Weatherall DJ, Clegg JB (1966) Polycythemia associated with a hemoglobinopathy. J Clin Invest 45:813–822

Chen Z, Notohamiprodjo M, Guan XY, Paietta E, Blackwell S, Stout K, Turner A, Richkind K, Trent JM, Lamb A, Sandberg AA (1998) Gain of 9p in the pathogenesis of polycythemia vera. Genes Chromosomes Cancer 22:321–324

Clegg JB, Naughton MA, Weatherball DJ (1966) Abnormal human haemoglobins. Separation and characterization of the alpha and beta chains by chromatography, and the determination of two new variants, hb Chesapeak and Hb J (Bangkok). J Mol Biol 19:91–108

Cockman ME, Masson N, Mole DR, Jaakkola P, Chang GW, Clifford SC, Maher ER, Pugh CW, Ratcliffe PJ, Maxwell PH (2000) Hypoxia inducible factor-alpha binding and ubiquitylation by the von Hippel-Lindau tumor suppressor protein. J Biol Chem 275:25733–25741

Constantinescu SN, Keren T, Socolovsky M, Nam H, Henis YI, Lodish HF (2001) Ligand-independent oligomerization of cell-surface erythropoietin receptor is mediated by the transmembrane domain. Proc Nat Acad Sci USA 98:4379–4384

Cormier-Regard S, Nguyen SV, Claycomb WC (1998) Adrenomedullin gene expression is developmentally regulated and induced by hypoxia in rat ventricular cardiac myocytes. J Biol Chem 273:17787–17792

Cramer T, Yamanishi Y, Clausen BE, Forster I, Pawlinski R, Mackman N, Haase VH, Jaenisch R, Corr M, Nizet V, Firestein GS, Gerber HP, Ferrara N, Johnson RS (2003) HIF-1 alpha is essential for myeloid cell-mediated inflammation. Cell 112:645–657

Curnutte JT, Hopkins PJ, Kuhl W, Beutler E (1992) Studying X inactivation. Lancet 339:749

De La Chapelle A, Sistonen P, Lehvaslaiho H, Ikkala E, Juvonen E (1993a) Familial erythrocytosis genetically linked to erythropoietin receptor gene. Lancet 341:82–84

De La Chapelle A, Traskelin AL, Juvonen E (1993b) Truncated erythropoietin receptor causes dominantly inherited benign human erythrocytosis. Proc Nat Acad Sci USA 90:4495–4499

Dietrich WF, Lander ES, Smith JS, Moser AR, Gould KA, Luongo C, Borenstein N, Dove W (1993) Genetic identification of Mom-1, a major modifier locus affecting Min-induced intestinal neoplasia in the mouse. Cell 75:631–639

Divoky V, Liu Z, Ryan TM, Prchal JF, Townes TM, Prchal JT (2001) Mouse model of congenital polycythemia: Homologous replacement of murine gene by mutant human erythropoietin receptor gene. Proc Nat Acad Sci USA 98:986–991

Eckhart AD, Yang N, Xin X, Faber JE (1997) Characterization of the alpha1B-adrenergic receptor gene promoter region and hypoxia regulatory elements in vascular smooth muscle. Proc Nat Acad Sci USA 94:9487–9492

Eckardt KU, Ratcliffe PJ, Tan CC, Bauer C, Kurtz A (1992) Age-dependent expression of the erythropoietin gene in rat liver and kidneys. J Clin Invest 89:753–760

Ema M, Hirota K, Mimura J, Abe H, Yodoi J, Sogawa K, Poellinger L, Fujii-Kuriyama Y (1999) Molecular mechanisms of transcription activation by HLF and HIF1alpha in response to hypoxia: their stabilization and redox signal-induced interaction with CBP/p300. EMBO J 18:1905–1914

Epstein AC, Gleadle JM, Mcneill LA, Hewitson KS, O'rourke J, Mole DR, Mukherji M, Metzen E, Wilson MI, Dhanda A, Tian YM, Masson N, Hamilton DL, Jaakkola P, Barstead R, Hodgkin J, Maxwell PH, Pugh CW, Schofield CJ, Ratcliffe PJ (2001) C. elegans EGL-9 and mammalian homologs define a family of dioxygenases that regulate HIF by prolyl hydroxylation. Cell 107:43–54

Erkelens DW, Statius Van Eps LW (1973) Bartter's syndrome and erythrocytosis. Am J Med 55:711–719

Feldser D, Agani F, Iyer NV, Pak B, Ferreira G, Semenza GL (1999) Reciprocal positive regulation of hypoxia-inducible factor 1alpha and insulin-like growth factor 2. Cancer Res 59:3915–3918

Fisher MJ, Prchal JF, Prchal JT, D'Andrea AD (1994) Anti-erythropoietin (EPO) receptor monoclonal antibodies distinguish EPO-dependent and EPO-independent erythroid progenitors in polycythemia vera. Blood 84:1982–1991

Fruchtman SM (2004) Treatment paradigms in the management of myeloproliferative disorders. Sem Hematol 41:18–22

Furukawa T, Narita M, Sakaue M, Otsuka T, Kuroha T, Masuko M, Azegami T, Kishi K, Takahashi M, Utsumi J, Koike T, Aizawa Y (1997) Primary familial polycythaemia associated with a novel point mutation in the erythropoietin receptor. Br J Haematol 99:222–227

Gerber HP, Condorelli F, Park J, Ferrara N (1997) Differential transcriptional regulation of the two vascular endothelial growth factor receptor genes. Flt-1, but not Flk-1/KDR, is up-regulated by hypoxia. J Biol Chem 272:23659–23667

Gordeuk VR, Sergueeva AI, Miasnikova GY, Okhotin D, Voloshin Y, Choyke PL, Butman JA, Jedlickova K, Prchal JT, Polyakova LA (2004) Congenital disorder of oxygen sensing: association of the homozygous Chuvash polycythemia VHL mutation with thrombosis and vascular abnormalities but not tumors. Blood 103:3924–3932

Gordeuk VR, Stockton DW, Prchal JT (2005) Congenital polycythemias/erythrocytoses. Haematologica 90:109–116

Gradin K, Mcguire J, Wenger RH, Kvietikova I, Whitelaw ML (1996) Functional interference between hypoxia and dioxin signal transduction pathways: competition for recruitement of the Arnt transcription factor. Mol Cell Biol 16:5221–5231

Gregg XT, Prchal JT (2005) Polycythemia vera and essential thrombocythemia. In: Young N (ed) Clinical hematology. Mosby, St. Louis, pp 470–485

Gregg XT, Liu Y, Prchal JT, Gartland GL, Cooper MD, Prchal JF (1996) Clonality in myeloproliferative disorders. Blood 88:1905a

Haase VH, Glickman JN, Socolovsky M, Jaenisch R (2001) Vascular tumors in livers with targeted inactivation of the von Hippel-Lindau tumor suppressor. Proc Nat Acad Sci U S A 98:1583–1588

Harano T, Harano K, Shibata S, Ueda S, Imai K, Seki M (1983) Hemoglobin Tokoname [alpha 139 (HC 1) Lys leads to Thr]: a new hemoglobin variant with a slightly increased oxygen affinity. Hemoglobin 7:85–90

Harano T, Harano K, Imai K, Terunuma S (1996) HB Swan River [alpha 6(A4)ASP → Gly] observed in a Japanese man. Hemoglobin 20:75–78

Hogenesch JB, Chan WK, Jackiw VH, Brown RC, Gu Y-Z (1997) Characterization of a subset of the basic helix-loop-helix-PAS superfamily that interacts with components of the dioxin signalling pathway. J Biol Chem 272:8581–8593

Hoyer JD, Wick MJ, Thibodeau SN, Viker KA, Conner R, Fairbanks VF (1998) Hb Tak confirmed by DNA analysis: not expressed as thalassemia in a Hb Tak/Hb E compound heterozygote. Hemoglobin 22:45–52

Hu J, Discher DJ, Bishopric NH, Webster KA (1998) Hypoxia regulates expression of the endothelin-1 gene through a proximal hypoxia-inducible factor-1 binding site on the antisense strand. Biochem Biophys Res Commun 245:894–899

Huang LE, Arany Z, Livingston DM, Bunn HF (1996) Activation of hypoxia-inducible transcription factor depends primarily upon redox-sensitive stabilization of its alpha subunit. J Biol Chem 271:32253–32259

Huang LE, Gu J, Schau M, Bunn HF (1998) Regulation of hypoxia-inducible factor 1alpha is mediated by and oxygen-dependent degradation domain via the ubiquitin-proteasome pathway. Proc Nat Acad Sci U S A 95:7987–7992

Huang LJ, Constantinescu SN, Lodish HF (2001) The N-terminal domain of Janus kinase 2 is required for Golgi processing and cell surface expression of erythropoietin receptor. Mol Cell 8:1327–1338

Ihle JN (1995) Cytokine receptor signalling. Nature 377:591–594

Ivan M, Kondo K, Yang H, Kim W, Valiando J, Ohh M, Salic A, Asara JM, Lane WS, Kaelin WG Jr. (2001) HIFalpha targeted for VHL-mediated destruction by proline hydroxylation: implications for O2 sensing [see comments]. Science 292:464–468

Iyer NV, Kotch LE, Agani F, Leung SW, Laughner E, Wenger RH, Gassmann M, Gearhart JD, Lawler AM, Yu AY, Semenza GL (1998) Cellular and developmental control of O2 homeostasis by hypoxia-inducible factor 1 alpha. Genes, Development 12:149–162

Jaakkola P, Mole DR, Tian YM, Wilson MI, Gielbert J, Gaskell SJ, Kriegsheim A, Hebestreit HF, Mukherji M, Schofield CJ, Maxwell PH, Pugh CW, Ratcliffe PJ (2001) Targeting of HIF-alpha to the von Hippel-Lindau ubiquitylation complex by O2-regulated prolyl hydroxylation. [see comments.]. Science 292:468–472

Jacobson LO, Goldwasser E, Fried W, Plzak L (2000) Role of the kidney in erythropoiesis. 1957. J Am Soc Nephrol 11:589–590

James C, Ugo V, Le Couedic JP, Staerk J, Delhommeau F, Lacout C, Garcon L, Raslova H, Berger R, Bennaceur-Griscelli A, Villeval JL, Constantinescu SN, Casadevall N, Vainchenker W (2005) A unique clonal JAK2 mutation leading to constitutive signalling causes polycythaemia vera. Nature 434:1144–1148

Jelinek J, Oki Y, Gharibyan V, Bueso-Ramos C, Prchal JT, Verstovsek S, Beran M, Estey E, Kantarjian HM, Issa JP (2005) JAK2 mutation 1849G → T is rare in acute leukemias but can be found in CMML, Philadelphia-chromosome negative CML and megakaryocytic leukemia. Blood 106:3370–3373

Jiang BH, Rue E, Wang GL, Roe R, Semenza GL (1996) Dimerization, DNA binding, and transactivation properties of hypoxia-inducible factor 1. J Biol Chem 271:17771–17778

Jiang BH, Zheng JZ, Leung SW, Roe R, Semenza GL (1997) Transactivation and inhibitory domains of hypoxia-inducible factor 1alpha. Modulation of transcriptional activity by oxygen tension. J Biol Chem 272:19253–19260

Jones AV, Kreil S, Zoi K, Waghorn K, Curtis C, Zhang L, Score J, Seear R, Chase AJ, Grand FH, White H, Zoi C, Loukopoulos D, Terpos E, Vervessou EC, Schultheis B, Emig M, Ernst T, Lengfelder E, Hehlmann R, Hochhaus A, Oscier D, Silver RT, Reiter A, Cross NC (2005) Widespread occurrence of the JAK2 V617F mutation in chronic myeloproliferative disorders. Blood 107:3339–33341

Kallio PJ, Okamoto K, O'Brien S, Carrero P, Makino Y, Tanaka H, Poellinger L (1998) Signal transduction in hypoxic cells: inducible nuclear translocation and recruitment of the CBP/p300 coactivator by the hypoxia-inducible factor-1alpha. EMBO J 17:6573–6586

Kietzmann T, Roth U, Jungermann K (1999) Induction of the plasminogen activator inhibitor-1 gene expression by mild hypoxia via a hypoxia response element binding the hypoxia-inducible factor-1 in rat hepatocytes. Blood 94:4177–4185

Kiger L, Kister J, Groff P, Kalmes G, Prome D, Galacteros F, Wajcman H (1996) Hb J-Europa [beta 62(E6)Ala → Asp]: normal oxygen binding properties in a new variant involving a residue located distal to the heme. Hemoglobin 20:135–140

Klingmuller U, Lorenz U, Cantley LC, Neel BG, Lodish HF (1995) Specific recruitment of SH-PTP1 to the erythropoietin receptor causes inactivation of JAK2 and termination of proliferative signals. Cell 80:729–738

Klippel S, Strunck E, Busse CE, Behringer D, Pahl HL (2002) Biochemical characterization of PRV-1, a novel hematopoietic cell surface receptor, which is overexpressed in polycythemia rubra vera. Blood 100:2441–2448

Knudson AG, Jr., Strong LC (1972) Mutation and cancer: neuroblastoma and pheochromocytoma. Am J Human Genet 24:514–532

Koury MJ, Bondurant MC (1990) Erythropoietin retards DNA breakdown and prevents programmed death in erythroid progenitor cells. Science 248:378–381

Kralovics R, Prchal JT (2000) Congenital and inherited polycythemia. Curr Opin Pediatr 12:29–34

Kralovics R, Prchal JT (2001) Genetic heterogeneity of primary familial and congenital polycythemia. Am J Hematol 68:115–121

Kralovics R, Sokol L, Prchal JF, Prchal JT (1995) Identification of putative molecular lesion of polycythemia vera phenotype. Blood 86:1066a

Kralovics R, Indrak K, Stopka T, Berman BW, Prchal JF, Prchal JT (1997 a) Two new EPO receptor mutations: truncated EPO receptors are most frequently associated with primary familial and congenital polycythemias. Blood 90:2057–2061

Kralovics R, Sokol L, Broxson EH, Jr., Prchal JT (1997 b) The erythropoietin receptor gene is not linked with the polycythemia phenotype in a family with autosomal dominant primary polycythemia. Proc Assoc Am Physicians 109:580–585

Kralovics R, Sokol L, Prchal JT (1998) Absence of polycythemia in a child with a unique erythropoietin receptor mutation in a family with autosomal dominant primary polycythemia. J Clin Invest 102:124–129

Kralovics R, Guan Y, Prchal JT (2002) Acquired uniparental disomy of chromosome 9p is a frequent stem cell defect in polycythemia vera. Exp Hematol 30:229–236

Kralovics R, Buser AS, Teo SS, Coers J, Tichelli A, Van Der Maas AP, Skoda RC (2003 a) Comparison of molecular markers in a cohort of patients with chronic myeloproliferative disorders. Blood 102:1869–1871

Kralovics R, Stockton DW, Prchal JT (2003 b) Clonal hematopoiesis in familial polycythemia vera suggests the involvement of multiple mutational events in the early pathogenesis of the disease. Blood 102:3793–3796

Kralovics R, Passamonti F, Buser AS, Teo SS, Tiedt R, Passweg JR, Tichelli A, Cazzola M, Skoda RC (2005) A gain-of-function mutation of JAK2 in myeloproliferative disorders. N Engl J Med 352:1779–1790

Kutti J, Ridell B (2001) Epidemiology of the myeloproliferative disorders: essential thrombocythaemia, polycythaemia vera and idiopathic myelofibrosis. Pathologie-Biologie (Paris) 49:164–166

Lando D, Peet DJ, Whelan DA, Gorman JJ, Whitelaw ML (2002) Asparagine hydroxylation of the HIF transactivation domain: a hypoxic switch. Science 295:858–861

Landolfi R, Marchioli R, Kutti J, Gisslinger H, Tognoni G, Patrono C, Barbui T (2004) Efficacy and safety of low-dose aspirin in polycythemia vera. N Engl J Med 350:114–124

Le Couedic JP, Mitjavila MT, Villeval JL, Feger F, Gobert S, Mayeux P, Casadevall N, Vainchenker W (1996) Missense mutation of the erythropoietin receptor is a rare event in human erythroid malignancies. Blood 87:1502–1511

Lee JW, Kim YG, Soung YH, Han KJ, Kim SY, Rhim HS, Min WS, Nam SW, Park WS, Lee JY, Yoo NJ, Lee SH (2006) The JAK2 V617F mutation in de novo acute myelogenous leukemias. Oncogene 25:1434–1436

Lee PJ, Jiang BH, Chin BY, Iyer NV, Alam J, Semenza GL, Choi AM (1997) Hypoxia-inducible factor-1 mediates transcriptional activation of the heme oxygenase-1 gene in response to hypoxia. J Biol Chem 272:5375–5381

Levine RL, Loriaux M, Huntly BJ, Loh ML, Beran M, Stoffregen E, Berger R, Clark JJ, Willis SG, Nguyen KT, Flores NJ, Estey E, Gattermann N, Armstrong S, Look AT, Griffin JD, Bernard OA, Heinrich MC, Gilliland DG, Druker B, Deininger MW (2005 a) The JAK2V617F activating mutation occurs in chronic myelomonocytic leukemia and acute myeloid leukemia, but not in acute lymphoblastic leukemia or chronic lymphocytic leukemia. Blood 106:3377–3379

Levine RL, Wadleigh M, Cools J, Ebert BL, Wernig G, Huntly BJ, Boggon TJ, Wlodarska I, Clark JJ, Moore S, Adelsperger J, Koo S, Lee JC, Gabriel S, Mercher T, D'andrea A, Frohling S, Dohner K, Marynen P, Vandenberghe P, Mesa RA, Tefferi A, Griffin JD, Eck MJ, Sellers WR, Meyerson M, Golub T, Lee SJ, Gilliland DG (2005 b) Activating mutation in the tyrosine kinase JAK2 in polycythemia vera, essential thrombocythemia, and myeloid metaplasia with myelofibrosis. Cancer Cell 7:387–397

Levine RL, Belisle C, Wadleigh M, Zahrieh D, Lee S, Chagnon P, Gilliland DG, Busque L (2006) X-inactivation based clonality analysis and quantitative JAK2V617F assessment reveals a strong association between clonality and JAK2V617F in PV but not ET/MMM, and identifies a subset of JAK2V617F negative ET and MMM patients with clonal hematopoiesis. Blood 24:24

Li J, Bench AJ, Vassiliou GS, Fourouclas N, Ferguson-Smith AC, Green AR (2004) Imprinting of the human L3MBTL gene, a polycomb family member located in a region of chromosome 20 deleted in human myeloid malignancies. Proc Nat Acad Sci USA 101:7341–7346

Liu E, Jelinek J, Pastore YD, Guan Y, Prchal JF, Prchal JT (2003) Discrimination of polycythemias and thrombocytoses by novel, simple, accurate clonality assays and comparison with PRV-1 expression and BFU-E response to erythropoietin. Blood 101:3294–3301

Liu E, Percy MJ, Amos CI, Guan Y, Shete S, Stockton DW, Mcmullin MF, Polyakova LA, Ang SO, Pastore YD, Jedlickova K, Lappin TR, Gordeuk V, Prchal JT (2004) The worldwide distribution of the VHL 598C>T mutation indicates a single founding event. Blood 103:1937–1940

Lok CN, Ponka P (1999) Identification of a hypoxia response element in the transferrin receptor gene. J Biol Chem 274:24147–24152

Luttun A, Carmeliet P (2003) Soluble VEGF receptor Flt1: the elusive preeclampsia factor discovered? J Clin Invest 111:600–602

Marine JC, Topham DJ, Mckay C, Wang D, Parganas E, Stravopodis D, Yoshimura A, Ihle JN (1999) SOCS1 deficiency causes a lymphocyte-dependent perinatal lethality. Cell 98:609–616

Masuhara M, Sakamoto H, Matsumoto A, Suzuki R, Yasukawa H, Mitsui K, Wakioka T, Tanimura S, Sasaki A, Misawa H, Yokouchi M, Ohtsubo M, Yoshimura A (1997) Cloning and characterization of novel CIS family genes. Biochem Biophys Res Commun 239:439–446

Maxwell PH, Pugh CW, Ratcliffe PJ (1993) Inducible operation of the erythropoietin 3′ enhancer in multiple cell lines: evidence for a widespread oxygen-sensing mechanism. Proc Nat Acad Sci U S A 90:2423–2427

Maxwell PH, Wiesener MS, Chang GW, Clifford C, Vaux EC, Cockman ME, Wykoff CC, Pugh CW, Maher ER, Ratcliffe PJ (1999) The tumour suppressor protein VHL targets hypoxia-inducible factors for oxygen-dependent proteolysis. Nature 399:271–275

Messinezy M, Westwood NB, El-Hemaidi I, Marsden JT, Sherwood RS, Pearson TC (2002) Serum erythropoietin values in erythrocytoses and in primary thrombocythaemia. Br J Haematol 117: 47–53

Michiels JJ, Thiele J (2002) Clinical and pathological criteria for the diagnosis of essential thrombocythemia, polycythemia vera, and idiopathic myelofibrosis (agnogenic myeloid metaplasia). Int J Hematol 76:133–145

Minamoto S, Ikegame K, Ueno K, Narazaki M, Naka T, Yamamoto H, Matsumoto T, Saito H, Hosoe S, Kishimoto T (1997) Cloning and functional analysis of new members of STAT induced STAT inhibitor (SSI) family: SSI-2 and SSI-3. Biochem Biophys Res Commun 237:79–83

Mitterbauer G, Winkler K, Gisslinger H, Geissler K, Lechner K, Mannhalter C (1999) Clonality analysis using X-chromosome inactivation at the human androgen receptor gene (Humara). Evaluation of large cohorts of patients with chronic myeloproliferative diseases, secondary neutrophilia, and reactive thrombocytosis. Am J Clin Pathol 112:93–100

Miura O, D'andrea A, Kabat D, Ihle JN (1991) Induction of tyrosine phosphorylation by the erythropoietin receptor correlates with mitogenesis. Mol Cell Biol 11:4895–4902

Moliterno AR, Hankins WD, Spivak JL (1998) Impaired expression of the thrombopoietin receptor by platelets from patients with polycythemia vera. N Engl J Med 338:572–580

Moo-Penn WF, Jue DL, Johnson MH, Therrell BL (1987) Hemoglobin Swan River [alpha 6(A4)Asp–Gly]. Hemoglobin 11:61–62

Mossuz P, Girodon F, Donnard M, Latger-Cannard V, Dobo I, Boiret N, Lecron JC, Binquet C, Barro C, Hermouet S, Praloran V (2004) Diagnostic value of serum erythropoietin level in patients with absolute erythrocytosis. Haematologica 89:1194–1198

Mrug M, Stopka T, Julian BA, Prchal JF, Prchal JT (1997) Angiotensin II stimulates proliferation of normal early erythroid progenitors. J Clin Invest 100:2310–2314

Mrug M, Julian BA, Prchal JT (2004) Angiotensin II receptor type 1 expression in erythroid progenitors: Implications for the pathogenesis of postrenal transplant erythrocytosis. Sem Nephrol 24:120–130

Mukhopadhyay CK, Mazumder B, Fox PL (2000) Role of hypoxia-inducible factor-1 in transcriptional activation of ceruloplasmin by iron deficiency. J Biol Chem 275:21048–1054

Najfeld V, Montella L, Scalise A, Fruchtman S (2002) Exploring polycythaemia vera with fluorescence in situ hybridization: additional cryptic 9p is the most frequent abnormality detected. Br J Haematol 119:558–566

Neubauer H, Cumano A, Muller M, Wu H, Huffstadt U, Pfeffer K (1998) Jak2 deficiency defines an essential developmental checkpoint in definitive hematopoiesis. Cell 93:397–409

Novy MJ, Edwards MJ, Metcalfe J (1967) Hemoglobin Yakina. II. High blood oxygen affinity associated with compensatory erythrocytosis and normal hemodynamics. J Clin Invest 46:1848–1854

Ohh M, Park CW, Ivan M, Hoffman MA, Kim TY, Huang LE, Pavletich N, Chau V, Kaelin WG (2000) Ubiquitination of hypoxia-inducible factor requires direct binding to the beta-domain of the von Hippel-Lindau protein. [see comments.]. Nat Cell Biol 2:423–427

Palmer LA, Semenza GL, Stoler MH, Johns RA (1998) Hypoxia induces type II NOS gene expression in pulmonary artery endothelial cells via HIF-1. Am J Physiol 274:L212–L219

Parganas E, Wang D, Stravopodis D, Topham DJ, Marine JC, Teglund S, Vanin EF, Bodner S, Colamonici OR, Van Deursen JM, Grosveld G, Ihle JN (1998) Jak2 is essential for signaling through a variety of cytokine receptors. Cell 93:385–395

Pearson TC (1997) Hemorheologic considerations in the pathogenesis of vascular occlusive events in polycythemia vera. Semin Thromb Hemost 23:433–439

Pearson TC, Wetherley-Mein G (1978) Vascular occlusive episodes and venous haematocrit in primary proliferative polycythaemia. Lancet 2:1219–1222

Percy MJ, Mcmullin MF, Roques AW, Westwood NB, Acharya J, Hughes AE, Lappin TR, Pearson TC (1998) Erythrocytosis due to a mutation in the erythropoietin receptor gene. Br J Haematol 100: 407–410

Perrotta S, Nobili B, Ferraro M, Migliaccio C, Borriello A, Cucciolla V, Martinelli V, Rossi F, Punzo F, Cirillo P, Parisi G, Zappia V, Rotoli B, Ragione F D (2006) Von Hippel-Lindau-dependent polycythemia is endemic on the island of Ischia: identification of a novel cluster. Blood 107:514–519

Perutz MF, Fermi G, Shih TB (1984) Structure of deoxyhemoglobin Cowtown [His HC3(146) beta–Leu]: origin of the alkaline Bohr effect and electrostatic interactions in hemoglobin. Proc Nat Acad Sci U S A 81:4781–4784

Phelan JT, II, Prchal JT (2001) Clonality studies in cancer based on X chromosome inactivation phenomena in molecular analysis of cancer. In: Jacqueline Boultwood, Carrie Fidler (eds) Humana, Totowa, pp 251–270

Poliakova LA (1974) [Familial erythrocytosis among the residents of the Chuvash ASSR]. [Russian]. Problemy Gematologii i Perelivaniia Krovi 19:30–33

Polyakova LA (1974) Familial erythrocytosis among inhabitants of the Chuvash ASSR. Problemy Gematologii i Perelivaniia Krovi 10

Polyakova LA (1977) Familial-hereditary erythrocytosis. Scientific Research Institute of Hematology and Blood, Moscow, Russia

Prchal JF, Axelrad AA (1974) Bone-marrow responses in polycythemia vera. N Engl J Med 290:1382 (letter)

Prchal JF, Prchal JT (1999) Molecular basis for polycythemia. Curr Opin Hematol 6:100–109

Prchal JT (1995) Primary polycythemias. Curr Opin Hematol 2:146–152

Prchal JT (2001 a) Molecular biology of polycythemias. Intern Med 40:681–687

Prchal JT (2001 b) Pathogenetic mechanisms of polycythemia vera and congenital polycythemic disorders. Semin Hematol 38:10–20

Prchal JT (2003) Classification and molecular biology of polycythemias (erythrocytoses) and thrombocytosis. Hematol Oncol Clin N Am 17:1151–1158:vi

Prchal JT (2005) Polycythemia vera and other primary polycythemias. Curr Opin Hematol 12:112–116

Prchal JT, Beutler E (2005a) Primary and Secondary Polycythemias (Erythrocytosis). In: Lichtman MA, Kipps TJ, Kaushansky K, Beutler E, Seligsohn U, Prchal JT (eds) Williams Hematology (7th edn), pp 779–803

Prchal JT, Gregg XT (2005b) Red cell enzymopathies. In: Hoffman R, Benz E (eds) Hematology: Basic Principles and Practices (4th edn), pp 861–876

Prchal JT, Guan YL (1993a) A novel clonality assay based on transcriptional analysis of the active X chromosome. Stem Cells 11:62–65

Prchal JT, Guan YL, Prchal JF, Barany F (1993b) Transcriptional analysis of the active X-chromosome in normal and clonal hematopoiesis. Blood 81:269–271

Prchal JT, Prchal JF, Belickova M, Chen S, Guan Y, Gartland GL, Cooper MD (1996) Clonal stability of blood cell lineages indicated by X-chromosomal transcriptional polymorphism. J Exp Med 183: 561–567

Pritchard MA, Baker E, Callen DF, Sutherland GR, Wilks AF (1992) Two members of the JAK family of protein tyrosine kinases map to chromosomes 1p31.3 and 9p24. Mamm Genome 3:36–38

Pugh CW, O'Rourke JF, Nagao M, Gleadle JM, Ratcliffe PJ (1997) Activation of hypoxia-inducible factor-1; definition of regulatory domains within the alpha subunit. J Biol Chem 272:11205–11214

Rahbar S, Rea C, Blume K, Seltzer D, Feiner R (1983) A second case of hemoglobin McKees Rocks (beta 145 Tyr leads to Term). A variant with premature termination of the beta-chain. Hemoglobin 7:97–104

Rahbar S, Louis J, Lee T, Asmerom Y (1985) Hemoglobin North Chicago (beta 36 [C2] proline–serine): a new high affinity hemoglobin. Hemoglobin 9:559–576

Reed RE, Winter WP, Rucknagel DL (1974) Haemoglobin inkster (alpha2 85aspartic acid leads to valine beta2) coexisting with beta-thalassaemia in a Caucasian family. Br J Haematol 26:475–484

Roberts AW, Robb L, Rakar S, Hartley L, Cluse L, Nicola NA, Metcalf D, Hilton DJ, Alexander WS (2001) Placental defects and embryonic lethality in mice lacking suppressor of cytokine signaling 3. Proc Nat Acad Sci USA 98:9324–9329

Roder S, Steimle C, Meinhardt G, Pahl HL (2001) STAT3 is constitutively active in some patients with Polycythemia rubra vera. Exp Hematol 29:694–702

Rolfs A, Kvietikova I, Gassmann M, Wenger RH (1997) Oxygen-regulated transferrin expression is mediated by hypoxia-inducible factor-1. J Biol Chem 272:20055–20062

Rosa R, Max-Audit I, Izrael V, Beuzard Y, Thillet J, Rosa J (1981) Hereditary pyruvate kinase abnormalities associated with erythrocytosis. Am J Hematol 10:47–55

Ryan HE, Lo J, Johnson RS (1998) HIF-1 alpha is required for solid tumor formation and embryonic vascularization. EMBO J 17: 3005–3015

Salceda S, Caro J (1997) Hypoxia-inducible factor 1 (HIF-1) protein is rapidly degraded by the ubiquitin-proteasome system under normoxic conditions. J Biol Chem 272:22642

Salkie ML, Gordon PA, Rigal WM, Lam H, Wilson JB, Headlee ME, Huisman TH (1982) Hb A2-Canada or alpha 2 delta 2 99(G1) Asp replaced by Asn, a newly discovered delta chain variant with increased oxygen affinity occurring in cis to beta-thalassemia. Hemoglobin 6:223–231

Saltzman A, Stone M, Franks C, Searfoss G, Munro R, Jaye M, Ivashchenko Y (1998) Cloning and characterization of human Jak-2 kinase: high mRNA expression in immune cells and muscle tissue. Biochem Biophys Res Commun 246:627–633

Sasaki A, Yasukawa H, Shouda T, Kitamura T, Dikic I, Yoshimura A (2000) CIS3/SOCS-3 suppresses erythropoietin (EPO) signaling by binding the EPO receptor and JAK2. J Biol Chem 275:29338–29347

Schneider RG, Bremner JE, Brimhall B, Jones RT, Shih TB (1979) Hemoglobin Cowtown (beta 146 HC3 His-Leu): a mutant with high oxygen affinity and erythrocytosis. Am J Clin Pathol 72:1028–1032

Schwaller J, Parganas E, Wang D, Cain D, Aster JC, Williams IR, Lee CK, Gerthner R, Kitamura T, Frantsve J, Anastasiadou E, Loh M L, Levy DE, Ihle JN, Gilliland DG (2000) Stat5 is essential for the myelo- and lymphoproliferative disease induced by TEL/JAK2. Mol Cell 6:693–704

Scott EM, Wright RC (1982) An alternate method for demonstration of bisphosphoglyceromutase (DPGM) on starch gels. Am J Hum Genet 34:1013–1015

Semenza GL (1999) Regulation of mammalian oxygen homeostasis by hypoxia-inducible factor 1. Ann Rev Cell Devel Biol 15:551–781

Semenza GL (2000a) Expression of hypoxia-inducible factor 1: mechanisms and consequences. Biochem Pharmacol 59:47–53

Semenza GL (2000b) HIF-1 and human disease: one highly involved factor. Genes Devel 14:1983–1991

Semenza GL (2000c) Hypoxia, clonal selection, and the role of HIF-1 in tumor progression. Crit Rev Biochem Mol Biol 35:71–103

Semenza GL, Wang GL (1992) A nuclear factor induced by hypoxia via de novo protein synthesis binds to the human erythropoietin gene enhancer at a site required for transcriptional activation. Mol Cell Biol 12:5447–5454

Semenza GL, Nejfelt MK, Chi SM, Antonarakis SE (1991) Hypoxia-inducible nuclear factors bind to an enhancer element located 3′ to the human erythropoietin gene. Proc Nat Acad Sci USA 88: 5680–5684

Semenza GL, Agani F, Feldser D, Iyer N, Kotch L, Laughner E, Yu A (2000) Hypoxia, HIF-1, and the pathophysiology of common human diseases. Adv Exp Med Biol 475:123–130

Sergeyeva A, Gordeuk VR, Tokarev YN, Sokol L, Prchal JF, Prchal JT (1997) Congenital polycythemia in Chuvashia. Blood 89:2148–2154

Shih LY, Huang JY, Lee CT (1999) Insulin-like growth factor I plays a role in regulating erythropoiesis in patients with end-stage renal disease and erythrocytosis. J Am Soc Nephrol 10:315–322

Silver RT (2003) Imatinib mesylate (Gleevec) reduces phlebotomy requirements in polycythemia vera. Leukemia 17:1186–1187

Sokol L, Prchal J F, D'Andrea A, Rado TA, Prchal JT (1994) Mutation in the negative regulatory element of the erythropoietin receptor gene in a case of sporadic primary polycythemia. Exp Hematol 22:447–453

Sokol L, Luhovy M, Guan Y, Prchal JF, Semenza GL, Prchal JT (1995) Primary familial polycythemia: a frameshift mutation in the erythropoietin receptor gene and increased sensitivity of erythroid progenitors to erythropoietin. Blood 86:15–22

Spivak JL, Silver RT (2004) Imatinib mesylate in polycythemia vera. Blood 103:3241; author reply 3241–3242

Starr R, Willson TA, Viney EM, Murray LJ, Rayner JR, Jenkins BJ, Gonda TJ, Alexander WS, Metcalf D, Nicola NA, Hilton DJ (1997) A family of cytokine-inducible inhibitors of signalling. Nature 387:917–921

Steensma DP, Dewald GW, Lasho TL, Powell HL, Mcclure RF, Levine RL, Gilliland DG, Tefferi A (2005) The JAK2 V617F activating tyrosine kinase mutation is an infrequent event in both "atypical" myeloproliferative disorders and the myelodysplastic syndrome. Blood 106:1207–1209

Tacchini L, Bianchi L, Bernelli-Zazzera A, Cairo G (1999) Transferrin receptor induction by hypoxia. HIF-1-mediated transcriptional activation and cell-specific post-transcriptional regulation. J Biol Chem 274:24142–24146

Takahashi Y, Takahashi S, Shiga Y, Yoshimi T, Miura T (2000) Hypoxic induction of prolyl 4-hydroxylase alpha (I) in cultured cells. J Biol Chem 275:14139–14146

Tanimoto K, Makino Y, Pereira T, Poellinger L (2000) Mechanism of regulation of the hypoxia-inducible factor-1 alpha by the von Hippel-Lindau tumor suppressor protein. EMBO J 19:4298–4309

Tazuke SI, Mazure NM, Sugawara J, Carland G, Faessen GH, Suen LF, Irwin JC, Powell DR, Giaccia AJ, Giudice LC (1998) Hypoxia stimulates insulin-like growth factor binding protein 1 (IGFBP-1) gene expression in HepG2 cells: a possible model for IGFBP-1 expression in fetal hypoxia. Proc Nat Acad Sci USA 95:10188–10193

Tefferi A, Lasho TL, Wolanskyj AP, Mesa RA (2004) Neutrophil PRV-1 expression across the chronic myeloproliferative disorders and in secondary or spurious polycythemia. Blood 103:3547–3548

Temerinac S, Klippel S, Strunck E, Roder S, Lubbert M, Lange W, Azemar M, Meinhardt G, Schaefer HE, Pahl HL (2000) Cloning of PRV-1, a novel member of the uPAR receptor superfamily, which is overexpressed in polycythemia rubra vera. Blood 95:2569–2576

Thiele J, Kvasnicka HM (2005) Diagnostic impact of bone marrow histopathology in polycythemia vera (PV). Hist Histopathol 20:317–328

Thiele J, Kvasnicka HM, Zankovich R, Diehl V (2001) The value of bone marrow histology in differentiating between early stage polycythemia vera and secondary (reactive) polycythemias. Haematologica 86:368–374

Thiele JM, Kvasnicka HM (2005) Diagnosis of polycythemia vera based on bone marrow pathology. Current Hematology Reports 4:218–223

Ugo V, Marzac C, Teyssandier I, Larbret F, Lecluse Y, Debili N, Vainchenker W, Casadevall N (2004) Multiple signaling pathways are involved in erythropoietin-independent differentiation of erythroid progenitors in polycythemia vera. Exp Hematol 32:179–187

Vogelstein B, Fearon ER, Hamilton SR, Feinberg AP (1985) Use of restriction fragment length polymorphisms to determine the clonal origin of human tumors. Science 227:642–645

Wagner KF, Katschinski DM, Hasegawa J, Schumacher D, Meller B, Gembruch U, Schramm U, Jelkmann W, Gassmann M, Fandrey J (2001) Chronic inborn erythrocytosis leads to cardiac dysfunction and premature death in mice overexpressing erythropoietin. Blood 97:536–542

Wajcman H, Kister J, M'Rad A, Soummer AM, Galacteros F (1994) Hb Cemenelum [alpha 92 (FG4) Arg → Trp]: a hemoglobin variant of the alpha 1/beta 2 interface that displays a moderate increase in oxygen affinity. Ann Hematol 68:73–76

Wajcman H, Riou J, Prome D, Kister J, Galacteros F (1999) Hb Brie Comte Robert [beta36(C2)Pro → Ala]: a new hemoglobin variant with high oxygen affinity and marked hydrophobic properties. Hemoglobin 23:281–286

Wang GL, Semenza GL (1993) General involvement of hypoxia-inducible factor 1 in transcriptional response of hypoxia. Proc Nat Acad Sci USA 90:4304–4308

Wang GL, Jiang BH, Rue EA, Semenza GL (1995) Hypoxia-inducible factor 1 is a basic-helix-loop-helix-PAS heterodimer regulated by cellular O2 tension. Proc Nat Acad Sci USA 92:5510–5514

Watowich SS, Xie X, Klingmuller U, Kere J, Lindlof M, Berglund S, De La Chapelle A (1999) Erythropoietin receptor mutations associated with familial erythrocytosis cause hypersensitivity to erythropoietin in the heterozygous state. Blood 94:2530–2532

Weatherall DJ, Clegg JB, Callender ST, Wells RM, Gale RE, Huehns ER, Perutz MF, Viggiano G, Ho C (1977) Haemoglobin Radcliffe (alpha2beta299(Gi)Ala): a high oxygen-affinity variant causing familial polycythaemia. Br J Haematol 35:177–191

Weinberg RS (1997) In vitro erythropoiesis in polycythemia vera and other myeloproliferative disorders. Semin Hematol 34: 64–69

Williamson D, Langdown JV, Myles T, Mason C, Henthorn JS, Davies SC (1992) Polycythaemia and microcytosis arising from the combination of a new high oxygen affinity haemoglobin (Hb Luton, alpha 89 His → Leu) and alpha thalassaemia trait. Br J Haematol 82:621–622

Williamson D, Beresford CH, Langdown JV, Anderson CC, Green AR (1994) Polycythaemia associated with homozygosity for the abnormal haemoglobin Sherwood Forest (beta 104 (G6)Arg → Thr). Br J Haematol 86:890–892

Wood SM, Wiesener MS, Yeates KM, Okada N, Pugh CW, Maxwell PH, Ratcliffe PJ (1998) Selection and analysis of a mutant cell line defective in the hypoxia-inducible factor-1 alpha-subunit (HIF-1alpha). Characterization of hif-1alpha-dependent and -independent hypoxia-inducible gene expression. J Biol Chem 273:8360–8368

Wu H, Liu X, Jaenisch R, Lodish HF (1995) Generation of committed erythroid BFU-E and CFU-E progenitors does not require erythropoietin or the erythropoietin receptor. Cell 83:59–67

Wykoff CC, Beasley NJ, Watson PH, Turner KJ, Pastorek J, Sibtain A, Wilson GD, Turley H, Talks KL, Maxwell PH, Pugh CW, Ratcliffe PJ, Harris AL (2000) Hypoxia-inducible expression of tumor-associated carbonic anhydrases. Cancer Res 60:7075–7083

Yoshimura A, Longmore G, Lodish HF (1990) Point mutation in the exoplasmic domain of the erythropoietin receptor resulting in hormone-independent activation and tumorigenicity. Nature 348:647–649

Yoshimura A, Ohkubo T, Kiguchi T, Jenkins NA, Gilbert DJ, Copeland NG, Hara T, Miyajima A (1995) A novel cytokine-inducible gene CIS encodes an SH2-containing protein that binds to tyrosine-phosphorylated interleukin 3 and erythropoietin receptors. EMBO J 14:2816–2826

Youssoufian H, Longmore G, Neumann D, Yoshimura A, Lodish HF (1993) Structure, function, and activation of the erythropoietin receptor. Blood 81:2223–2236

Yu AY, Frid MG, Shimoda LA, Wiener CM, Stenmark K, Semenza GL (1998) Temporal, spatial, and oxygen-regulated expression of hypoxia-inducible factor-1 in the lung. Am J Physiol 275:L818–L826

Zhao R, Xing S, Li Z, Fu X, Li Q, Krantz SB, Zhao ZJ (2005) Identification of an acquired JAK2 mutation in polycythemia vera. J Biol Chem 280:22788–22792

Essential Thrombocythemia

Ayalew Tefferi

Contents

Abstract. Essential thrombocythemia (ET) was first described in 1934, classified as a myeloproliferative disorder (MPD) in 1951, and accepted as a distinct clinicopathologic entity in 1960. Formal diagnostic criteria were established in the 1970s and in 1981; ET was recognized as a clonal stem cell disorder. In 2005, an activating *JAK2* mutation (Jak2^{V617F}) was demonstrated in a spectrum of MPDs, including ET where the mutational frequency is estimated at 50%. In ET, Jak2^{V617F} has been associated with higher levels of hemoglobin and leukocyte count, higher risk of transformation into polycythemia vera (PV), and advanced age at diagnosis. In contrast, it is currently not clear if the specific mutation has an effect on survival, thrombosis risk, or leukemic transformation rate. Life expectancy in ET is significantly shorter than the control population but the difference may not be apparent in the first 10 years. The 20-year risk of both leukemic and fibrotic transformation is less than 10%. Clinical course is usually indolent with a minority of the patients experiencing thrombohemorrhagic complications. There is increasing evidence regarding the thrombogenic role of neutrophils in ET and this might partly explain the superior overall performance by hydroxyurea, compared to anagrelide, in a recent randomized study.

18.1 Introduction

Essential thrombocythemia (ET) currently lacks an ET-specific clinical or laboratory marker. Instead, it is defined as a persistent thrombocythemic state that is neither reactive nor associated with an otherwise defined chronic myeloid disorder such as chronic myeloid leukemia (CML), polycythemia vera (PV), myelofibrosis with myeloid metaplasia (MMM), and the myelodysplastic syndrome (MDS) (Tefferi and Gilliland 2005 a). In most patients, the disease is believed to represent a stem-cell-derived clonal myeloproliferation that is the common biological link for most, if not all, chronic myeloid disorders (Fialkow 1990). However, the primary oncogenic mutation(s) in ET has not been identified and there are both clinical and laboratory evidence that "ET" represents more than one disease (Harrison et al. 1999 a).

Clinically, ET is characterized by a near-normal life expectancy, frequent occurrence of microvascular disturbances such as headaches and acral paresthesia, and an age- and thrombosis-history-dependent increased risk of thromboembolic complications (Cortelazzo et al. 1990; Tefferi et al. 2001). In addition, 5–10% of patients might experience disease transformation into acute myeloid leukemia (AML), MMM, or PV in the first two decades of their disease (De Sanctis et al. 2003; Passamonti et al. 2004 b; Tefferi et al. 2001). The majority of patients with ET do not require treatment and drug therapy has not been shown to either prolong life or prevent leukemic transformation (Barbui et al. 2004). At present, treatment is considered to either prevent thrombohemorrhagic events in high-risk disease (Cortelazzo et al. 1995 a) or alleviate microvascular symptoms such as headaches and erythromelalgia (Michiels et al. 1985, 1993 a). The former is accomplished by the use of cytoreductive agents and the latter by aspirin (Finazzi and Barbui 2005).

18.2 Epidemiology

Reported incidence figures for ET range from 0.2 to 2.5/100,000 with point prevalence rates of above 10/100,000 (Chaiter et al. 1992; Heudes et al. 1989; Jensen et al. 2000 b; Johansson et al. 2004; McNally et al. 1997; Mesa et al. 1999; Ridell et al. 2000). However, true incidence rates are probably higher because of the indolent nature of the disease that increases the proportion of unrecognized cases (Ruggeri et al. 2003) as well as the fact that traditional diagnostic criteria exclude patients whose presenting platelet counts are below 600,000/L (Lengfelder et al. 1998; Murphy et al. 1986). The former point is supported by recent epidemiological studies that disclosed an increasing trend in incidence attributed to the more frequent use of automated platelet counts (Jensen et al. 2000 b; Johansson et al. 2004). Large retrospective studies indicate a median age at diagnosis of 55 years (Passamonti et al. 2004 b) although the figure is substantially higher in population-based studies (Mesa et al. 1999). Approximately 20% of the patients are diagnosed before age 40 years (Gugliotta 1997; McNally et al. 1997). A female preponderance (1.5–3 : 1) exists, especially in younger patients, whereas the disease is extremely rare in children (Hasle 2000; Jensen et al. 2000 b; McNally et al. 1997). On the latter point, there are well-documented cases of ET in children although some of the reported cases may have represented familial thrombocytosis (Dror et al. 1999; Randi et al. 2000). There is currently no good evidence that links environmental risk factors to the development of ET although the usual suspects, including long-term use of dark hair dye, have been implicated (Falcetta et al. 2003; Mele et al. 1996).

18.3 Historical Perspective

The first description of ET is credited to Emil Epstein and Alfred Goedel, who in 1934 published a case report of what they termed "hemorrhagic thrombocythemia" (Epstein and Goedel 1934). In 1951, ET (then referred to as megakaryocytic leukemia) was classified by Dameshek as a "myeloproliferative disorder (MPD)" along with CML, PV, MMM, and erythroleukemia (Dameshek

1951). Initial descriptions of the latter MPD antedated that of ET; CML was first described in 1845 (Virchow 1845), PV in 1892 (Vaquez 1892), MMM in 1879 (Heuck 1879), and erythroleukemia in 1917 (Di Guglielmo 1917). By 1960, ET was generally accepted as a distinct clinicopathologic entity (Gunz 1960) and strict diagnostic criteria were established later in the 1970s by the polycythemia vera study group (PVSG) (Murphy et al. 1986). In 1981, Fialkow and colleagues utilized G-6-PD isoenzyme analysis to demonstrate that ET represented a stem-cell-derived clonal myeloproliferation (Fialkow et al. 1981). In 2005, an activating *JAK2* mutation (Jak2^{V617F}) was demonstrated in MPD (James et al. 2005 a) and it was shown to be present in approximately half of the patients with ET (Baxter et al. 2005; Kralovics et al. 2005; Levine et al. 2005). However, the pathogenetic relevance of the latter observation remains to be defined (Goldman 2005).

18.4 Disease Classification

At present, classification of myeloid disorders, including ET, is in general based on a constellation of clinical, bone marrow histological, cytochemical, chromosomal, and immunophenotypic features (Jaffe et al. 2001). Accordingly, the World Health Organization (WHO) system for classification of myeloid neoplasms classifies chronic myeloid disorders into four separate categories; MPD, MDS/MPD, MDS, and systemic mastocytosis (SM) (Vardiman et al. 2002). The WHO MPD category includes the four classic (i.e., Dameshek's) MPD (CML, ET, PV, MMM) and in addition chronic neutrophilic leukemia (CNL), chronic eosinophilic leukemia (CEL), hypereosinophilic syndrome (HES), and unclassified MPD (UMPD). The WHO MDS/MPD category includes chronic myelomonocytic leukemia (CMML), juvenile myelomonocytic leukemia (JMML), and "atypical" CML.

However, most chronic myeloid disorders, including MDS, classic MPD, and atypical MPD, have now been shown to represent a clonal stem cell process (Adamson et al. 1976; Bain 2003; Barr and Fialkow 1973; Fialkow et al. 1967, 1977, 1978 a, 1981; Flotho et al. 1999; Froberg et al. 1998; Fugazza et al. 1995; Gilliland et al. 1991; Jacobson et al. 1978; Martin et al. 1980; Pardanani et al. 2003 a, 2003 c; Reeder et al. 2003; Tefferi et al. 1990; Yavuz et al. 2002) and the primary, disease-causing molecular events have been described for the minority of the disease subcategories including CML (BCR-ABL) (Daley et al. 1990; de Klein et al. 1982; Groffen et al. 1984; Heisterkamp et al. 1985; Kelliher et al. 1990; Lugo et al. 1990; McLaughlin et al. 1987; Nowell and Hungerford 1960; Pendergast et al. 1991; Sattler et al. 1996; Voncken et

Table 18.1. A semimolecular classification of chronic myeloid disorders (with permission from Tefferi and Gilliland 2005 a)

- Myelodysplastic syndrome
- Myeloproliferative disorders
  - Classic myeloproliferative disorders
    - Molecularly-defined
      - Chronic myeloid leukemia (*Bcr/Abl+*)
    - Clinicopathologically-assigned
      (Bcr/Abl– and frequently associated with JAK2^{V617F} mutation)
      - Essential thrombocythemia
      - Polycythemia vera
      - Myelofibrosis with myeloid metaplasia
  - Atypical myeloproliferative disorders
    - Molecularly-defined
      - PDGFRA-rearranged eosinophilic/mast cell disorders (e.g., *FIP1L1-PDGFRA*)
      - *PDGFRB*-rearranged eosinophilic disorders (e.g., *TEL/ETV6-PDGFRB*)
      - Systemic mastocytosis associated with *c-kit* mutation (e.g., *c-kit^{D816V}*)
      - *8p11* Myeloproliferative syndrome (e.g., *ZNF198/FIM/RAMP-FGFR1*)
    - Clinicopathologically-assigned
      - Chronic neutrophilic leukemia
      - Chronic eosinophilic leukemia, molecularly not defined
      - Hypereosinophilic syndrome
      - Chronic basophilic leukemia
      - Chronic myelomonocytic leukemia
      - Juvenile myelomonocytic leukemia (associated with recurrent mutations of RAS signaling pathway molecules including *PTPN11* and *NF1)*
      - Systemic mastocytosis, molecularly not defined
      - Unclassified myeloproliferative disorder

al. 1995) SM (either *FIP1L1-PDGFRA* or Kit^{D816V} mutation) (Buttner et al. 1998; Cools et al. 2003; Furitsu et al. 1993; Longley et al. 1999; Nagata et al. 1995; Pardanani et al. 2003b, 2004), CEL (rearrangements of *PDGFRB)* (Abe et al. 1997; Apperley et al. 2002; Baxter et al. 2003; Golub et al. 1994; Grand et al. 2004b; Granjo et al. 2002; Gupta et al. 2002; Kulkarni et al. 2000; Magnusson et al. 2001; Ross et al. 1998; Schwaller et al. 2001; Steer and Cross 2002; Wilkinson et al. 2003), and stem cell leukemia/lymphoma syndrome (rearrangements of *FGFR1)* (Aguiar et al. 1995; Belloni et al. 2005; Chaffanet et al. 1998; Fioretos et al. 2001; Grand et al. 2004a; Guasch et al. 2003; Kulkarni et al. 1999; Nakayama et al. 1996; Popovici et al. 1998, 1999; Reiter et al. 1998; Rosati et al. 2002; Smedley et al. 1998a; Smedley et al. 1998b; Sohal et al. 2001; Still et al. 1997; van den Berg et al. 1996; Vizmanos et al. 2004; Xiao et al. 1998). Furthermore, molecular phenotypes of a yet-to-be-determined relevance are being described involving JMML (*PTPN11, NF1*) (Gitler et al. 2004; Largaespada et al. 1996; Loh et al. 2004; Side et al. 1998; Tartaglia et al. 2003), and both classic and atypical MPD (Jak2^{V617F}) (Baxter et al. 2005; James et al. 2005b; Jones et al. 2005; Kralovics et al. 2005; Levine et al. 2005; Steensma et al. 2005; Zhao et al. 2005). Based on such progress, a new, semimolecular classification system for chronic myeloid disorders has been proposed (Table 18.1) (Tefferi and Gilliland 2005a).

18.5 Pathogenesis

18.5.1 Clonal Origin

It is now well established that most patients that fulfill current diagnostic criteria for ET display clonal hematopoiesis that involves both myeloid and lymphoid lineage in some instances (Anger et al. 1990; Elkassar et al. 1997; Fialkow et al. 1981; el Kassar et al. 1995; Raskind et al. 1985; Shih et al. 2001; Tsukamoto et al. 1994). The initial studies in this regard utilized G-6-PD isoenzyme analysis and the more recent studies used X-linked DNA as well as RNA analysis for determination of clonality (Fialkow et al. 1978b; Gilliland et al. 1991; Prchal and Guan 1993). However, X-linked clonal assays have revealed both polyclonal hematopoiesis in a substantial minority of patients with ET (Harrison et al. 1999a) and "monoclonal" hematopoiesis in normal elderly controls (Champion et al. 1997). Furthermore, in some cases, the clonal process in ET was shown to include lymphocytes (Raskind et al. 1985) or be restricted to megakaryocytes (Elkassar et al. 1997). Based on some of these observations, some investigators have promoted the existence of "monoclonal" vs. "polyclonal" ET based on X chromosome inactivation patterns derived from granulocyte and T lymphocytes (Chiusolo et al. 2001; Harrison et al. 1999a). Several studies in this regard have suggested clinical relevance of this particular concept by demonstrating a difference in thrombosis risk (Chiusolo et al. 2001; Harrison et al. 1999a; Vannucchi et al. 2004) but the validity of this particular observation is undermined by the lack of information from prospective studies.

The primary molecular abnormality in ET remains elusive and it is likely that it consists of more than one mutation to explain the heterogeneity of the disease in terms of both clinical behavior and laboratory features. Cytogenetic studies in ET are seen in less than 5% of patients at diagnosis (Bacher et al. 2005; Sessarego et al. 1989; Steensma and Tefferi 2002). Both structural and numerical abnormalities involving many individual chromosomes, including trisomies 9 and 8, long arm deletions of chromosomes 5, 7, 13, 17, and 20 have been associated with ET but none have enough specificity to be particularly useful in either diagnosis or providing pathogenetic insight (Steensma and Tefferi 2002).

18.5.2 Jak2 and Essential Thrombocythemia

MPD-relevant cytoplasmic protein tyrosine kinases include the Janus family of kinases (Jaks) including Jak2 (Rane and Reddy 2000; Yamaoka et al. 2004), the Src family of kinases (Roskoski 2004), and Abl kinase (Pendergast 2002; Rane and Reddy 2002; Wang 2000). Jak2 is structurally characterized by the presence of two homologous kinase domains; Jak homology 1 (JH1), which is functional, and JH2, which lacks kinase activity (i.e., pseudo-kinase) (Rane and Reddy 2000, 2002; Yeh and Pellegrini 1999). The JH2 domain interacts with the JH1 domain to inhibit kinase activity (Saharinen et al. 2003). Jak2 mediates signaling downstream of cytokine receptors by phosphorylating signal transducers and activators of transcription (STAT) proteins. The Jak/STAT signal transduction pathway plays a major role in both cellular proliferation and cell survival and is regulated at multiple levels through distinct mechanisms including direct dephosphorylation of Jak2 by specific tyrosine phosphatases (e.g., SHP-1), proteolytic degradation of Jak2 through binding to a family of suppressors of cytokine signaling (e.g., SOCS-1), and inhibition of DNA binding of STAT by protein inhibitors of activated STAT (PIAS) (Sasaki et al. 2000; Shuai and Liu 2003; Starr and Hilton 1999; Stofega et al. 2000).

Abnormalities affecting either members of the Jak/STAT signaling pathway or its regulatory elements have been associated with various tumor phenotypes including hematologic malignancies. For example, *JAK2* has been identified as a fusion partner of both *ETV6/TEL* in t(9; 12)(p24; p13), which is associated with both T and pre-B acute lymphoid leukemia and atypical CML in transformation (Lacronique et al. 1997; Peeters et al. 1997) and *PCM1-JAK2*-associated acute or chronic myeloid disorder associated with eosinophilia (Reiter et al. 2005). Several lines of evidence have previously implicated the Jak/STAT pathway in the pathogenesis as well as the phenotype of Epo independence and/or hypersensitivity in MPD (Golde et al. 1977; Prchal and Axelrad 1974; Zanjani et al. 1977). For example, activating mutations of EpoR have been associated with constitutive phosphorylation of Jak2 and STAT5 (Arcasoy et al. 1999) and the failure to negatively regulate Jak2, in moth-eaten mice lacking SHP-1 expression, produces myeloid cell Epo hypersensitivity (Klingmuller et al. 1995; Shultz et al. 1997).

Several studies have recently reported on the association of Jak2^{V617F} with both classic and atypical MPDs (Baxter et al. 2005; James et al. 2005b; Jones et al. 2005; Kralovics et al. 2005; Levine et al. 2005; Steensma et al. 2005; Zhao et al. 2005). The newly identified somatic point mutation is a G-C to T-A transversion, at nucleotide 1849 of exon 12, resulting in the substitution of valine by phenylalanine at codon 617. The Jak2^{V617F} occurs within the JH2 domain and interferes with its autoinhibitory function (Feener et al. 2004; Lindauer et al. 2001; Saharinen and Silvennoinen 2002; Saharinen et al. 2000). The reported mutational frequency in ET ranges from 23 to 57% and homozygosity for the mutant allele is rare in ET (James et al. 2005b; Kralovics et al. 2005; Levine et al. 2005). In vitro, Jak2^{V617F} was associated with constitutive phosphorylation of Jak2 and its downstream effectors as well as induction of Epo hypersensitivity (James et al. 2005b; Levine et al. 2005; Zhao et al. 2005). In vivo, murine bone marrow transduced with a retrovirus containing Jak2^{V617F}-induced erythrocytosis in the transplanted mice (James et al. 2005b). Taken together, these observations suggest a pathogenetic relevance for the particular mutation in MPD.

Consistent with the above-mentioned laboratory observation, a study of 150 patients with ET who were followed for a median of 11.4 years disclosed a significant association between the presence of the Jak2^{V617F} mutation and certain parameters at diagnosis including advanced age and higher counts of both hemoglobin and leukocytes. Furthermore, during follow-up, patients with the mutation were more likely to transform into PV but the incidences of AML, MMM, or thrombotic events were similar between patients with and without the mutation. Multivariate analysis did not identify the presence of Jak2^{V617F} as independent predictor of inferior survival. On the other hand, ET patients with the mutation displayed a higher level of neutrophil PRV-1 expression (Tefferi et al. 2005). Therefore, although the presence of Jak2^{V617F} in ET appears to promote a PV phenotype, it does not appear to carry treatment-relevant information (Wolanskyj et al. 2005).

18.5.3 Myeloid Colony Growth and Cytokine Response

ET shares a spectrum of biological features with PV including clonal myelopoiesis (Fialkow et al. 1981), in vitro growth factor independence/hypersensitivity of both erythroid and megakaryocyte progenitor cells (Axelrad et al. 2000; Juvonen et al. 1993), low serum erythropoietin level (Messinezy et al. 2002), altered megakaryocyte/platelet Mpl expression (Harrison et al. 1999b; Yoon et al. 2000), increased neutrophil PRV-1 expression (Passamonti et al. 2004a; Tefferi et al. 2004), and decreased platelet serotonin content (Koch et al. 2004). Laboratory studies in ET have demonstrated myeloid growth factor hypersensitivity to IL-3 (Kobayashi et al. 1993) as well as TPO (Axelrad et al. 2000). Growth factor independence of myeloid progenitor cells in ET and related MPD has not been attributed to mutations in ligand receptor (Hess et al. 1994; Taksin et al. 1999) or receptor-associated signal transducer molecules (Asimakopoulos et al. 1997). In particular, the genes for the receptors of both EPO (Hess et al. 1994; Lecouedic et al. 1996; Mittelman et al. 1996) and TPO (Harrison et al. 1998; Taksin et al. 1999) have been examined in patients with MPD and found to be intact. However, in patients with ET (Wang et al. 1998), PV (Cerutti et al. 1997), and MMM (Wang et al. 1997) serum TPO levels are usually normal or elevated despite an increased megakaryocyte mass. This has been attributed to the markedly decreased megakaryocyte/platelet expression of Mpl in PV and other related MPD (Harrison et al. 1999b; Horikawa et al. 1997; Moliterno et al. 1998; Yoon et al. 2000). While the specific trait may be used to complement morphological diagnosis in PV and ET, its pathogenetic relevance remains unclear (Mesa et al. 2002; Tefferi et al. 2000 c).

18.5.4 Pathogenetic Mechanisms of Thrombosis, Bleeding, and Vasomotor Symptoms Associated with Essential Thrombocythemia

Bleeding diathesis in ET is currently believed to involve an acquired von Willebrand syndrome (AVWS) that becomes apparent in the presence of extreme thrombocytosis (Budde and van Genderen 1997; Budde et al. 1993; Sato 1988). The mechanism of AVWS in ET is currently believed to involve a platelet count-dependent increased proteolysis of high molecular weight VWF by the ADAMTS13 cleaving protease (Budde et al. 1984, 1986; Levy et al. 2001; Lopez-Fernandez et al. 1987; Tsai 1996). A spectrum of other qualitative platelet defects are also seen in ET and include prolonged bleeding time (Murphy et al. 1978), defects in epinephrine-, collagen-, and ADP-induced platelet aggregation (Boneu et al. 1980; Waddell et al. 1981), decreased ATP secretion (Lofvenberg and Nilsson 1989), altered thromboxane generation (Zahavi et al. 1991), increased spontaneous whole blood platelet aggregation (Balduini et al. 1991), acquired storage pool deficiency that results from abnormal ex vivo platelet activation, and decreased platelet membrane GP Ib and GP IIb/IIIa receptor expression (Burstein et al. 1984; Faurschou et al. 2000; Gersuk et al. 1989; Jensen et al. 2000 a; Kaywin et al. 1978; Le Blanc et al. 1998; Mazzucato et al. 1989; Wehmeier et al. 1989, 1990, 1991). However, none of these abnormalities is currently implicated as a risk factor for bleeding although the use of aspirin is known to exacerbate the bleeding diathesis of patients with either ET or PV, possibly through a mechanism that involves the lipoxygenase pathway (Cortelazzo et al. 1998).

Thrombocytosis per se has not been correlated with thrombosis risk in ET (Barbui et al. 2004). However, specific defects in arachidonic acid metabolism have been described and might result in abnormal thromboxane A_2 (TX A_2) generation (Landolfi et al. 1992; Rocca et al. 1995 a; Schafer 1982). Accordingly, the recent demonstration of antithrombotic activity in a controlled study of aspirin use in PV might be attributed in part to the drug's interference with TX A_2 synthesis (Landolfi et al. 2004 b). However, the latter possibility is more likely to play a role in aspirin-induced alleviation of microcirculatory symptoms which are believed to be linked to small vessel-based abnormal platelet-endothelial interactions (Michiels et al. 1985; van Genderen et al. 1995, 1996). Alternatively, the antithrombotic property of hydroxyurea (Cortelazzo et al. 1995 a) in ET that is not shared by anagrelide (Green et al. 2004) suggests a thrombophilic role for granulocytes and monocytes and would be consistent with in vitro data in patients with MPD who show alterations in several neutrophil activation parameters, markers of both endothelial damage and thrombophilic state, and the presence of circulating platelet-leukocyte aggregates (Falanga et al. 2000, 2005; Jensen et al. 2001).

18.6 Clinical Features

The increasing use of automated cell counters has resulted in the diagnosis of ET in many asymptomatic individuals (Besses et al. 1999). When symptoms are present, they can be either not life threatening (vasomotor symptoms also known as microcirculatory symptoms) or potentially fatal (thrombosis, bleeding, disease transformation into either MMM or AML) (Barbui et al. 2004; Harrison 2005 b; Passamonti et al. 2004 b). Non-life-threatening events in ET include microcirculatory

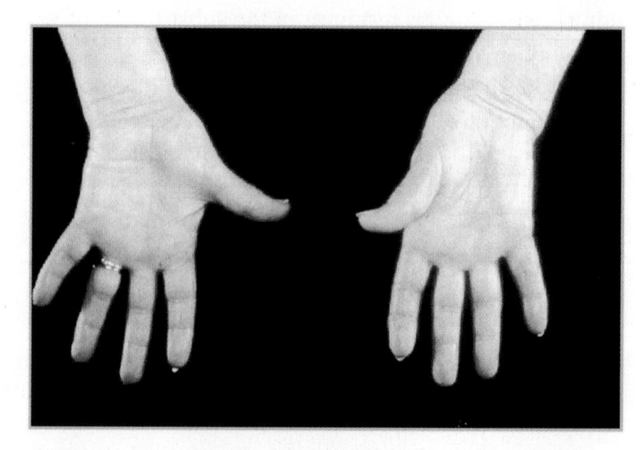

Fig. 18.1. Erythromelalgia in a patient with essential thrombocythemia

symptoms (headache, visual symptoms, lightheadedness, atypical chest pain, acral dysesthesia, erythromelalgia) (Besses et al. 1999; Fenaux et al. 1990; Tefferi et al. 2001) which occur in approximately a third of the patients and an increased risk of first trimester miscarriages that occurs in 30–40% of pregnant women with ET (Elliott and Tefferi 2003; Harrison 2005a; Wright and Tefferi 2001). Accordingly, ET should be in the differential diagnosis of a patient that is being evaluated for either the aforementioned list of microcirculatory disturbances or recurrent miscarriages. Erythromelalgia is a vasomotor symptom that is defined as acral dysesthesia and erythema that is responsive to low-dose aspirin (Fig. 18.1) (Michiels et al. 1985, 1996). The mechanism of erythromelalgia is believed to involve abnormal platelet-endothelium interaction and histopathological studies demonstrate platelet-rich arteriolar microthrombi with endothelial inflammation and intimal proliferation (Michiels et al. 1985, van Genderen et al. 1996). A similar mechanism might be involved in ET-associated transient neurologic and visual disturbances that are responsive to aspirin therapy (Michiels et al. 1993b).

Thrombohemorrhagic complications and clonal evolution are the major life threatening events in ET. Tables 18.2 and 18.3 list the incidences of both thrombotic and hemorrhagic events in ET that show the higher prevalence of both major thrombotic events (as opposed to major bleeding episodes) and arterial (as opposed to venous) thrombosis (Elliott and Tefferi 2005). Patients with either ET or PV have an increased risk of abdominal large vessel thrombosis that is seen in approximately 10% of patients (Anger et al. 1989a, b; Bazzan et al. 1999a; Lengfelder et al. 1998). Therefore, a MPD must be in the differential diagnosis of a major abdominal vein thrombosis and the possibility of latent disease should be considered in the absence of overtly abnormal blood counts (Teofili et al. 1992). Other atypical sites of thrombosis in ET include the cerebral sinuses (Kesler et al. 2000; Mohamed et al. 1991) and retinal vessels (Imasawa and Iijima 2002; Tache et al. 2005). Fortunately, disease transformation into either AML or MMM is infrequent in ET (Andersson et al. 2000; De Sanctis et al. 2003; Passamonti et al. 2004b).

Table 18.2. Thrombotic and hemorrhagic events in essential thrombocythemia reported at diagnosis (with permission modified from Elliott & Tefferi, 2005)

	n	Platelet $\times 10^9$/L (median/mean)	Asymptomatic (%)	Major thrombosis (%)	Major arterial thrombosis* (%)	Major venous thrombosis* (%)	MVD (%)	Total bleeds (%) (major)
Bellucci et al. (1986)	94	1200	67	22	81	19	43	37 (3·2)
Fenaux et al. (1990)	147	1150	36	18	83	17	34	18 (4)
Cortelazzo et al. (1990)	100	1135	34	11	91	9	30	9 (3)
Colombi et al. (1991)	103	1200	73	23·3	87·5	12·5	33	3·6 (1·9)
Besses et al. (1999)	148	898	57	25	NA	NA	29	6·1 (NA)
Jensen et al. (2000a)	96	1102	52	14	85	15	23	9 (5·2)

MVD, microvascular disturbances; NA, not available

* Percentage of total major thrombotic events.

Table 18.3. Thrombotic and hemorrhagic events in essential thrombocythemia reported at follow-up (with permission modified from Elliott & Tefferi, 2005)

	n	Major thrombosis (%)	Major arterial thrombosis (%)*	Major venous thrombosis (%)*	MVD (%)	Total bleeds (%) (major)	Percentage of deaths from hemorrhage (%)	Percentage of deaths from thrombosis (%)
Bellucci et al. (1986)	94	17	62·5	37·5	17	14 (3·2)	0	0
Fenaux et al. (1990)	147	13·6	86	14	4·1	NA (0·7)	0	25
Cortelazzo et al. (1990)	100	20	71	29	NA	NA (1)	0	100 one pt (IAVT)
Colombi et al. (1991)	103	10·6	91	9	33	8·7 (5·8)	0	27·3
Besses et al. (1999)	148	22·3	94	6	27·7	11·5 (4·1)	0	13·3
Jensen et al. (2000a)	96	16·6	69	31	16·7	13·6 (7·3)	3·3	16·7

MVD, microvascular disturbances; IAVT, intra-abdominal venous thrombosis

* Percentage of total major thrombotic events.

18.7 Evaluation of Thrombocytosis

The normal platelet count in both sexes as well as across different ethnic backgrounds is estimated to be less than 400×10^9/L (Brummitt and Barker 2000; Gevao et al. 1996; Lozano et al. 1998; Ross et al. 1988; Ruocco et al. 2001). Therefore, ET must be considered in the presence of a platelet count above 400×10^9/L. In an individual patient, however, a biologically relevant increase in platelet count might occur without exceeding the population reference range and this possibility has to be taken into consideration when evaluating a clinical occurrence that is characteristic of a MPD (Lengfelder et al. 1998; Sacchi et al. 2000).

Figure 18.2 outlines a step-by-step approach to the patient with thrombocytosis. The first step is to entertain the possibility of reactive thrombocytosis (RT). The distinction between ET and RT is clinically relevant because the former and not the latter are associated with an increased risk of thrombohemorrhagic complications (Buss et al. 1985; Griesshammer et al. 1999; Randi et al. 1991; Valade et al. 2005). An incomplete list of conditions that are associated with RT is presented in Table 18.4 (Tefferi et al. 1994a). The absence of comorbid conditions associated with a previously documented persistent increase in platelet count strongly suggests ET or a related MPD as opposed to RT. The same holds true when thrombocytosis is accompanied by vasomotor symptoms, splenomegaly, acral dysesthesia, pruritus, or any thrombohemorrhagic event.

18.7.1 Step 1 Rule Out Reactive Thrombocytosis

In general, patient history and physical findings are adequate to either diagnose or exclude the possibility of RT. In this regard, the value of old records that would help determine the duration of thrombocytosis cannot be overemphasized. The hematology data (complete blood count, white blood cell differential, red blood cell indices) and the peripheral blood smear provide information that is complementary to the clinical picture. The degree of thrombocytosis per se cannot distinguish RT from ET whereas both quantitative and qualitative abnormalities of the red cells and leucocytes provide important clues (Buss et al. 1994; Schilling 1980). For ex-

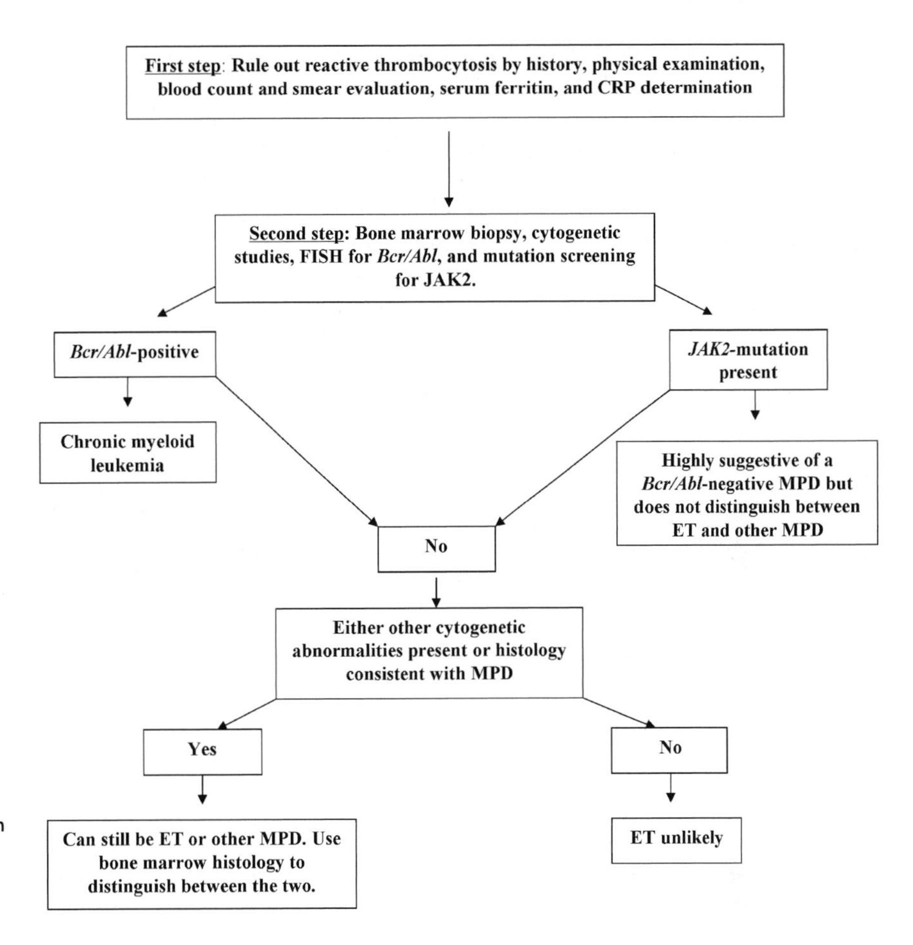

Fig. 18.2. A diagnostic algorithm for essential thrombocythemia (ET). MPD, myeloproliferative disorder; CRP, C-reactive protein

Table 18.4. Causes of thrombocytosis (Buss et al. 1994, Chen et al. 1999, Chuncharunee et al. 2000, Robbins and Barnard 1983, Santhosh-Kumar et al. 1991, Yohannan et al. 1994)

Primary thrombocytosis	Reactive thrombocytosis
Essential thrombocythemia	Infection
Polycythemia vera	Tissue damage
Myelofibrosis with myeloid metaplasia (overt)	Chronic inflammation
Myelofibrosis with myeloid metaplasia (cellular phase)	Malignancy
Chronic myeloid leukemia	Rebound thrombocytosis
Myelodysplastic syndrome	Renal disorders
Acute leukemia	Hemolytic anemia
Polycythemia vera	Post-splenectomy
	Blood loss

ample, RT-associated abnormalities include microcytosis, presence of Howell-Jolly bodies, and rouleaux formation that are associated with iron deficiency anemia, hyposplenism, and an inflammatory condition, respectively.

In addition to hematology group and blood smear, initial laboratory tests should include the measurement of serum ferritin concentration and C-reactive protein (CRP) levels. A normal serum ferritin level excludes the possibility of iron deficiency anemia-associated RT. However, a low serum ferritin level does not exclude the possibility of ET. The measurement of CRP is helpful in attending to the possibility of an occult inflammatory or malignant process (Tefferi et al. 1994a). Similarly, levels of other acute phase features including erythrocyte sedimentation rate (Espanol et al. 1999), plasma fibrinogen (Messinezy et al. 1994), and plasma IL-6 levels (Tefferi et al. 1994a) have been shown to be increased during RT. However, although the finding of normal values for these parameters argues against RT, abnormal values do not exclude the possibility of ET. Plasma TPO levels are not helpful in distinguishing ET from RT (Hou et al. 1998; Uppenkamp et al. 1998; Wang et al. 1998). Similarly, the diagnostic value of platelet indices (mean volume, size distribution width) as well as platelet function tests are undermined by either excess overlap in the measured values between RT and ET or a high degree of expertise in test performance and result interpretation (Osselaer et al. 1997; Sehayek et al. 1988; Small and Bettigole 1981).

18.7.2 Step 2 Distinguish Essential Thrombocythemia from Another Myeloid Disorder

If clinical and laboratory evaluation does not suggest RT, then the possibility of either ET or a related MPD becomes stronger and bone marrow examination would be the next step to confirm the diagnosis. Such an action is necessary especially in the presence of MPD-associated abnormalities including increased hematocrit, macrocytosis, and leukoerythroblastic smear suggesting PV, MDS, and MMM, respectively. However, before pursuing bone marrow examination, the rare possibility of a genetically-defined process (e.g., activating mutation of the *MPL* gene) (Ding et al. 2004) must be kept in mind while evaluating a patient with either life-long history of thrombocytosis or a family history of the same (Florensa et al. 2004).

Clonal thrombocytosis is an integral feature of ET but it also occurs in approximately 50% of patients with either PV or MMM (Griesshammer et al. 1999; Thiele et al. 1999). Similarly, an increased platelet count might be seen in as many as 35% of patients with CML (Thiele et al. 1999). The incidence of thrombocytosis is much lower in both MDS and atypical MPD (Cabello et al. 2005). In MDS, thrombocytosis has been associated with certain cytogenetic abnormalities including trisomy 8 (Patel and Kelsey 1997), deletion of the long arm of chromosome 5 (5q-gap syndrome) (Brusamolino et al. 1988; Tefferi et al. 1994b), and abnormalities of chromosome 3 (Jenkins et al. 1989; Jotterand Bellomo et al. 1992) as well as the presence of ringed sideroblasts (Cabello et al. 2005; Gupta et al. 1999). Furthermore, MPD-associated bone marrow histologic abnormalities can be subtle and some patients with CML (Michiels et al. 2004a; Stoll et al. 1988), MDS (Gupta et al. 1999; Koike et al. 1995), or cellular phase of AMM (Thiele et al. 1999) can present with isolated thrombocytosis that is difficult to distinguish from ET. Therefore, the role of bone marrow examination is not only to confirm the diagnosis of ET but also to exclude other causes of clonal thrombocythemia. Accordingly, bone marrow biopsy should be accompanied by karyotype analysis, FISH for *BCR-ABL*, and mutation screening for Jak2^{V617F} (Fig. 18.2).

Bone marrow histology is normal appearing in RT without the presence of either megakaryocyte clusters or abnormal cellular morphology. In contrast, clonal thrombocythemia is often associated with increased number of megakaryocytes and other myeloid cells, abnormality in cellular morphology, presence of megakaryocyte clusters (Fig. 18.3), and variable degrees of reticulin fibrosis (Annaloro et al. 1999; Buss et al. 1991; Thiele et al. 1999). Although detailed analysis of megakaryocyte morphology might assist in distinguishing CML (dwarf megakaryocytes and not too many clusters) from ET (giant megakaryocytes with cluster formation), cytogenetic studies and FISH for *BCR-ABL* should accompany bone marrow examination to rule out the possibility of CML (Fig. 18.2) (Stoll et al. 1988). Similarly, the detection of the Jak2^{V617F} mutation strongly argues against RT since the mutant allele has so far not been reported in either normal controls (Baxter et al. 2005; James et al. 2005b; Kralovics et al. 2005; Levine et al. 2005) or patients with secondary erythrocytosis (James

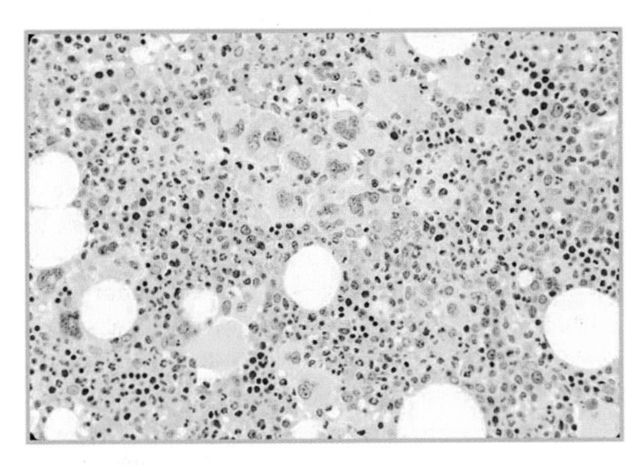

Fig. 18.3. Megakaryocyte clusters in essential thrombocythemia

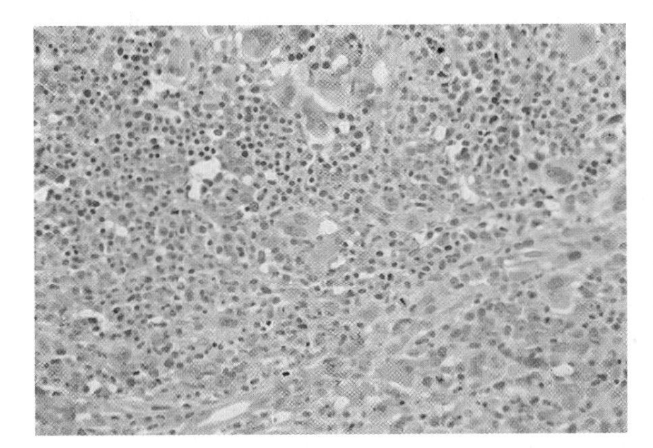

Fig. 18.4. Cellular phase myelofibrosis with myeloid metaplasia

et al. 2005b; Jones et al. 2005; Kralovics et al. 2005). However, peripheral blood mutation screening cannot substitute for bone marrow histology because $Jak2^{V617F}$ is absent in almost half of the patients with ET and its presence cannot distinguish ET from other MPDs (Jones et al. 2005; Kralovics et al. 2005; Levine et al. 2005; Tefferi and Gilliland 2005b).

Bone marrow histology should be carefully scrutinized for the presence of both trilineage dysplasia that would suggest MDS and intense marrow cellularity accompanied by atypical megakaryocytic hyperplasia that would suggest cellular phase AMM (Fig. 18.4). The latter and not ET is often accompanied by elevated levels of serum lactate dehydrogenase level, increased peripheral blood CD34 cell count, and a leukoerythroblastic peripheral blood smear (Arora et al. 2005; Tefferi and Elliott 2004). Mild reticulin fibrosis is detected in approximately 14% of patients with ET at diagnosis and does not portend an unusual outcome (Tefferi et al. 2001). Clonal cytogenetic lesions in ET are detected in $<5\%$ of the cases and are diagnostically nonspecific (Steensma and Tefferi 2002).

18.7.3 The Role of Additional Specialized Assays

There are several research-based assays that might complement the clinical and pathology-based distinction between ET and RT. For example, many studies have demonstrated markedly decreased TPO receptor (Mpl) surface expression in both megakaryocytes (Yoon et al. 2000) and platelets of patients with ET (Horikawa et al. 1997). However, more recent studies have demonstrated the limited value of Mpl-based assays for the evaluation of thrombocytosis (Harrison et al. 1999b). Other specialized tests that may be utilized to distinguish ET from RT include in vitro myeloid colony assays (both spontaneous and TPO-hypersensitive megakaryocyte growth is seen in ET but not in RT) (Axelrad et al. 2000; Rolovic et al. 1995) and Prv-1 expression assay in peripheral blood granulocytes (high level in ET and not detectable in RT) (Teofili et al. 2002a). In regards to the former, the assay is available only in research laboratories and may not be suitable for widespread use at the present time. In regards to the neutrophil Prv-1 assay, not only does it lack diagnostic accuracy that is adequate enough for use in routine clinical practice (Sirhan et al. 2005), but increased neutrophil Prv-1 expression clusters with the presence of both an increased leukocyte alkaline phosphatase score and the presence of the $Jak2^{V617F}$ mutation and is therefore effectively replaced by these latter tests (Goerttler et al. 2005b; Sirhan et al. 2005; Tefferi and Gilliland 2005c). Finally, it is underscored that none of the currently available specialized tests including mutation screening $Jak2^{V617F}$, endogenous erythroid colony formation, or the Prv-1 assay are capable of distinguishing ET from PV (Tefferi 2003; Tefferi and Gilliland 2005c).

18.8 Prognosis

18.8.1 Life Expectancy and Clonal Evolution

Most patients with ET can expect a normal life expectancy in the first decade of the disease (Barbui et al. 2004; Passamonti et al. 2004b; Rozman et al. 1991; Tefferi et al. 2001). Information regarding survival beyond the first decade is limited but a slight shortening of survival is expected because of delayed occurrences of clonal evolution (Barbui et al. 2004; Wolanskyj et al. 2003). Regarding the latter point, in a recent retrospective study of 435 patients with ET, the 15-year cumulative risk of clonal evolution into either AML or MMM was 2% and 4%, respectively, and was not influenced by single agent drug therapy including the use of hydroxyurea (Passamonti et al. 2004b). A leukemic transformation rate of 5.5% was reported by another recent study of 164 ET patients uniformly treated with pipobroman for a median of approximately 13 years (De Sanctis et al. 2003). Furthermore, such clonal evolution is believed to represent a natural progression of the disease and can occur in the absence of cytoreductive therapy (Andersson et al. 2000).

18.8.2 Thrombosis Risk Stratification

Most investigators agree that age ≥60 years and history of thrombosis significantly increase the risk of thrombosis in ET (Bazzan et al. 1999a; Bellucci et al. 1986; Besses et al. 1999; Watson and Key 1993a). The particular consensus is supported by many retrospective studies of which only one was controlled (Tables 18.2 and 18.3) (Barbui et al. 2004; Cortelazzo et al. 1990). Accordingly, the presence of either one of the two adverse features defines a high-risk disease category (Table 18.5). In the absence of these two adverse features, patients are assigned to either a low-risk or indeterminate-risk (a.k.a. intermediate-risk) disease category based on the presence or absence of either extreme thrombocytosis (platelet count 1 million/μL) or cardiovascular risk factors (Table 18.5) (Barbui et al. 2004; Bazzan et al. 1999a; Cortelazzo et al. 1990; Watson and Key 1993a). However, not everyone subscribes to this risk stratification model. Other investigators include patients with history of hemorrhage, hypertension, diabetes, or extreme thrombocytosis in the high-risk category and patients with the age range between 40 and 60 years in an intermediate-risk category, based on limited and uncontrolled data that are not always constant across different studies (*vide infra*) (Barbui et al. 2004; Cortelazzo et al. 1990; Harrison 2005b).

Table 18.5. Risk stratification in essential thrombocythemia

Low-risk	Age below 60 years, *and* No history of thrombosis, *and* Platelet count below 1 million/μL, *and* Absence of cardiovascular risk factors (smoking, hypertension, hyperlipidemia, diabetes)
Indeterminate-risk	Neither low-risk nor high-risk
High-risk	Age 60 years or older, *or* A positive history of thrombosis

To date, there is no controlled study that correlates the degree of thrombocytosis in young asymptomatic patients with an increased risk of thrombosis. If anything, there are carefully conducted prospective cohort studies that did not show any significant correlation (Barbui et al. 2004; Ruggeri et al. 1998b). Therefore, there is no rationale to consider such patients as being at high-risk for thrombosis. A similar argument can be made regarding cardiovascular risk factors (smoking, hypertension, diabetes, and hypercholesterolemia) and risk of thrombosis in ET. First of all, anyone with cardiovascular risk factors is prone to an excess risk of thrombosis and it is not clear if the patient with ET has an even higher risk as a result of the underlying MPD (Ganti et al. 2003). Unfortunately, none of the currently available studies have adequately addressed the specific question and instead different studies have arrived at different conclusions, with most studies not showing correlation between vascular risk factors and thrombosis risk in ET (Barbui et al. 2004; Bazzan et al. 1999b; Besses et al. 1999; Cortelazzo et al. 1990; Ganti et al. 2003; Jantunen et al. 2001; Randi et al. 1998; Watson and Key 1993b).

What then is the rationale to assign young (age <60 years) asymptomatic (no history of thrombosis) patients with either extreme thrombocytosis or cardiovascular risk factors into the indeterminate- rather than low-risk disease category? First, too few patients with extreme thrombocytosis were included in many of the aforementioned studies to allow valid conclusion regarding their thrombosis risk. In addition, it is now well established that some patients with extreme thrombocytosis have associated AVWS and may be at risk for abnormal bleeding and their placement in a disease category that is separate from low-risk disease allows specific attention given to the particular problem (Fabris et al. 1986). For example, while aspirin therapy is encouraged in low-risk disease, one has to rule out the possibility of clinically significant AVWS before allowing its use in indeterminate-risk disease that is associated with extreme thrombocytosis.

18.8.3 Risk Factors Other than Age, Thrombosis History, and Vascular Risk Factors

Several recent studies have explored the contribution of hereditary and acquired causes of thrombophilia to the occurrence of thrombotic events in MPD and the findings have so far been inconsistent. For example, two prospective studies found no difference in the allele frequencies of factor V Leiden, prothrombin G20210A; and MTHFR mutations among ET patients with and without thrombotic complications (Afshar-Kharghan 2001; Dicato MA 1999) whereas another retrospective study suggested an increase in the prevalence of the Factor V Leiden mutation in patients with a history of venous thrombotic events (Ruggeri et al. 2002). Similarly, although several studies have demonstrated elevated levels of homocysteine among patients with MPD (Amitrano et al. 2003; Faurschou et al. 2000; Gisslinger et al. 1999), the clinical relevance of the particular observation, as it relates to arterial thrombosis, is suggested by one (Amitrano et al. 2003) but not other studies (Faurschou et al. 2000; Gisslinger et al. 1999). An increased prevalence of antiphospholipid antibodies in patients with ET has also been described but its clinical relevance remains to be carefully evaluated before making any assumptions (Harrison et al. 2002; Jensen et al. 2002). Finally, the presence of increased neutrophil Prv-1 expression, monoclonal hematopoiesis, or decreased megakaryocyte Mpl expression has been implicated as being thrombogenic by some (Goerttler et al. 2005a; Johansson et al. 2003; Shih et al. 2002; Teofili et al. 2002b) but not other (Goerttler et al. 2005a; Vannucchi et al. 2004) investigators.

18.9 Treatment

18.9.1 The Goal of Therapy

Before considering any form of specific therapy for the patient with ET, one must define the goal of therapy as well as produce the evidence that supports such an action. If the goal is to alleviate microvascular symptoms such as headaches or erythromelalgia, then the use of low-dose aspirin (40–100 mg/day) is appropriate after excluding the possibility of clinically significant AVWS in patients with extreme thrombocytosis (Elliott and Tefferi 2005; McCarthy et al. 2002). However, not all patients with vasomotor symptoms respond to aspirin therapy and some may require platelet cytoreduction in order to obtain relief (Regev et al. 1997b). In asymptomatic cases of ET-associated AVWS, prophylactic cytoreduction is advised only in the presence of a clinically relevant reduction in VW protein function (e.g., ristocetin cofactor activity <20%) (Elliott and Tefferi 2005). In symptomatic patients, in contrast, cytoreductive therapy is indicated and the target platelet count would be the one that corrects the laboratory abnormality. In general, cytoreductive therapy is never instituted in ET to either prolong life or prevent clonal evolution into AML (Passamonti et al. 2004b). The usual current indication for such therapy is to prevent thrombohemorrhagic events and only when dictated by the presence of defined risk factors for thrombosis (Table 18.5) (Tefferi and Murphy 2001).

18.9.2 Management of Low-Risk Disease

Patients with low-risk disease (Table 18.5) should not be treated with cytoreductive agents because drug therapy in such an instance might not carry a favorable risk to benefit profile (Barbui et al. 2004; Bazzan et al. 1999a; Besses et al. 1999; Cortelazzo et al. 1990, 1995a; Fenaux et al. 1990; Ruggeri et al. 1998a,b; Tefferi et al. 2000b). Instead, aspirin therapy is often sought to either alleviate microvascular disturbances (e.g., headache, lightheadedness, acral paresthesia, erythromelalgia, atypical chest pain) or provide some degree of protection from thrombotic complications as has been observed in a controlled study involving patients with PV (Landolfi et al. 2004a; Michiels et al. 1985). Unlike the case with higher doses (500 mg or higher per day), low-dose aspirin (81–325 mg/day) may not increase bleeding diathesis (Landolfi et al. 2004a; van Genderen et al. 1997b). The low-risk pregnant patient should not receive any cytoreductive agent and the use of aspirin is optional and may not influence outcome of pregnancy (Beressi et al. 1995).

18.9.3 Management of High-Risk Disease

There is currently universal agreement regarding the need to use cytoreductive therapy in high-risk patients with ET (Barbui et al. 2004; Elliott and Tefferi 2005; Harrison 2005b). This is because of not only the well-known increased risk of thrombosis in such patients, but also because of the proven benefit of cytoreductive therapy (Finazzi et al. 2000). The antithrombotic value of cytoreductive therapy in high-risk ET has been addressed by two randomized treatment trials (Cortelazzo et al. 1995a; Green et al. 2004). In the first study, treatment with hydroxyurea was compared to observation alone and the risk of thrombosis was significantly less in the treated group (3.6% vs. 24%) (Cortelazzo et al. 1995a). The second study did not have an untreated arm and instead compared hydroxyurea to anagrelide, both in combination with low-dose aspirin therapy (Green et al. 2004). The results of this study were published only in an abstract form, at the time of this writing, and revealed an unequivocal superiority for hydroxyurea over anagrelide (Green et al. 2004). After a median follow-up of 39 months, the composite risk of both thrombosis and bleeding was favorably affected by hydroxyurea treatment (36 vs. 55 events in the anagrelide arm) and the drug was much better tolerated than anagrelide (Harrison 2005b). In addition, the study showed a higher risk of fibrotic transformation but a lower risk of venous thrombosis in patients whose treatment included anagrelide as compared to those treated with hydroxyurea and aspirin. The results from the aforementioned two studies are the basis for recommending hydroxyurea as the first-line drug of choice for high-risk patients with ET (Table 18.6).

In addition to treatment with hydroxyurea, high-risk patients would probably benefit from aspirin therapy (Table 18.6) (Falanga et al. 2005; Finazzi and Barbui 2005; Michiels et al. 2004b; van Genderen et al. 1999). Aspirin therapy in ET is believed to reduce abnormal thromboxane synthesis (Rocca et al. 1995b; van Genderen et al. 1999) as well as inhibit platelet-neutrophil microaggregate formation (Falanga et al. 2005). In a patient who either does not tolerate hydroxyurea or is refractory to the drug (Demircay et al. 2002), interferon-α is a reasonable alternative (Saba et al. 2005) and is the drug of choice during pregnancy (Alvarado et al. 2003; Elliott and Tefferi 1997; Martinelli et al. 2004). When both hydroxyurea and interferon-α are not tolerated, other drugs including anagrelide and pipobroman might be considered (Table 18.7) (Barbui et al. 2004; Finazzi and Barbui 2005; Harrison 2005b). Once cytoreductive therapy is initiated, the therapeutic goal in terms of platelet count, based on anecdotal evidence of optimal thrombosis control, is $<400\times10^9$/L (Regev et al. 1997a; Storen and Tefferi 2001).

18.9.4 Indeterminate-Risk Disease

The use of cytoreductive therapy in indeterminate-risk patients with ET is controversial. In general, I recommend the use of low-dose aspirin in the absence of clinically relevant AVWS (ristocetin cofactor activity of <20%) that

Table 18.6. Treatment algorithm in essential thrombocythemia

Risk category	Age <60 years	Age ≥60 years	Women of childbearing age
Low-risk	Low-dose aspirin*	Not applicable	Low-dose aspirin*
Indeterminate-risk**	Low-dose aspirin*	Not applicable	Low-dose aspirin*
High-risk	Hydroxyurea *and* Low-dose aspirin	Hydroxyurea *and* Low-dose aspirin	Interferon alfa *and* Low-dose aspirin

* In the absence of a contraindication including evidence for acquired von Willebrand syndrome, i.e., a ristocetin co-factor activity of less than 50%.

** The decision to use cytoreductive agents in indeterminate-risk patients should be made on an individual basis (please see text for elaboration).

Table 18.7. Clinical properties of platelet-lowering agents

Drug (class)	Hydroxyurea[1]	Anagrelide[2]	Interferon alpha[3]	Phosphorus-32[4]	Pipobroman[5]
	Myelosuppressive	Unknown	Myelosuppressive	Myelosuppressive	Myelosuppressive
Mechanism of action	Antimetabolite	Unknown	Biologic agent	Radionuclide	Alkylating agent
Pharmacology	Half-life ≅ 5 h, renal excretion	Half-life ≅ 1.5 h, renal excretion	Kidney is main site of metabolism	Half-life ≅ 14 days	Insufficient information
Starting dose	500 mg PO BID	0.5 mg PO TID	5 million units SC TIW	2.3 mCi/m2 IV	1 mg/kg/day PO
Onset of action	≅ 3–5 days	≅ 6–10 days	1–3 weeks	4–8 weeks	≅ 16 days
Frequent side effects	Leukopenia, oral ulcers, anemia, hyperpigmentation, nail discoloration, xerodermia	Headache, palpitations, diarrhea, fluid retention, anemia	Flu-like syndrome, fatigue, anorexia, weight loss, lack of ambition, alopecia	Transient mild cytopenia	Nausea, abdominal pain, diarrhea
Infrequent side effects	Leg ulcers, alopecia, skin atrophy	Arrhythmias	Confusion, depression, autoimmune thyroiditis, myalgia, arthritis	Prolonged pancytopenia in elderly patients	Leukopenia, thrombocytopenia, hemolysis
Rare side effects	Fever, cystitis, platelet oscillations	Cardiomyopathy	Pruritus, hyperlipidemia, transaminasemia	Leukemogenic	
Cost*	Annual = $1,714, for 500 mg TID dose.	Annual = $8500, for 0.5 mg QID dose .	Annual = $10,500, for 3 million units 5 days/week	Approximately $1,025 for 4 mCi	Not available in USA

PO, oral; BID, twice-a-day; TID, thrice-a-day; QID, four times-a-day; SC, subcutaneous; TIW, three times-a-week; IV, intravenous. *Current cost to patient in US dollars

[1]Best et al. 1998; Daoud et al. 1997; Kennedy et al. 1975; Lossos and Matzner 1995; Najean and Rain 1997; Nguyen and Margolis 1993; Stevens 1999; Tefferi et al. 2000a; Yarbro 1992; [2]Anonymous 1992; Jurgens et al. 2004; Mazur 1992; Silverstein et al. 1988; Solberg et al. 1997; Spencer and Brogden 1994; Storen and Tefferi 2001; Tefferi et al. 1997; [3]Elliott and Tefferi 1997; Gilbert 1998; Gugliotta 1989; Lengfelder et al. 2000; Quesada et al. 1986; [4]Arthur 1967; Roberts and Smith 1997; Wagner et al. 1989; [5]Anonymous 1967; Mazzucconi et al. 1986; Najean and Rain 1997; Najman et al. 1982; Passamonti et al. 2000

may occur in a minority of patients with extreme thrombocytosis (Anonymous 1994). In addition, it is reasonable to consider cytoreductive treatment in patients with extreme thrombocytosis (platelet count over 1000×10^9/L) that is associated with either a clinically overt bleeding diathesis or aspirin-resistant microvascular symptoms. The target platelet count in this instance is the level that results in symptom relief or correction of the bleeding diathesis. There is the factor of anxiety that comes into play when managing a patient with extreme thrombocytosis and one has to temper the temptation to use cytoreductive agents in asymptomatic patients with the awareness that long-term use of such drugs could be detrimental (De Benedittis et al. 2004; Jurgens et al. 2004).

18.9.5 The Issue of Drug Leukemogenicity

Physicians in practice are often confronted with the possibility of leukemia arising from the use of hydroxyurea, which is the current choice of initial cytoreductive therapy in ET. This represents an unsubstantiated fear that unfortunately led to the use of alternative drugs without any controlled evidence of antithrombotic efficacy and with the potential for long-term side effects including anagrelide-associated cardiomyopathy (Jurgens et al. 2004) and interferon-associated neuropathy (Vardizer et al. 2003). The most recent demonstration of increased fibrotic transformation and suboptimal control of thrombosis and bleeding seen in anagrelide-treated patients with ET compared to those treated with hydroxyurea is yet another example of the danger associated with wide-spread use of new drugs without the backing of properly designed controlled studies (Green et al. 2004; Storen and Tefferi 2001).

The physician treating an individual patient must first have a good understanding of the natural history of ET that features a leukemic transformation rate that seldom exceeds 5% in the first 15 years (Passamonti et al. 2004b; Wolanskyj et al. 2003). Second, none of either large retrospective (Finazzi et al. 2004; Passamonti et al. 2004b) or prospective controlled studies (Harrison et al. 2005c) has ever shown an association between hydroxyurea use and AML in ET. Furthermore, in a recent large study of 1,638 patients with PV (Finazzi et al. 2005), among the 22 patients who developed either AML or MDS, five were exposed to either phlebotomy treatment alone or in combination with interferon-α (denominator = 669) and six to hydroxyurea alone (denominator = 742) for a rather intriguing hazard ratio of 0.86 in favor of hydroxyurea. This remarkably low incidence of AML in hydroxyurea-treated patients, despite the fact that the drug is usually administered to patients who are vulnerable to clonal evolution because of either aggressive disease phenotype or advanced age, should dispel the unsubstantiated fear of drug leukemogenicity associated with hydroxyurea use (Tefferi 2005a).

18.9.6 Management of Disease Complications

ET-associated acute thrombosis should be managed with both systemic anticoagulation and concomitant cytoreductive therapy (Cortelazzo et al. 1995b). In addition, although the use of aspirin in combination with oral anticoagulant therapy is discouraged in most instances, it is not unreasonable to consider such combination therapy in individual cases when indicated. Similarly, there is no controlled evidence that supports the use of platelet apheresis in any situation. Regardless, I currently recommend platelet apheresis for the acute management of hemorrhage or thrombosis that is accompanied by a platelet count of above 1000×10^9/L along with the prompt institution of cytoreductive therapy (Adami 1993). Other current indications include ET-associated AVWS associated with major hemorrhage and as a prophylactic measure before major surgery (Adami 1993; Budde et al. 1984; Greist 2002; Grima 2000; van Genderen et al. 1997a). In regards to symptomatic ET-associated AVWS, there is usually no need for the application of therapeutic approaches that are used in the management of congenital VWD.

18.9.7 Management of the Pregnant Patient

There are currently no controlled studies that provide evidence-based guidelines for the management of the pregnant patient with ET. Therefore, current recommendations are based on large retrospective studies and anecdotal reports (Harrison 2005a; Niittyvuopio et al. 2004; Wright and Tefferi 2001). First-trimester spontaneous abortion rate in ET (37%) is significantly higher than the 15% rate expected in the control population and does not appear to be influenced by specific treatment (Wright and Tefferi 2001). Late obstetric complications as well as maternal thrombohemorrhagic events are relatively infrequent. Neither the platelet count nor treatment with aspirin appears to affect either maternal morbidity or pregnancy outcome. In fact, several studies have shown a spontaneous lowering of platelet counts during pregnancy in ET. Therefore, cytoreductive treatment is currently not recommended for low-risk women with ET who are either pregnant or wish to be pregnant. In contrast, high-risk women require cytoreductive therapy to minimize the risk of recurrent thrombosis and anecdotal evidence of safety has encouraged a preference for the use of interferon-α in case of pregnancy in such patients (Elliott and Tefferi 1997).

18.10 Conclusion

There has been recent progress in both the science (James et al. 2005a) and treatment (Green et al. 2004) of ET with a relatively apparent impact in routine clinical practice. A new activating mutation of the Jak2 tyrosine kinase (Jak2^{V617F}) has been identified as a molecule of interest and its clinical relevance is being defined (Tefferi and Gilliland 2005b, c). A recent trial has demonstrated the superiority of hydroxyurea over anagrelide in the treatment of patients with high-risk ET and this has already resulted in a dramatic decline in the overall use of anagrelide (Green et al. 2004). For now, the practical value of mutation screening for Jak2^{V617F} is limited to disease diagnosis since the natural history as well as the incidence of life-threatening complications does not appear to be influenced by the presence of the mutation. Furthermore, Jak2^{V617F} is also found in other MPDs and it is unlikely that it represents a disease-causing mutation in ET.

The indolent natural history of ET is a true challenge for drug development (Tefferi 2005b). Because the survival in ET might not be inferior to an age- and sex-matched control population (Barbui et al. 2004; Passamonti et al. 2004b; Rozman et al. 1991; Tefferi et al. 2001), it is next to impossible to show a survival advantage attached to a "new" drug. It is equally statistically challenging to demonstrate the value of a new drug in the control of disease-related complications because of the low baseline rates seen with hydroxyurea therapy (Passamonti et al. 2004b). It is therefore reasonable to question the value of additional randomized treatment trials in ET. Instead, it might be more cost effective to direct resources and effort towards basic and translational research that focuses on disease pathogenesis and leads to curative therapy.

References

Abe A, Emi N, Tanimoto M, Terasaki H, Marunouchi T, Saito H (1997) Fusion of the platelet-derived growth factor receptor beta to a novel gene CEV14 in acute myelogenous leukemia after clonal evolution. Blood 90:4271–4277

Adami R (1993) Therapeutic thrombocytapheresis: a review of 132 patients. Int J Artif Organs 16 Suppl 5:183–184

Adamson JW, Fialkow PJ, Murphy S, Prchal JF, Steinmann L (1976) Polycythemia vera: stem-cell and probable clonal origin of the disease. N Engl J Med 295:913–916

Afshar-Kharghan VLA, Gray L, Padilla A, Borthakur G, Roberts S, Pruthi R, Tefferi A (2001) Hemostatic gene polymorphisms and the prevalence of thrombohemorrhagic complications in polycythemia vera and essential thrombocythemia. Blood 98:471a

Aguiar RC, Macdonald D, Mason PJ, Cross NC, Goldman JM (1995) Myeloproliferative disorder associated with 8p11 translocations. Blood 86:834–835

Alvarado Y, Cortes J, Verstovsek S, Thomas D, Faderl S, Estrov Z, Kantarjian H, Giles FJ (2003) Pilot study of pegylated interferon-alpha 2b in patients with essential thrombocythemia. Cancer Chemother Pharmacol 51:81–86

Amitrano L, Guardascione MA, Ames PR, Margaglione M, Antinolfi I, Iannaccone L, Annunziata M, Ferrara F, Brancaccio V, Balzano A (2003) Thrombophilic genotypes, natural anticoagulants, and plasma homocysteine in myeloproliferative disorders: relationship with splanchnic vein thrombosis and arterial disease. Am J Hematol 72:75–81

Andersson PO, Ridell B, Wadenvik H, Kutti J (2000) Leukemic transformation of essential thrombocythemia without previous cytoreductive treatment. Ann Hematol 79:40–42

Anger B, Janssen JW, Schrezenmeier H, Hehlmann R, Heimpel H, Bartram CR (1990) Clonal analysis of chronic myeloproliferative disorders using X-linked DNA polymorphisms. Leukemia 4:258–261

Anger BR, Seifried E, Scheppach J, Heimpel H (1989a) Budd-Chiari syndrome and thrombosis of other abdominal vessels in the chronic myeloproliferative diseases. Klin Wochenschr 67:818–825

Anger BR, Seifried E, Scheppach J, Heimpel H (1989b) Budd-Chiari syndrome and thrombosis of other abdominal vessels in the chronic myeloproliferative diseases. Klin Wochenschr 67:818–825

Annaloro C, Lambertenghi Deliliers G, Oriani A, Pozzoli E, Lambertenghi Deliliers D, Radaelli F, Faccini P (1999) Prognostic significance of bone marrow biopsy in essential thrombocythemia. Haematologica 84:17–21

Anonymous (1967) Evaluation of two antineoplastic agents: Pipobroman (Vercyte) and thioguanine. J Am Med Assoc 200:619–620

Anonymous (1992) Anagrelide, a therapy for thrombocythemic states: experience in 577 patients. Anagrelide Study Group. Am J Med 92:69–76

Anonymous (1994) Antiplatelet trialist's collaboration collaborative overview of randomised trials of antiplatelet therapy-1. Br Med J 308:81–106

Apperley JF, Gardembas M, Melo JV, Russell-Jones R, Bain BJ, Baxter EJ, Chase A, Chessells JM, Colombat M, Dearden CE, Dimitrijevic S, Mahon FX, Marin D, Nikolova Z, Olavarria E, Silberman S, Schultheis B, Cross NC, Goldman JM (2002) Response to imatinib mesylate in patients with chronic myeloproliferative diseases with rearrangements of the platelet-derived growth factor receptor beta. N Engl J Med 347:481–487

Arcasoy MO, Harris KW, Forget BG (1999) A human erythropoietin receptor gene mutant causing familial erythrocytosis is associated with deregulation of the rates of Jak2 and Stat5 inactivation. Exp Hematol 27:63–74

Arora B, Sirhan S, Hoyer JD, Mesa RA, Tefferi A (2005) Peripheral blood CD34 count in myelofibrosis with myeloid metaplasia: a prospective evaluation of prognostic value in 94 patients. Br J Haematol 128:42–48

Arthur K (1967) Radioactive phosphorus in the treatment of polycythaemia. A review of ten years' experience. Clin Radiol 18:287–291

Asimakopoulos FA, Hinshelwood S, Gilbert JGR, Delibrias CC, Gottgens B, Fearon DT, Green AR (1997) The gene encoding hematopoietic cell phosphatase (Shp-1) is structurally and transcriptionally intact in polycythemia vera. Oncogene 14:1215–1222

Axelrad AA, Eskinazi D, Correa PN, Amato D (2000) Hypersensitivity of circulating progenitor cells to megakaryocyte growth and development factor (PEG-rHu MGDF) in essential thrombocythemia. Blood 96:3310–3321

Bacher U, Haferlach T, Kern W, Hiddemann W, Schnittger S, Schoch C (2005) Conventional cytogenetics of myeloproliferative diseases other than CML contribute valid information. Ann Hematol 84:250–257

Bain BJ (2003) Cytogenetic and molecular genetic aspects of eosinophilic leukaemias. Br J Haematol 122:173–179

Balduini CL, Bertolino G, Noris P, Piletta GC (1991) Platelet aggregation in platelet-rich plasma and whole blood in 120 patients with myeloproliferative disorders. Am J Clin Pathol 95:82–86

Barbui T, Barosi G, Grossi A, Gugliotta L, Liberato LN, Marchetti M, Mazzucconi MG, Rodeghiero F, Tura S (2004) Practice guidelines for the therapy of essential thrombocythemia. A statement from the Italian Society of Hematology, the Italian Society of Experimental Hematology and the Italian Group for Bone Marrow Transplantation. Haematologica 89:215–232

Barr RD, Fialkow PJ (1973) Clonal origin of chronic myelocytic leukemia. N Engl J Med 289:307–309

Baxter EJ, Kulkarni S, Vizmanos JL, Jaju R, Martinelli G, Testoni N, Hughes G, Salamanchuk Z, Calasanz MJ, Lahortiga I, Pocock CF, Dang R, Fidler C, Wainscoat JS, Boultwood J, Cross NC (2003) Novel translocations that disrupt the platelet-derived growth factor receptor beta (PDGFRB) gene in BCR-ABL-negative chronic myeloproliferative disorders. Br J Haematol 120:251–256

Baxter EJ, Scott LM, Campbell PJ, East C, Fourouclas N, Swanton S, Vassiliou GS, Bench AJ, Boyd EM, Curtin N, Scott MA, Erber WN, Green AR (2005) Acquired mutation of the tyrosine kinase JAK2 in human myeloproliferative disorders. Lancet 365:1054–1061

Bazzan M, Tamponi G, Schinco P, Vaccarino A, Foli C, Gallone G, Pileri A (1999 a) Thrombosis-free survival and life expectancy in 187 consecutive patients with essential thrombocythemia. Ann Hematol 78:539–543

Bazzan M, Tamponi G, Schinco P, Vaccarino A, Foli C, Gallone G, Pileri A (1999 b) Thrombosis-free survival and life expectancy in 187 consecutive patients with essential thrombocythemia. Ann Hematol 78:539–543

Belloni E, Trubia M, Gasparini P, Micucci C, Tapinassi C, Confalonieri S, Nuciforo P, Martino B, Lo-Coco F, Pelicci PG, Di Fiore PP (2005) 8p11 myeloproliferative syndrome with a novel t(7;8) translocation leading to fusion of the FGFR1 and TIF1 genes. Genes Chromosomes Cancer 42:320–325

Bellucci S, Janvier M, Tobelem G, Flandrin G, Charpak Y, Berger R, Boiron, M (1986) Essential thrombocythemias. Clinical evolutionary and biological data. Cancer 58:2440–2447

Beressi AH, Tefferi A, Silverstein MN, Petitt RM, Hoagland HC (1995) Outcome analysis of 34 pregnancies in women with essential thrombocythemia. Arch Inter Med 155:1217–1222

Besses C, Cervantes F, Pereira A, Florensa L, Sole F, Hernandez-Boluda, JC, Woessner S, Sans-Sabrafen J, Rozman C, Montserrat E (1999) Major vascular complications in essential thrombocythemia: a study of the predictive factors in a series of 148 patients. Leukemia 13:150–154

Best PJ, Daoud MS, Pittelkow MR, Petitt RM (1998) Hydroxyurea-induced leg ulceration in 14 patients. Ann Inter Med 128:29–32

Boneu B, Nouvel C, Sie P, Caranobe C, Combes D, Laurent G, Pris J, Bierme R (1980) Platelets in myeloproliferative disorders. I. A comparative evaluation with certain platelet function tests. Scand J Haematol 25:214–220

Brummitt DR, Barker HF (2000) The determination of a reference range for new platelet parameters produced by the Bayer ADVIA120 full blood count analyser. Clin Lab Haematol 22:103–107

Brusamolino E, Orlandi E, Morra E, Bernasconi P, Pagnucco G, Colombo A, Lazzarino M, Bernasconi C (1988) Hematologic and clinical features of patients with chromosome 5 monosomy or deletion (5q). Med Pediatr Oncol 16:88–94

Budde U, Schaefer G, Mueller N, Egli H, Dent J, Ruggeri Z, Zimmerman T (1984) Acquired von Willebrand's disease in the myeloproliferative syndrome. Blood 64:981–985

Budde U, Dent JA, Berkowitz SD, Ruggeri ZM, Zimmerman TS (1986) Subunit composition of plasma von Willebrand factor in patients with the myeloproliferative syndrome. Blood 68:1213–1217

Budde U, Scharf RE, Franke P, Hartmann-Budde K, Dent J, Ruggeri ZM (1993) Elevated platelet count as a cause of abnormal von Willebrand factor multimer distribution in plasma. Blood 82:1749–1757

Budde U, van Genderen PJ (1997) Acquired von Willebrand disease in patients with high platelet counts. Sem Thromb Hemost 23:425–431

Burstein SA, Malpass TW, Yee E, Kadin M, Brigden M, Adamson JW, Harker LA (1984) Platelet factor-4 excretion in myeloproliferative disease: implications for the aetiology of myelofibrosis. Br J Haematol 57:383–392

Buss DH, Stuart JJ, Lipscomb GE (1985) The incidence of thrombotic and hemorrhagic disorders in association with extreme thrombocytosis: an analysis of 129 cases. Am J Hematol 20:365–372

Buss DH, O'Connor ML, Woodruff RD, Richards F, Brockschmidt JK (1991) Bone marrow and peripheral blood findings in patients with extreme thrombocytosis. A report of 63 cases. Arch Pathol Lab Med 115:475–480

Buss DH, Cashell AW, O'Connor ML, Richards F, 2nd, Case LD (1994) Occurrence, etiology, and clinical significance of extreme thrombocytosis: a study of 280 cases. Am J Med 96:247–253

Buttner C, Henz BM, Welker P, Sepp NT, Grabbe J (1998) Identification of activating c-kit mutations in adult-, but not in childhood-onset indolent mastocytosis: a possible explanation for divergent clinical behavior. J Invest Dermatol 111:1227–1231

Cabello AI, Collado R, Ruiz MA, Martinez J, Navarro I, Ferrer R, Sosa AM, Carbonell F (2005) A retrospective analysis of myelodysplastic syndromes with thrombocytosis: reclassification of the cases by WHO proposals. Leuk Res 29:365–370

Cerutti A, Custodi P, Duranti M, Noris P, Balduini, CL (1997) Thrombopoietin levels in patients with primary and reactive thrombocytosis. Br J Haematol 99:281–284

Chaffanet M, Popovici C, Leroux D, Jacrot M, Adelaide J, Dastugue N, Gregoire MJ, Hagemeijer A, Lafage-Pochitaloff M, Birnbaum D, Pebusque MJ (1998) t(6;8), t(8;9) and t(8;13) translocations associated with stem cell myeloproliferative disorders have close or identical breakpoints in chromosome region 8p11–12. Oncogene 16:945–949

Chaiter Y, Brenner B, Aghai E, Tatarsky I (1992) High incidence of myeloproliferative disorders in Ashkenazi Jews in northern Israel. Leuk Lymphoma 7:251–255

Champion KM, Gilbert JG, Asimakopoulos FA, Hinshelwood S, Green AR (1997) Clonal haemopoiesis in normal elderly women: implications for the myeloproliferative disorders and myelodysplastic syndromes. Br J Haematol 97:920–926

Chen HL, Chiou SS, Sheen JM, Jang RC, Lu CC, Chang TT (1999) Thrombocytosis in children at one medical center of southern Taiwan. Acta Paediatr Taiwan 40:309–313

Chiusolo P, La Barbera EO, Laurenti L, Piccirillo N, Sora F, Giordano G, Urbano R, Mazzucconi MG, De Stefano V, Leone G, Sica S (2001) Clonal hemopoiesis and risk of thrombosis in young female patients with essential thrombocythemia. Exp Hematol 29:670–676

Chuncharunee S, Archararit N, Ungkanont A, Jootar S, Angchaisuksiri P, Bunyaratavej A, Rojanasthein S, Atichartakarn V (2000) Etiology and incidence of thrombotic and hemorrhagic disorders in Thai patients with extreme thrombocytosis. J Med Assoc Thailand 83 Suppl 1:95–100

Cools J, DeAngelo DJ, Gotlib J, Stover EH, Legare RD, Cortes J, Kutok J, Clark J, Galinsky I, Griffin JD, Cross NC, Tefferi A, Malone J, Alam R, Schrier SL, Schmid J, Rose M, Vandenberghe P, Verhoef G, Boogaerts M, Wlodarska I, Kantarjian H, Marynen P, Coutre SE, Stone R, Gilliland DG (2003) A tyrosine kinase created by fusion of the PDGFRA and FIP1L1 genes as a therapeutic target of imatinib in idiopathic hypereosinophilic syndrome. N Engl J Med 348: 1201–1214

Cortelazzo S, Viero P, Finazzi, GADE, Rodeghiero F, Barbui T (1990) Incidence and risk factors for thrombotic complications in a historical cohort of 100 patients with essential thrombocythemia. J Clin Oncol 8:556–562

Cortelazzo S, Finazzi G, Ruggeri M, Vestri O, Galli M, Rodeghiero F, Barbui T (1995 a) Hydroxyurea for patients with essential thrombocythemia and a high risk of thrombosis. N Engl J Med 332: 1132–1136

Cortelazzo S, Finazzi G, Ruggeri M, Vestri O, Galli M, Rodeghiero F, Barbui T (1995 b) Hydroxyurea for patients with essential thrombocythemia and a high risk of thrombosis. N Engl J Med 332: 1132–1136

Cortelazzo S, Marchetti M, Orlando E, Falanga A, Barbui T, Buchanan MR (1998) Aspirin increases the bleeding side effects in essential thrombocythemia independent of the cyclooxygenase pathway: role of the lipoxygenase pathway. Am J Hematol 57:277–282

Daley GQ, Van Etten RA, Baltimore D (1990) Induction of chronic myelogenous leukemia in mice by the P210bcr/abl gene of the Philadelphia chromosome. Science 247:824–830

Dameshek W (1951) Some speculations on the myeloproliferative syndromes. Blood 6:372–375

Daoud MS, Gibson LE, Pittelkow MR (1997) Hydroxyurea dermopathy: a unique lichenoid eruption complicating long-term therapy with hydroxyurea. J Am Acad Dermatol 36:178–182

De Benedittis M, Petruzzi M, Giardina C, Lo Muzio L, Favia G, Serpico R (2004) Oral squamous cell carcinoma during long-term treatment with hydroxyurea. Clin Exp Dermatol 29:605–607

de Klein A, van Kessel AG, Grosveld G, Bartram CR, Hagemeijer A, Bootsma D, Spurr NK, Heisterkamp N, Groffen J, Stephenson JR (1982) A cellular oncogene is translocated to the Philadelphia chromosome in chronic myelocytic leukaemia. Nature 300:765–767

De Sanctis V, Mazzucconi MG, Spadea A, Alfo M, Mancini M, Bizzoni L, Peraino M, Mandelli F (2003) Long-term evaluation of 164 patients with essential thrombocythaemia treated with pipobroman: occurrence of leukaemic evolution. Br J Haematol 123: 517–521

Demircay Z, Comert A, Adiguzel C (2002) Leg ulcers and hydroxyurea: report of three cases with essential thrombocythemia. Int J Dermatol 41:872–874

Di Guglielmo G (1917) Richerche di ematologia. I. Un caso di eritroleucemia. Megacariociti in circolo e loro funzione piastrinopoietico. Folia Med (Pavia) 13:386

Dicato MASB, Berchem GJ et al (1999) V Leiden mutations, prothromin and methylene-tetrahydrofolate reductase are not risk factors for thromboembolic disease in essential thrombocythemia. Blood 94:111a

Ding J, Komatsu H, Wakita A, Kato-Uranishi M, Ito M, Satoh A, Tsuboi K, Nitta M, Miyazaki H, Iida S, Ueda R (2004) Familial essential thrombocythemia associated with a dominant-positive activating mutation of the c-MPL gene, which encodes for the receptor for thrombopoietin. Blood 103:4198–4200

Dror Y, Zipursky A, Blanchette VS (1999) Essential thrombocythemia in children. J Pediatr Hematol Oncol 21:356–363

El Kassar N, Hetet G, Li Y, Briere J, Grandchamp B (1995) Clonal analysis of haemopoietic cells in essential thrombocythaemia. Br J Haematol 90:131–137

El Kassar N, Hetet G, Briere J, Grandchamp B (1997) Clonality analysis of hematopoiesis in essential thrombocythemia – advantages of studying T lymphocytes and platelets. Blood 89:128–134

Elliott MA, Tefferi A (1997) Interferon-alpha therapy in polycythemia vera and essential thrombocythemia. Sem Thromb Hemost 23:463–472

Elliott MA, Tefferi A (2003) Thrombocythaemia and pregnancy. Baillieres Best Pract Res Clin Haematol 16:227–242

Elliott MA, Tefferi A (2005) Thrombosis and haemorrhage in polycythaemia vera and essential thrombocythaemia. Br J Haematol 128:275–290

Epstein E, Goedel A (1934) Hämorrhagische Thrombozythämie bei vasculärer Schrumpfmilz (Hemorrhagic thrombocythemia with a vascular, sclerotic spleen). Virchows Arch A Pathol Anat Histopathol 293:233

Espanol I, Hernandez A, Cortes M, Mateo J, Pujol-Moix N (1999) Patients with thrombocytosis have normal or slightly elevated thrombopoietin levels. Haematologica 84:312–316

Fabris F, Casonato A, Grazia del Ben M, De Marco L, Girolami A (1986) Abnormalities of von Willebrand factor in myeloproliferative disease: a relationship with bleeding diathesis. Br J Haematol 63:75–83

Falanga A, Marchetti M, Evangelista V, Vignoli A, Licini M, Balicco M, Manarini S, Finazzi G, Cerletti C, Barbui T (2000) Polymorphonuclear leukocyte activation and hemostasis in patients with essential thrombocythemia and polycythemia vera. Blood 96:4261–4266

Falanga A, Marchetti M, Vignoli A, Balducci D, Barbui T (2005) Leukocyte-platelet interaction in patients with essential thrombocythemia and polycythemia vera. Exp Hematol 33:523–530

Falcetta R, Sacerdote C, Bazzan M, Pollio B, Ciocca Vasino MA, Ciccone G, Vineis P (2003) [Occupational and environmental risk factors for essential thrombocythemia: a case-control study]. G Ital Med Lav Ergon 25 Suppl:9–12

Faurschou M, Nielsen OJ, Jensen MK, Hasselbalch HC (2000) High prevalence of hyperhomocysteinemia due to marginal deficiency of cobalamin or folate in chronic myeloproliferative disorders. Am J Hematol 65:136–140

Feener EP, Rosario F, Dunn SL, Stancheva Z, Myers MG Jr (2004) Tyrosine phosphorylation of Jak2 in the JH2 domain inhibits cytokine signaling. Mol Cell Biol 24:4968–4978

Fenaux P, Simon M, Caulier MT, Lai JL, Goudemand J, Bauters F (1990) Clinical course of essential thrombocythemia in 147 cases. Cancer 66:549–556

Fialkow PJ (1990) Stem cell origin of human myeloid blood cell neoplasms. Verh Dtsch Ges Pathol 74:43–47

Fialkow PJ, Gartler SM, Yoshida A (1967) Clonal origin of chronic myelocytic leukemia in man. Proc Natl Acad Sci USA 58:1468–1471

Fialkow PJ, Jacobson RJ, Papayannopoulou T (1977) Chronic myelocytic leukemia: clonal origin in a stem cell common to the granulocyte, erythrocyte, platelet and monocyte/macrophage. Am J Med 63:125–130

Fialkow PJ, Denman AM, Jacobson RJ, Lowenthal MN (1978a) Chronic myelocytic leukemia. Origin of some lymphocytes from leukemic stem cells. J Clin Invest 62:815–823

Fialkow PJ, Denman AM, Singer J, Jacobson RJ, Lowenthal MN (1978b) Human myeloproliferative disorders: clonal origin in pluripotent stem cells, pp 131–144. In: Clarkson B et al (ed) Differentiation of normal and neoplastic hematopoietic cells. Cold Spring Harbor Laboratory, Cold Spring Harbor 5:131–144

Fialkow PJ, Faguet GB, Jacobson RJ, Vaidya K, Murphy S (1981) Evidence that essential thrombocythemia is a clonal disorder with origin in a multipotent stem cell. Blood 58:916–919

Finazzi G, Barbui T (2005) Risk-adapted therapy in essential thrombocythemia and polycythemia vera. Blood Rev 19:243–252

Finazzi G, Ruggeri M, Rodeghiero F, Barbui T (2000) Second malignancies in patients with essential thrombocythaemia treated with busulphan and hydroxyurea: long-term follow-up of a randomized clinical trial. Br J Haematol 110:577–583

Finazzi G, Caruso V, Marchioli R, Capnist G, Chisesi T, Finelli C, Gugliotta L, Landolfi R, Kutti J, Gisslinger H, Marilus R, Patrono C, Pogliani EM, Randi ML, Villegas A, Tognoni G, Barbui T (2005) Acute leukemia in polycythemia vera. An analysis of 1,638 patients enrolled in a prospective observational study. Blood 105:2664–2670

Fioretos T, Panagopoulos I, Lassen C, Swedin A, Billstrom R, Isaksson M, Strombeck B, Olofsson T, Mitelman F, Johansson B (2001) Fusion of the BCR and the fibroblast growth factor receptor-1 (FGFR1) genes as a result of t(8;22)(p11;q11) in a myeloproliferative disorder: the first fusion gene involving BCR but not ABL. Genes Chromosomes Cancer 32:302–310

Florensa L, Besses C, Zamora L, Bellosillo B, Espinet B, Serrano S, Woessner S, Sole F (2004) Endogenous erythroid and megakaryocytic circulating progenitors, HUMARA clonality assay, and PRV-1 expression are useful tools for diagnosis of polycythemia vera and essential thrombocythemia. Blood 103:2427–2428

Flotho C, Valcamonica S, Mach-Pascual S, Schmahl G, Corral L, Ritterbach J, Hasle H, Arico M, Biondi A, Niemeyer CM (1999) RAS mutations and clonality analysis in children with juvenile myelomonocytic leukemia (JMML). Leukemia 13:32–37

Froberg MK, Brunning RD, Dorion P, Litz CE, Torlakovic E (1998) Demonstration of clonality in neutrophils using FISH in a case of chronic neutrophilic leukemia. Leukemia 12:623–626

Fugazza G, Bruzzone R, Dejana, AM, Gobbi M, Ghio R, Patrone F, Rattenni S, Sessarego M (1995) Cytogenetic clonality in chronic myelomonocytic leukemia studied with fluorescence in situ hybridization. Leukemia 9:109–114

Furitsu T, Tsujimura T, Tono T, Ikeda H, Kitayama H, Koshimizu U, Sugahara H, Butterfield JH, Ashman LK, Kanayama Y et al (1993) Identification of mutations in the coding sequence of the proto-oncogene c-kit in a human mast cell leukemia cell line causing ligand-independent activation of c-kit product. J Clin Invest 92:1736–1744

Ganti AK, Potti A, Koka VK, Pervez H, Mehdi SA (2003) Myeloproliferative syndromes and the associated risk of coronary artery disease. Thromb Res 110:83–86

Gersuk GM, Carmel R, Pattengale PK (1989) Platelet-derived growth factor concentrations in platelet-poor plasma and urine from patients with myeloproliferative disorders. Blood 74:2330–2334

Gevao SM, Pabs-Garnon E, Williams AC (1996) Platelet counts in healthy adult Sierra Leoneans. W Afr J Med 15:163–164

Gilbert HS (1998) Long term treatment of myeloproliferative disease with interferon-alpha-2b – feasibility and efficacy. Cancer 83:1205–1213

Gilliland DG, Blanchard KL, Levy J, Perrin S, Bunn HF (1991) Clonality in myeloproliferative disorders: analysis by means of the polymerase chain reaction. Proc Natl Acad Sci USA 88:6848–6852

Gisslinger H, Rodeghiero F, Ruggeri M, Heis-Vahidi Fard N, Mannhalter C, Papagiannopoulos M, Rintelen C, Lalouschek W, Knobl P, Lechner K, Pabinger I (1999) Homocysteine levels in polycythaemia vera and essential thrombocythaemia. Br J Haematol 105:551–555

Gitler AD, Kong Y, Choi JK, Zhu Y, Pear WS, Epstein JA (2004) Tie2-Cre-induced inactivation of a conditional mutant Nf1 allele in mouse results in a myeloproliferative disorder that models juvenile myelomonocytic leukemia. Pediat Res 55:581–584

Goerttler PL, Marz E, Johansson PL, Andreasson B, Kutti J, Moliterno AR, Marchioli R, Spivak JL, Pahl HL (2005a) Thrombotic and bleeding complications in four subpopulations of patients with essential thrombocythemia defined by c-Mpl protein expression and PRV-1 mRNA levels. Haematologica 90:851–853

Goerttler PS, Steimle C, Marz E, Johansson PL, Andreasson B, Griesshammer M, Gisslinger H, Heimpel H, Pahl HL (2005b) The Jak2V617F mutation, PRV-1 overexpression and EEC formation define a similar cohort of MPD patients. Blood 106:2862–2864

Golde DW, Bersch N, Cline MJ (1977) Polycythemia vera: hormonal modulation of erythropoiesis in vitro. Blood 49:399–405

Goldman JM (2005) A unifying mutation in chronic myeloproliferative disorders. N Engl J Med 352:1744–1746

Golub TR, Barker GF, Lovett M, Gilliland DG (1994) Fusion of PDGF receptor beta to a novel ets-like gene, tel, in chronic myelomonocytic leukemia with t(5;12) chromosomal translocation. Cell 77: 307–316

Grand EK, Grand FH, Chase AJ, Ross FM, Corcoran MM, Oscier DG, Cross NC (2004a) Identification of a novel gene, FGFR1OP2, fused to FGFR1 in 8p11 myeloproliferative syndrome. Genes Chromosomes Cancer 40:78–83

Grand FH, Burgstaller S, Kuhr T, Baxter EJ, Webersinke G, Thaler J, Chase AJ, Cross NC (2004b) p53-Binding protein 1 is fused to the platelet-derived growth factor receptor beta in a patient with a t(5;15)(q33;q22) and an imatinib-responsive eosinophilic myeloproliferative disorder. Cancer Res 64:7216–7219

Granjo E, Lima M, Lopes JM, Doria S, Orfao A, Ying S, Barata LT, Miranda M, Cross NC, Bain BJ (2002) Chronic eosinophilic leukaemia presenting with erythroderma, mild eosinophilia and hyper-IgE: clinical, immunological and cytogenetic features and therapeutic approach. A case report. Acta Haematol 107:108–112

Greist A (2002) The role of blood component removal in essential and reactive thrombocytosis. Ther Apher 6:36–44

Griesshammer M, Bangerter M, Sauer T, Wennauer R, Bergmann L, Heimpel H (1999) Aetiology and clinical significance of thrombocytosis: analysis of 732 patients with an elevated platelet count. J Inter Med 245:295–300

Grima KM (2000) Therapeutic apheresis in hematological and oncological diseases. J Clin Apher 15:28–52

Groffen J, Stephenson JR, Heisterkamp N, de Klein A, Bartram CR, Grosveld G (1984) Philadelphia chromosomal breakpoints are clustered within a limited region, bcr, on chromosome 22. Cell 36:93–99

Guasch G, Popovici C, Mugneret F, Chaffanet M, Pontarotti P, Birnbaum D, Pebusque MJ (2003) Endogenous retroviral sequence is fused to FGFR1 kinase in the 8p12 stem-cell myeloproliferative disorder with t(8;19)(p12;q13.3). Blood 101:286–288

Gugliotta LEA (1989) In vivo and in vitro inhibitory effect of alpha-interferon on megakaryocyte colony growth in essential thrombocythemia. Br J Haematol 71:177–181

Gugliotta LEA (1997) Epidemiological, diagnostic, therapeutic, and prognostic aspects of essential thrombocythemia in a retrospective study of the GIMMC group in two thousand patients. Blood 90:348a (abstract no 1551)

Gunz FW (1960) Hemorrhagic thrombocythemia: a critical review. Blood 15:706–723

Gupta R, Abdalla SH, Bain BJ (1999) Thrombocytosis with sideroblastic erythropoiesis: a mixed myeloproliferative myelodysplastic syndrome. Leuk Lymphoma 34:615–619

Gupta R, Knight CL, Bain BJ (2002) Receptor tyrosine kinase mutations in myeloid neoplasms. Br J Haematol 117:489–508

Harrison C (2005a) Pregnancy and its management in the Philadelphia negative myeloproliferative diseases. Br J Haematol 129:293–306

Harrison CN (2005b) Essential thrombocythaemia: challenges and evidence-based management. Br J Haematol 130:153–165

Harrison CN, Gale RE, Wiestner AC, Skoda RC, Linch DC (1998) The activating splice mutation in intron 3 of the thrombopoietin gene is not found in patients with non-familial essential thrombocythaemia. Br J Haematol 102:1341–1343

Harrison CN, Gale RE, Machin SJ, Linch DC (1999a) A large proportion of patients with a diagnosis of essential thrombocythemia do not have a clonal disorder and may be at lower risk of thrombotic complications. Blood 93:417–424

Harrison CN, Gale RE, Pezella F, Mire-Sluis A, MacHin SJ, Linch DC (1999b) Platelet c-mpl expression is dysregulated in patients with essential thrombocythaemia but this is not of diagnostic value. Br J Haematol 107:139–147

Harrison CN, Donohoe S, Carr P, Dave M, Mackie I, Machin SJ (2002) Patients with essential thrombocythaemia have an increased prevalence of antiphospholipid antibodies which may be associated with thrombosis. Thromb Haemost 87:802–807

Harrison CN, Campbell PJ, Buck G, Wheatley K, East CL, Bareford D, Wilkins BS, van der Walt JD, Reilly JT, Grigg AP, Revell P, Woodcock BE, Green AR (2005c) United Kingdom Medical Research Council Primary Thrombocythemia 1 Study. Hydroxyurea compared with anagrelide in high-risk essential thrombocythemia. N Engl J Med 353:85–86

Hasle H (2000) Incidence of essential thrombocythaemia in children. Br J Haematol 110:751

Heisterkamp N, Stam K, Groffen J, de Klein A, Grosveld G (1985) Structural organization of the bcr gene and its role in the Ph' translocation. Nature 315:758–761

Hess G, Rose P, Gamm H, Papadileris S, Huber C, Seliger B (1994) Molecular analysis of the erythropoietin receptor system in patients with polycythaemia vera. Br J Haematol 88:794–802

Heuck G (1879) Zwei Fälle von Leukämie mit eigenthümlichem Blut- resp. Knochenmarksbefund (Two cases of leukemia with peculiar blood and bone marrow findings, respectively). Arch Pathol Anat Physiol Virchows 78:475–496

Heudes D, Carli PM, Bailly F, Milan C, Mugneret F, Petrella T (1989) Myeloproliferative disorders in the department of Cote d'Or between 1980 and 1986. Nouv Rev Fr Hematol 31:375–378

Horikawa Y, Matsumura I, Hashimoto K, Shiraga M, Kosugi S, Tadokoro S, Kato T, Miyazaki H, Tomiyama Y, Kurata Y, Matsuzawa Y, Kanakura Y (1997) Markedly reduced expression of platelet C-Mpl receptor in essential thrombocythemia. Blood 90:4031–4038

Hou M, Carneskog J, Mellqvist UH, Stockelberg D, Hedberg M, Wadenvik H, Kutti J (1998) Impact of endogenous thrombopoietin levels on the differential diagnosis of essential thrombocythaemia and reactive thrombocytosis. Eur J Haematol 61:119–122

Imasawa M, Iijima H (2002) Multiple retinal vein occlusions in essential thrombocythemia. Am J Ophthalmol 133:152–155

Jacobson RJ, Salo A, Fialkow PJ (1978) Agnogenic myeloid metaplasia: a clonal proliferation of hematopoietic stem cells with secondary myelofibrosis. Blood 51:189–194

Jaffe ES, Harris NL, Stein H, Vardiman JW (eds) (2001) WHO classification of tumors: Tumors of the hematopoietic and lymphoid tissues. IARC press, Lyon

James C, Ugo V, Le Couedic JP, Staerk J, Delhommeau F, Lacout C, Garcon L, Raslova H, Berger R, Bennaceur-Griscelli A, Villeval JL, Constantinescu SN, Casadevall N, Vainchenker W (2005a) A unique clonal JAK2 mutation leading to constitutive signalling causes polycythaemia vera. Nature 434:1144–1148

James C, Ugo V, Le Couedic JP, Staerk J, Delhommeau F, Lacout C, Garcon L, Raslova H, Berger R, Bennaceur-Griscelli A, Villeval JL, Constantinescu SN, Casadevall N, Vainchenker W (2005b) A unique clonal JAK2 mutation leading to constitutive signalling causes polycythemia vera. Nature (in press)

Jantunen R, Juvonen E, Ikkala E, Oksanen K, Anttila P, Ruutu T (2001) The predictive value of vascular risk factors and gender for the development of thrombotic complications in essential thrombocythemia. Ann Hematol 80:74–78

Jenkins RB, Tefferi A, Solberg LA Jr, Dewald GW (1989) Acute leukemia with abnormal thrombopoiesis and inversions of chromosome 3. Cancer Genet Cytogenet 39:167–179

Jensen MK, de Nully Brown P, Lund BV, Nielsen OJ, Hasselbalch HC (2000a) Increased platelet activation and abnormal membrane glycoprotein content and redistribution in myeloproliferative disorders [see comment]. Br J Haematol 110:116–124

Jensen MK, de Nully Brown P, Nielsen OJ, Hasselbalch HC (2000b) Incidence, clinical features and outcome of essential thrombocythaemia in a well defined geographical area. Eur J Haematol 65:132–139

Jensen MK, de Nully Brown P, Lund BV, Nielsen OJ, Hasselbalch HC (2001) Increased circulating platelet-leukocyte aggregates in myeloproliferative disorders is correlated to previous thrombosis, platelet activation and platelet count. Eur J Haematol 66:143–151

Jensen MK, de Nully Brown P, Thorsen S, Hasselbalch HC (2002) Frequent occurrence of anticardiolipin antibodies, Factor V Leiden mutation, and perturbed endothelial function in chronic myeloproliferative disorders. Am J Hematol 69:185–191

Johansson P, Ricksten A, Wennstrom L, Palmqvist L, Kutti J, Andreasson B (2003) Increased risk for vascular complications in PRV-1 positive patients with essential thrombocythaemia. Br J Haematol 123: 513–516

Johansson P, Kutti J, Andreasson B, Safai-Kutti S, Vilen L, Wedel H, Ridell B (2004) Trends in the incidence of chronic Philadelphia chromosome negative (Ph-) myeloproliferative disorders in the city of Goteborg, Sweden, during 1983–99. J Inter Med 256:161–165

Jones AV, Kreil S, Zoi K, Waghorn K, Curtis C, Zhang L, Score J, Seear R, Chase AJ, Grand FH, White H, Zoi C, Loukopoulos D, Terpos E, Vervessou EC, Schultheis B, Emig M, Ernst T, Lengfelder E, Hehlman R, Hochhaus A, Oscier D, Silver RT, Reiter A, Cross NCP (2005) Widespread occurrence of the JAK2 V617F mutation in chronic myeloproliferative disorders. Blood First Edition Paper epub 5/26/05

Jotterand Bellomo M, Parlier V, Muhlematter D, Grob, JP, Beris P (1992) Three new cases of chromosome 3 rearrangement in bands q21 and q26 with abnormal thrombopoiesis bring further evidence to the existence of a 3q21q26 syndrome. Cancer Genet Cytogenet 59:138–160

Jurgens DJ, Moreno-Aspitia A, Tefferi A (2004) Anagrelide-associated cardiomyopathy in polycythemia vera and essential thrombocythemia. Haematologica 89:1394–1395

Juvonen E, Ikkala E, Oksanen K, Ruutu T (1993) Megakaryocyte and erythroid colony formation in essential thrombocythaemia and reactive thrombocytosis: diagnostic value and correlation to complications. Br J Haematol 83:192–197

Kaywin P, McDonough M, Insel PA, Shattil SJ (1978) Platelet function in essential thrombocythemia. Decreased epinephrine responsiveness associated with a deficiency of platelet alpha-adrenergic receptors. N Eng J Med 299:505–509

Kelliher MA, McLaughlin J, Witte ON, Rosenberg N (1990) Induction of a chronic myelogenous leukemia-like syndrome in mice with v-abl and BCR/ABL. Proc Natl Acad Sci USA 87:6649–6653

Kennedy BJ, Smith LR, Goltz RW (1975) Skin changes secondary to hydroxyurea therapy. Arch Dermatol 111:183–187

Kesler A, Ellis MH, Manor Y, Gadoth N, Lishner M (2000) Neurological complications of essential thrombocytosis (ET). Acta Neurol Scand 102:299–302

Klingmuller U, Lorenz U, Cantley LC, Neel BG, Lodish HF (1995) Specific recruitment of SH-PTP1 to the erythropoietin receptor causes inactivation of JAK2 and termination of proliferative signals. Cell 80:729–738

Kobayashi S, Teramura M, Hoshino S, Motoji T, Oshimi K, Mizoguchi H (1993) Circulating megakaryocyte progenitors in myeloproliferative disorders are hypersensitive to interleukin-3. Br J Haematol 83:539–544

Koch CA, Lasho TL, Tefferi A (2004) Platelet-rich plasma serotonin levels in chronic myeloproliferative disorders: evaluation of diagnostic use and comparison with the neutrophil PRV-1 assay. Br J Haematol 127:34–39

Koike T, Uesugi Y, Toba K, Narita M, Fuse I, Takahashi M, Shibata A (1995) 5q-syndrome presenting as essential thrombocythemia: myelodysplastic syndrome or chronic myeloproliferative disorders? Leukemia 9:517–518

Kralovics R, Passamonti F, Buser AS, Soon-Siong T, Tiedt R, Passweg JR, Tichelli A, Cazzola M, Skoda RC (2005) A gain of function mutation in Jak2 is frequently found in patients with myeloproliferative disorders. N Eng J Med 352:1779–1790

Kulkarni S, Reiter A, Smedley D, Goldman JM, Cross NC (1999) The genomic structure of ZNF198 and location of breakpoints in the t(8;13) myeloproliferative syndrome. Genomics 55:118–121

Kulkarni S, Heath C, Parker S, Chase A, Iqbal S, Pocock CF, Kaeda J, Cwynarski K, Goldman JM, Cross NC (2000) Fusion of H4/D10S170 to the platelet-derived growth factor receptor beta in BCR-ABL-negative myeloproliferative disorders with a t(5;10) (q33;q21). Cancer Res 60:3592–3598

Lacronique V, Boureux A, Valle VD, Poirel H, Quang CT, Mauchauffe M, Berthou C, Lessard M, Berger R, Ghysdael J, Bernard OA (1997) A TEL-JAK2 fusion protein with constitutive kinase activity in human leukemia. Science 278:1309–1312

Landolfi R, Ciabattoni G, Patrignani P, Castellana MA, Pogliani E, Bizzi B, Patrono C (1992) Increased thromboxane biosynthesis in patients with polycythemia vera: evidence for aspirin-suppressible platelet activation in vivo. Blood 80:1965–1971

Landolfi R, Marchioli R, Kutti J, Gisslinger H, Tognoni G, Patrono C, Barbui T (2004a) Efficacy and safety of low-dose aspirin in polycythemia vera. N Engl J Med 350:114–124

Landolfi R, Marchioli R, Kutti J, Gisslinger H, Tognoni G, Patrono C, Barbui T, European Collaboration on Low-Dose Aspirin in Polycythemia Vera I (2004b) Efficacy and safety of low-dose aspirin in polycythemia vera. N Engl J Med 350:114–124

Largaespada DA, Brannan CI, Jenkins NA, Copeland NG (1996) Nf1 deficiency causes Ras-mediated granulocyte/macrophage colony stimulating factor hypersensitivity and chronic myeloid leukaemia. Nat Genet 12:137–143

Le Blanc K, Lindahl T, Rosendahl K, Samuelsson J (1998) Impaired platelet binding of fibrinogen due to a lower number of GPIIB/IIIA receptors in polycythemia vera. Thromb Res 91:287–295

Lecouedic JP, Mitjavila MT, Villeval JL, Feger F, Gobert S, Mayeux P, Casadevall N, Vainchenker W (1996) Missense mutation of the erythropoietin receptor is a rare event in human erythroid malignancies. Blood 87:1502–1511

Lengfelder E, Hochhaus A, Kronawitter U, Hoche D, Queisser W, Jahn-Eder M, Burkhardt R, Reiter A, Ansari H, Hehlmann R (1998) Should a platelet limit of 600 x 10(9)/l be used as a diagnostic criterion in essential thrombocythaemia? An analysis of the natural course including early stages. Br J Haematol 100:15–23

Lengfelder E, Berger U, Hehlmann R (2000) Interferon alpha in the treatment of polycythemia vera [In Process Citation]. Ann Hematol 79:103–109

Levine RL, Wadleigh M, Cools J, Ebert BL, Wernig G, Huntly BJ, Boggon TJ, Wlodarska I, Clark JJ, Moore S, Adelsperger J, Koo S, Lee JC, Gabriel S, Mercher T, D'Andrea A, Frohling S, Dohner K, Marynen P, Vandenberghe P, Mesa RA, Tefferi A, Griffin JD, Eck MJ, Sellers WR, Meyerson M, Golub TR, Lee SJ, Gilliland DG (2005) Activating mutation in the tyrosine kinase JAK2 in polycythemia vera, essential thrombocythemia, and myeloid metaplasia with myelofibrosis. Cancer Cell 7:387–397

Levy GG, Nichols WC, Lian EC, Foroud T, McClintick JN, McGee BM, Yang AY, Siemieniak DR, Stark KR, Gruppo R, Sarode R, Shurin SB, Chandrasekaran V, Stabler, SP, Sabio H, Bouhassira EE, Upshaw, JD Jr, Ginsburg D, Tsai HM (2001) Mutations in a member of the ADAMTS gene family cause thrombotic thrombocytopenic purpura. Nature 413:488–494

Lindauer K, Loerting T, Liedl KR, Kroemer RT (2001) Prediction of the structure of human Janus kinase 2 (JAK2) comprising the two carboxy-terminal domains reveals a mechanism for autoregulation. Protein Eng 14:27–37

Lofvenberg E, Nilsson TK (1989) Qualitative platelet defects in chronic myeloproliferative disorders: evidence for reduced ATP secretion. Eur J Haematol 43:435–440

Loh ML, Vattikuti S, Schubbert S, Reynolds MG, Carlson E, Lieuw KH, Chen, JW, Lee CM, Stokoe D, Bonifas JM, Curtiss NP, Gotlib J, Meshinchi S, Le Beau MM, Emanuel PD, Shannon KM (2004) Mutations in PTPN11 implicate the SHP-2 phosphatase in leukemogenesis. Blood 103:2325–2331

Longley BJ Jr, Metcalfe DD, Tharp M, Wang X, Tyrrell L, Lu SZ, Heitjan D, Ma Y (1999) Activating and dominant inactivating c-KIT catalytic domain mutations in distinct clinical forms of human mastocytosis. Proc Natl Acad Sci U S A 96:1609–1614

Lopez-Fernandez M F, Lopez-Berges C, Martin R, Pardo A, Ramos FJ, Battle J (1987) Abnormal structure of von Willebrand factor in myeloproliferative syndrome is associated to either thrombotic or bleeding diathesis. Thromb Haemost 58:753–757

Lossos IS, Matzner Y (1995) Hydroxyurea-induced fever: case report and review of the literature. Ann Pharmacother 29:132–133

Lozano M, Narvaez J, Faundez A, Mazzara R, Cid J, Jou JM, Marin JL, Ordinas A (1998) Platelet count and mean platelet volume in the Spanish population. Med Clin (Barc) 110:774–777

Lugo TG, Pendergast AM, Muller AJ, Witte ON (1990) Tyrosine kinase activity and transformation potency of bcr-abl oncogene products. Science 247:1079–1082

Magnusson MK, Meade KE, Brown KE, Arthur DC, Krueger LA, Barrett AJ, Dunbar CE (2001) Rabaptin-5 is a novel fusion partner to platelet-derived growth factor beta receptor in chronic myelomonocytic leukemia. Blood 98:2518–2525

Martin PJ, Najfeld V, Hansen JA, Penfold GK, Jacobson RJ, Fialkow PJ (1980) Involvement of the B-lymphoid system in chronic myelogenous leukaemia. Nature 287:49–50

Martinelli P, Martinelli V, Agangi A, Maruotti GM, Paladini D, Ciancia R, Rotoli B (2004) Interferon alfa treatment for pregnant women affected by essential thrombocythemia: case reports and a review. Am J Obstet Gynecol 191:2016–2020

Mazur EMEA (1992) Analysis of the mechanism of anagrelide-induced thrombocytopenia in humans. Blood 79:1931–1937

Mazzucato M, De Marco L, De Angelis V, De Roia D, Bizzaro N, Casonato A (1989) Platelet membrane abnormalities in myeloproliferative disorders: decrease in glycoproteins Ib and IIb/IIIa complex is associated with deficient receptor function. Br J Haematol 73:369–374

Mazzucconi MG, Francesconi M, Chistolini A, Falcione E, Ferrari A, Tirindelli MC, Mandelli F (1986) Pipobroman therapy of essential thrombocythemia. Scand J Haematol 37:306–309

McCarthy L, Eichelberger L, Skipworth E, Danielson C (2002) Erythromelalgia due to essential thrombocythemia. Transfusion 42:1245

McLaughlin J, Chianese E, Witte ON (1987) In vitro transformation of immature hematopoietic cells by the P210 BCR/ABL oncogene product of the Philadelphia chromosome. Proc Natl Acad Sci U S A 84:6558–6562

McNally RJ, Rowland D, Roman E, Cartwright RA (1997) Age and sex distributions of hematological malignancies in the UK. Hematol Oncol 15:173–189

Mele A, Visani G, Pulsoni A, Monarca B, Castelli G, Stazi MA, Gentile G, Mandelli F (1996) Risk factors for essential thrombocythemia: A case-control study. Italian Leukemia Study Group. Cancer 77: 2157–2161

Mesa RA, Silverstein MN, Jacobsen SJ, Wollan PC, Tefferi A (1999) Population-based incidence and survival figures in essential thrombocythemia and agnogenic myeloid metaplasia: An Olmsted County study, 1976–1995. Am J Hematol 61:10–15

Mesa RA, Hanson CA, Li CY et al (2002) Diagnostic and prognostic value of bone marrow angiogenesis and megakaryocyte c-Mpl expression in essential thrombocythemia. Blood 99:4131–4137

Messinezy M, Westwood N, Sawyer B, Grace R, Holland LJ, Lawrie AS, Pearson TC (1994) Primary thrombocythaemia: a composite approach to diagnosis. Clin Lab Haematol 16:139–148

Messinezy M, Westwood NB, El-Hemaidi I, Marsden JT, Sherwood RS, Pearson TC (2002) Serum erythropoietin values in erythrocytoses and in primary thrombocythaemia. Br J Haematol 117:47–53

Michiels JJ, Abels J, Steketee J, van Vliet HH, Vuzevski VD (1985) Erythromelalgia caused by platelet-mediated arteriolar inflammation and thrombosis in thrombocythemia. Ann Inter Med 102:466–471

Michiels JJ, Koudstaal PJ, Mulder AH, van Vliet HH (1993 a) Transient neurologic and ocular manifestations in primary thrombocythemia. Neurology 43:1107–1110

Michiels JJ, Koudstaal PJ, Mulder AH, van Vliet HH (1993 b) Transient neurologic and ocular manifestations in primary thrombocythemia. Neurology 43:1107–1110

Michiels JJ, van Genderen PJ, Lindemans J, van Vliet HH (1996) Erythromelalgic, thrombotic and hemorrhagic manifestations in 50 cases of thrombocythemia. Leuk Lymphoma 1:47–56

Michiels J, Berneman Z, Schroyens W, Kutti J, Swolin B, Ridell B, Fernando P, Zanetto U (2004 a) Philadelphia (Ph) chromosome-positive thrombocythemia without features of chronic myeloid leukemia in peripheral blood: natural history and diagnostic differentiation from Ph-negative essential thrombocythemia. Ann Hematol 83:504–512

Michiels JJ, Berneman ZN, Schroyens W, Van Vliet HH (2004b) Pathophysiology and treatment of platelet-mediated microvascular disturbances, major thrombosis and bleeding complications in essential thrombocythaemia and polycythaemia vera. Platelets 15:67–84

Mittelman M, Gardyn J, Carmel M, Malovani H, Barak Y, Nir U (1996) Analysis of the Erythropoietin Receptor Gene in Patients With Myeloproliferative and Myelodysplastic Syndromes. Leuk Res 20:459–466

Mohamed A, McLeod JG, Hallinan J (1991) Superior sagittal sinus thrombosis. Clin Exp Neurol 28:23–36

Moliterno AR, Hankins WD, Spivak JL (1998) Impaired expression of the thrombopoietin receptor by platelets from patients with polycythemia vera. N Engl J Med 338:572–580

Murphy S, Davis JL, Walsh PN, Gardner FH (1978) Template bleeding time and clinical hemorrhage in myeloproliferative disease. Arch Inter Med 138:1251–1253

Murphy S, Iland H, Rosenthal D, Laszlo J (1986) Essential thrombocythemia: an interim report from the polycythemia vera study group. Semin Hematol 23:177–182

Nagata H, Worobec AS, Oh CK, Chowdhury BA, Tannenbaum S, Suzuki Y, Metcalfe DD (1995) Identification of a point mutation in the catalytic domain of the protooncogene c-kit in peripheral blood mononuclear cells of patients who have mastocytosis with an associated hematologic disorder. Proc Natl Acad Sci U S A 92:10560–10564

Najean Y, Rain JD (1997) Treatment of polycythemia vera – the use of hydroxyurea and pipobroman in 292 patients under the age of 65 years. Blood 90:3370–3377

Najman A, Stachowiak J, Parlier Y, Gorin NC, Duhamel G (1982) Pipobroman therapy of polycythemia vera. Blood 59:890–894

Nakayama H, Inamitsu T, Ohga S, Kai T, Suda M, Matsuzaki A, Ueda K (1996) Chronic myelomonocytic leukaemia with t(8;9) (p11;q34) in childhood: an example of the 8p11 myeloproliferative disorder? Br J Haematol 92:692–695

Nguyen TV, Margolis DJ (1993) Hydroxyurea and lower leg ulcers. Cutis 52:217–219

Niittyvuopio R, Juvonen E, Kaaja R, Oksanen K, Hallman H, Timonen T, Ruutu T (2004) Pregnancy in essential thrombocythaemia: experience with 40 pregnancies. Eur J Haematol 73:431–436

Nowell PC, Hungerford DA (1960) A minute chromosome in human chronic granulocytic leukemia. J Natl Cancer Inst 25:85

Osselaer JC, Jamart J, Scheiff JM (1997) Platelet distribution width for differential diagnosis of thrombocytosis. Clin Chem 43: 1072–1076

Pardanani A, Reeder T, Li CY, Tefferi A (2003a) Eosinophils are derived from the neoplastic clone in patients with systemic mastocytosis and eosinophilia. Leuk Res 27:883–885

Pardanani A, Reeder TL, Kimlinger TK, Baek JY, Li CY, Butterfield JH, Tefferi A (2003b) Flt-3 and c-kit mutation studies in a spectrum of chronic myeloid disorders including systemic mast cell disease. Leuk Res 27:739–742

Pardanani AD, Morice WG, Hoyer JD, Tefferi A (2003c) Chronic basophilic Leukemia: a distinct clinico-pathologic entity? Eur J Haematol 71:18–22

Pardanani A, Brockman SR, Paternoster SF, Flynn HC, Ketterling RP, Lasho TL, Ho CL, Li CY, Dewald GW, Tefferi A (2004) FIP1L1-PDGFRA fusion: prevalence and clinicopathologic correlates in 89 consecutive patients with moderate to severe eosinophilia. Blood 104:3038–3045

Passamonti F, Brusamolino E, Lazzarino M, Barate C, Klersy C, Orlandi E, Canevari A, Castelli G, Merante S, Bernasconi C (2000) Efficacy of pipobroman in the treatment of polycythemia vera: long-term results in 163 patients. Haematologica 85:1011–1018

Passamonti F, Pietra D, Malabarba L, Rumi E, Della Porta MG, Malcovati L, Bonfichi M, Pascutto C, Lazzarino M, Cazzola M (2004a) Clinical significance of neutrophil CD177 mRNA expression in Ph-negative chronic myeloproliferative disorders. Br J Haematol 126: 650–656

Passamonti F, Rumi E, Pungolino E, Malabarba L, Bertazzoni P, Valentini M, Orlandi E, Arcaini L, Brusamolino E, Pascutto C, Cazzola M, Morra E, Lazzarino M (2004b) Life expectancy and prognostic factors for survival in patients with polycythemia vera and essential thrombocythemia. Am J Med 117:755–761

Patel K, Kelsey P (1997) Primary acquired sideroblastic anemia, thrombocytosis, and trisomy 8. Ann Hematol 74:199–201

Peeters P, Raynaud SD, Cools J, Wlodarska I, Grosgeorge J, Philip P, Monpoux F, Van Rompaey L, Baens M, Van den Berghe H, Marynen P (1997) Fusion of TEL, the ETS-variant gene 6 (ETV6), to the receptor-associated kinase JAK2 as a result of t(9;12) in a lymphoid and t(9;15;12) in a myeloid leukemia. Blood 90:2535–2540

Pendergast AM (2002) The Abl family kinases: mechanisms of regulation and signaling. Adv Cancer Res 85:51–100

Pendergast AM, Muller AJ, Havlik MH, Maru Y, Witte ON (1991) BCR sequences essential for transformation by the BCR-ABL oncogene bind to the ABL SH2 regulatory domain in a non-phosphotyrosine-dependent manner. Cell 66:161–171

Popovici C, Adelaide J, Ollendorff V, Chaffanet M, Guasch G, Jacrot M, Leroux D, Birnbaum D, Pebusque MJ (1998) Fibroblast growth factor receptor 1 is fused to FIM in stem-cell myeloproliferative disorder with t(8;13). Proc Natl Acad Sci U S A 95:5712–5717

Popovici C, Zhang B, Gregoire MJ, Jonveaux P, Lafage-Pochitaloff M, Birnbaum D, Pebusque MJ (1999) The t(6;8)(q27;p11) translocation in a stem cell myeloproliferative disorder fuses a novel gene, FOP, to fibroblast growth factor receptor 1. Blood 93:1381–1389

Prchal JF, Axelrad AA (1974) Letter: Bone-marrow responses in polycythemia vera. N Engl J Med 290:1382

Prchal JT, Guan YL (1993) A novel clonality assay based on transcriptional analysis of the active X chromosome. Stem Cells 11 Suppl 1:62–65

Quesada JR, Talpaz M, Rios A, Kurzrock R, Gutterman JU (1986) Clinical toxicity of interferons in cancer patients: a review. J Clin Oncol 4:234–243

Randi ML, Stocco F, Rossi C, Tison T, Girolami A (1991) Thrombosis and hemorrhage in thrombocytosis: evaluation of a large cohort of patients (357 cases). J Med 22:213–223

Randi ML, Fabris F, Cella G, Rossi C, Girolami A (1998) Cerebral vascular accidents in young patients with essential thrombocythemia: relation with other known cardiovascular risk factors. Angiology 49:477–481

Randi ML, Putti MC, Fabris F, Sainati L, Zanesco L, Girolami A (2000) Features of essential thrombocythaemia in childhood: a study of five children. Br J Haematol 108:86–89

Rane SG, Reddy EP (2000) Janus kinases: components of multiple signaling pathways. Oncogene 19:5662–5679

Rane SG, Reddy EP (2002) JAKs, STATs and Src kinases in hematopoiesis. Oncogene 21:3334–3358

Raskind WH, Jacobson R, Murphy S, Adamson JW, Fialkow PJ (1985) Evidence for the involvement of B lymphoid cells in polycythemia vera and essential thrombocythemia. J Clin Invest 75:1388–1390

Reeder TL, Bailey RJ, Dewald GW, Tefferi A (2003) Both B and T lymphocytes may be clonally involved in myelofibrosis with myeloid metaplasia. Blood 101:1981–1983

Regev A, Stark P, Blickstein D, Lahav M (1997 a) Thrombotic complications in essential thrombocythemia with relatively low platelet counts. Am J Hematol 56:168–172

Regev A, Stark P, Blickstein D, Lahav M (1997 b) Thrombotic complications in essential thrombocythemia with relatively low platelet counts. Am J Hematol 56:168–172

Reiter A, Sohal J, Kulkarni S, Chase A, Macdonald DH, Aguiar RC, Goncalves C, Hernandez JM, Jennings BA, Goldman JM, Cross NC (1998) Consistent fusion of ZNF198 to the fibroblast growth factor receptor-1 in the t(8;13)(p11;q12) myeloproliferative syndrome. Blood 92:1735–1742

Reiter A, Walz C, Watmore A, Schoch C, Blau I, Schlegelberger B, Berger U, Telford N, Aruliah S, Yin JA, Vanstraelen D, Barker HF, Taylor PC, O'Driscoll A, Benedetti F, Rudolph C, Kolb HJ, Hochhaus A, Hehlmann R, Chase A, Cross NC (2005) The t(8;9)(p22;p24) is a recurrent abnormality in chronic and acute leukemia that fuses PCM1 to JAK2. Cancer Res 65:2662–2667

Ridell B, Carneskog J, Wedel H, Vilen L, Hogh Dufva I, Mellqvist UH, Brywe N, Wadenvik H, Kutti J (2000) Incidence of chronic myeloproliferative disorders in the city of Goteborg, Sweden 1983–1992. Eur J Haematol 65:267–271

Robbins G, Barnard DL (1983) Thrombocytosis and microthrombocytosis: a clinical evaluation of 372 cases. Acta Haematol 70: 175–182

Roberts BE, Smith AH (1997) Use of radioactive phosphorus in haematology. Blood Rev 11:146–153

Rocca B, Ciabattoni G, Tartaglione R, Cortelazzo S, Barbui T, Patrono C, Landolfi R (1995 a) Increased thromboxane biosynthesis in essential thrombocythemia. Thromb Haemost 74:1225–1230

Rocca B, Ciabattoni G, Tartaglione R, Cortelazzo S, Barbui T, Patrono C Landolfi R (1995 b) Increased thromboxane biosynthesis in essential thrombocythemia. Thromb Haemost 74:1225–1230

Rolovic Z, Basara N, Gotic M, Sefer D, Bogdanovic A (1995) The determination of spontaneous megakaryocyte colony formation is an unequivocal test for discrimination between essential thrombocythaemia and reactive thrombocytosis. Br J Haematol 90:326–331

Rosati R, La Starza R, Veronese A, Aventin A, Schwienbacher C, Vallespi T, Negrini M, Martelli MF, Mecucci C (2002) NUP98 is fused to the NSD3 gene in acute myeloid leukemia associated with t(8;11)(p11.2;p15). Blood 99:3857–3860

Roskoski R Jr (2004) Src protein-tyrosine kinase structure and regulation. Biochem Biophys Res Commun 324:1155–1164

Ross DW, Ayscue LH, Watson J, Bentley SA (1988) Stability of hematologic parameters in healthy subjects. Intraindividual versus interindividual variation. Am J Clin Pathol 90:262–267

Ross TS, Bernard OA, Berger R, Gilliland DG (1998) Fusion of Huntingtin interacting protein 1 to platelet-derived growth factor beta receptor (PDGFbetaR) in chronic myelomonocytic leukemia with t(5;7)(q33;q11.2). Blood 91:4419–4426

Rozman C, Giralt M, Feliu E, Rubio D, Cortes MT (1991) Life expectancy of patients with chronic nonleukemic myeloproliferative disorders. Cancer 67:2658–2663

Ruggeri M, Finazzi G, Tosetto A, Riva S, Rodeghiero F, Barbui T (1998 a) No treatment for low-risk thrombocythaemia: results from a prospective study. Br J Haematol 103:772–777

Ruggeri M, Finazzi G, Tosetto A, Riva S, Rodeghiero F, Barbui T (1998 b) No treatment for low-risk thrombocythaemia: results from a prospective study. Br J Haematol 103:772–777

Ruggeri M, Gisslinger H, Tosetto A, Rintelen C, Mannhalter C, Pabinger I, Heis N, Castaman G, Missiaglia E, Lechner K, Rodeghiero F (2002) Factor V Leiden mutation carriership and venous thromboembolism in polycythemia vera and essential thrombocythemia. Am J Hematol 71:1–6

Ruggeri M, Tosetto A, Frezzato M, Rodeghiero F (2003) The rate of progression to polycythemia vera or essential thrombocythemia in patients with erythrocytosis or thrombocytosis. Ann Inter Med 139:470–475

Ruocco L, Del Corso L, Romanelli AM, Deri D, Pentimone F (2001) New hematological indices in the healthy elderly. Minerva Med 92:69–73

Saba R, Jabbour E, Giles F, Cortes J, Talpaz M, O'Brien S, Freireich EJ, Garcia-Manero G, Kantarjian H, Verstovsek S (2005) Interferon alpha therapy for patients with essential thrombocythemia. Cancer 103:2551–2557

Sacchi S, Vinci G, Gugliotta L, Rupoli S, Gargantini L, Martinelli V, Baravelli S, Lazzarino M, Finazzi G (2000) Diagnosis of essential thrombocythemia at platelet counts between 400 and $600 \times 10(9)$/L. Gruppo Italiano Malattie Mieloproliferative Croniche (GIMMC). Haematologica 85:492–495

Saharinen P, Takaluoma K, Silvennoinen O (2000) Regulation of the Jak2 tyrosine kinase by its pseudokinase domain. Mol Cell Biol 20:3387–3395

Saharinen P, Silvennoinen O (2002) The pseudokinase domain is required for suppression of basal activity of Jak2 and Jak3 tyrosine kinases and for cytokine-inducible activation of signal transduction. J Biol Chem 277:47954–47963

Saharinen P, Vihinen M, Silvennoinen O (2003) Autoinhibition of Jak2 tyrosine kinase is dependent on specific regions in its pseudokinase domain. Mol Biol Cell 14:1448–1459

Santhosh-Kumar CR, Yohannan MD, Higgy KE, al-Mashhadani SA (1991) Thrombocytosis in adults: analysis of 777 patients. J Inter Med 229:493–495

Sasaki A, Yasukawa H, Shouda T, Kitamura T, Dikic I, Yoshimura A (2000) CIS3/SOCS-3 suppresses erythropoietin (EPO) signaling by binding the EPO receptor and JAK2. J Biol Chem 275:29338–29347

Sato K (1988) Plasma von Willebrand factor abnormalities in patients with essential thrombocythemia. Keio J Med 37:54–71

Sattler M, Salgia R, Okuda K, Uemura N, Durstin MA, Pisick E, Xu G, Li JL, Prasad KV, Griffin JD (1996) The proto-oncogene product p120CBL and the adaptor proteins CRKL and c-CRK link c-ABL, p190BCR/ABL and p210BCR/ABL to the phosphatidylinositol-3′ kinase pathway. Oncogene 12:839–846

Schafer AI (1982) Deficiency of platelet lipoxygenase activity in myeloproliferative disorders. N Engl J Med 306:381–386

Schilling RF (1980) Platelet millionaires. Lancet 2:372–373

Schwaller J, Anastasiadou E, Cain D, Kutok J, Wojiski S, Williams IR, LaStarza R, Crescenzi B, Sternberg DW, Andreasson P, Schiavo R, Siena S, Mecucci C, Gilliland DG (2001) H4(D10S170), a gene frequently rearranged in papillary thyroid carcinoma, is fused to the platelet-derived growth factor receptor beta gene in atypical chronic myeloid leukemia with t(5;10)(q33;q22). Blood 97:3910–3918

Sehayek E, Ben-Yosef N, Modan M, Chetrit A, Meytes D (1988) Platelet parameters and aggregation in essential and reactive thrombocytosis. Am J Clin Pathol 90:431–436

Sessarego M, Defferrari R, Dejana AM, Rebuttato AM, Fugazza G, Salvidio E, Ajmar F (1989) Cytogenetic analysis in essential thrombocythemia at diagnosis and at transformation. A 12-year study. Cancer Genet Cytogenet 43:57–65

Shih LY, Lin TL, Dunn P, Wu JH, Tseng CP, Lai CL, Wang PN, Kuo MC (2001) Clonality analysis using X-chromosome inactivation patterns by HUMARA-PCR assay in female controls and patients with idiopathic thrombocytosis in Taiwan. Exp Hematol 29:202–208

Shih LY, Lin TL, Lai CL, Dunn P, Wu JH, Wang PN, Kuo MC, Lee LC (2002) Predictive values of X-chromosome inactivation patterns and clinicohematologic parameters for vascular complications in female patients with essential thrombocythemia. Blood 100:1596–1601

Shuai K, Liu B (2003) Regulation of JAK-STAT signalling in the immune system. Nat Rev Immunol 3:900–911

Shultz LD, Rajan TV, Greiner DL (1997) Severe defects in immunity and hematopoiesis caused by SHP-1 protein-tyrosine-phosphatase deficiency. Trends Biotechnol 15:302–307

Side LE, Emanuel PD, Taylor B, Franklin J, Thompson P, Castleberry RP, Shannon KM (1998) Mutations of the NF1 gene in children with juvenile myelomonocytic leukemia without clinical evidence of neurofibromatosis, type 1. Blood 92:267–272

Silverstein MN, Petitt RM, Solberg LA Jr, Fleming JS, Knight RC, Schacter LP (1988) Anagrelide: a new drug for treating thrombocytosis. N Engl J Med 318:1292–1294

Sirhan S, Lasho TL, Elliott MA, Tefferi A (2005) Neutrophil polycythemia rubra vera-1 expression in classic and atypical myeloproliferative disorders and laboratory correlates. Haematologica 90:406–408

Small BM, Bettigole RE (1981) Diagnosis of myeloproliferative disease by analysis of the platelet volume distribution. Am J Clin Pathol 76:685–691

Smedley D, Hamoudi R, Clark J, Warren W, Abdul-Rauf M, Somers G, Venter D, Fagan K, Cooper C, Shipley J (1998a) The t(8;13)(p11;q11–12) rearrangement associated with an atypical myeloproliferative disorder fuses the fibroblast growth factor receptor 1 gene to a novel gene RAMP. Hum Mol Genet 7:637–642

Smedley D, Somers G, Venter D, Chow CW, Cooper C, Shipley J (1998b) Characterization of a t(8;13)(p11;q11–12) in an atypical myeloproliferative disorder. Genes Chromosomes Cancer 21:70–73

Sohal J, Chase A, Mould S, Corcoran M, Oscier D, Iqbal S, Parker S, Welborn J, Harris RI, Martinelli G, Montefusco V, Sinclair P, Wilkins BS, van den Berg H, Vanstraelen D, Goldman JM, Cross NC (2001) Identification of four new translocations involving FGFR1 in myeloid disorders. Genes Chromosomes Cancer 32:155–163

Solberg LA, Tefferi A, Oles KJ, Tarach JS, Petitt RM, Forstrom LA, Silverstein MN (1997) The effects of anagrelide on human megakaryocytopoiesis. Br J Haematol 99:174–180

Spencer CM, Brogden RN (1994) Anagrelide. A review of its pharmacodynamic and pharmacokinetic properties, and therapeutic potential in the treatment of thrombocythaemia. Drugs 47:809–822

Starr R, Hilton DJ (1999) Negative regulation of the JAK/STAT pathway. Bioessays 21:47–52

Steensma DP, Dewald GW, Lasho TL, Powell HL, McClure RF, Levine RL, Gilliland DG, Tefferi A (2005) The JAK2 V617F activating tyrosine kinase mutation is an infrequent event in both "atypical" myeloproliferative disorders and the myelodysplastic syndrome. Blood epub 4/28/05

Steensma DP, Tefferi A (2002) Cytogenetic and molecular genetic aspects of essential thrombocythemia. Acta Haematol 108:55–65

Steer EJ, Cross NC (2002) Myeloproliferative disorders with translocations of chromosome 5q31–35: role of the platelet-derived growth factor receptor Beta. Acta Haematol 107:113–122

Stevens MR (1999) Hydroxyurea: an overview. J Biol Reg Homeost Agents 13:172–175

Still IH, Chernova O, Hurd D, Stone RM, Cowell JK (1997) Molecular characterization of the t(8;13)(p11;q12) translocation associated with an atypical myeloproliferative disorder: evidence for three discrete loci involved in myeloid leukemias on 8p11. Blood 90:3136–3141

Stofega MR, Herrington J, Billestrup N, Carter-Su C (2000) Mutation of the SHP-2 binding site in growth hormone (GH) receptor prolongs GH-promoted tyrosyl phosphorylation of GH receptor, JAK2, and STAT5B. Mol Endocrinol 14:1338–1350

Stoll DB, Peterson P, Exten R, Laszlo J, Pisciotta AV, Ellis JT, White P, Vaidya K, Bozdech M, Murphy S (1988) Clinical presentation and natural history of patients with essential thrombocythemia and the Philadelphia chromosome. Am J Hematol 27:77–83

Storen EC, Tefferi A (2001) Long-term use of anagrelide in young patients with essential thrombocythemia. Blood 97:863–866

Tache JE, Saffra N, Marshak H, Aithal S, Novetsky A, Huang YW (2005) Retinal vein thrombosis as the presenting symptom of essential thrombocythemia. Am J Med Sci 329:139–140

Taksin AL, Couedic JPL, Dusanter-Fourt I, Masse A, Giraudier S, Katz A, Wendling F, Vainchenker W, Casadevall N, Debili N (1999) Autonomous megakaryocyte growth in essential thrombocythemia and idiopathic myelofibrosis is not related to a c-mpl mutation or to an autocrine stimulation by Mpl-L. Blood 93:125–139

Tartaglia M, Niemeyer CM, Fragale A, Song X, Buechner J, Jung A, Hahlen K, Hasle H, Licht JD, Gelb BD (2003) Somatic mutations in PTPN11 in juvenile myelomonocytic leukemia, myelodysplastic syndromes and acute myeloid leukemia. Nat Genet 34:148–150

Tefferi A (2003) Polycythemia vera: a comprehensive review and clinical recommendations. Mayo Clin Proc 78:174–194

Tefferi A (2005a) Hydroxyurea vindicated: lack of drug leukemogenicity in polycythemia vera. Curr Hematol Rep 4:211–212

Tefferi A (2005b) The indolent natural history of essential thrombocythemia: a challenge to new drug development. Mayo Clin Proc 80:97–98

Tefferi A, Elliott MA (2004) Schistocytes on the peripheral blood smear. Mayo Clin Proc 79:809

Tefferi A, Gilliland DG (2005a) Classification of myeloproliferative disorders: from Dameshek towards a semi-molecular system. Best Pract Res Clin Haematol (in press)

Tefferi A, Gilliland DG (2005b) JAK2 in Myeloproliferative disorders is not just another kinase. Cell Cycle 4:1053–1056

Tefferi A, Gilliland DG (2005 c) The JAK2 V617F tyrosine kinase mutation in myeloproliferative disorders: Status report and immediate implications for disease classification and diagnosis. Mayo Clin Proc 80:947–958

Tefferi A, Murphy S (2001) Current opinion in essential thrombocythemia: pathogenesis, diagnosis, and management. Blood Rev 15: 121–131

Tefferi A, Thibodeau SN, Solberg LA Jr (1990) Clonal studies in the myelodysplastic syndrome using X-linked restriction fragment length polymorphisms. Blood 75:1770–1773

Tefferi A, Ho TC, Ahmann GJ, Katzmann JA, Greipp PR (1994 a) Plasma interleukin-6 and C-reactive protein levels in reactive versus clonal thrombocytosis. Am J Med 97:374–378

Tefferi A, Mathew P, Noel P (1994 b) The 5q- syndrome: a scientific and clinical update. Leuk Lymphoma 14:375–378

Tefferi A, Silverstein MN, Petitt RM, Mesa RA, Solberg LA (1997) Anagrelide as a new platelet-lowering agent in essential thrombocythemia: Mechanism of action, efficacy, toxicity, current indications. Sem Thromb Hemost 23:379

Tefferi A, Elliott MA, Kao PC, Yoon S, El-Hemaidi I, Pearson TC (2000 a) Hydroxyurea-induced marked oscillations of platelet counts in patients with polycythemia vera. Blood 96:1582–1584

Tefferi A, Solberg LA, Silverstein MN (2000 b) A clinical update in polycythemia vera and essential thrombocythemia. Am J Med 109: 141–149

Tefferi A, Yoon SY, Li CY (2000 c) Immunohistochemical staining for megakaryocyte c-mpl may complement morphologic distinction between polycythemia vera and secondary erythrocytosis. Blood 96:771–772

Tefferi A, Fonseca R, Pereira DL, Hoagland HC (2001) A long-term retrospective study of young women with essential thrombocythemia. Mayo Clin Proc 76:22–28

Tefferi A, Lasho TL, Wolanskyj AP, Mesa RA (2004) Neutrophil PRV-1 expression across the chronic myeloproliferative disorders and in secondary or spurious polycythemia. Blood 103:3547–3548

Tefferi A, Sirhan S, Lasho TL, Schwager SM, Li CY, Dingli D, Wolanskyj AP, Steensma DP, Mesa R, Gilliland DG (2005) Concomitant neutrophil JAK2 mutation screening and PRV-1 expression analysis in myeloproliferative disorders and secondary polycythaemia. Br J Haematol 131:166–171

Teofili L, De Stefano V, Leone G, Micalizzi P, Iovino MS, Alfano G, Bizzi B (1992) Hematological causes of venous thrombosis in young people: high incidence of myeloproliferative disorder as underlying disease in patients with splanchnic venous thrombosis. Thromb Haemost 67:297–301

Teofili L, Martini M, Luongo M, Di Mario A, Leone G, De Stefano V, Larocca LM (2002 a) Overexpression of the polycythemia rubra vera-1 gene in essential thrombocythemia. J Clin Oncol 20:4249–4254

Teofili L, Pierconti F, Di Febo A, Maggiano N, Vianelli N, Ascani S, Rossi E, Pileri S, Leone G, Larocca LM, De Stefano V (2002 b) The expression pattern of c-mpl in megakaryocytes correlates with thrombotic risk in essential thrombocythemia. Blood 100:714–717

Thiele J, Kvasnicka HM, Diehl V, Fischer R, Michiels JJ (1999) Clinicopathological diagnosis and differential criteria of thrombocythemias in various myeloproliferative disorders by histopathology, histochemistry and immunostaining from bone marrow biopsies. Leuk Lymphoma 33:207–218

Tsai HM (1996) Physiologic cleavage of von Willebrand factor by a plasma protease is dependent on its conformation and requires calcium ion. Blood 87:4235–4244

Tsukamoto N, Morita K, Maehara T, Okamoto K, Sakai H, Karasawa M, Naruse T, Omine M (1994) Clonality in chronic myeloproliferative disorders defined by X-chromosome linked probes: demonstration of heterogeneity in lineage involvement. Br J Haematol 86:253–258

Uppenkamp M, Makarova E, Petrasch S, Brittinger G (1998) Thrombopoietin serum concentration in patients with reactive and myeloproliferative thrombocytosis. Ann Hematol 77:217–223

Valade N, Decailliot F, Rebufat Y, Heurtematte Y, Duvaldestin P, Stephan F (2005) Thrombocytosis after trauma: incidence, aetiology, and clinical significance. Br J Anaesth 94:18–23

van den Berg H, Kroes W, van der Schoot CE, Dee R, Pals ST, Bouts TH, Slater RM (1996) A young child with acquired t(8;9)(p11;q34): additional proof that 8p11 is involved in mixed myeloid/T lymphoid malignancies. Leukemia 10:1252–1253

van Genderen PJ, Michiels JJ, van Strik R, Lindemans J, van Vliet HH (1995) Platelet consumption in thrombocythemia complicated by erythromelalgia: reversal by aspirin. Thromb Haemost 73: 210–214

van Genderen PJ, Lucas IS, van Strik R, Vuzevski VD, Prins FJ, van Vliet HH, Michiels JJ (1996) Erythromelalgia in essential thrombocythemia is characterized by platelet activation and endothelial cell damage but not by thrombin generation. Thromb Haemost 76: 333–338

van Genderen PJ, Leenknegt H, Michiels JJ (1997 a) The paradox of bleeding and thrombosis in thrombocythemia: is von Willebrand factor the link? Sem Thromb Hemost 23:385–389

van Genderen PJ, Mulder PG, Waleboer M, van de Moesdijk D, Michiels JJ (1997 b) Prevention and treatment of thrombotic complications in essential thrombocythaemia: efficacy and safety of aspirin. Br J Haematol 97:179–184

van Genderen PJ, Prins FJ, Michiels JJ, Schror K (1999) Thromboxane-dependent platelet activation in vivo precedes arterial thrombosis in thrombocythaemia: a rationale for the use of low-dose aspirin as an antithrombotic agent. Br J Haematol 104:438–441

Vannucchi AM, Grossi A, Pancrazzi A, Antonioli E, Guglielmelli P, Balestri F, Biscardi M, Bulgarelli S, Longo G, Graziano C, Gugliotta L, Bosi A (2004) PRV-1, erythroid colonies and platelet Mpl are unrelated to thrombosis in essential thrombocythaemia. Br J Haematol 127:214–219

Vaquez MH (1892) Sur une forme speciale de cyanose s'accompagnant d'hyperglobulie excessive et persistante (On a special form of cyanosis accompanied by excessive and persistent erythrocytosis). C R Soc Biol (Paris) 44:384–388

Vardiman JW, Harris NL, Brunning RD (2002) The World Health Organization (WHO) classification of the myeloid neoplasms. Blood 100:2292–2302

Vardizer Y, Linhart Y, Loewenstein A, Garzozi H, Mazawi N, Kesler A (2003) Interferon-alpha-associated bilateral simultaneous ischemic optic neuropathy. J Neuroophthalmol 23:256–259

Virchow R (1845) Weisses Blut. Frorieps Notizen 36:151–156

Vizmanos JL, Hernandez R, Vidal MJ, Larrayoz MJ, Odero MD, Marin J, Ardanaz MT, Calasanz MJ, Cross NC (2004) Clinical variability of patients with the t(6;8)(q27;p12) and FGFR1OP-FGFR1 fusion: two further cases. Hematol J 5:534–537

Voncken JW, Kaartinen V, Pattengale PK, Germeraad WT, Groffen J, Heisterkamp N (1995) BCR/ABL P210 and P190 cause distinct leukemia in transgenic mice. Blood 86:4603–4611

Waddell CC, Brown JA, Repinecz YA (1981) Abnormal platelet function in myeloproliferative disorders. Arch Pathol Lab Med 105:432–435

Wagner S, Waxman J, Sikora K (1989) The treatment of essential thrombocythaemia with radioactive phosphorus. Clin Radiol 40:190–192

Wang JC, Chen C, Lou LH, Mora M (1997) Blood thrombopoietin, IL-6 and IL-11 levels in patients with agnogenic myeloid metaplasia. Leukemia 11:1827–1832

Wang JC, Chen C, Novetsky AD, Lichter SM, Ahmed F, Friedberg NM (1998) Blood thrombopoietin levels in clonal thrombocytosis and reactive thrombocytosis. Am J Med 104:451–455

Wang JY (2000) Regulation of cell death by the Abl tyrosine kinase. Oncogene 19:5643–5650

Watson KV, Key N (1993 a) Vascular complications of essential thrombocythaemia: a link to cardiovascular risk factors. Br J Haematol 83:198–203

Watson KV, Key N (1993 b) Vascular complications of essential thrombocythaemia: a link to cardiovascular risk factors. Br J Haematol 83:198–203

Wehmeier A, Scharf RE, Fricke S, Schneider W (1989) Bleeding and thrombosis in chronic myeloproliferative disorders: relation of platelet disorders to clinical aspects of the disease. Haemostasis 19:251–259

Wehmeier A, Fricke S, Scharf RE, Schneider W (1990) A prospective study of haemostatic parameters in relation to the clinical course of myeloproliferative disorders. Eur J Haematol 45:191–197

Wehmeier A, Tschope D, Esser J, Menzel C, Nieuwenhuis HK, Schneider W (1991) Circulating activated platelets in myeloproliferative disorders. Thromb Res 61:271–278

Wilkinson K, Velloso ER, Lopes LF, Lee C, Aster JC, Shipp MA, Aguiar RC (2003) Cloning of the t(1;5)(q23;q33) in a myeloproliferative disorder associated with eosinophilia: involvement of PDGFRB and response to imatinib. Blood 102:4187–4190

Wolanskyj AP, Lasho TL, Schwager SM, McClure RF, Wadleigh M, Lee SJ, Gary Gilliland D, Tefferi A (2005) JAK2 mutation in essential thrombocythaemia: clinical associations and long-term prognostic relevance. Br J Haematol 131:208–213

Wolanskyj AP, Segovis CM, Schwager SM, Larson DR, Ayalew T (2003) Essential thrombocythemia: Beyond the first decade. Blood 102:920 a

Wright CA, Tefferi A (2001) A single institutional experience with 43 pregnancies in essential thrombocythemia. Eur J Haematol 66:152–159

Xiao S, Nalabolu SR, Aster JC, Ma J, Abruzzo L, Jaffe ES, Stone R, Weissman SM, Hudson TJ, Fletcher JA (1998) FGFR1 is fused with a novel zinc-finger gene, ZNF198, in the t(8;13) leukaemia/lymphoma syndrome. Nat Genet 18:84–87

Yamaoka K, Saharinen P, Pesu M, Holt VE 3rd, Silvennoinen O, O'Shea JJ (2004) The Janus kinases (Jaks). Genome Biology 5:253

Yarbro JW (1992) Mechanism of action of hydroxyurea. Semin Oncol 19:1–10

Yavuz AS, Lipsky PE, Yavuz S, Metcalfe DD, Akin C (2002) Evidence for the involvement of a hematopoietic progenitor cell in systemic mastocytosis from single-cell analysis of mutations in the c-kit gene. Blood 100:661–665

Yeh TC, Pellegrini S (1999) The Janus kinase family of protein tyrosine kinases and their role in signaling. Cell Mol Life Sci 55:1523–1534

Yohannan MD, Higgy KE, al-Mashhadani SA, Santhosh-Kumar CR (1994) Thrombocytosis. Etiologic analysis of 663 patients. Clin Pediatr (Phila) 33:340–343

Yoon SY, Li CY, Tefferi A (2000) Megakaryocyte c-Mpl expression in chronic myeloproliferative disorders and the myelodysplastic syndrome: immunoperoxidase staining patterns and clinical correlates. Eur J Haematol 65:170–174

Zahavi J, Zahavi M, Firsteter E, Frish B, Turleanu R, Rachmani R (1991) An abnormal pattern of multiple platelet function abnormalities and increased thromboxane generation in patients with primary thrombocytosis and thrombotic complications. Eur J Haematol 47:326–332

Zanjani ED, Lutton JD, Hoffman R, Wasserman LR (1977) Erythroid colony formation by polycythemia vera bone marrow in vitro. Dependence on erythropoietin. J Clin Invest 59:841–848

Zhao R, Xing S, Li Z, Fu X, Li Q, Krantz SB, Zhao ZJ (2005) Identification of an acquired JAK2 mutation in Polycythemia vera. J Biol Chem 280:22788–22792

Subject Index

A

B

C

D

E

F

G

H

I

J

L

M

N

O

P

Q

R

S

T

V

W

Z